BASIC GYNECOLOGY

for Postgraduate Students

BASIC GYNECOLOGY
for Postgraduate Students

Tripti Rani Das
MBBS FCPS (Obs & Gyne) MS (Obs & Gyne)
Professor
Department of Obstetrics and Gynecology
Bangladesh Medical University
Shahbagh, Dhaka, Bangladesh

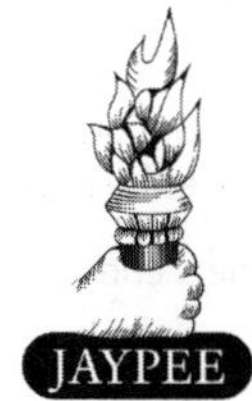

JAYPEE BROTHERS MEDICAL PUBLISHERS
The Health Sciences Publisher
New Delhi | London

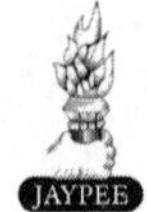

Jaypee Brothers Medical Publishers (P) Ltd

Headquarters
EMCA House, 23/23-B
Ansari Road, Daryaganj
New Delhi 110 002, India
Landline: +91-11-23272143, +91-11-23272703
+91-11-23282021, +91-11-23245672
e-mail: jaypee@jaypeebrothers.com

Corporate Office
4838/24, Ansari Road, Daryaganj
New Delhi 110 002, India
Phone: +91-11-43574357
Fax: +91-11-43574314
e-mail: jaypee@jaypeebrothers.com

Overseas Office
JP Medical Ltd.
83, Victoria Street, London
SW1H 0HW (UK)
Phone: +44-20 3170 8910
e-mail: info@jpmedpub.com

EU GPSR Authorised Representative
Logos Europe, 9 rue Nicolas Poussin
17000, La Rochelle, France
Phone: +33 (0) 6 67 93 73 78
e-mail: contact@logoseurope.eu

Website: www.jaypeebrothers.com
Website: www.jaypeedigital.com

Inquiries for bulk sales may be solicited at: jaypee@jaypeebrothers.com

Basic Gynecology for Postgraduate Students

First Edition: **2026**

ISBN: 978-93-7545-473-1

Printed at: Samrat Offset Pvt. Ltd.

Dedicated to
My parents and my brother

Preface

True to its title, this work is intended to facilitate the preparation of postgraduate candidates for their summative and formative evaluations. Beyond the acquisition of medical knowledge, this book emphasizes the strategic techniques necessary to excel in a high-stakes examination environment.

The final examination comprises theory examination followed by practical and oral examination for postgraduates. The written examination covers two papers followed by practical examination. Written examination covers basic surgical skills and both gynecology and obstetrics.

This book offers a unique and in-depth approach to gynecology by covering the full spectrum of information needed for both theoretical and practical assessments. By adopting a question-and-answer format, the book simulates the actual examination environment.

The book is divided into 32 chapters, and each chapter covers the main important materials that will be sufficient to know the details about the particular topics.

Success in gynecology requires more than just memorization; it demands the ability to apply clinical reasoning under pressure. This book is designed to bridge the gap between textbook learning and bedside performance. By engaging with the case studies and structured questions provided here, you are not just studying—you are practicing the very skills that will define your career as a specialist. We encourage you to use this text as a companion during your clinical rotations to reinforce the link between theory and practice.

Tripti Rani Das

Acknowledgments

First and foremost, I would like to express my deepest gratitude to all those who have contributed to the completion of this book. It would not have been possible without the support and guidance of many individuals.

My heartfelt thanks to my mentors and colleagues in the field of Gynecology, where expertise, advice, and encouragement have been invaluable throughout this journey.

I am indebted to Professor Sultana Razia Begum, Former Chairperson, Department of Obstetrics and Gynecology, Bangabandhu Sheikh Mujib Medical University (BSMMU), Dhaka, Bangladesh, for constant support and encouragement in my professional life. Special thanks to my students and all of my friends for their insightful feedback and for generously sharing their knowledge and experience, which significantly shaped the direction of this work.

I am also deeply grateful to my family and especially my only daughter Janhvi Joyeta, a medical student whose patience, understanding, and unbelievable support provided the foundation I needed to dedicate myself to this book and also content encouragement and belief in me were a source of strength. Thank you for being by my side in every step on the way.

I would also like to extend my appreciation to the medical professionals, my researchers and patients whose experiences and contributions to the field have informed the discussions in this book. Their courage, dedication, and commitment to advancing women's health are truly inspiring.

Finally, my sincere thanks to M/s Jaypee Brothers Medical Publishers (P) Ltd, New Delhi, India, for their professionalism and dedication in bringing their work to fruition.

Tripti Rani Das

Contents

CHAPTER 1

Female Genital Organs Anatomy

Includes
- External Genital Organ
- Internal Genital Organ
- Accessory reproductive organ

SHORT ANSWER TYPE QUESTIONS OF EXTERNAL GENITALIA

Q1. External Genitalia of female.
- Mons Veneris
- Labia majora
- Labia Minora
- Clitoris
- Vestibule
- Perineum

Q2. What are components of Vulva?

Components of Vulva are
- Mons pubis
- Labia majora
- Labia minora
- Hymen
- Clitoris
- Vestibule
- Urethra and Skene's glands
- Bartholin's glands and vestibular bulbs

Q3. What is the boundary of Vulva?
- Anteriorly – Mons pubis
- Posteriorly – Rectum
- Laterally – Genitocrural folds

The hair pattern (escutcheon) in the majority of women is triangular, with the base facing upward.

Q4. Composition of Labia Majora?

The labia majora are covered in hair and consist of squamous epithelium, containing apocrine, sebaceous, and sweat glands. They meet medially to form the posterior commissure, located in front of the anus. Essentially, the labia majora are formed by the elevation of skin and subcutaneous tissue on either side. In males, the scrotum is homologous to the labia majora in females.

Q5. Composition of Labia Minora?

The labia minora are two thin folds of skin that lack fat, hair follicles, and sweat glands. They contain numerous blood vessels, nerve endings, erectile muscle, and many sebaceous glands. The labia minora enclose the clitoris at the front. The lower portion of the labia minora fuses at the midline to create a fold of skin called the fourchette. In males, the penile urethra and part of the skin of the penis are homologous to the labia minora in females.

Q6. Composition of Clitoris?

The clitoris is made up of a cylindrical erectile body that measures approximately 1.5 to 2 cm in length and is located at the top of the vestibule. The glans of the clitoris is highly innervated and vascularized. It has two crura that are connected to the underside of the pubic symphysis by the suspensory ligament. In males, the penis is homologous to the clitoris in females.

Q7. Composition of Vestibule?

It is triangular space bounded

Anteriorly – clitoris

Posteriorly – fourchette

On either side – labia minora.

Openings into the vestibule

a. Urethral opening
b. Vaginal orifice and hymen
c. Opening of Bartholin's ducts
d. Skene's glands

a. Urethral opening: Located 1-1.5 cm beneath the pubic arch, positioned anterior to the vaginal orifice. Paraurethral ducts open directly into the vestibule or on the posterior wall of the urethral opening.
b. Vaginal Orifice and Hymen: The vaginal orifice is located at the posterior end of the vestibule. The hymen is partially covered by a septum made of mucous membrane.
c. The Bartholin's ducts, which are small and pea-sized, appear yellowish-white in color. The lining epithelium of the glands is cuboidal, the ducts are lined with columnar epithelium, and the opening is lined with stratified squamous epithelium. In males, the bulb of the penis is equivalent to Bartholin's glands in females. Bartholin's glands are located superficial perineal pouch.
d. Skene's glands: These are paraurethral glands equivalent to the male prostate. Two Skene's ducts open on each side of the external urethral meatus within the vestibule.

Q8. Composition of Perineum?

Development of external genitalia

Embryonic structure	Derivatives
Labioscrotal swelling	Labia majora
Urogenital folds	Labia minora
Genital tubercle	Clitoris
Urogenital sinus	• Urinary bladder, urethra • Urethral and paraurethral glands • Vagina • Bartholin's glands • Vestibule
Paramesonephric duct (Mullerian duct)	Uterus, cervix, fallopian tubes, vagina (muscular wall), hydatid of Morgagni

Contd...

Contd...

Mesonephric duct (Wolffian duct)	• Duct of epoophoron • Gartner's duct, part of bladder and urethra
Mesonephric tubules	• Epoophoron • Paroophoron
Undifferentiated gonad	Ovary
Cortex	Ovarian follicles
Medulla	Rete ovarii (medulla)
Gubernaculum	• Ovarian ligament • Round ligament
Mullerian tubercle	Hymen
Primordial germ cells	Ova

Internal Genitalia organs

- Vagina
- Uterus
- Fallopian tubes
- Ovaries

Vagina: The vagina is a fibromuscular membranous structure with significant elasticity, as demonstrated during childbirth. It consists of an anterior wall, a posterior wall, and two lateral walls.

Anterior wall - 7 cm

Posterior wall - 9 cm

Lateral wall - stiffer at its middle and looks 'H" shaped on transverse section.

Vaginal fornices: Clefts formed due to the projection of the uterine cervix through the anterior vaginal wall.

Fornices are:

Anterior - 1 (most shallow)

Posterior - 1 (deeper)

Lateral - 2

Vaginal pH changes with estrogenic activity and ranges between 4 and 5.

Development of the vagina

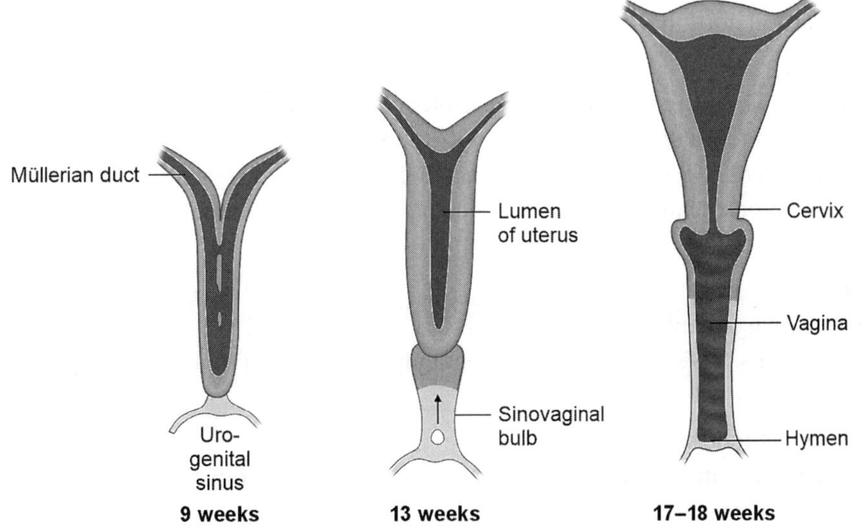

The vagina is developed from the following's sources:

a. The upper four-fifths, located above the hymen, consists of a mucous membrane of endodermal origin from the canalized sinovaginal bulbs, while the muscle layer is derived from the mesoderm of two fused Mullerian ducts.
b. The lower one-fifth in the region below the hymen is derived from endoderm of the urogenital sinus.
c. The external vaginal orifice is made from the genital folds ectoderm after the urogenital membrane has been breached.

Arterial Supply of the Vagina

- Main supply: Vaginal artery, a branch of the internal iliac artery.
- Upper part: Cervicovaginal branch of the uterine artery.
- Lower part: From middle rectal and internal pudendal artery

Venous Drainage of vagina: The vaginal venous plexus of veins is drained by the internal iliac veins.

Lymphatic Drainage

- Upper one-third: External iliac nodes.
- Middle one-third: Internal iliac nodes.
- Lower one-third: Medial group of superficial inguinal nodes.

Nerve Supply

- Lower one-third: Pudendal nerve.
- Upper two-thirds: Sympathetic L1, 2 and parasympathetic S2-S4. Supplied by the inferior hypogastric and uterovaginal plexuses.

Nerves from the sympathetic system cause vasoconstriction, while the parasympathetic nerves in the region are vasodilators.

Uterus: The uterus sits in the pelvis, with the bladder in front and the rectum behind.

Position: Dextrorotated

Parts of the uterus:
The uterus can be divided into three parts:

- Body: Extends from fundus to isthmus—Fundus top part of the uterus situated above the insertion of the two fallopian tubes. It is a part of body of uterus.
- Isthmus: It is the area between the body and cervix. It is actually a short area of constriction.
- Cervix: Lies below the isthmus and divided into two parts, a supravaginal portion superior to the limits of the vaginal and a vaginal portion which projects into the cavity of the vagina.

Ligaments of uterus

Peritoneal Ligaments: These are simply peritoneal folds that do not offer any support to the uterus.

1. The anterior ligament is made up of the uterovesical fold of peritoneum.
2. The posterior ligament is formed by the rectovaginal fold, which creates the rectovaginal pouch of peritoneum.
3. The right and left broad ligaments are peritoneal folds that connect the uterus to the lateral pelvic wall.

Ligaments

1. Round ligaments
2. Transverse cervical ligaments
3. Uterosacral ligaments. These are discussed separately under the section titled 'supports' of the uterus.

Arterial Supply

The uterus receives its blood supply:

1. Primarily from the two uterine arteries, which significantly enlarge during pregnancy.
2. Partially from the ovarian arteries.

Blood Supply of Uterus

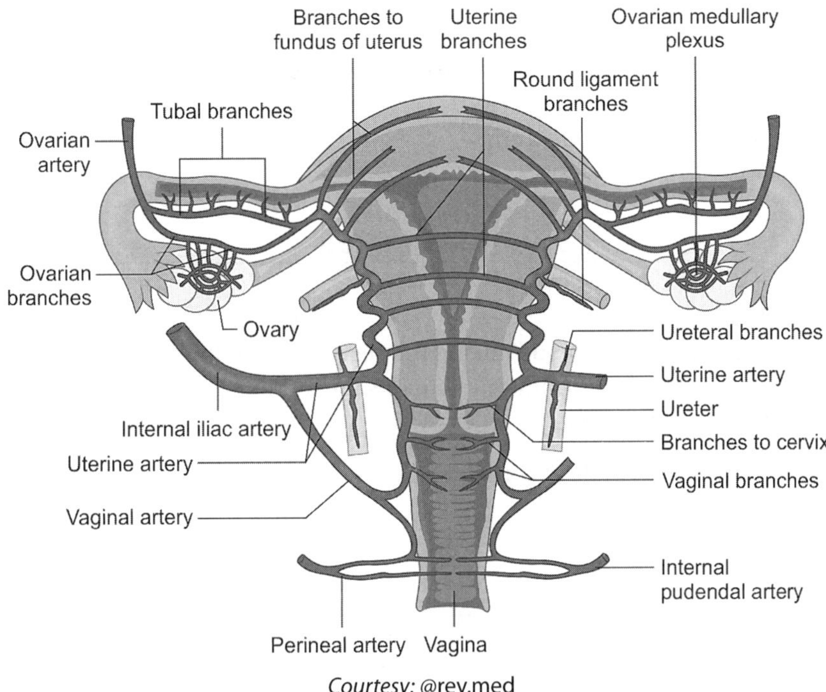

Courtesy: @rev.med

The uterine artery is the main blood supply of uterus which is branch of anterior division of internal iliac artery. The ovarian artery also supply the uterus which is a branch of the abdominal aorta. The arteries anastomose alone the fallopian tube.

Venous Drainage

The veins establish a plexus along the lateral edge of the uterus, which drains into the internal iliac vein through the uterine, ovarian, and vaginal veins.

Lymphatic Drainage

The upper lymphatics from the fundus and upper section of the body primarily drain into the aortic nodes, with only a partial drainage to the uterus.

Middle lymphatics from the lower region of the body flow into the external iliac lymph nodes.

The cervical lower lymphatics drain into the sacral and internal iliac nodes

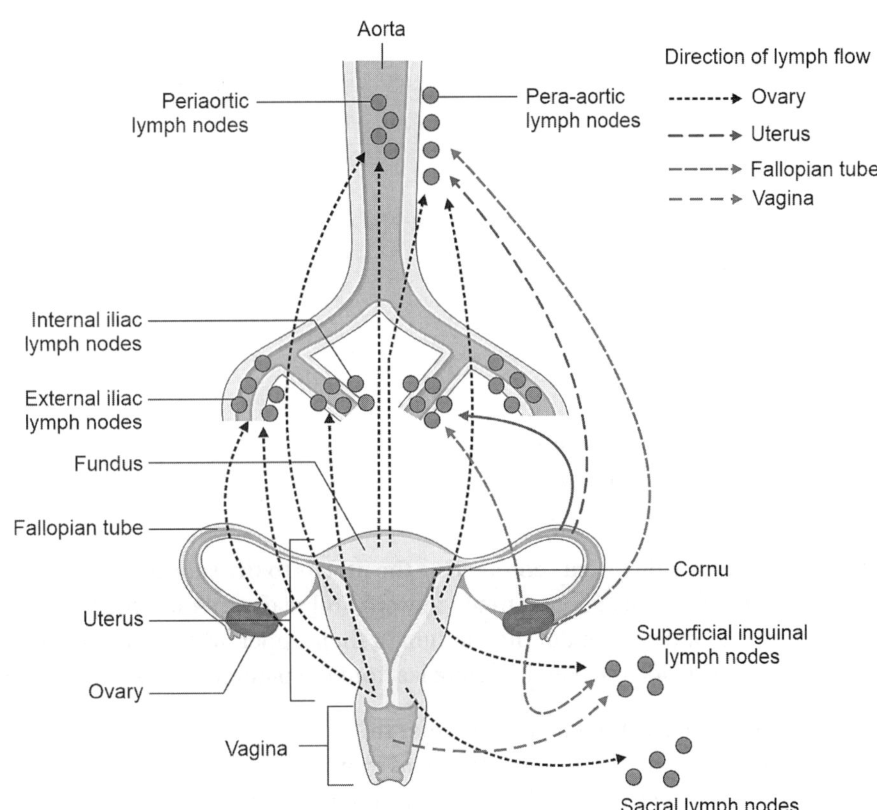

Q1. What is the uterine relationship other pelvic organs?

- Anteriorly – Urinary bladder and uterovesical fold of peritoneum.
- Posteriorly – pouch of Douglas and coils of intestine.
- Laterally – parametrium and Uterine artery crosses over the ureter (water under the bridge) 2 cm lateral to the cervix.
- Superiorly – coils of intestine and omentum.
- Inferiorly – the vagina.

SHORT NOTES

Supports of the Uterus

The levator ani muscles and the connective tissue linking the cervix walls to the pelvic walls. The interaction between the levator ani muscles and connective tissue primarily supports the uterus and cervix. Which is clinically known as the cardinal ligament and the uterosacral ligament.

Q1. What are the ligaments of uterus and cervix?

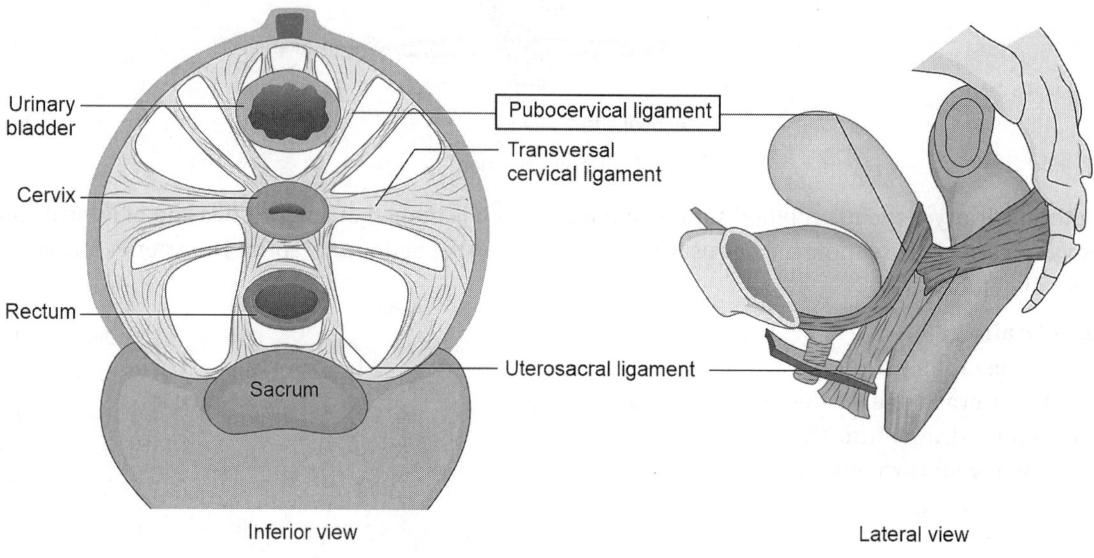

Source: Physiopedia

- Round ligaments
- Ovarian ligaments
- Broad ligaments
- Mackenrodt ligaments
- Uterosacral ligaments
- Pubocervical ligaments

Q2. What are the ligaments connecting the uterus to the sacrum?

The uterosacral ligaments stretch upward and rearward from the posterior aspect of the cervix to the lateral part of the second segment of the sacrum. In their upper area, they narrow down into subtle peritoneal folds. These ligaments divide the pouch of Douglas from the pararectal fossa on either side.

Q3. What do the cardinal ligaments refer to?

Cardinal ligaments (often referred to as transverse cervical ligaments or Mackenrodt ligaments) provide the most robust support for the uterus. These ligaments are primarily made of dense connective tissue that extends from the pelvic sidewalls to the genital region, encircling the cervix and the upper part of the vagina. They extend upward and backward toward the origin of the internal iliac vessels. This elastic and fibrous tissue, along with certain smooth muscle fibers, is occasionally referred to collectively as the parametrium.

Q4. Pubocervical ligaments

Pubocervical ligaments run from the cervix to the pubic bones along the lower lateral surface of the bladder. They are comprised of two slender fibrous bands. These ligaments draw the cervix forwards, opposing the backward pull of the uterosacral ligaments.

Q5. Round ligaments and Broad ligaments.

Round ligaments: These maintain the forward position of the uterus and help preserve its anteflexed posture.

Broad ligaments: These encompass the blood vessels that supply the uterus and fallopian tubes. The levator ani muscles serve as a support for the pelvic floor and help prevent uterine prolapse. Surgical significance: Although it is uncommon (0.3-0.5%), there is a possibility of ureteral injury occurring during gynecological procedures.

Pelvic ureters and surgical importance

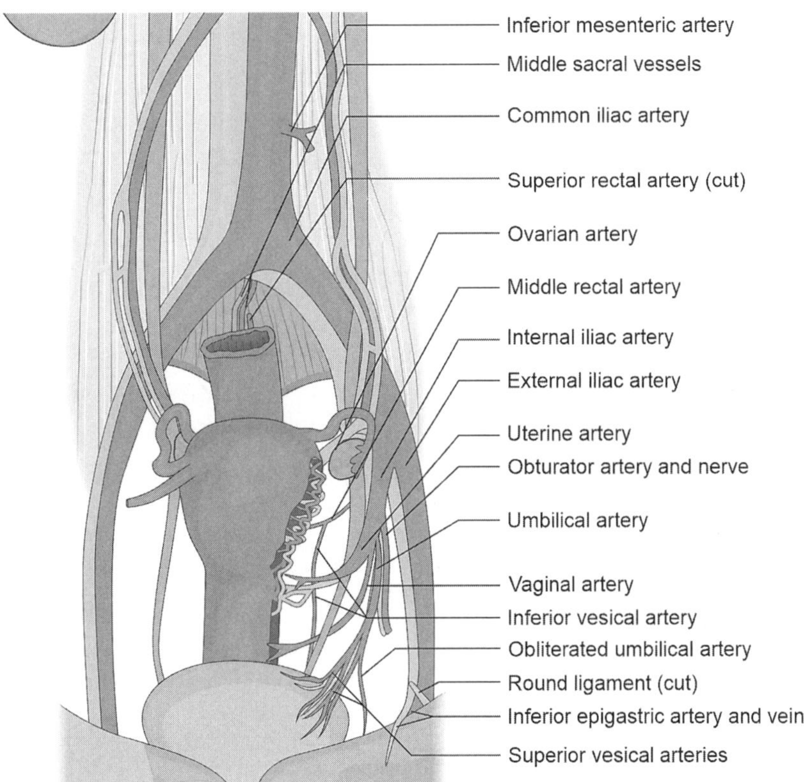

Pelvic ureter pathway: The pelvic segment of the ureter starts as it crosses the pelvic brim below the ovarian vessels and close to the splitting of the common iliac artery. It moves medial to the ovarian vessels and subsequently anterior to the bifurcation of the hypogastric and external iliac arteries. The ureter subsequently moves slightly in front of the hypogastric artery until it nears the ischial spine level, at which point it passes medial to the hypogastric artery's anterior division and lateral to the uterosacral ligament. The ureter subsequently enters the cardinal ligament "tunnel," goes beneath the uterine artery ("water under the bridge") 1.5-2 cm lateral to the cervix at the internal cervical os level, and moves medially over the anterior vaginal fornix. Traveling forward, it closely approaches the lateral fornix of the vagina, occurring 8-12 mm from the cervix and vaginal wall before arriving at the bladder. The ureters are approximately 5 cm apart when they enter the bladder. They travel through the bladder wall at an angle (approximately 2 cm long) and in a forward, inward, and downward manner. The ureters enter the bladder through two slit-like openings, the urethral orifices, which are approximately 2.5 cm apart when the bladder is not filled. Within the pelvis, the ureter features a unique connective tissue covering that connects to the medial layer of the broad ligament. Consequently, upon accessing the retroperitoneal space in the pelvis, the ureter can be located within the medial layer of the broad ligament.

Surgical significance: While uncommon (0.3-0.5%), ureteral damage can happen during gynecological procedures.

CHAPTER

Development of Female Genital Organs and its Congenital Anomalies

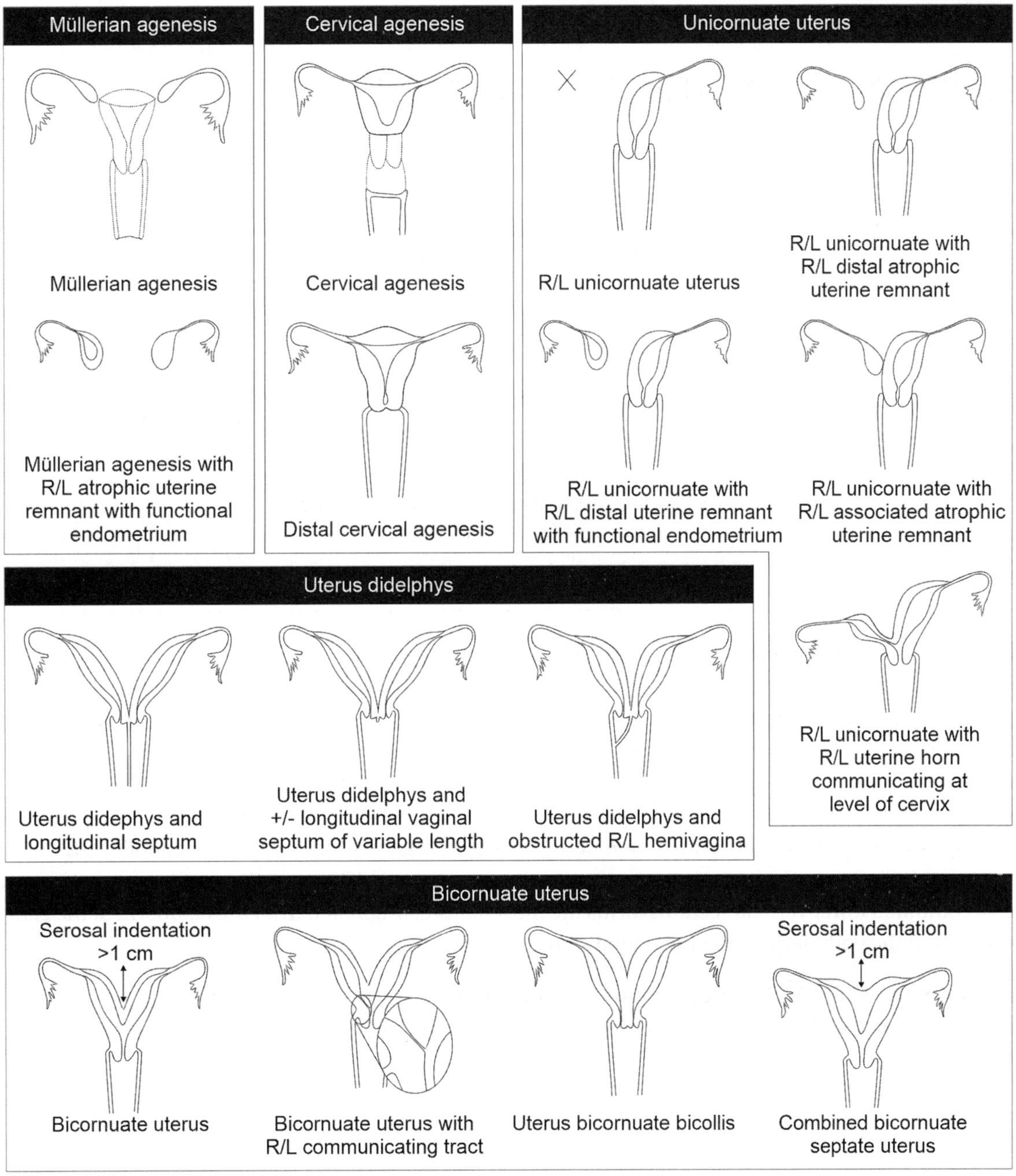

Müllerian agenesis

Müllerian agenesis

Müllerian agenesis with R/L atrophic uterine remnant with functional endometrium

Cervical agenesis

Cervical agenesis

Distal cervical agenesis

Unicornuate uterus

R/L unicornuate uterus

R/L unicornuate with R/L distal atrophic uterine remnant

R/L unicornuate with R/L distal uterine remnant with functional endometrium

R/L unicornuate with R/L associated atrophic uterine remnant

R/L unicornuate with R/L uterine horn communicating at level of cervix

Uterus didelphys

Uterus didephys and longitudinal septum

Uterus didelphys and +/- longitudinal vaginal septum of variable length

Uterus didelphys and obstructed R/L hemivagina

Bicornuate uterus

Serosal indentation >1 cm

Bicornuate uterus

Bicornuate uterus with R/L communicating tract

Uterus bicornuate bicollis

Serosal indentation >1 cm

Combined bicornuate septate uterus

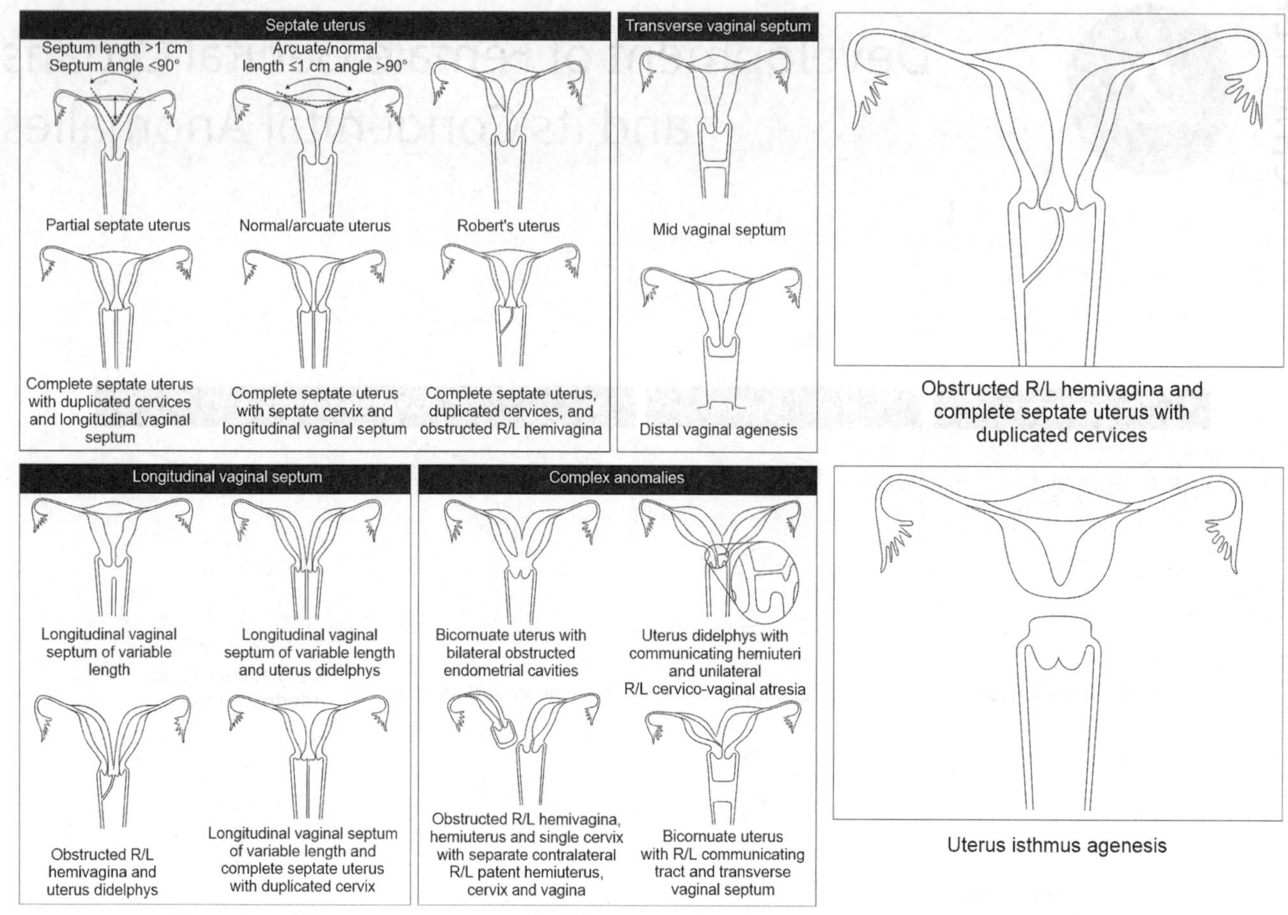

ASRM 2021 Classification of Mullerian anomalies
Source: Pfeifer, Samantha M. et al.

SHORT NOTES

Q1. Write down the development of the female internal genital organs.

The fallopian tubes were formed from the cervical vertical and the majority of the intermediate horizontal segments of the corresponding paramesonephric duct. The uterus originated from the cephalic portion of the uterovaginal canal, which is created when the vertical segments of the two paramesonephric ducts fuse together. Additionally, portions of the paramesonephric duct's horizontal sections support the uterine fundus. The vagina's upper four-fifths, lower one-fifth (down below the hymen), and external vaginal orifice (vaginal introitus) were primarily formed by the Mullerian ducts and partially by the urogenital sinus. From the endoderm of the canalized sinovaginal bulb (urogenital sinus), a mucous membrane is formed. The mesoderm of the two paramesonephric ducts' combined lower vertical sections forms the musculature. originated from the ectoderm of the genitalia and evolved from the endoderm of the urogenital sinus.

Q2. Write down the ASRM Mullerian anomalies classification.

The task force of ASRM and SRS classifies Mullerian anomalies into nine categories:

- Mullerian agenesis
- Cervical agenesis
- Unicornuate uterus
- Bicornuate uterus

- Uterus didelphys
- Septate uterus
- Longitudinal vaginal septum
- Transverse vaginal septum
- Complex anomalies

Q3. Write down different type of developmental anomalies of uterus and its incidence?

Female internal genital mainly develops from Mullerian duct anomaly is classified as by "American Fertility society" as follows

Types of fusion anomalies (incidence)	*Developmental defects*
Class – I (Agenesis/hypoplasia)	a. Vaginal b. Cervical c. Fundal d. Tubal e . Combined
Class – II (Unicornuate uterus) (10%)	Failure of development of one Mullerian duct
Class – III (Didelphys)-Didelphys (8%)	There is complete lack of fusion of the mullerian ducts with a double uterus, double cervix and a double vagina
Class – IV • Bicornuate uterus (26%) • Uterus bicornis bicollis • Uterus bicornis unicollis	• There is varying degrees of fusion failure of the muscle walls of the two ducts • There are two uterine cavities with double cervix with or without vaginal septum • There are two uterine cavities with one cervix. The horns may be equal or one horn may be rudimentary and may have no communication with the developed horn
Class – V • Septate uterus (35%)	The two Mullerian ducts are fused together but there is persistence of septum in between the two either partially (subseptate) or completely
Class – VI • Arcuate (18%)	The cornual parts of the uterus remains departed. Arcuate/Normal uterus has depth of indentation ≤ or equal to 1 cm and the angle is >90°
Class VII (DES related) – DES related	• Vaginal adenosis • Adenocarcinoma • Cervical – Cockscomb cervix – Cervical collar • Uterus – Hypoplasia – T shaped cavity

a. Category I -II: Developmental failure.
b. Category III -IV: Failure of midline fusion
c. Category V -VI: Failure of resorption.

Abnormalities of fallopian tube:

- Whole or part is absent
- Not well developed
- Atresia—congenital
- Length more than normal
- Duplication
- Accessory tube
- Diverticula
- Accessory ostia

Abnormalities of the ovaries:

1. Streak gonads/gonadal dysgenesis:
   - Usually associated with errors in sex chromosomal pattern.

2. Accessory ovary.
3. Super numerary ovaries.
4. Failure of descent:
   - May stay at the pelvic brim level/or even close to the kidney's lower pole
   - Can be seen in hernial sec sometimes

Abnormalities of the vagina:

1. Absence:
   - May be completely absent/more often the Mullerian portion.
2. Vaginal hypoplasia.
3. Septate and subseptate vagina.
4. Double vagina (Duplication).

Q4. Please outline the clinical significance of uterine anomalies.

The significance is contingent upon the severity of the abnormality.

Gynecological

1. Women with uterine agenesis may experience primary amenorrhea.
2. Primary amenorrhea accompanied by pelvic pain, which is frequently caused by complete obstruction of the genital tract (at the levels of the vagina, cervix, or lower uterus).
3. Menstrual disorders: Hematometra can occur in cases of obstructive anomalies.
4. Menorrhagia may be present in a bicornuate uterus, along with abnormal uterine bleeding (AUB) due to increased surface area.
5. Dysmenorrhea associated with pelvic pain (either cyclic or noncyclic) may arise from a unilateral obstructive anomaly.
6. Obstructive anomalies can result in retrograde menstruation and endometriosis.
7. Infertility and dyspareunia may be seen due to presence of a vaginal septum.

Obstetrical

1. Adverse obstetrical outcomes: The risk of recurrent pregnancy loss (RPL) varies from 6 to 38%.
2. Midtrimester miscarriages, which may occur repeatedly.
3. A higher incidence of malpresentation—transverse lie in arcuate or subseptate uterus, breech presentation in bicornuate, unicornuate, or complete septate uterus/preterm labor, fetal growth restriction, and intrauterine demise (IUD).
4. Prolonged labor due to incoordinate uterine action.
5. Obstructed labor caused by the nongravid horn of the bicornuate uterus or a rudimentary horn.
6. Pregnancy in a rudimentary horn.
7. An increased rate of cesarean deliveries.
8. Retained placenta and postpartum hemorrhage.

Q5. What methods will you employ to diagnose Mullerian duct abnormalities?

The female internal genital organs, including the uterus and fallopian tubes, as well as the upper three-fifths of the vagina, develop from the Mullerian duct.

Diagnosis: Utilizing a comprehensive approach that includes: -

- Detailed medical history
- Thorough clinical examination
- Relevant investigations

History:

1. Age: Patients typically present with primary amenorrhea or various reproductive issues such as subfertility or recurrent pregnancy loss (RPL), usually between the ages of 14 and 20.
2. Symptom analysis: Primary amenorrhea with or without cyclical lower abdominal pain.

3. Symptoms of frequency, urgency, and dysuria due to outflow tract obstruction: Urinary retention.
4. Infertility.
    - Dyspareunia
    - Recurrent pregnancy loss

Physical examination:
General:
- BMI normal (normal female structure)
- Well developed breast.
- Well-developed secondary sexual characteristics like.
    - Normal growth of pubic and axillary hair.
- Female configuration.

Per-abdominal:
- Lower abdominal mass (Outflow tract obstruction)).

Prevaginal examination:
Inspection:
- Short/blind vagina (Mullerian Agenesis)
- Imperforate hymen-Bluish bulge membrane
- Transvaginal septum: Pink septum

Digital examination:
- Admits tip of finger. (usually little finger)
- Blind vagina (Mullerian agenesis)

P/R/E:
- Uterus may be absent/ (Mullerian agenesis).
- Uterus may be bulky (Due to Hematometra and hematocolpos in imperforated hymen).
- Tender adnexal mass due to chocolate cyst in outflow tract obstruction

Investigation:
A. Imaging: Finding depends on type of anomalies
    1. USG of lower abdomen and pelvis [preferably TVS or 3D TVS (Gold standard)]
        - Uterus may be absent
        - Double uterus, cervix
        - Chocolate cyst.
        - Collection within uterus/vagina.
        - Renal anomalies usually present in 40% cases which is diagnosed by USG of whole abdomen
    2. Hysteroscopy:
        - Septate uterus may be seen
    3. Hysterography/Hysterosalpingography:
        - Double uterus
        - Arcuate.
        - Septate
        - Bicornuate.
    4. MRI of abdomen and pelvis

B. Karyotyping 46 XX
    - Mullerian anomalies.

Treatment
The treatment subphases are categorized into three sections: (a) Medical (b) dilatation, (c) surgical. Surgical intervention for the correction of Mullerian anomalies is intricate and should be conducted by expert surgeons. A

multidisciplinary team (MDT) approach, including radiologists, gynecologists, urologists, and pediatric surgeons, is advised. Temporary medical management may be necessary if surgery needs to be postponed. Medical management aims to suppress menstruation to avert collection and associated discomfort. Dilatation is utilized for nonsurgical vaginal lengthening, achieving success rates of up to 90%. The surgical approach is tailored to rectify each anomaly, in conjunction with the MDT. The mere presence of any uterine malformation does not warrant surgical intervention; however, women with obstructive anomalies require surgery. Reproductive outcomes indicate a better obstetric prognosis in cases of septate uterus (86%) and bicornuate uterus (50%) following surgical correction. Conversely, unicornuate uterus is associated with a poor pregnancy outcome of 40%, and no treatment has proven generally effective. Uterus didelphys presents the highest likelihood of successful pregnancy at 64%. Unification operations are typically unnecessary, and other factors contributing to infertility or recurrent fetal loss must be ruled out. Rudimentary horns should be excised to mitigate the risk of ectopic pregnancy, which stands at 8%. Unification operations in cases of bicornuate uterus are indicated in otherwise unexplained instances of uterine malformation. Abdominal metroplasty is performed through a unification operation (Strassman, Jones, and Jones), with a high success rate of 85% in terms of live births. Hysteroscopic metroplasty is more frequently employed in cases of septate uterus, where the resection of the septum can be accomplished using a resectoscope, scissors, or laser. The advantages include: (a) A high success rate (80-89%); (b) a short hospital stay; (c) reduced postoperative morbidity (such as infection or adhesions); and (d) a higher subsequent chance of vaginal delivery compared to abdominal metroplasty, where cesarean section is obligatory.

CHAPTER 3

Gynecological Examination

Case Taking

Gynecological

1. Identification:
   - Date of admission
   - Date of examination
   - Name
   - Age
   - Religion
   - Address
   - Marital status
   - Parity
   - Social status
2. Chief complaints
3. Present illness history
4. Menstrual history
   - Menarche age
   - LMP
   - Menstrual cycle length: Days
   - Regularity of cycle: Regular/irregular
   - Duration of flow
   - Amount of flow: Scanty/average/heavy
   - Associated symptoms? Present/absent
   - Associated pain: Yes/No
   - Intermenstrual bleeding or discharge per vaginal

   If the patient is postmenopausal:
   - Age of onset menopause
   - Menopausal symptoms, if any
   - Previous menstrual pattern
5. Obstetric history

Obstetric history.

Number	Date and year	Event during Pregnancy	Events during labor	Mode of delivery	Puerperium	Baby: Living or not, duration of breastfeeding/ immunization status
1	2019	Uneventful	Nonprogress of labor	Lower segment cesarean section (LSCS)	Uneventful	Male/living/ breastfed/ immunized

6. Past medical history
7. Past surgical history
8. Family history
9. Social history
10. Personal history
11. Sexual history
12. General examination: (i) Build - obese/thin/average, (ii) Nutrition - well-nourished/malnourished, (iii) Height, (iv) Weight, (v) pallor - absent/mild/moderate/severe, (vi) Pulse rate, (vii) Blood pressure, (viii) Respiratory rate, (ix) Edema, (x) Temperature, (xi) jaundice (xii) Cyanosis, (xiii) Neck veins and (xiv) Neck glands
13. Systemic examination: (i) Cardiac examination (ii) Pulmonary examination, and (iii) Gastrointestinal examination - liver/spleen
14. Examination of breast
15. Abdominal examination: (i) Inspection, (ii) palpation, (iii) Percussion, and (iv) Auscultation
16. Pelvic examination: (i) Inspection, (ii) Speculum examination, (iii) Bimanual examination, (iv) Rectal examination in selected cases, and (v) Rectovaginal examination in selected cases. Note that for undergraduate student's speculum examination, bimanual examination, and rectal and rectovaginal are not allowed.
17. Case summary
18. Provisional & Differential diagnosis
19. Investigation suggested.

Q1. Name the different components of gynecological examination.
The gynecological examinations include examination of breast, abdomen, and pelvic examinations.

Q2. Name the prerequisites to be fulfilled prior gynecological examination.
(i) Verbal consent, (ii) A female attendant, (iii) Patient should be asked to empty her bladder, (iv) Patient should be properly positioned with adequate exposure under good light sourcing, (v) Patient's privacy should be maintained by covering the other areas apart from examination area with a sheet or gown, (vi) patients is examined standing on right side, (vii) Equipment such as gloves, speculum of proper size and water soluble lubricants should be available prior hand.

Q3. How breast is examined?
Inspection—asymmetry in shape and size, nipple inversion, bulging and dimpling
Palpation—with the patient seated and again with the patient supine, the ipsilateral arm above the head and a pillow under the ipsilateral shoulder, the patient presses both hands against the hips or the palms together in front of the forehead. The breast is palpated with the palmar surfaces of the 2nd, 3rd, and 4th fingers, moving systematically in a small circular pattern from the nipple to the periphery. The axillary and supraclavicular lymph nodes are most easily examined with the patient seated or standing outer edges. Supporting the patient's arm during the axillary examination allows the arm to be filly relaxed so that nodes deep within the axilla can be palpated.

Q4. Name the points you note at the time of inspection of abdomen.
(i) Contour of the abdomen (ii) Skin subcutaneous tissue - condition of the skin, scar marks, linea nigra, striae gravidarum, engorged veins, (iii) Presence of swelling in relation to anatomical regions, (iv) Position of umbilicus, and (v) Movements.

Q5. What are the components of superficial palpation?
(i) Temperature and (ii) Tenderness.

Q6. Which points you record at the time of palpation of a pelvic lump?
(i) Site of swelling, (ii) Size (iii) Shape, (iv) Surface, (v) Consistency, (vi) Margin, (vii) Movements, (viii) Parietal or intra-abdominal (ix) Is the swelling pulsatile or not? And (x) Expansible impulse on coughing and reducibility (in cases of hernia).

Q7. Described the methods of percussion.

Shifting dullness: Percussion should be stated from the center of the abdomen and is carried down to one flank. At the point where dullness starts the finger is kept in its position and the patient is asked to turn to opposite side. That particular area is again percussed after waiting for a few minutes to allow the fluid to gravitate down. If the area becomes resonant, indicate presence of free fluid in abdomen.

Fluid thrill: Ask the patient to position her hand in midline of abdomen and flick the abdomen to test for transmitted thrill. In presence of ascites, a fluid thrill can be demonstrated but in presence of ovarian cyst fluid thrill is absent.

Q8. How do you carry out speculum examination?

The speculum examination include entry, positioning, opening, use and removal.

The speculum is moistened with warm water before insertion. The labia are gently separated with gloved left hand to expose the introitus. Then, the speculum is inserted with the blades closed nearly in the vertical plane (at about 1 and 7 o'clock) and thereby avoiding pressure over sensitive urethra. The speculum is fully inserted toward the cervix, then rotated by almost 90° so that the handle is down, and gently opened; it is pulled back as needed to visualize the cervix.

The vaginal and cervix are inspected for lesions. Before the metal speculum is removed, the screw should be loosened so the speculum blades can partially close. The speculum should gradually partially close upon withdrawal. The examiner should take care to keep a finger between the two metal blades to prevent complete apposition, which could pinch the patient's mucosa.

Q9. How do you perform a bimanual examination?

Patient is placed in lithotomy position or dorsal position with thighs flexed and knees apart. The labia are separated and gloved, lubricated index and middle fingers of the dominant hand are inserted into the vagina to just below the cervix. The other hand is placed just above the pubic symphysis position, and gently presses down to determine the size, consistency of the uterus. Tenderness with lateral movement of the cervix (cervical motion tenderness) is assessed along with its consistency, size, and contour. The adnexa are palpated. Any masses that are appreciated are assessed for size, location, mobility, tenderness, and contour. The posterior cul-de-sac and uterosacral ligaments are checked for nodularity and masses.

Q10. How do you perform rectovaginal examination?

In rectovaginal examination the examiner inserts an index finger into the vagina, and utilizing lubricant, inserts the middle finger into the rectum. The examiner palpates the rectovaginal septum and again places the opposite hand on the patient's lower abdomen to palpate the previously assessed structures. The uterosacral ligaments may be palpated more easily with the rectovaginal examination than the bimanual examination. The rectum is assessed for masses.

A. General examination:
- Appearance—Healthy or ill looking
- Body built—average/short stature/tall stature. Weight can be calculated as body mass index (BMI). BMI is calculated on the basis of height and weight (weight in kg divided by height in m^2). Normal range of BMI is 19–24. When BMI < 18.5 it is considered as obese.
- Nutrition: Average/good/poor.
  Nutrition can be assessed by:
  a. Measurement of the skin fold thickness between the index or middle finger
  b. By measuring the mid arm circumference (<22 cm – malnourished, >30 cm – likely obese)
  c. Measuring mid-thigh circumference
  d. Examining the features of any vitamin deficiency.
- Anemia—clinically can be categorized as mild, moderate and severe

- Primary sites to see anemia are:
  1. Lower palpebral conjunctiva

  Other site:
  1. Tongue-dorsum
  2. Palate-soft
  3. Nail beds
  4. Palm and sole
  5. Skin
- Jaundice—present/absent.

  Sites to detect jaundice:
  1. Conjunctiva—upper bulbar
  2. Tongue—undersurface
  3. Palate—soft
  4. Sole and palm
  5. Skin

  Jaundice should be checked in sunlight near an open window.
- Cyanosis: Absent/Present.
- Sites to detect cyanosis are as follows:

  Peripheral:
  - Nose-tip
  - Ear-lobule
  - Lips outer surface, cheek and chin
  - Tips of fingers and toes
  - Inner surface of lips
  - Gun, soft palate, cheeks.

  Edema:

  Primary sites to examine edema:
  1. Above the medial malleolus by pressing with tip of thumb for at least 15 seconds.
  2. Lower third of shin bones—anterior surface
  3. Foot—dorsum
- Tongue, teeth, gum and tonsils:
- Examination of secondary sexual characters:
  - Hair, axillary, breast and pubic region

These are important in primary amenorrhea and intersex.

- For face and skin: Acne, Hirsutism, acanthosis nigricans are features of androgen excess commonly PCOS.
- Neck veins: Engorged or not.
- Neck glands: Thyroid gland inspected and palpated for any enlargement or any other pathology.
- Pulse: Radial pulse is palpated at the wrist, lateral to the flexor carpi radialis tendon by the palp of three fingers with the patient's forearm semi pronated and wrist slightly flexed. Following points of the pulse are to be noted:
  1. Rate
  2. Rhythm
  3. Volume
  4. Any special character
  5. Upper and lower limb pulse differences.
- Respiration: Beats/min
- Temperature: By thermometer.
- Blood pressure: Blood pressure is mentioned as systolic/ diastolic in mm Hg. Patient must take rest at least for 5 minutes before the measurement of blood pressure. Blood pressure can be measured either in sitting

or lying down posture in relax attitude supporting the patient's arm comfortably at the level of heart. The sphygmomanometer cuff is applied over the upper arm, with the center on brachial artery.

- Systolic pressure is first assessed roughly by palpation of radial pulse or brachial pulse after inflating the cuff till it becomes impalpable. In auscultation technique, diaphragm of the stethoscope is placed gently over the brachial pulses which is situated medical to the biceps brachii tendon over the elbow joint. The cuff is initially inflated to a pressure 20–30 mm Hg higher than the estimated systolic pressure determined by palpation.
- Then the cuff is deflated 2 mm/sec until a regular tapping sound is heard.
  For the assessment of diastolic pressure the cuff is deflating slowly unit the sounds disappear. The pressure is recorded as diastolic pressure at which the sound completely disappears.

B. Systemic examination:
- Cardiovascular system:
  - Palpation of precordium and auscultation of heart sounds are done in different areas.
  - If any lesion is detected or suspected detailed examination of different areas is done and noted.
- Respiratory system:
  1. Trachea position
  2. Palpation: Both sides
  3. Percussion: Done on both sides
  4. Auscultation: Done on both sides.
- GI system: Liver and spleen should be palpated

C. Gynecological examination:
1. Examination of Breasts: This should be a routine to detect any breast pathology.
   A. Self-breast examination (SBE) is done by the patient herself.
   B. Clinical breast examination (CBE) is done by a skilled profession. CBE includes visual inspection combined with palpation of the breasts and axilla (ACOG 2011).
      - Skin, areola, nipple, sizes of breasts and local swelling in different positions should be inspected
        a. Arms resting on thighs
        b. Arms pressing on hips
        c. Arms over the head and
        d. Learning.
      - Breast are palpated in lying down positing. With head on one pillow and patient's hand under the head on the side to be examined.
      - Each breast should be palpated systematically in all the quadrants from outwards towards the nipple. Presence of any lump and tenderness is noted. If there is any lump its characteristics are noted (size, position, consistency, fixity, surface, margins and tenderness). The nipple should be palpated for any abnormality or discharge- watery, bloody or milky (galactorrhea). The axilla should be palpated for any extension of breast (axillary tail) between thumb and finger and presence of nodes. The supra-clavicular lymph node should also be palpated.
      - In case of primary amenorrhea, development of breast is staged according to Tanner's staging.
2. Abdominal examination:
   Prerequisites:
   - Bladder should be empty.
   - Presence of a female attendant/chaperone for the support of the patient and physician.
   - The physician should examine from right side of the patient.
   - The patient should be explained properly what the physician are going to do.
   - Informed consent of the patient should be taken.
   - The patient is to lie flat on the table on dorsal supine position. Head can be supported by a small pillow, partial flexion of knees and things facilitate relation of abdominal muscles.

Regions of abdomen: 9 regions of abdomen should be examined.

Inspection:

- Contour
- Skin condition
- Umbilicus: Everted/flushed/inverted.
- Presence of any scar.
- Presence of any lump of fullness of the abdomen.
- Inguinal lymph nodes should be palpated

Palpation: Palpation is performed by flat of the hand and movements must be gentle and from metacarpophalangeal joints.

Superficial palpation: By superficial palpation temperature, tenderness, parietal edema, localized lump, fluid thrill are elicited.

Deep palpation: With flat of the dominant hand as well as the fingers abdomen is palpated deeply by asking the patient to breathe quietly. All the surgical areas of the abdomen are palpated systemically either clockwise or anticlockwise. The tender region should be palpated at the end. Difficult palpation in obesity and ascites the left hand is placed over right hand to feel deeply.

Liver and spleen are palpated. Patient is asked to take deep breath during palpation.

- Palpation of Kidney: The site of kidney is palpated and renal angle is elicited keeping hand behind near the junction of lateral border of erector spinae and lower border of 12th rib.
- Palpation of all surgical areas to see presence of any lump, tenderness, rigidity and muscle guard.
- Rebound tenderness is elicited
- If any mass is present I lower abdomen its site, size, shape, consistency, surface, margins, mobility from side to side and from above to down, tenderness are to be noted. Whether the lower border of the lump can be reached or not should be elicited. In general, border cannot be reached in pelvic tumor, but in ovarian tumor with a long pedicle one can go below the lower pole. If the tumor is cystic and huge, one can exhibit a fluid thrill felt with a flat hand placed on one side of the tumor when the cyst is tapped on the other side of the tumor with the other hand.

Q11. How would you determine a lump is retroperitoneal or intra-abdominal?

Knee elbow position to rule but retroperitoneal lump. In intra-abdominal lump it will be prominent and in case of retroperitoneal mass, it will become not prominent.

Percussion: Percussion can differentiate abdominal mass and ascites.

A pelvic tumor is usually dull on percussion with resonance on the flanks. However, if there are intestinal adhesions or the tumor is retroperitoneal, it will be resonant.

In presence of ascites, the flanks will be dull on percussion and the shifting dullness, if elicited, if elicited, confirm the diagnosis of free fluid in the peritoneal cavity.

If ovarian cyst is associated with gross ascites the midline will be resonant, flank is dull and shifting dullness becomes positive.

Demonstration of shifting dullness: In supine position, percussion should be started from the mid line out to the flanks. Any changes from resonant to dull is noted along with the areas of dullness and resonance. Finger on the site of dullness is kept and patient is asked to turn on to her side and a pause of 10–30 seconds is given. Then again percussion is done. If the dull and tympanic areas are reversed shifting dullness is said to be positive.

Demonstration of fluid thrill: It is done when abdomen is tensely distended. The palm of the left hand is placed against the left side of the patient's abdomen. The patient or an assistant is asked to place of the edge of hand on the midline of abdomen. The right side of the abdomen is flicked by a finger of right hand, ripple is felt against left hand "Fluid thrill" is said to be present.

Auscultation: Auscultation reveals the intestinal sounds. Hyperactive bowel sounds are found in paralytic ileus, bowel sound is absent in peritonitis, Hyperactive bowel sounds may be due to intestinal obstruction. The uterine souffle may be heard over a pregnant uterus or vascular fibroid, which is synchronous with the patient's pulse.

3. Pelvic Examination:
   Pelvic examination includes:
   - Inspection of the external genitalia
   - Vaginal examination:
     1. Inspection of the cervix and vaginal walls.
     2. Speculum examination
     3. Palpation of the vagina and vaginal cervix by digital examination.
     4. Bimanual examination of the pelvic organs.
   - Rectal examination
   - Recto vaginal examination.

Prerequisites:
1. The patient's bladder must be empty. The exception being a case of stress incontinence.
2. A female attendant should be present by her side.
3. Inform consent from the patient should be taken.
4. To examine a minor or unmarried girl, a consent from parent or guardian is required.
5. Proper privacy should be maintained.
6. Lower bowel should preferably be empty.
7. Good light source should be available.
8. Sterile gloves, sterile lubricant, speculum, sponge holding forceps and required.

Positions of the patient:
1. The patient is commonly examined in dorsal position with the knees flexed and thighs abducted. This position gives better view of the external genitalia and the bi manual pelvic examination can be effectively performed. Gynecological examinations is performed in different positions which are:
2. Dorsal lithotomy position.
3. Sim's semi prone position.
4. Left lateral position.

Inspection of external genitalia:
1. The following structures should be visually inspected in the vulva:
   - Labia minora and majora
   - Clitoris
   - Urethra
   - Fourchette
   - Vaginal introitus
   - Bartholin's gland
   - Anus
   - Gynecological perineum.
2. To note any anatomical abnormality starting from the pubic hair, clitoris, labia and perineum.
3. If there is any vaginal discharge to see the character of the discharge.
4. To separate the labia using fingers of the left hand to note external urethral meatus, visible openings of the Bartholin's duct and character of the hymen.
5. To ask the patient to strain to elicit:
   - Stress incontinence—urine comes out through ureteral meatus.
   - Genital prolapse and the structures involved: Anterior vaginal wall, uterus or posterior vaginal wall.
   - To look for hemorrhoids, anal fissure, and fistula or perineal tear.

Palpation of external genitalia and vagina: For any vulvar or vaginal lesion—digital examination is done.
Urethra and Bartholin gland are squeezed to see any discharge.
Bartholin gland is situated in posterior third of introitus deep to bulbospongiosus on two lateral sides.
In prolapse cervix is dragged. The degree of prolapse is determined, perineal body and levator ani are palpated to assess the tone.

Speculum examination: Speculum examination is usually done in dorsal position with a Cusco's bivalve self-retaining speculum or Sim's single- or double-bladed speculum before bimanual examination.

Q12. How to introduce Cusco's speculum?

- Once the labia are parted using the left thumb and index finger, lubricated transverse blades of Cusco's speculum are inserted in anteroposterior direction and then rotated 90 degrees to position the blades transversely.
- One should be careful during the introduction to ensure that the speculum does not roughly contact the ureteral meatus, as it is very sensitive.
- Once the blades are opened, the cervix is clearly visible. If the speculum does not show the cervix.
- The Cusco's speculum handle can be positioned anteriorly, aiding in optimal cervix visualization. The retaining screw can be secured to enable the speculum to be self-holding without assistance

Insertion of Sim's speculum:

- To visualize the anterior vaginal speculum, either single-bladed or double-bladed, it is most effective in Sim's semi-prone left lateral position, though it can also be performed in a dorsal supine position if the patient's back is positioned at the edge of the table.
- This instrument allows for the visualization of the anterior vaginal wall, lateral vaginal wall, and cervix.
    - In cases of cystocele, the anterior vaginal wall retractor is used to pull it back for clear visualization of the cervix and vaginal vault

Normal findings of cervix on inspection and speculum examination: The cervix is examined for its color, any discharge, the appearance of the external os, tears, hypertrophy, cervicitis, erosion, ectropion, cervical polyps, mucus or fibroids, cysts, Nabothian cysts, and any growths.

A healthy cervix is a deep shade of pink. The external os is pinhole or round in individuals who have never given birth, while it appears as a transverse slit in those who have given birth multiple times. The squamocolumnar junction is located close to the external os during reproductive age. Pre-ovulatory cervical mucus is clear, transparent, plentiful, and elastic.

Cervical smear for PAP smear is taken from the surface of cervix by using Ayer's spatula and from the endocervix by cyto-brush. In case of any discharge it should be collected for microscopic examination. The sample by Pap smear should be taken before performing vaginal examination.

Bimanual examination: With gloves on and lubricant applied, the index and middle fingers of the right hand are carefully inserted into the vagina until the cervix can be felt, while the labia minora are retracted using the left thumb and index finger.

- In anteverted uterus cervix should be directed posteriorly so that anterior lip is touched first.
- In case of uterus in mid position both lips of cervix cannot be touched together
- Introverted uterus cervix is directed anterior due to which posterior lip palpated first.

The cervix is examined through palpation first. The other hand is positioned on the patient's abdomen in the suprapubic area to conduct the bimanual examination, allowing the palpation of the uterus and fornices to observe the findings.

Bimanual examination should be methodical, gentle but purposeful.
The following information can be obtained bimanual examination:

1. Uterus is palpated
2. Uterine appendages can be palpated
3. Pouch of Douglas can be examined

Normal uterus is anteverted/retroverted, anteflexed, pear shaped, firm and mobile in all directions.
The normal fallopian tubes cannot be palpated.
Pouch of Douglas can be examined
Identification of a mass felt on bimanual examination:

Uterine tumor: Uterus is not separated from the mass.
Movements of the mass felt on abdomen are transmitted to the cervix and vice versa, The exception being one of sub-serosal pedunculated fibroid.

Adnexal mass:

- The uterus is separated from the mass.
- The mass's movement does not transfer to the cervix, except in one case: If the mass is anchored to the uterus

Rectal examination: Rectal examination (recto abdominal)—Rectal examination is done by wearing gloves and using lubricant in index finger indications. In gynecology for rectal examination are:

- Cancer cervix
- Posterior vaginal wall prolapses: To differentiate the enterocele and rectocele.
- Endometriosis
- Ovarian malignancy
- Adolescent girl
- Primary amenorrhea
- Vagina stenosis

Rectovaginal examination: The procedure is done by introducing the index finger in the vaginal and the middle finger in the rectum.
Rectovaginal examination: Is done to palpate recto vaginal septum, POD, posterior surface of uterus, fornices and utero-sacral ligaments. Growth if present in rectovaginal septum.

Checklist for per vaginal examination:

- Greetings
- Self-introduction
- Taking consent of patient
- Evacuation of bladder
- Privacy maintenance
- Use of light source
- Instruments checking
- Wearing of gloves properly
- Inspection of vulva and perineum
- Per speculum examination with lubricant
- Bimanual examination
- Per rectal examination when indicated
- Drop of instruments for decontamination
- Reassurance and thanks.

CHAPTER 4

Puberty and its Abnormalities

Puberty Menorrhagia

Excessive blood loss during menstruation from menarche to 20 years is called puberty menorrhagia.

Incidence:

14-16% of DUB patients are adolescent girls.

Causes: Puberty menorrhagia is mostly due to unopposed estrogen stimulation from anovulatory cycles.

Probable causes of AUB:

1. DUB—95%
2. Endocrine dysfunction:
    - Polycystic ovarian syndrome
    - Hypo-or hyperthyroidism
    - Hyperprolactinemia
3. Pelvic tumors:
    - Fibroid uterus
    - Sarcoma
    - Estrogen-producing ovarian tumor
4. Hematological:
    - ITP (Idiopathic Thrombocytopenic Purpura)
    - Von Willebrand's disease
    - Leukemia
5. Pregnancy complications (abortion)

Evaluation:

From history:

1. History of bleeding from another site of the body—gum bleeding, epistaxis.
2. History of sudden weight gain or loss.
3. History of taking any drugs.
4. If sexually active, pregnancy complication should be excluded.

Examination:

1. Height, weight, BMI
2. Pulse
3. Blood pressure
4. Enlargement of thyroid gland
5. Features of bleeding disorder:
    - Petechiae
    - Purpura

P/A/E:

Usually not done unless sexually active.

Investigation
- CBC (Complete Blood Count)
- Blood grouping and Rh typing
- Coagulation profile- BT (Bleeding Time), CT (Clotting Time), PT (prothrombin Time), APTT (Activated Partial Thromboplastin Time)
- Serum FS (Ferritin), LH (Luteinizing Hormone), and estradiol
- Serum prolactin
- Blood sugar after 75 gm glucose
- Imaging—USG (Ultrasonography), MRI (Magnetic Resonance Imaging) to exclude pelvic pathology if needed
- If no cause found, endometrial sampling (EUA) and, if not responsive to medical treatment, curettage for histopathological examination (HPE) may be needed.

Management puberty menorrhagia:
Initial step of management is assurance and explanation to the patient and patient's guardian.

Mild anemia:
- Iron with vitamin supplementation
- Weight reduction
- Nutrition
- Re-evaluation after 3-6 months.

Moderate anemia:
- Progesterone therapy:
  - Tab medroxyprogesterone Acetate (10 mg) 1+1+1 from 16th to 25th day.
- Re- evaluation after 3 months.

Severe anemia:
- Hospitalization
- Bed rest
- Blood transfusion
- Norethisterone (5 mg) 1+1+1 for 21 days for 3-6 cycles.
- Tranexamic acid
- Treatment of other causes.
- Re-evaluation up to 12 months.

Definition:
The term precocious puberty is reserved for girls who exhibit any secondary sexual characteristics before the age of 8 (before the age of 7 in Whites) or menstruate before the age of 10.

Cause of precocious puberty:
GnRH - dependent (central or true):
- Constitutional - most common
- Juvenile primary hypothyroidism
- CNS lesions - trauma, tumor, infection (TB, encephalitis)

Incomplete:
- Premature thelarche
- Premature pubarche
- Premature menarche

GnRH - independent:
- Precocious puberty of peripheral origin:
  - Ovary: Granulosa cell tumor, Theca cell tumor, Leydig cell tumor, choriocarcinoma, androblastoma, McCune - Albright syndrome.

- Adrenal: Hyperplasia, Tumor
- Liver: Hepatoblastoma
- Iatrogenic: Estrogen or androgen intake

Etiopathology:

- Constitutional: Due to premature activation of hypothalamic-pituitary-ovarian axis
- Intracranial lesions: Meningitis, Encephalitis, Craniopharyngioma, Neurofibroma, hypothalamic tumor
- Other causes: Choriocarcinoma, Hepatoblastoma.

Diagnosis: Meticulous history taking and physical examination are essential.

History:

- History of early menarche in mother and sisters
- Sequence of pubertal changes
- Often no cause detected

Examination: Tanner staging

Investigations:

1. Serum:
   - hCG
   - FSH
   - LH
   - Prolactin
2. Thyroid profile (TSH, T4)
3. Serum estradiol, testosterone, 17-OH progesterone, dehydroepiandrosterone (DHEA)
4. USG, CT scan, MRI of abdomen and pelvis to rule out ovarian, adrenal, and uterine pathology
5. Skull X-ray, CT scan, or MRI brain to exclude intracranial lesions
6. Electroencephalogram
7. X-ray of hand and wrist
8. GnRH stimulation test

Treatment:

1. Counseling
2. GnRH agonist therapy:
   - Medroxyprogesterone acetate
   - Danazol
3. Treatment according to the causes

Other:

SN—Mention the secondary sexual characteristics of females with clinical significance

- Delayed puberty
- Tanner staging.

Menopause: permanent cessation of, menstruation at the end if reproductive life due to loss of ovarian follicular activity. The clinical diagnosis is confirmed following cessation of menstruation (amenorrhea) for twelve consecutive months without any other pathology. It is characterized by amenorrhea, hypoestrogenemia, and FSH > 40 IU.L. The age at which menopause occurs is genetically predetermined, ranging between 45 and 55 years, with an average being 50 years.

Menopausal symptoms:

1. **Ovarian symptoms:**
   - Hot flushes characterized by sudden feeling of heat followed by profuse sweating, coinciding with GnRH pulse secretion and increased LH levels. May last for 1-10 minutes.

- Perspiration and cutaneous vasodilation.
- Palpitations, fatigue, weakness, and sleep disturbance.

2. **Urogenital:**
    - Atrophic epithelial changes in the urinary bladder, urethra, and vagina.
    - Urgency, dysuria, recurrent UTIs, stress incontinence.
    - Vaginal infections, dryness, pruritus, leucorrhea, dyspareunia.
    - Decreased sexual desire.
3. **Osteoporosis and fractures:**
    - Decreased collagen bone matrix, primarily affecting trabecular and cortical bones.
    - Osteoporosis may lead to back pain, loss of height, kyphosis and joint pain.
    - Fractures may involve the vertebral body, femoral neck and distal forearm.
4. **Cardiovascular and cerebrovascular effects:**
    - Central obesity.
    - Atherosclerosis
    - Increased insulin resistance
    - Increased risk of ischemic heart disease and coronary artery disease.
    - Increase risk of stroke.

Psychological:

- Anxiety
- Headaches
- Insomnia
- Irritability
- Depression, dementia.
- Mood swings, inability to concentrate.

Skin and hair:

- Decreased collagen content, loss of elasticity, and wrinkling of the skin.
- "Purse string" Wrinkling around the mouth, crow's feet around the eyes.
- Loss of axillary and public hair, slight balding.

Diagnose menopause:

1. Cessation of menstruation for consecutive 12 months during climacteric.
2. Average age is 50 years.
3. Appearance of menopausal symptoms – hot flushes and night sweats.
4. Serum estradiol level < 20 pg/mL.
5. Serum FSH and LH > 40 mIU/mL (3 values at weekly intervals are required).
6. Vaginal cytology showing a maturation index of at least 10/85/5.

Delayed Puberty

Q1. Define delayed puberty.

Delayed puberty: When the breast tissue and /or pubic hair have not appeared by 13-14 years or menarche appears as late as 16 years.

The normal upper age limit of menarche is 15 years.

Q2. What are the causes of delayed puberty?

Causes of delayed puberty

A. Hypergonadotropic hypogonadism
    1. Gonadal dysgenesis, 45XO
    2. Pure gonadal dysgenesis 46XX, 46XY
    3. Ovarian failure, 46XX

B. Hypogonadotropic hypogonadism
   1. Constitutional delay
   2. Chronic illness, malnutrition
   3. Primary hypothyroidism
   4. Isolated gonadotrophin deficiency (Kallmann's syndrome)
   5. Intracranial lesions-tumors: Craniopharyngioma, pituitary adenomas

Eugonadism
1. Anatomical causes
   a. Müllerian agenesis
   b. Imperforate hymen
   c. Transverse vaginal septum
2. Androgen insensitivity syndrome

PCOS

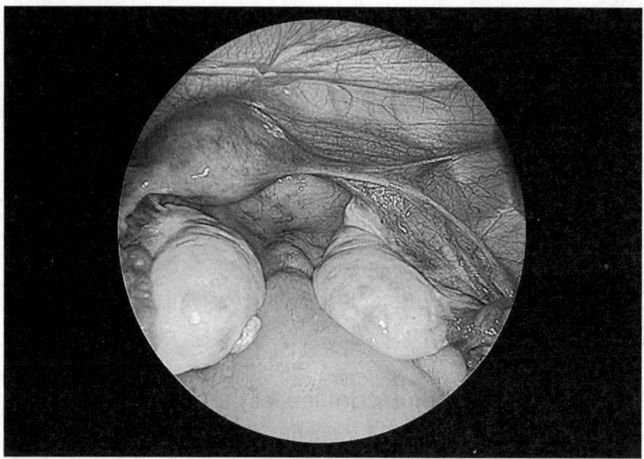

PCOS-Laparoscopic view

Q1. What do you mean by PCOS?

PCOS is a multifactorial and polygenic condition. It is a syndrome manifested by
- Amenorrhea
- Hirsutism
- Obesity
- Associated with
- Enlarged polycystic ovaries due to excessive androgen production

Q2. What is diagnostic criteria ASRM/ESHRE?

Presence of any 2 of the following 3 criteria:
- Oligo and or anovulation
- Hyperandrogenism (clinical and or biochemical)
- PCO

Q3. What is the incidence of PCOS?
- 4-8% in general population
- 15% among infertile, i.e., more common among infertile women
- 50% in south - Asian ethnicity
- Prevent in young reproductive age group (20-30%)

- 20% in normal women
- Dominant mode of inheritance is about 50% of 1st degree relatives have PCOS.

Q4. What are the USG finding of PCOS?

- Ovaries are enlarged (Ovarian volume is ≥10cm^3)
- Stroma is increased
- Capsule is thickened
- Pearly white in color
- Presence of multiple (≥12). Peripherally arranged follicle measuring about 2-9 mm in diameter are found crowded around the cortex.

Q5. What are the histological features?

- Thickening of tunica albuginea
- Cysts are follicles at varying stages of maturation and atresia.
- Theca cell hypertrophy (stromal hyperthecosis)

Q6. Clinical features of patient with PCOS.

Increasing obesity (abdominal – central) Menstrual abnormalities (70%)

- Oligomenorrhea
- Amenorrhea
- DUB Infertility Hirsutism
- Virilism (rare)
- Acanthosis nigricans is characterized by specific skin changes due to insulin resistance [the skin is thickened and pigmented (Gray brown)]

HAIR-AN syndrome: IT is triad of patients with PCOS present with hyperandrogenism, insulin resistance and acanthosis nigricans.

Q7. How you will investigate her?

If age >30 years with infrequent cycle

1. D2 FSH and LH – LH : FSH. 2:1
2. USG Preferably TVS in obese patient is useful. Ovaries are enlarged in volume (10 cm^3) >12 peripherally arranged follicle
3. High estradiol and estrone
4. SHBG is decreased.
5. Hyperandrogenism – androstenedione is increased (mainly from ovary less from adrenals)
6. Serum testosterone is increased > 150 ng/dL
7. DHEAS may be marginally elevated.
8. Insulin resistance (IR):
   Fasting insulin levels > 25 micro IU/mL
   Fasting glucose /insulin ratio < 4.5 (suggest IR 50%)
9. Insulin is increased (> 300 micro IU/mL)
10. Laparoscopy – Bilateral polycystic ovaries are characteristics to PCOS.

Q8. What is the consequences of PCOS?

Long-term consequences:

- Excess androgen (mainly androstenedione)
- Diminished SHBG
- Cumulative excess unbound E2 and estrone. Thus, results in a tonic hyperestrogenic state
- Endometrial hyperplasia late sequelae of PCOS:
- DM (15%) due to IR

- Endometrial Ca due to
  - Persistently elevated level of estrogen
  - Estrogen effects are not opposed by progesterone due to chronic anovulatory state
- HTN
- CVD and dyslipidemia (decrease HDL, increased TG, increase LDH)
- Obstructive sleep apnea

Q9. What are the biochemical abnormalities associated with PCOS?

- Hyperandrogenemia
- Hyperinsulinemia
- Hyperlipidemia
- High serum estrogen (estradiol, estrone)
- Androgenic follicular environment
- Hyperprolactinemia
- Insulin resistance
- Hyper secretion of LH
- Low serum SHBG
- Low FSH
- Low serum progesterone

Q10. What are the criteria of metabolic syndrome (diagnostic criteria)?

- TG levels ≥ 150
- HDL - cholesterol <50 mg/dL
- Blood pressure ≥130/85 mm Hg
- Fasting glucose ≥100 mg/dL
- Abdominal obesity (waist circumference >88 cm)

Q11. How you will manage a patient with PCOS?

Management depends on patients clinical symptoms like:

- Menstrual abnormality
- Subfertility
- Obesity
- Hirsutism
- Combined symptoms

1. Weight reduction: It is first line treatment in obese patient.
   - BMI should be <25 kg/m^2 which will improve menstrual disorders, infertility, impaired glucose tolerance (insulin resistance).
   - Weight reduction (2-5%) improves the metabolic syndrome and may also improve hirsutism.
2. Correction of metabolic syndrome may improve hirsutism.
   Antiandrogen (cyproterone acetate, spironolactone, flutamide are used for hirsutism)
3. For metabolic syndrome and hyperinsulinemia: Insulin sanitizers that is:
   - Metform 500 mg three times daily mainly are used other sensitizer
   - Pioglitazone
   - Rosiglitazone
4. For management of hyperandrogenemia:
   a. If fertility is not desired - combined oral contraceptive pill (Progestin suppresses LH and estrogen improve SHBG, reducing free testosterone.) Newer progestins - Dydrogesterone is best suited.
   b. If fertility is desired: chronic anovulation is common cause. So, ovulation induction can be achieved

By

- Clomiphene citrate
- Letrozole
- If unresponsive then pure FSH or HMG along with HCG with follicular monitoring is crucial because more chance of OHSS

5. For endometrial hyperplasia: endometrial biopsy may have to be done. LNG-IUS COCP and continues progesterone is the treatment of choice to prevent endometrial hyperplasia and abnormal bleeding.
6. Surgery: laparoscopic ovarian drilling (LOD) is done
   - For cases found resistant to medical therapy
   - For morbidly obese women – bariatric surgery
   - Wedge resection of ovary was previously done. But it is not done now a days because it causes periovarian adhesions and decreases ovarian reserve.

CHAPTER 5

Menstruation

SHORT ANSWER TYPE QUESTIONS

Q1. Define menstruation.

Menstruation is indeed a complex physiological process that involves the shedding of the endometrial lining of the uterus, which occurs in response to hormonal fluctuations throughout the menstrual cycle. This cycle is regulated by the hypothalamic-pituitary-ovarian axis, which coordinates the release of hormones that govern the various phases of the cycle.

Key Components of the Menstrual Cycle:

1. Hypothalamus: The hypothalamus releases gonadotropin-releasing hormone (GnRH), which stimulates the pituitary gland.
2. Pituitary Gland: In response to GnRH, the anterior pituitary secretes two key hormones:
   - Follicle-Stimulating Hormone (FSH): Promotes the growth and maturation of ovarian follicles.
   - Luteinizing Hormone (LH): Triggers ovulation and stimulates the corpus luteum to produce progesterone.
3. Ovaries: The ovaries produce estrogen and progesterone in response to FSH and LH.
   - Estrogen: Levels rise during the follicular phase, leading to the thickening of the endometrium.
   - Progesterone: Produced by the corpus luteum during the luteal phase, it stabilizes the endometrial lining in preparation for a potential pregnancy.
4. Menstruation: If fertilization does not occur, the corpus luteum degenerates, leading to a drop in progesterone and estrogen levels. This hormonal decline triggers the breakdown of the endometrial lining, resulting in menstruation, which typically lasts 3–7 days.

Phases of the Menstrual Cycle:

1. Menstrual Phase: Shedding of the endometrial lining occurs, marking the start of the cycle.
2. Follicular Phase: FSH stimulates the growth of follicles, and estrogen levels rise, leading to the thickening of the endometrium.
3. Ovulation: A surge in LH causes the release of a mature egg from the ovary.
4. Luteal Phase: The corpus luteum forms and secretes progesterone, preparing the endometrium for potential implantation.

Q2. Name the hormones involved in regulation of menstrual cycle.

- GnRH
- FSH
- LH
- Estrogen
- Progesterone

Q3. Composition of menstrual blood.

- Dark altered colored blood
- Mucous
- Epithelial cells of vagina
- Endometrial fragments
- Prostaglandins
- Bacteria and enzymes

Q4. Important information about menstruation.

- Menarche: Between 11 and 15 years, mean 13 years
- Menstrual cycle: 24–38 days, mean 28 days
- Menstrual period: 4–5 days
- Amount: 20–80 mL, mean 35 mL
- Menopause: 45–55 years, average 51.3 years

Q5. Cycle-ovarian

- Follicles-recruitment
- Selection and maturation of dominant follicle
- Ovulation
- Corpus luteum formation
- Demise of the corpus luteum

Q6. Structures of mature Graafian follicle

The fully mature Graafian follicle measures about 20 mm, and is composed of the following structures from outside inward.

- Theca externa
- Theca interna
- Membrana granulosa (limitans)
- Granulosa cell layer

Approximate 3 months for the follicle to grow and mature for ovulation

Q7. Endometrial cycle: Two zone

- **Basal zone (Stratum basalis)**
  - Inner one-third of the total depth of endometrium
  - Measures about 1 mm
  - Consists of stromal cells
  - Supplied by the basal arteries
  - Uninfluenced by hormone
- **Functional zone**
  - Influenced by hormones
  - Has two layers:
    a. Stratum compactum
    b. Stratum spongiosum
  - Divided into four stages
    1. Regenerative phase
    2. Proliferative phase: Estrogen
    3. Secretory phase: Progesterone
    4. Menstrual phase

Q8. Mechanism of menstrual bleeding.

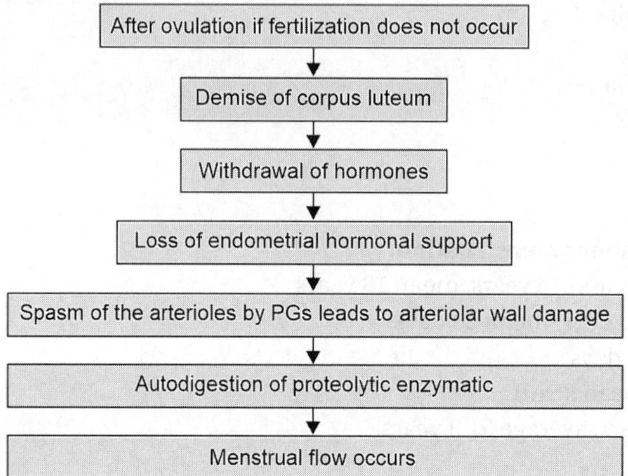

Q9. How menstrual blood flow stops.

The menstrual flow stops due to combined effect of prolonged vasoconstriction, myometrial contraction and local aggregation of platelets with deposition of fibrin around them. Resumption of estrogen secretion leads to clot formation over the decapitated stumps of endometrial vessels.

Q10. Premenstrual symptoms

- Irritability, lethargy, and constipation
- Acne
- Pelvic discomfort
- Excess weight gain
- Breast tenderness

Q11. Ovulatory symptoms

Abdominal pain on right or left iliac fossa

- Slight pervaginal bleeding
- Mucoid discharge from vagina

Q12. What structural similarity is present between LH and FSH?

Both LH and FSH are glycoproteins and structures of α-subunits is identical and differs only in the structures of β-subunits.

Q13. What are the function of FSH in menstrual cycle?

- FSH stimulates granulosa cells to produce estrogen and inhibin
- It induces the expression of LH receptors on granulosa cells.

Q14. What are the function of LH in menstrual cycle?

- LH stimulates theca cells for androgen synthesis which transport to granulosa cells for conversion into estrogen by aromatase enzyme.
- LH surge results ovulation.

Q15. What are the function of estradiol in menstrual cycle?

- Induction of FSH and LH receptors on granulosa cells
- It exert negative feedback at low levels and positive feedback at high levels to FSH and LH.
- It induces proliferation of endometrial glands.

Q16. What is two-cell-two gonadotropin theory?

The theory states that the ovary has two cellular compartments, theca and granulosa cells that are controlled by two gonadotropin, LH and FSH. LH influences theca cells and generates androgen from cholesterol. FSH influences granulosa cells to generate estrogen from androgens

Q17. Important events and time of ovulation

- Ovulation occurs around D14 of a regular 28 days cycle
- Ovulation occurs 34–36 hours after onset of LH surge
- 12–16 hours after LH peak
- 83 hours after E2 rise
- Ovulation is preceded by completion of 1st meiotic division.
- Extrusion of 1st polar body in perivitelline space
- Granulosa cells luteinized
- Corpus luteum formation
- Progesterone synthesis
- Beginning of secretory phase endometrium

Q18. What are the stage of corpus luteum?

- Proliferation
- Vascularization
- Maturation
- Regression

Q19. What is the fate of corpus luteum in normal menstrual cycle?

- Corpus luteum undergoes atresia and begins evolving into corpus albicans.

Q20. When progesterone secretion reaches its peak?

- Between D5 and D7 of postovulation.

Q21. When proliferative phase begins and ends?

- Begins at the end of menstruation and ends with onset of ovulation.

Q22. When secretory phase begins and ends?

- Begins at ovulation and ends with onset of next menstrual cycle.

SHORT NOTES

Q1. Describe the endocrinology of ovulation.

The following are potential explanations that may occur individually or in combination:

LH Surge: A prolonged elevation of estradiol at 200 pg/mL for 24–48 hours in the late follicular phase initiates an LH surge because of a positive feedback mechanism. This increase prompts the finishing of the oocyte's reduction division and starts the luteinization of granulosa cells, resulting in the production of progesterone and prostaglandins. Furthermore, the LH surge triggers acute inflammatory responses, leading to the secretion of cytokines, collagenases, and plasminogen activator or plasmin, which ultimately result in follicle rupture and the formation of the corpus luteum

FSH Increase: The preovulatory elevation of 17-alpha-hydroxyprogesterone boosts estrogen's capacity to trigger an FSH surge. The elevation of FSH results in an increase of plasminogen activator, which transforms plasminogen into plasmin, facilitating the breakdown of the follicle wall.

Therefore, the simultaneous increase in LH and FSH midcycle is accountable for the follicle's final maturation phase, the conclusion of the oocyte's first meiotic division with the release of the first polar body, and the release of the oocyte (ovulation).

Q2. How normal menstruation can be postponed by using medicines?

To delay menstruation, hormones like combined oral contraceptive pills (taken as two tablets daily) or progestogens such as norethisterone (5 mg taken twice daily) can be utilized. These drugs must be ingested at least 3–6 days prior to the anticipated start of menstruation and maintained until the issue is settled. Menstruation is anticipated to happen 2–3 days following the cessation of the medication.

Q3. Menstrual symptoms

In most cases, no signs of vaginal bleeding. At first, it starts as pink discharge, but on days 2 and 3, it turns dark red. In adolescents or those who have never given birth, there may be manageable colicky pain at the onset due to uterine contractions. Premonitory symptoms such as pelvic discomfort, lower back pain, breast fullness, or mastalgia may occur just before menstruation. A headache or depression might occur.

Q4. Menstrual hygiene

Caring and sensitive treatment of young girls going through their first menstruation is crucial. This should be accomplished by them further clarifying the physiological and other related changes that occur during the period. The girls ought to proceed with their usual routine.

The everyday bathing routine must not be interrupted. In the first few cycles, the girl might find sanitary pads suitable, but with experience, she may choose to switch to tampons if she wishes.

Q5. Anovular menstruation

In an anovulatory cycle, the follicles grow without any selection of dominant follicle. The estrogen is secreted in increasing amount. There may be imbalance between estrogen and FSH or because of temporary unresponsiveness of the hypothalamus to the rising estrogen GnRH is inhibited → ovulation does not occur. The overall result is uninterrupted secretion of estrogen as long as the follicles remain. The endometrium stays in a proliferative or occasionally hyperplastic condition. The structural stromal support is insufficient, and the endometrium stays delicate. As the estrogen levels decline, there is a lack of synchronization in the shedding of the endometrium and menstrual cycle. The bleeding can be extensive, lasting longer than expected and occurring inconsistently.

This kind of bleeding is commonly seen during puberty, after giving birth, following an abortion, and in the premenopausal phase.

Q6. Changes in menstrual cycle

	Menstrual	*Proliferative*	*Secretory*
Day	1–5	6–14	15–28
Layer thickness	1–2 mm	10–12 mm	12–14 mm
Glands	Epithelial regeneration	Straight Few coiled	Corkscrew-shaped glands Dilatation Subnuclear vacuolation Luminal secretion Saw tooth glandular epithelium Marked spiraling of vessels
Stroma	Shedding	Cell proliferation Loose stroma	Stromal edema
Estrogen/progesterone	Low	Estrogen ↑	Progesterone ↑
FSH/LH	Low	FSH ↑	LH ↑

Q7. Changes in cervical cycle

Cervical characteristics	*Follicular phase*	*Luteal phase*
Cervical mucous	Thin and watery (copious)	Thick and viscid(scanty)
Stretchability	Increased to beyond 10 cm	Lost
Fern tree pattern	Present	Lost
Glycoprotein network	Parallel, facilitating sperm penetration	Interlacing bridges, preventing sperm penetration
Internal os	Funnel-shaped	Tightly closed

CHAPTER 6

Disorders of Menstruation: Abnormal Uterine Bleeding

Case Taking

History

Age:

- Common around menarche and perimenopause.

Menstrual history:

- Age at menarche
- Menstrual cycle
- Menstrual period
- Menstrual flow
- Last menstrual period
- Dysmenorrhea
- Intermenstrual bleeding and post coital bleeding

Obstetric history: Number of pregnancies and mode of delivery

Medical history: Coagulopathies, malignancy and endocrine disorders.

Drug history: Anticoagulant.

General examination: BMI, anemia, BP, thyroid gland, bruising or petechiae.

Systemic examination:
Cardiorespiratory system.
Abdominal examination**:** Any mass or organomegaly

Pelvic examination:
Inspection
Per speculum examination: Structural lesion on cervix and vagina.
Bimanual examination: Structural lesion on uterus.
Per rectal examination: If suspicion of malignancies.

Case discussion

AUB-P

A 40-year-old, P1(VD) + 0, women has presented with a history of intermenstrual bleeding for last 6 month. On general examination, she is clinically anemic. On P/S/E—a polypoidal mass is coming out through external os, on B/M/E—uterus is bulky.

Q1. What is her provisional diagnosis?

- AUB-P (endometrial or cervical polyp)

Q2. What are the differential diagnosis?

- Submucous fibroid
- Retained products of conception

- Endometrial hyperplasia
- Cervical carcinoma
- Endometrial carcinoma

Q3. What are the risk factors?
- DM, HTN, obesity and increased age (uncontrolled endometrial hyperplasia due to unopposed estrogen)

Q4. Name of investigations to diagnose the case?
- TVS
- SIS (saline infusion sonography)
- Hysteroscopy

Q5. How will you treat the case?
- Polypectomy and D&C followed by histopathology.

AUB-A

A 42-year-old, P2(VD) + 2 MR, women has presented with a history of heavy menstrual bleeding for last 2 years and severe dysmenorrhea for 2 years. On general examination, she is clinically anemic. On abdominal and B/M/E—uterus is 12 weeks size, soft to firm in consistency.

Q1. What is her provisional diagnosis?
- AUB-A

Q2. What are the differential diagnosis?
- Submucous fibroid uterus
- PID
- Endometriosis

Q3. Name of investigations to diagnose the case?
- TVS
  - Irregular or blurred endomyometrial junction
  - Multiple cystic or honeycomb appearance of myometrium.
  - Inhomogeneous myometrium
  - Increased vascularity of myometrium on Doppler
- MRI (if diagnosis is uncertain)

Q4. How will you treat the case?
- Hysterectomy with prophylactic bilateral salpingectomy and preservation of ovaries if they are found healthy.

Q5. What are the histological findings of adenomyosis?
- Endometrial glands and stroma surrounded by myometrium.
- Hemosiderin-laden macrophages.

AUB-L

A 38-year-old, P1(c/s) + 0, women has presented with a history of heavy menstrual bleeding for last 2 years and feeling of heaviness for 6 months. On general examination, she is clinically anemic. On abdominal and B/M/E—uterus is 18 weeks size, firm in consistency, nodular surface.

Q1. What is her provisional diagnosis?
- AUB-L

Q2. What are the differential diagnosis?
- Adenomyosis
- Ovarian tumor (if subserous pedunculated fibroid)

Q3. Name of investigations to diagnose the case?

- USG of whole abdomen
  - Size, site, number of fibroid and endometrial thickness.
- Hysteroscopy (diagnostic and therapeutic).
- MRI (if diagnostic dilemma)

Q4. What conditions are associated with fibroid uterus?

- Follicular cyst of ovary
- Endometrial hyperplasia
- Endometrial carcinoma
- Endometriosis

Q5. How will you treat the case?

- As patient is 38 years and have fertility concern, myomectomy is preferable for her.

SHORT ANSWER TYPE QUESTIONS

Q1. What are different types of menstrual disorders?

- Abnormal uterine bleeding
- Dysmenorrhea
- Premenstrual syndrome
- Premenstrual dysphoric disorder

Q2. Define abnormal uterine bleeding.

Any uterine bleeding outside the normal volume, duration, regularity, or frequency is considered abnormal uterine bleeding (AUB).

Q3. Types of abnormal uterine bleeding.

Acute: An episode of bleeding in a women who require immediate intervention.

Chronic: Bleeding which is abnormal in duration, volume and/or frequency and majority cases present for the last 6 months.

Q4. Classification of AUB.

Structural causes (PALM)

P—Polyp

A—Adenomyosis

L—Leiomyoma (submucosal and intramural)

M—Malignancy and hyperplasia

Nonstructural systemic causes (COEIN)

C—Coagulopathy

O—Ovulatory dysfunction

E—Endometrial

I—Iatrogenic (OCP, IUCDs including LNG-IUCD)

N—Not yet identified (Infection, PID, tuberculosis, cervicitis, Asherman syndrome, foreign bodies, arteriovenous malformations).

Q5. Patterns of AUB.

- **Heavy menstrual bleeding (HMB):** Blood loss >80 mL, if interferes with woman's physical, emotional, social and psychological quality.
- **Prolonged bleeding:** Bleeding continued for >8 days.
  (Women may have combined heavy and prolonged bleeding).

- **Frequent bleeding:** Menses <24 days intervening
- **Infrequent bleeding:** Menses >38 days intervening.
- **Amenorrhea:** Absence of menses over 90 days.
- **Regular cycle:** Variation of cycle length from cycle to cycle ≤7–9 days.
- **Irregular cycle:** Cycle length vary from cycle to cycle ≥10 days.
- **AUB-O (Ovulatory dysfunction):** AUB-O is defined as a state of abnormal uterine bleeding without any clinically detectable organic, systemic, and iatrogenic cause (pelvic pathology, e.g., tumor, inflammation, or pregnancy is excluded).
- **Intermenstrual bleeding:** Occurs between normal menses
  - Pre- and postmenstrual spotting
  - Postcoital bleeding.
- **Metrorrhagia:** Intermenstrual bleeding is defined as irregular, acyclic bleeding from the uterus.
- **Breakthrough bleeding** is related to hormone administration.
- **Withdrawal bleeding:** Due to abrupt decline in progesterone level.
- **Postmenopausal bleeding.**

Q6. Old versus New terminology.

Old	*New*
Menorrhagia	Heavy menstrual bleeding (HMB)
Polymenorrhea	Frequent bleeding
Oligomenorrhea	Infrequent bleeding
Metrorrhagia	Intermenstrual bleeding
Menometrorrhagia	Heavy and prolonged bleeding (HPMB)
DUB	AUB-O
Hypomenorrhea	Light menstruation

Q7. Old versus New normal limits.

Menstrual cycle characteristics	*Old*	*New*
Duration of cycle (days)	21–35	24–38
Duration of flow	Normal 3–5 days Prolonged >7 days Shortened <2 days	Normal <8 days Prolonged >8 days
Volume	Normal 20–60 mL Heavy >80 mL Light <5 mL	Normal 5–80 mL Heavy >80 mL or sufficient to hampers quality of life Light <5 mL

Q8. Define and common causes of HMB.

Heavy menstrual bleeding is defined as a bleeding that interferes with woman's physical, emotional, social and maternal quality of life.

Causes:

- Fibroid uterus
- Adenomyosis
- Pelvic endometriosis
- Chronic tuba-ovarian mass

Q9. Common causes of contact bleeding.

- **Benign conditions:**
  - Urogenital atrophy
  - Cervical or endometrial polyps
  - Cervical ectropion
- **Infection:**
  - Vulvovaginitis (candidiasis or trichomonas)
  - Cervicitis (chlamydia or gonorrhea)
  - Endometritis in presence of IUCD
- **Vulval:**
  - Lichen sclerosus
  - Genital warts
  - Genital herpes
  - Chancroid
  - Syphilis
  - Lymphogranuloma venereum
- **Malignancy:**
  - Vaginal
  - Cervical
- **Others:**
  - Trauma
  - Bleeding disorders
  - Foreign bodies
  - Sexual abuse
  - Pregnancy-related

Q10. Common causes of acyclical bleeding.

- DUB-usually during adolescence, following childbirth and abortion and preceding menopause
- Submucous fibroid
- Uterine polyp
- Carcinoma cervix
- Endometrial carcinoma

Q11. Common causes of intermenstrual bleeding.

Apart from the causes of contact bleeding, other causes are:

- Urethral caruncle
- Ovulatory dysfunction
- Breakthrough bleeding in pill use
- IUCD in utero
- Decubitus ulcer
- Postcoital bleeding
- Progesterone only contraceptive use

Q12. Common causes of infrequent bleeding.

- Age-related-during adolescence and preceding menopause
- Weight-related-obesity
- HPO axis dysregulation: Stress, anorexia, extreme exercise
- Endocrine disorder-PCOS (most common), hyperthyroidism, POF

- Androgen producing tumors-ovarian, adrenal
- Tubercular endometritis-late cases, uterine synechiae
- Drugs**:** Phenothiazines, cimetidine, methyldopa

Q13. Define light menstruation and causes of it.

When the menstrual bleeding is unduly scanty (<5 mL) and lasts for less than 2 days, it is called light menstruation.

Causes:

- Local: Uterine synechiae or endometrial tuberculosis
- Endocrine: Oral contraceptives, thyroid dysfunction, and premenopausal period
- Systemic: Malnutrition

Q14. High risk cases for coagulopathies.

- HMB since menarche
- One of the following:
  - PPH
  - Dental bleed
  - Surgical bleed
- Two or more of the following symptoms
  - Bruising 1 to 2 times per month
  - Epistaxis 1 to 2 times per month
  - Frequent gum bleeding
  - Family history of bleeding disorders

Q15. Investigations for coagulopathies.

- CBC—Platelet count
- Coagulation profile
  - BT, CT
  - PT
  - APTT
  - Fibrinogen
  - FDP
  - D-dimer

Q16. Investigations for AUB.

- **Transvaginal sonography (TVS) and color Doppler**
  - Endometrial thickness >12 mm—endometrial hyperplasia
  - Hyperechoic and regular outline
  - Angiogenesis and neovascular signal study
  - Endometrial thickness: <3 mm suggests atrophic endometrium
  - Fibroid, adenomyosis and adnexal pathology
- **Saline infusion sonography (SIS)**
  - Endometrial polyps,
  - Submucous fibroids and
  - Intrauterine abnormality (septate/subseptate uterus).
- **Magnetic resonance imaging (MRI)**
- **Hysteroscopy**
  - Evaluation of endometrial lesion (polyp and submucous fibroid)
- **Hysteroscopy and directed biopsy (H and B)**
  - Can be performed as an outpatient basis.
  - H and B has replaced conventional D&C.

- **Endometrial sampling**
  - Women >45 years can be done as an outpatient basis by Pipelle sampler
- **Laparoscopy:**
  - Pelvic pathology: Endometriosis, PID or ovarian tumor (granulosa cell tumor) if associated with pelvic pain.
- **Endometrial biopsy (EB)**
- To exclude the organic lesions in the endometrium
  - Incomplete abortion, endometrial polyp, tubercular endometritis or endometrial carcinoma.
  - Quickest way to stop acute bleeding for women >35 years.

Q17. Indications of endometrial biopsy.

- Persistent IMB or persistent irregular bleeding,
- Obese
- PCOS
- Women taking tamoxifen
- Where treatment for HMB has failed.

Q18. How will you treat AUB?

AUB-P: Polypectomy and D&C

AUB-A:

- Medical: LNG-IUCD
- Surgical: Adenomyomectomy, hysterectomy

AUB-L:

Medical:

- Tranexamic acid with NSAIDs
- SPRM (ulipristal acetate)
- OCP
- Progesterone (continuous or cyclical)
- GnRH agonists

Surgical:

Conservative:

- Myomectomy
- UAE
- MRgUS
- Endometrial ablation

Definite:

- Hysterectomy

AUB-M: Surgery ± adjuvant therapy

AUB-C: Tranexamic acid, desmopressin

AUB-O:

- Lifestyle modification—Obesity, PCOS
- Cabergoline—Hyperprolactinemia
- Levothyroxine—Hypothyroidism

AUB-I: Stop the offending drug.

AUB-N: Treatment according to cause.

CHAPTER 7

Premenstrual Syndrome

Q1. What is PMS?

Premenstrual syndrome is a cyclical luteal phase condition characterized by physical, psychological, and behavioral changes of sufficient severity that hamper normal quality of life.

Q2. When during menstrual cycle does PMS occur?

During the luteal phase of menstrual cycle.

Q3. In which age group it is common?

Premenstrual syndrome affects women in all ages from adolescence till menopause. Women in their fourth decade of life tend to be affected most severely.

Q4. Name the symptoms of PMS.

Common premenstrual symptoms.	
Psychological symptoms	***Somatic symptoms***
Irritability, labile mood, or depressed mood, anger, oversensitivity, social withdrawal, insomnia, difficulty in concentrating, subjective memory difficulties, anxiety, subjective sense of feeling overwhelmed, or out of control	Abdominal bloating, food craving, breast tenderness, headaches, fatigue, gastrointestinal upset, muscles stiffness, joint pain, generalized aches, appetite changes, acne, and edema

Q5. What is the difference between premenstrual symptoms and PMS?

Up to 75% of women with regular menses describe a few symptoms during the luteal phase but may not interfere with day-to-day activity and thus may not meet the criteria for PMS. Clinically, significant cluster of premenstrual.

Q6. What is the difference between PMS and PMDD?

Premenstrual dysphoric disorder is viewed as a severe subtype of PMS. If the mental symptoms predominate, are very severe, and are associated with impairment, then the patient is classified as having PMDD (premenstrual dysmorphic disorder).

Q7. Classification of PMS.

1. Premenstrual exacerbation of an underlying disorder
2. Nonovulatory PMDS
3. Progestogens-induced PMDS
4. PMDS with absent menstruation

Q8. Write down the management of PMS.

Therapeutic management of PMS.

1. Consider CBT (cognitive behavioral therapy) as a treatment option.
2. Hormonal medical management of PMS:
   Drospirenone-containing COCP—1st line.
   Contraceptive pill continuously rather than cyclically.

Hormonal medical management of PMS.
Percutaneous estradiol + cyclical progestogen (in case of physical and psychological symptoms of sever PMS)
Alternative contraption copper coil/barrier

LNG-IUS.
(Micronized progesterone is better than LNG-IUS)
Percutaneous estradiol cyclical 10–12 days + progesterone/LNG-LUS
To prevent endometrial hyperplasia
Low dose danazol (200 mg twice daily) + contraception (in case breast symptoms).

3. GnRH analog only for severe case or treatment failure
   If GnRH used for >6 months add-back therapy combined HRT/tibolone.
   Women on long-term GnRH
   BMD (bone mineral density)—every year.
4. Nonhormonal medical management of PMS:
   SSRI-1st line
   Severe PMS
   Either luteal or continuous dosing with SSRIs can be recommended
   SSRIs should be discontinued gradually to avoid withdrawal symptoms, if given on a continuous basis.

Side effect of SSRI:
- Nausea
- Insomnia
- Somnolence
- Fatigue, reduction in libido
- Spironolactone can be used to treat physical symptoms
- Discontinue SSRI before pregnancy

Severe PMS—hysterectomy TAH with BLSO use HRT if age <45.

Why not only BLSO?

Bilateral oophorectomy alone (without removal of the uterus) will necessitate the use of a progestogen as part of any subsequent HRT regime and this carries a risk of reintroduction of PMS like symptoms.

When treating women with PMS. Surgery GnRH analogs should be used as a test of cure and to ensure that HRT is tolerated.

Algorithm of management of PMS:
1. 1st line → CBT, vitamin B_6, COC
   SSRT (low dose)
   Citalopram/escitalopram 10 mg.
2. 2nd line → Estradiol patches (100 micrograms)
   + micronized Progesterone (100 mg or 200 mg)
   (Day 17–28) or LNG - IUS 52 mg, higher dose SSRIS continuously on luteal phase, e.g., citalopram/esitalph. 20–40 mg.
3. 3rd - line → GnRH analog + add-back
   (continuous combined estrogen + progesterone
   50–100 micrograms estradiol patches or 2 to 4 doses of estradiol gel combined with micronized progesterone 100 mg/day or tibolone 2.5 mg.
4. Fourth line - surgical treatment + HRT

DYSMENORRHEA: SHORT ANSWER QUESTIONS

Q1. Define dysmenorrhea.

Painful menstruation of sufficient magnitude so as to incapacitate day to day activities.

Q2. What are the types of dysmenorrhea?

- Primary
- Secondary

Q3. What is primary dysmenorrhea (spasmodic)?

The primary dysmenorrhea is one where there is no identifiable pelvic pathology.

Q4. What is incidence of primary dysmenorrhea (spasmodic)?

15–20%

Q5. What are the causes of pain?

Dysrhythmic uterine contractions and uterine hypoxia.

- Psychosomatic factors of tension and anxiety during adolescence, lower the pain threshold.
- Abnormal anatomical and functional aspect of myometrium.

Q6. Mechanisms of primary dysmenorrhea.

- Dysperistalsis
- Hyperactivity of the uterine JZ
- Imbalance in the autonomic nervous control of uterine muscle
- Role of prostaglandins: PGF2α, PGE2, **and** PGF2α are strong vasoconstrictors, which cause ischemia (angina) of the myometrium.
- Role of vasopressin: It causes uterine hyperactivity and dysrhythmic contractions → ischemia and hypoxia with which causes pain.
- Endothelins causes myometrial smooth muscle contractions, especially in the endomyometrial JZ and also can induce PGF2α.
- Platelet activating factor (PAF)
- Leukotrienes and PAFs are vasoconstrictors and stimulate myometrial contractions.

Q7. Clinical differentiating points between primary and secondary dysmenorrhea.

Primary	***Secondary***
No identifiable pelvic pathology	Secondary to pelvic pathology
Mostly in adolescents	Elderly/parous women
Confined to ovulatory cycle Starts with the onset or just before the men's	Pain starts 7–10 days before the onset of menstruation
Normal pelvic examination	No systemic discomfort Intermenstrual period not completely free of pain
Normal on laboratory tests and imaging	Presence of pelvic pathology

Q8. What are the characteristics of pain in primary dysmenorrhea?

- The pain begins a few hours before or just with the onset of menstruation.
- The severity of pain usually lasts for few hours, may extend to 24 hours but seldom persists beyond 48 hours.
- The pain is spasmodic and confined to lower abdomen; may radiate to the back and medial aspect of thighs.
- Systemic discomforts like nausea, vomiting, fatigue, diarrhea, headache and tachycardia may be associated.
- It may be accompanied by vasomotor changes causing pallor, cold sweats and occasional fainting. Rarely, syncope and collapse in severe cases may be associated.

Q9. How will you diagnosis primary dysmenorrhea?

- Abdominal or pelvic (rectal) examination: No abnormal findings.
- Ultrasound/MRI, laparoscopy: For detection and exclusion of any pelvic abnormalities
- If risk of PID, tests for *Chlamydia trachomatis* and gonorrhea.

Q10. How will you treat primary dysmenorrhea?

- **Nonpharmacologic measures**
  - Assurance
  - To keep bowels empty
  - Exercise
  - Heat therapy
  - Behavioral
  - Low fat, vegetarian diet, vitamin B_1, B_6, E
- **Nonhormonal:** Prostaglandin synthetase inhibitors
  - Mefenamic acid: 250–500 mg 8 hourly
  - Ibuprofen 400 mg 8 hourly
  - Naproxen 250 mg 6 hourly
  - COX-2 inhibitors: Celecoxib 200 mg twice daily
- **Hormones**
  - Combined oral contraceptive pills: 1 tablet daily (3–6 cycles)
  - Oral progestins (dydrogesterone): D5–D25
  - LNG-IUS (50% reduce pain)
  - Nexplanon or implant
- **Surgical management**
  - Laparoscopic uterine nerve ablation (LUNA)
  - Laparoscopic presacral neurectomy (LPSN)

Q11. What are the factors of primary dysmenorrhea?

Reducing the risk	*Increasing the risk*
Physical exercise	Age younger (<30 years)
Used of COCs	BMI <20 kg/m^2
Younger age of the first childbirth	Prolonged duration of menses
Higher parity	Irregular or heavy menses
	Sterilization
	Family history

Secondary Dysmenorrhea (Congestive)

Q12. What is secondary dysmenorrhea?

Secondary dysmenorrhea is normally considered to be menstruation-associated pain occurring in the presence of pelvic pathology.

Q13. Why pain occur in secondary dysmenorrhea?

Due to premenstrual pelvic congestion or increased vascularity in the pelvic organs.

Q14. What are the causes of pain in secondary dysmenorrhea?
Common causes of secondary dysmenorrhea.

- Endometriosis—70–80%
- Adenomyosis
- IUCD in utero
- Obstruction due to mullerian anomalies
- Cervical stenosis
- Pelvic adhesions
- Uterine fibroid/polyp

- Pelvic congestion
- Ovarian cyst/mass
- Chronic pelvic infection
- Interstitial cystitis

Q15. What are the causes of unilateral dysmenorrhea?

- Ovarian dysmenorrhea
- Bicornuate uterus
- Unilateral location of pelvic endometriosis
- Small fibroid polyp near one cornu
- Right ovarian vein syndrome
- Colonic or cecal spasm

Q16. What are the patient profile of secondary dysmenorrhea?

- The patients are usually in their thirties
- More often parous
- Unrelated to any social status.

Q17. What are the clinical features of secondary dysmenorrhea?

- The pain is dull, situated in the back and in front without any radiation.
- It usually appears 3–5 days prior to the period
- Relieves with the onset of bleeding.
- There is no systemic discomfort but may have some discomfort in between periods.
- Patient may present with dyspareunia, dysuria, abnormal uterine bleeding and infertility.
- Abdominal and vaginal examinations usually reveal the pathology.

Q18. What are the investigations to diagnose secondary dysmenorrhea?

- **Transvaginal sonography:** Leiomyoma, adenomyosis.
- **Saline infusion sonography:** Submucous fibroid, polyps.
- **Laparoscopy:** Endometriosis, PID
  (useful for both diagnostic and therapeutic purposes)
- **Hysteroscopy:** Submucous fibroid, polyps
  (useful for both diagnostic and therapeutic purposes).

Q19. How to treat secondary dysmenorrhea?

Treatment: Treatment depends on the diagnosis, severity, age and parity of the patient.

Q20. What is right ovarian vein syndrome?

Right ovarian vein crosses the ureter at right angle. During premenstrual period, due to pelvic congestion or increased blood flow, there may be marked engorgement in the vein → pressure on ureter → stasis → infection → pyelonephritis → pain. This is an important cause of unilateral dysmenorrhea.

Q21. How cervical stenosis causes dysmenorrhea?

Cervical stenosis may cause obstruction to the menstrual flow → causing increase intrauterine pressure → retrograde menstrual flow through the fallopian tube in the peritoneal cavity → pelvic endometriosis → dysmenorrhea.

Q22. What are the causes of cervical stenosis?

- May be congenital
- Injury to the cervix
- Electrocautery or cauterization.

Q23. How will you diagnose cervical stenosis?

Diagnosis is made during while passing on uterine sound or dilators through the internal OS and is confirmed by hysteroscopy or HSG.

Q24. How will you treat cervical stenosis?

Dilatation of the cervix under anesthesia with or without use of misoprostol prior to dilatation.

Pelvic Congestion Syndrome

Q25. What is pelvic congestion syndrome?

The patient has a congestive type of dysmenorrhea without any demonstrable pelvic pathology.

Q26. What is pathogenesis of pelvic congestion syndrome?

Chronic pelvic pain, sensation of heaviness and pelvic pressure are due to the congested and tortuous ovarian and pelvic veins. This is mainly due to incompetent valves in the veins to cause retrograde flow and stasis. Estrogen may causes venous dilatation in addition to the mechanical factors.

Q27. How will you diagnose and treat pelvic congestion syndrome?

Chief complains:
- Vague disorders such as backache and pelvic pain with long standing position
- Dyspareunia
- Menorrhagia or metrorrhagia.

Examination:
- Tenderness at the junction of the middle and lateral third of a line drawn between the symphysis and the anterior superior iliac spine.
- Ovarian tenderness may be found.
- The uterus may feel bulky and boggy.

Investigations:
- Doppler scan, duplex ultrasound scans
- CT
- MRI
- Pelvic venography
- Angiography

Dilated tortuous ovarian vein with diameter >6 mm is seen.

Treatment:
- Hormonal suppression
- Local sclerotherapy
- Ovarian vein embolization or
- Hysterectomy with bilateral salpingo-oophorectomy (in parous women with advancing age)

Medroxyprogesterone acetate (MPA) 50 mg daily for 4 months or with GnRH agonist was found effective.

Premenstrual Syndrome (PMS) and Premenstrual Dysphoric Disorder (PMDD)

Q28. What is premenstrual syndrome (PMS)?

Is a psychoneuroendocrine disorder of unknown etiology, often noticed just prior to menstruation.

Q29. What are the symptoms of PMS?

Affective symptoms
- Depression
- Angry outburst
- Irritability

- Confusion
- Fatigue and social
- Withdrawal

Somatic symptoms

- Breast tenderness
- Bloating
- Headache
- Swollen extremities

Q30. How will you diagnose PMS?

According to the American Psychiatric Association (2013) Diagnostic and Statistical Manual (DSM) recommends symptoms to be confirmed by prospective patient mood charting for at least two menstrual cycles.

Q31. In which time the symptoms appear?

There is cyclic appearance of a large number of symptoms during the last 7–10 days of the menstrual cycle.

Q32. What is the pathophysiology of PMS and PMDD?

The exact cause is not known but the following hypothesis are postulated:

- Change in ovarian steroids (estrogen and progesterone) with ovulation → alteration in ovarian neurohormones and neurotransmitters → reduction of serotonergic function during luteal phase of the cycle → manifestation of PMS and PMDD.
- **Neuroendocrine factors:**
  - **Serotonin:** During the luteal phase, decreased synthesis of serotonin is observed in women suffering from PMS.
  - **Endorphins:** The symptom complex of PMS is thought to be due to the withdrawal of endorphin.

  Others several biological factors alteration like
  - Estrogen
  - Progesterone
  - Gamma aminobutyric acid (GABA)
  - Renin-angiotensin-aldosterone system (RAAS) are thought to be involved.
  - Common psychiatric conditions such as depression and anxiety disorders are associated.
  - Idiopathic

Q33. What are the diagnostic criteria for premenstrual dysphoric disorder (PMDD)?

PMDD does not need any somatic symptoms:

A. **Presence of symptoms (at least 5 or more must occur):** Occur in most cycles during the week before menses and improve within a few days after the onset of menses and diminish in the week postmenses.

B. **One (or more) of the following symptoms must be present:**
   - Marked affective lability (mood swings, tearful, rejection)
   - Marked irritability or anger or increased interpersonal conflicts
   - Marked depressed moods, feelings of hopelessness, or self-deprecating thoughts
   - Marked anxiety, tension

C. **One (or more) of the following symptoms must also be present:**
   - Decreased interest in usual activities (school)
   - Difficulty in concentrating
   - Easy fatigability, low energy, lethargy
   - Hypersomnia or insomnia; overeating, food cravings
   - Physical symptoms such as breast tenderness, muscle or joint aches, "bloating" or weight gain

D. **Symptoms are associated with:** Significant distress or interferences with work, school, or relationships

Q34. What are the types of PMS?

1. Core PMS
2. Variant PMS:
   - Premenstrual exacerbation underlying disorder
   - Nonovulatory PMS
   - Progestogen induced PMS
   - PMS with absent menstruation.

Q35. What are the clinical features of PMS?

- PMS is more common in women aged 30–45.
- It may be related to childbirth or a disturbing life event.
- There are no abnormal pelvic findings excepting features of pelvic congestion.

Q36. How will you manage PMS or PMDD?

General:

1. Lifestyle modification
2. Cognitive behavior therapy
3. Group psychoeducation and relaxation therapy

Specific: Management of severe PMS (according to the RCOG Green Top Guideline 48 + Dutta)

First line:

- Lifestyle modification:
  a. Assurance, yoga, stress management, diet manipulation
  b. Avoidance of salt, caffeine and alcohol especially in second half of cycle
- Aerobic exercise: 30 minutes in most days of the week, including the luteal phase.
- Cognitive behavioral therapy
- Vitamin B_6 combined new-generation pill, such as Yasmin, Cilest (cyclically or continuously)
- Continuous or luteal phase (day 15–28)—low dose SSRI

Second line:

- Estradiol patches (100 micrograms) + oral progestogen such as Duphaston 10 mg D17–D280 or Mirena.
- Higher-dose SSRIs continuously or luteal phase.

Third line:

GnRH analogs + addback HRT
(continuous combined estrogen + progestogen or tibolone)

Fourth line:

Total abdominal hysterectomy and bilateral oophorectomy + HRT (including testosterone)
If luteal phase treatment is not effective, after 3 months, continuous SSRIs is started.
Psychoactive drugs are very effective (60%) for PMS and PMDD.

- Nonhormonal medications:
  - Pyridoxine 100 mg twice daily is helpful by correcting tryptophan metabolism.
  - Diuretics in the second half of the cycle—furosemide 20 mg daily for consecutive 5 days a week reduces fluid retention.

CHAPTER 8

Primary Amenorrhea

Q1. Define primary amenorrhea.

Primary amenorrhea is the absence of menstruation by 15 years of age in the presence of normal secondary sexual characteristics, or by 13 years of age if secondary sexual characteristics have not developed.

Q2. What are the causes of primary amenorrhea?

Causes of primary amenorrhea:

1. Development abnormality of the genital tract
   a. Imperforate hymen
   b. Vaginal septum
   c. Absence of the vagina
   d. Vaginal atresia
   e. Mullerian agenesis
2. Chromosomal abnormality
   a. Turner's syndrome (45 X0)
   b. Androgen insensitivity syndrome (46 XY)
3. Systemic disease
   a. Congenital adrenogenital syndrome
   b. Juvenile diabetes
   c. Cretinism
   d. Tuberculosis
4. Disorder of the hypothalamopituitary ovarian axis
   a. Hypogonadotropic hypogonadism
   b. Hypergonadotropic hypogonadism
5. Unresponsive endometrium: Congenital uterine synechiae.

Q3. How will you diagnose and manage a case of primary amenorrhea?

Management of primary amenorrhea

- Diagnosis
  1. History
     - Age
     - Family history of primary amenorrhea
     - Medical diseases such as genital TB or diabetes
     - Abnormal loss or gain in weight within short period of time.
  2. Clinical features
     a. Symptoms: No menstruation by 16 years
     b. Signs:
        - Stature
        - Weight

- Personality
- Webbing in neck
- Secondary sex character
- Mental retardation
- Examination of the genitalia
- Any abdominal lump or tenderness
- Bimanual examination to exclude any pathology in vagina, cervix and uterus.

3. Investigations
   1. Blood:
      - Hb%, TC, DC and ESR
      - Blood sugar
      - T_3, T_4, TSH
      - FSH, LH, prolactin
      - Testosterone
   2. Karyotyping
   3. Ultrasonography
   4. Laparoscopy
   5. Hysteroscopy
   6. Endometrial biopsy
   7. Gonadal biopsy
   8. X-ray chest
   9. Mantoux test
   10. Progesterone challenge test
   11. CT scan or MRI

Treatment

Scope of therapeutic success is very limited and treatment according to cause.

1. Developmental anomalies
   a. Complete agenesis of vagina: Vaginal reconstruction.
   b. Mullerian agenesis
      i. Counseling (menstruation and conception will never happen but can have coital function)
      ii. Vaginoplasty operation (to correct dyspareunia).
2. Chromosomal abnormalities
   a. Turner's or other type of gonadal dysgenesis
      Short-term use of combined estrogen and progesterone therapy at least for breast development.
   b. XY GONADAL dysgenesis: Counseling and gonads to be removed
   c. Androgen insensitivity syndrome: Ectopic gonads are to be removed after development of secondary sex character.
3. Hypothalamopituitary ovarian axis defect:
   i. Gross defect: Nothing to do
   ii. Mild form: Gonadotrophins or GnRH analogs (to induce ovulation and menstruation)
   iii. Isolated gonadotrophin deficiency:
      - Pulsatile administration of GnRH (induction of ovulation)
      - Estrogen and progesterone therapy (for menstruation)
   iv. CNS tumors: Surgical excision or radiotherapy
4. Thyroid and adrenal dysfunction
   i. Mild hypothyroidism: Thyroxin
   ii. Adrenogenital syndrome with enlarged clitoris: Surgical removal of clitoris and prolonged corticosteroid therapy.

5. Metabolic and nutritional: DM and TB are to be treated accordingly.
6. Unresponsive endometrium: Uterine synechiae of tubercular origin should be treated by antitubercular drugs supplemented by adhesiolysis and IUCD insertion.

Q4. How will you approach a girl with primary amenorrhea who lacks a normal vagina but having well developed breast?

If the girl is having absence of vagina first step is to know whether the girl is having cryptomenorrhea (imperforate hymen, transverse vaginal septum, or cervicovaginal agenesis) or true vaginal absence with absence of uterus. Clinical examination (history of cyclic abdominal pain, P/A mass in lower abdomen, P/R mass felt through anterior rectal wall) with ultrasound examination will help to exclude cryptomenorrhea. Once cryptomenorrhea is excluded, possibilities are Mayer-Rokitansky-Küster-Hauser (MRKH) syndrome and AIS.

If no uterus is present in ultrasonography along with absence of pubic and axillary hairs, AIS is likely. Further evaluation would include karyotyping (which would be 46 XY karyotyping) and serum testosterone which will be normal male range.

In MRKH syndrome, it is important to screen for anomalies of kidneys by ultrasonography and intravenous pyelogram (IVP) of kidneys and skeletal abnormalities of kidneys by ultrasonography and intravenous pyelogram (IVP) of kidneys and skeletal abnormalities by X-ray of dorsolumbar spine.

Q5. How will you investigate a girl with normal reproductive tract with primary amenorrhea?

If the normal reproductive tract is confirmed, first step is to investigate the patient's estrogen status. If the breasts are developed, she is exposed to estrogen for some time at least in the past. The possibilities are constitutional delay in puberty or resistant ovary syndrome.

If normal reproductive tract is present but there is no evidence of breast development, the patient has never been exposed to estrogen. The cause of which is likely to be ovarian failure or failure of gonadotropin production due to hypothalamus/pituitary abnormality.

Next step is to do an endocrine evaluation with estimation of LH, FSH, TSH, prolactin, and serum estradiol. Low or absent estrogen production is either due to an abnormal ovary or low gonadal stimulation of a normal ovary.

If LH and FSH are raised in menopausal range, likely causes are gonadal dysgenesis or ovarian failure in absence of breast development. Turner syndrome is the most common form of gonadal dysgenesis and a karyotyping will be required to confirm Turner syndrome and other form of gonadal dysgenesis. A 46, XY karyotype will typically diagnose Swyer syndrome. To confirm resistant ovary syndrome, an ovarian biopsy will be required to show multiple follicles.

Low LH and FSH level may be due to delay in progression of normal maturation (delayed puberty) or an inability to secrete adequate amount of gonadotropins (hypothalamic/pituitary abnormalities). A constitutional delay in puberty is often associated with family history of delayed onset of puberty. A delayed puberty is often indistinguishable from hypothalamic/pituitary failure but following features help in distinguishing between the two:

- Increased prolactin and increased TSH level often suppress GnRH secretion thereby causing hypogonadotropic hypogonadism.
- Hypogonadotropic hypogonadism due to Kallmann syndrome is associated with anosmia.
- MRI of brain may detect pituitary tumor or empty sella syndrome where pituitary is significantly affected resulting in decreased gonadotropin secretion.
- Bone age radiograph (X-ray of nondominant hand)—distinguishes from constitutional delay in puberty from permanent from constitutional delay in puberty from permanent hypogonadotropic hypogonadism.
- In presence of hyperandrogenism, serum testosterone, 17-hydroxyprogesterone, and DHEAS should be measured to assess androgen secreting tumor of ovary, congenital adrenal hyperplasia (CAH), and adrenal tumor.

Q6. Which patients with primary amenorrhea are treated with surgical intervention?

- Anatomic obstruction of outflow tract may require drainage of hematocolpos, excision of vaginal septum, and vaginoplasty. Women with MRKH syndrome may require vaginoplasty.
- In patients with Y chromosome, e.g., Swyer syndrome, AIS gonadectomy is performed to prevent development of gonadoblastoma. In AIS, gonadectomy is delayed until after puberty to ensure proper breast development due to aromatization peripheral testosterone to estradiol in liver.
- Primary amenorrhea due to androgen secreting tumor of ovary or adrenal will required surgical intervention.
- In some women with virilization due to partial androgen sensitivity syndrome or CAH may require reduction clitoroplasty in presence of clitoromegaly.

Q7. How do you investigate a case of primary amenorrhea?

Investigations will vary widely depending on the abnormalities found during clinical examination. One can divided primary amenorrhea into three general categories:

1. Patient with good secondary sex character development
2. Patient with poor/no secondary sex character development
3. Patient with heterosexual secondary sex character developments.

Patient with Good Secondary Sex Character Development

Differential diagnosis includes:

- Congenital and anatomical abnormalities (imperforate hymen, transverse vaginal septum, vaginal agenesis, cervical agenesis with vaginal dysgenesis, and MRKH syndrome)
- Androgen insensitivity syndrome
- Resistant ovary syndrome
  - Imperforate hymen, transverse vaginal septum, vaginal agenesis, and cervical agenesis with vaginal dysgenesis: All these conditions will present as cryptomenorrhea. Differentiating features are cyclic lower abdominal pain and swelling in lower abdomen; on vulval inspection: A tense bulging and bluish membrane may be seen; on rectal examination: A large bulging mass is felt. USG-hematometra and hematocolpos.
  - Mayer-Rokitansky-Küster-Hauser syndrome: Normal breast, pubic, axillary hairs development, absent vaginal canal, and absent or rudimentary uterus on per rectal examination. USG—absence of uterus; FSH, estradiol—normal; testosterone—female range, karyotype 46, XX.
  - Androgen insensitivity syndrome: Large breast with juvenile nipple, absent pubic, and axillary hairs, absent vaginal canal, testes may be felt in labia or inguinal canal, absent uterus, FSH—increased, testosterone—male range, karyotype 46, XY>
  - Resistant ovary syndrome: Normal secondary sexual characteristics elevated plasma FSH and LH—in the menopausal range, 46, XX karyotype, multiple follicles are seen on ovarian biopsy.

Patient with Poor/No Secondary Sex Character Development

The differential diagnosis includes:

- Hypothalamic amenorrhea
- Pituitary amenorrhea
- Ovarian causes of amenorrhea
- Constitutional delay in puberty
  - Hypothalamic amenorrhea: History of anosmia, sever chronic disease, rapid weight loss, malnutrition, depression or other psychiatric disorders anorexia nervosa, recreational drug abuse and psychotropic drug use. Absent secondary sex character; vagina, uterus present; FSH, LH low (5 IU/L), estradiol low, normal TSH, prolactin, karyotype 46, XX.
  - To differentiate between hypothalamic or pituitary origin perform a GnRH test—if there is an appropriate LH response following the administration of exogenous GnRH the diagnosis of hypothalamic failure to produce or secrete adequate GnRH is made. If no response after priming the pituitary with a 10-day course of GnRH, the diagnosis of pituitary failure is made.

- Pituitary amenorrhea: History of galactorrhea, headaches, or reduces peripheral vision (prolactinoma/ craniopharyngioma); traumatic head injury or infection; visual-field defects; absent secondary sex character; vagina, uterus present; FSH, LH low (< IU/L), estradiol low, normal TSH, prolactin may be increased in hyperprolactinemia, MRI brain may be abnormal in pituitary tumor, karyotype 46, XX.
- Ovarian causes of amenorrhea: Turner syndrome, Mosaic Turner, pure gonadal dysgenesis, and XY gonadal dysgenesis Swyer's syndrome)
  - Turner syndrome: Short stature, poor breast development, broad chest (shield chest), and widely spaced nipples, low hairline. Low-set ears, shortened metacarpal IV, webbed neck from cystic hygroma in infancy, cubitus valgus; vagina, uterus present; FSH, LH high (menopausal range), estradiol low, karyotype 45, X0.
  - Mosaic Turner: Classic physical features of Turner's syndrome are absent. FSH, LH high, estradiol low, karyotype 45, X, 46, XX, or 45X, 46, XY.
  - Pure gonadal dysgenesis: Normal appearance, taller than 150 cm, vagina, uterus present; FSH, LH high; estradiol low; Gonads–streak. Karyotype 46, XX.

- Constitutional delay in puberty: History of delayed puberty in family, history of chronic systemic illness, e.g., chronic renal failure, malnutrition, etc., absent secondary sex character; vagina, uterus present; FSH, LH low (<5 IU/L), estradiol low normal TSH, normal prolactin, karyotyping 46, XX, MRI brain normal, bone age is <14.5 years. Diagnosis is by exclusion of other causes

Patient with Heterosexual Development of Secondary Sex Character

- If secondary sexual development in heterosexual, the diagnosis may be (production of estrogen and excess testosterone):
  - Congenital adrenal hyperplasia
  - Adrenal tumor
  - Masculinizing ovarian tumor
  - One of the forms of XY female
  - Cushing's syndrome

Congenital adrenal hyperplasia: Clitoral enlargement, presence of vagina with normal internal genital organs (uterus, ovaries), increased production of cortisol precursor, 17-hydroxyprogesterone, increased androgens and ACTH level. The elevated level of androgens results into varying degree of masculinization. MRI, CT scan, and ultrasound can be judiciously used if androgenic tumors are suspected.

Other causes: Incomplete AIS (XY female) may present with female phenotype and genital ambiguity. Other possibilities which must be considered are presence of an ovarian masculinizing tumor, an adrenal adenoma or carcinoma or a pituitary lesion giving rise to the features of Cushing's syndrome.

CRYPTOMENORRHEA

Q1. Define cryptomenorrhea.

Cryptomenorrhea is a condition where there is periodic shedding of the endometrium and bleeding but the menstrual blood fails to come out from the genital tract due to obstruction in the passage.

Q2. What are the causes of cryptomenorrhea?

Causes of cryptomenorrhea

1. Congenital (common)
   a. Imperforate hymen
   b. Transverse vaginal septum
   c. Atresia of the vaginal

2. Acquired
   a. Cervical stenosis following:
      - Amputation of the cervix
      - Deep cauterization
      - Conization of the cervix
      - Post MR
      - Following obstructed labor
   b. Vulvovaginitis of infancy leading to labial adhesion
   c. Vaginal stenosis

Nice to know

Pathophysiology of cryptomenorrhea

- Periodic shedding of endometrium and bleeding but the menstrual blood fails to come out from the genital tract due to obstruction
- With each monthly discharge, the vagina fills with blood but some of its water content is absorbed, so the blood becomes inspissated
- The amount gradually increases and in the course of months and years it distends, first the vagina (hematocolpos), then the uterus (hematometra) and finally the tubes (hematosalpinx)
- The altered blood causes inflammation of the tube, so its outer end gets closed and results in hematosalpinx
- If the tubes remain open, pelvic endometriosis is a possible complication

Q3. Write down the management of cryptomenorrhea.

Management of cryptomenorrhea

- Diagnosis
  - Clinical features
    1. Age: 13–15 (Congenital type)
    2. Amenorrhea dated back from the events
    3. Periodic lower abdominal pain
    4. Retention of urine (hematocolpos)
    5. Abdominal examination reveals a uniform globular mass in the hypogastrium
    6. Pelvic examination reveals:
       - Offending lesion either in the vagina or cervix
       - The uterus is symmetrically enlarged

Treatment:

1. Cruciate incision of the hymen and drainage of blood
2. Dilatation of the cervix in stenosis
3. In cases of secondary atresia of the vagina, reconstructive surgery is to be performed to maintain patency.

Q4. Write short notes on cryptomenorrhea.

Cryptomenorrhea refers to concealed menstruation where cyclical endometrial shedding takes place, but menstrual blood is retained inside the genital tract because of a physical blockage preventing its passage outside the body.

Q5. What do you mean by Asherman's syndrome?

Asherman's syndrome/uterine synechiae

Formation of adhesions following postabortal and puerperal curettage and also following diagnostic curettage in dysfunctional uterine bleeding.

- Clinical features
  1. Hypomenorrhea
  2. Oligomenorrhoea
  3. Amenorrhea

- Investigations
  1. Progesterone challenge test: Negative
  2. Hysterosalpingography: Shows honeycomb appearance
  3. Hysteroscopy: Reveals the extent of adhesions directly
- Treatment
  1. Lysis of the intrauterine adhesions by sounding or hysteroscopy followed by insertion of IUCD for 3 months to prevent adhesion of the uterine walls.
  2. Combined oral contraceptive pills or conjugated estrogen for 3 cycles to regenerate endometrium.

CHAPTER 9

Secondary Amenorrhea

Q1. Define secondary amenorrhea.

Secondary amenorrhea is the absence of menstruation for three normal cycles or for 6 months.

Or

Absence of menstruation for about 6 months in a woman during the reproductive phase who had normal menstrual cycles before.

Q2. What are the causes of secondary amenorrhea?

Causes of secondary amenorrhea

A. Physiological cause
   1. Pregnancy
   2. Lactation
   3. Post-menarche
   4. Pre-menopausal

B. Pathological cause
   1. Hypothalamic cause
      a. Hypothalamic dysfunction
      b. Stress
      c. Drugs: Oral pills, injectable contraceptives, phenothiazine, reserpine, etc.
      d. Simple weight loss > 20% of ideal body weight
      e. Anorexia nervosa
      f. Diseases: Craniopharyngioma, encephalitis, trauma, etc.
      g. Hyperprolactinemia
   2. Pituitary cause
      a. Sheehan's syndrome
      b. Pituitary tumor
   3. Ovarian cause
      a. Premature ovarian failure
      b. Resistant ovarian syndrome
      c. Oophoritis
      d. Post-radiation and chemotherapy
      e. Polycystic ovary syndrome
   4. Uterine cause
      a. TB endometritis
      b. Asherman's syndrome
      c. Surgical removal

Q3. How will you manage a case of secondary amenorrhea?

Management of secondary amenorrhea

- Diagnosis

  History
  1. Age (post-menarche, pre-menopausal)
  2. Period of amenorrhea
  3. Mode of onset (sudden or following oligomenorrhoea)
  4. Pregnancy symptoms
  5. Any stressful condition
  6. Significant weight loss or gain
  7. Acne, hirsutism, milk secretion
  8. Headache, visual disturbance
  9. Hot flushes, vaginal dryness, dyspareunia
  10. Obstetric history:
      - Recent delivery, abortion, MR
      - Breastfeeding
      - Severe PPH
      - Post-partum or post-abortal D&C
      - Amenorrhea following caesarean section (caesarean hysterectomy)
  11. Drug history: Oral pills injectable contraceptives, phenothiazines, reserpine, etc.
  12. Family history
  13. Medical history of TB or contact, liver disease, renal disease etc.
  14. History of radiotherapy or chemotherapy.
- General examination
  1. Appearance: Ill health, overweight, acne, hirsutism, central obesity or goiter
  2. Weight: Weight loss > 20% of ideal body weight is significant
  3. Breast: Atrophied, normal, milk secretion
- Abdominal examination: To see any mass in the abdomen
- Vaginal examination
  1. Vulva: Atrophied, normal clitoral enlargement
  2. Vagina: Rugosed, smooth, dry
  3. Cervix: Secretion abundant or absent
  4. Adnexa: Any swelling
- Investigation
  - General investigation
    1. Blood for TC, DC, ESR
    2. X-ray chest and Mantoux test to exclude TB
    3. Urine for pregnancy test
    4. X-ray skull (to exclude pituitary tumor)
    5. USG (to exclude pregnancy, ovarian tumor, etc.)
    6. Estimation of prolactin, TSH, T_3 and T_4 (to exclude hyperprolactinemia and thyroid disorder)
  - Special investigation
    1. Progesterone challenge test
    2. Combined estrogen and progesterone test
    3. Serum FSH and LH estimation
    4. Ovarian biopsy
    5. Hysterosalpingography

6. Hysteroscopy
7. D and C
8. Endometrial biopsy

Treatment:

Before treatment pregnancy, lactation, post-menarcheal amenorrhea should be excluded.

1. No abnormality detected
   No treatment, assurance only
2. Hypothalamic origin
   a. Anxiety and stress : Assurance
   b. Drugs causing amenorrhea should be stopped
   c. Simple weight loss : Improved diet
   d. Anorexia nervosa : Improved diet and psychotherapy
   e. Hyperprolactinemia : Bromocriptine/cabergoline for 6-9 months
3. Pituitary origin
   a. Sheehan's syndrome : Hormone replacement therapy
   b. Pituitary adenoma : Surgery or radiotherapy
4. Ovarian origin
   a. Premature ovarian failure
      - No satisfactory treatment
      - HRT (to prevent osteoporosis)
      - Ovum donation (treatment of infertility)
   b. Autoimmune oophoritis : Corticosteroids
   c. PCOD : Clomiphene citrate
   d. Virilizing tumor of ovary : Surgical removal of ovary.
5. Uterine origin:
   a. Asherman's syndrome : Adhesiolysis (by D&C or hysteroscopy) followed by IUCD insertion for 3 months and OCP for 3 cycles.
   b. Tubercular endometritis : Anti-tubercular drugs
6. Other causes
   a. Hypothyroidism : Thyroxin
   b. Adrenal tumor : Adrenalectomy
   c. Adrenal hyperplasia : Corticosteroid

Q4. Progesterone challenge test in secondary amenorrhea.

- Medroxyprogesterone 10 mg is to be given orally daily for 10 days
- The test is called positive if vaginal bleeding occurs after withdrawal of the drug and it indicate:
- Endometrium is functioning
- Endogenous estrogen at least more than 40 pgm/mL is present
- Hypothalamic-pituitary-ovarian axis is normal
- FSH and LH levels are not normal enough to produce folliculogenesis and ovulation
- So, FSH, LH, and estrogen levels are to be estimated.

Q5. Write a short note on Sheehan's syndrome.

Sheehan's syndrome may be defined as decreased functioning of the pituitary gland caused by necrosis due to blood loss and hypovolemic shock during and after child birth.

Clinical features

1. History of severe postpartum hemorrhage, shock or severe infection

2. Failing lactation
3. Loss of pubic and axillary hair, lethargy, hypotension, secondary amenorrhea and atrophy of the breasts and genitalia.

Investigations

1. Serum FSH, LH, TSH and ACTH level
2. CT scan of pituitary region

Treatment

1. Replacement therapy with appropriate hormones including corticosteroids and thyroxine are needed
2. Fertility can be achieved in these women with hMG and hCG.

Q6. Outline the investigation of a case of secondary amenorrhea.

Flowchart: Diagnostic scheme for evaluating secondary amenorrhea.

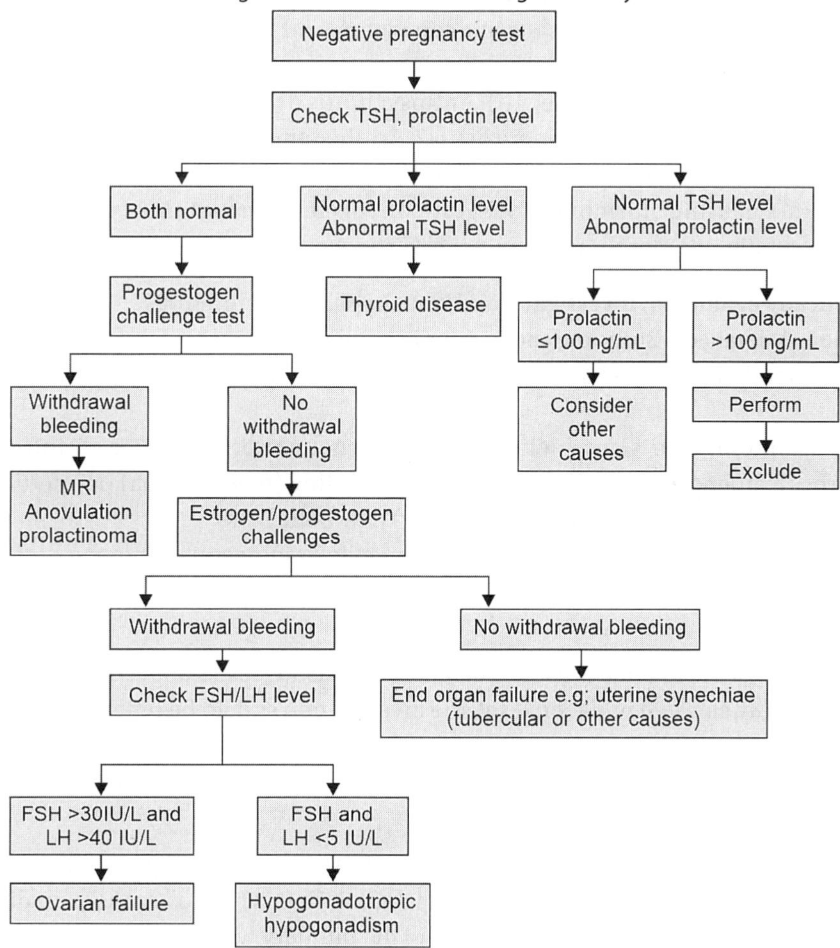

Q7. Define hyperprolactinemia. Describe its pathophysiology. What are its causes?

Hyperprolactinemia is a condition characterized by an elevated serum prolactin (PRL) level in the blood. Normal PRL levels in women are 25 ug/L (500 mU/L) and in men are 20 ug/L (400 mU/L).

Causes: The causes of hyperprolactinemia can be divided into physiological, pathological and pharmacological causes.

- Physiological causes: Pregnancy, nipple stimulation, lactation, exercise, stress (hypoglycemia, myocardial infarction, surgery), seizures, sleep, neonatal period, and sexual intercourse.
- Pathological causes:
  - Pituitary diseases: Prolactinoma, acromegaly, Cushing disease, macroadenoma (compressive), macroprolactinemia.
  - Hypothalamic disease: Stalk damage due to tumors like craniopharyngioma, suprasellar pituitary mass extension, meningioma, dysgerminoma, granulomas (sarcoidosis, tuberculosis), infiltrative disease (histiocytosis disease).
  - Systemic causes: Primary hypothyroidism, chronic renal failure, liver cirrhosis, polycystic ovarian disease.
  - Reflex causes: Chest wall trauma, surgery, herpes zoster.
  - Genetic cause: Inactivating prolactin receptor mutation.
  - Ectopic secretion: Induction: bronchogenic carcinoma, and hypernephromas.
- Pharmacological causes: (i) Antiemetic drugs: Dopamine receptor blocking agents; Metoclopramide, domperidone, and prochlorperazine; (ii) Antipsychotic drugs: Dopamine receptor blocking agents: risperidone, haloperidol, fluphenazine; (iii) H2 Antihistamines: Cimetidine, ranitidine; (iv) Tricyclic antidepressant, selective serotonin receptor inhibitor: Amitriptyline, clomipramine, fluoxetine; (v) Thyrotropin-releasing hormone, (vi) Anticonvulsant: Phenytoin; (vii) Antihypertensive drugs: Methadone, morphine, apomorphine, heroin; (viii) Estrogen therapy; (ix) Cholinergic agent: physostigmine.

Q8. How do you clinically evaluated, investigate, and treat hyperprolactinemia?

Clinical evaluation: A detailed history and meticulous examination are to be done in relation to sign symptoms of hyperprolactinemia and to exclude causes of hyperprolactinemia (physiological, pharmacological, and systemic causes).

- For women, symptoms and signs include: (i) Menstrual abnormalities, e.g.; infrequent menstruation (oligomenorrhea), amenorrhea, heavy menstruation bleeding (menorrhagia) or infertility; (ii) Galactorrhea: may not always be present; (iii) Decreased libido; (iv) Low bone mass.
- For men, symptoms and signs are decreased libido, erectile dysfunction. Impotence, infertility, gynecomastia, oligospermia, galactorrhea (rare), and low bone mass.

Investigations:

Serum prolactin: Hyperprolactinemia is usually diagnosed as fasting levels above 20 ng/ mL in men and above 25 ng/mL women. In mildly elevated prolactin level, the investigation should be repeated.

If serum prolactin is elevated, the next steps are: (i) Exclusion of physiological causes; (ii) Exclusion of pharmacological causes; (iii) Radiological imaging of the hypothalamic-pituitary region to find out the cause.

Further investigations may include:

- (i) Pregnancy test; (ii) Thyroid function test; (iii) Renal function test; (iv) Insulin- like growth factor-1 (IGF-1); (v) adrenocorticotrophic hormone (ACTH); (vi) LH, (vii) FSH, (viii) Testosterone/estradiol.
- Imaging test: The preferred imaging study is MRU of the pituitary with contrast.
- Visual field testing should be done in cases of macroadenoma and tumors that are adjacent to/or compressing to optic chiasma.
- In instances where other causes pf hyperprolactinemia have been excluded and no adenoma can be visualized with MRI, the hyperprolactinemia is referred to as "Idiopathic".

Treatment: the treatment of hyperprolactinemia can be broadly divided into three group: (i) Treatment of idiopathic hyperprolactinemia or microadenoma. These cases can be managed only with medicines; (ii) Treatment of macroadenoma: This group needs management with drugs and surgery or radiotherapy; (iii) Hyperprolactinemia due to a known cause, e.g.; pharmacologic or systemic causes; treating underline cause brings back prolactin to normal.

- Group 1: Idiopathic hyperprolactinemia; Dopamine agonist such as bromocriptine, cabergoline are the mainstay of treatment. Once the normal serum prolactin level is achieved the dosage is adjusted so that lowest dose is used to maintain normal prolactin level. If the normal prolactin level is maintained with lowest dosage for 2 years the drug can be discontinued.
- Group 2: Macroadenoma – It has medical, surgical, and radiation treatments.
  Medical treatment: Endocrine society guideline recommends dopamine agonist therapy for symptomatic women with microadenomas or macroadenomas. Cabergoline is preferred to other dopamine agonists because of its better efficacy. Dopamine agonist therapy decreases tumor size, prolactin level and normalize menstrual function. The therapy can be tapered and can be discontinued after 2 years of normal serum prolactin level and no adenoma is visible on MRI
  Surgery or radiotherapy: Surgery and radiotherapy are indicated for women who do not respond to medical treatment with dopamine agonists. Endoscopic endonasal trans-sphenoidal surgery is the surgical method of choice. For large prolactinoma with visual field defects during pregnancy prophylactic surgery can be considered. In case of residual tumor following surgery adjuvant radiation therapy can be considered. Gamma knife stereotactic radiosurgery can be considered if prolactinoma is resistant or intolerant to the treatment of dopamine agonist.
- Group 3: Hyperprolactinemia due to a known cause: (i) Hypothyroidism: Treated with thyroid replacement therapy; (ii) Drug-induced hyperprolactinemia: Drug can be stopped or replaced if there is troublesome galactorrhea, hypogonadism or osteoporosis; (iii) hypothalamic disease: Stalk damage: Treatment of the cause should be considered first. If not possible, hyperprolactinemia is treated with the dopamine agonist; (iv) Renal Failure: correction of the renal failure by transplantation results in normal prolactin levels.
  An outline of management of hyperprolactinemia is shown below.

Q9. Define premature ovarian insufficiency/primary ovarian insufficiency. What ae its causes? Described its pathophysiology.

Premature ovarian insufficiency (POI) is a clinical condition characterized by ovarian follicle depletion, which leads to hypoestrogenism and amenorrhea, before the age of 40 years. In this condition, there is deficient sex hormone production and decreased ovarian follicles, which accelerate the onset of menopause.

Causes:

- Genetic: (i) Turner syndrome (45 XO) or mosaic Turner (45X/46 XX), Trisomy X (47 XXX or mosaic; (ii) Fragile X premutation; (iii) Galactosemia (galactose – 1- phosphate uridyltransferase deficiency); (iv) Autoimmune polyglandular syndrome (types 1 and 2); (v) FSH receptor mutations; (vi) 17 α-hydroxylase deficiency; (vii) Aromatase deficiency; (viii) Blepharophimosis, ptosis, and epicanthus inversus syndrome; (ix) bloom syndrome; (x) Ataxia telangiectasia; and (xi) Fanconi anemia.
- Autoimmune ovarian damage
- Infections: (i) Mumps oophoritis; (ii) Tuberculosis (iii) Malaria; (iv) Cytomegalovirus; (v) Varicella; and (vi) Shigella.
- Induced: (a) Iatrogenic: bilateral oophorectomy, bilateral ovarian cystectomies, chemotherapy (Primarily, alkylating agents, and anthracyclines), Radiation external bean or intracavitary, uterine artery embolization; (b) Environmental toxins.
- Idiopathic

Pathophysiology:

The primordial follicles begins to develop in utero and reaches its peak number at 6-7 million by 20 weeks of gestation. Thereafter, the follicles rapidly undergo atresia, at birth, the number of oocytes reaches approximately 1-2 million, and by the time puberty is reached, only 3,00,000-400000 oocytes remain. Out of these, only 400-500 are ovulated during reproductive life of the women. This follicular atresia is regulated by interaction of various molecules. While androgens, TNF alfa and Fas ligand favors atresia of the follicles, estrogen. Gonadotropins, and nitric oxide inhibits atretic process. Thus, attrition of follicles from the beginning, (ii) a faster atretic rate or (iii) impaired recruitment of the follicles. However, the precise pathophysiology of POI is not clearly understood as this disease is variable in nature.

Q10. Describe the clinical presentation, investigations and management of premature ovarian insufficiency/ primary ovarian insufficiency.

Clinical presentation:

- Menstrual history: (a) infrequent menses followed by amenorrhea; (b) Sudden onset of secondary amenorrhea; (c) Primary amenorrhea.
- Family history: Should include maternal age at menopause and family history of POI in first -or second-degree relatives. Family history of any known autoimmune or genetic disorders also to be inquired.
- Symptoms POI: Vasomotor symptoms like palpitation, hot flushes and night sweats; vulvovaginal atrophy, vaginal dryness, dyspareunia, insomnia, mood disturbances, cognitive problems e.g.; memory issues, tiredness, loss of libido; and weight gain.
- Infertility.
- Autoimmune: Vitiligo, hyperpigmentation, adrenal insufficiency etc.

Investigations: Diagnosis: (i) Elevated serum follicle-stimulating hormone (FSH) levels (25 IU/L) on two separate occasions at least one month apart, with concomitant low estradiol (E2) levels (< 50 pg/ mL); amenorrhea for at least 4 months in women younger than 40 years of age.
However, the lower FSH cutoff for diagnosis of POI varies; the widely accepted lower limit of FSH is > 40 IU/L, > 30 IU/L (UK National Institute for Health and Care Excellence), > 25 IU/L (European Society of Human Reproduction and Embryology (ESHRE).

Other investigations to support the diagnosis: (i) AMH: Low or undetectable, marker of ovarian reserve; (ii) Pelvic ultrasound (TVS): Low antral follicle count (<5) and thin endometrial echo (<4 mm) with small ovarian volume; (iii) Inhibin: Low inhibin, marker of ovarian reserve.

Investigations to find out the etiology: (i) Genetic Screening referral for genetic counseling/testing; Karyotyping; and Fragile X mental retardation 1 (FMR1) premutation; (ii) Immunologic causes: adrenal function test with 21 hydroxylase antibody test; thyroid function test, and TPO antibody; whether antibody positive or negative; (iii) Ultrasonography and MRI to assess the presence or absence of ovarian tissue for congenital and surgical reasons e.g.; dysgenesis, endometriosis surgery; (iv) Infectious disease screen guided by history and examination; (v) Toxin screen guided by history; (vi) Metabolic screen guided by clinical examination and family history e.g.; GALT enzyme or genetic (autosomal recessive) testing; (vii) Investigation for iatrogenic causes, guided by medical and surgical history.

Treatment: Treatment modalities are:

- Counseling and emotional support: The diagnosis of POI is associated with a higher level of depression. Women may be upset because of permanent loss of reproductive function. They should be offered psychological support to cope with the emotional consequences of POI.
- Hormone therapy: All women with POI should receive hormone therapy with estrogen and progestogen to relieve the symptoms of estrogen deficiency and to maintain bone density.
- A few women may require hormone therapy even before amenorrhea develops due to estrogen deficiency symptoms.
- Estrogen: Estrogen is prescribed orally or trans-dermally, continuously or cyclically 21 days on, 7 days off).
- Progestogen: Progestins is administered cyclically, 10-14 days each month, to counter unopposed estrogen effects on endometrium.
- Hormone therapy does not prevent ovulation in these patients; in fact it may improve the chance of pregnancy theoretically by lowering LH levels and luteinization of the remaining follicles. So the patient should be instructed to obtain a prompt pregnancy test if menstrual bleeding fails to appears when expected.

- The COC pill is not considered a first line approach for these women.
- Androgen replacement with oral or injectable testosterone may be carefully considered in selected group of women who have persistent fatigue, low libido, and poor wellbeing in spite of adequate estrogen replacement therapy.

The dosage and different hormonal formulations are given below:

- Estrogens: 17-E2 2-4 mg orally or CEE 0.625-1.25 mg orally, or 17 β-E2 50-100 μg transdermally, and topical vaginal estrogens when vulvovaginal atrophy is diagnosed.
- Progestogens (women with an intact uterus only) Natural progesterone orally, 200 mg cyclically or 100 mg continuously; Dydrogesterone, 10-20 mg orally; Norethisterone, 1-5 mg orally; or Norethisterone, 0.25 mg transdermally.
- Androgens: Oral methyltestosterone 1.2-2.5 mg/d, injectable testosterone esters 50 mg every 6 weeks intramuscularly, or subcutaneous testosterone pellet implants 50 mg every 3-6 months.

Fertility treatment: (i) Unproven treatments to restore fertility should be avoided; (ii) Fertility is possible with donor oocyte; (iii) Autologous intraovarian platelet rich plasma therapy has been shown to increase AMH while reducing FSH levels. However, therapy remains experimental.

CHAPTER 10

Reproductive Tract Infection and Genital Tuberculosis

Q1. Describe the female defense mechanism?

The infection from one pelvic organ to other spreads frequently due to free anastomosis between the lymphatics and blood vessel and there is an open pathway of peritoneal cavity to exterior through vagina but defense mechanism helps to lower the ascending infection.

Defense mechanism of

1. **Vulva**

   Anatomical:
   - Apposition of cleft by labia
   - Compound racemose type of Bartholin's gland

   Physiological:
   - Apocrine gland: fungicidal action
   - Natural high resistance to infection
2. **Vagina**

   Anatomical:
   - Apposition of anterior and posterior wall
   - Stratified epithelium resistance to infection

   Physiological:
   - Maintained by estrogen
   - Stratified squamous epithelium resistant to infection
   - Vaginal acidity
   - Flora: The G positive Doderlein's bacilli splits glycogen into lactic acid

   Defense of vagina in relation to age

	Newborn (0-10 day)s	*Up to puberty*	*Childbearing*	*Postmenopausal*
Epithelium	Multilayered	Thin	Multilayered	Thin
Glycogen	++	(-)	++	(-)
Doderlein's bacillus	+	(-)	++	(-)
pH	Acidic (4-5)	Neutral or alkaline	Acidic (4-5)	Neutral (6-7)

3. **Cervix:** Closed by bacteriolytic cervical mucus
4. **Uterus:** Periodic shedding of endometrium during menstruation eliminates infection

Q2. What are the phases of life where defense is lost?

- From 10 days of life till puberty
- During reproductive period
  - During menstruation:
    - Vaginal acidity lowered
    - Fall of estrogen

- Following abortion and childbirth
  - Favors bacterial growth due to raw placental site, tear of cervix, bruising of vagina.
- During menopause

Q3. Write down the pH of vagina according to age?

Age	*pH*
0–10 days of life	Acidic (4–5)
Up to puberty	Neutral or alkaline (6–8)
Childbearing period	Acidic (4–5)
Postmenopausal	Neutral (6–7)

Q4. What do you mean by pelvic infection and classify it?

Infection including uterus, uterine tubes, adjacent parametrium and overlying peritoneum is said to be pelvic infection.

It can be classified as:

Acute pelvic infections

- Pelvic Inflammatory disease (PID)
- Following delivery and abortion
- Following gynecological procedures
- Following intrauterine devices (IUD)
- Secondary to other infections

Sexually transmitted Infection (STI)

Q5. What do you mean by sexually transmitted infection (STI)?

STIs include those infections which are predominantly transmitted through sexual contact from an infected partner.

Q6. What are the common STIs?

1. **Bacterial:**

Disease	*Agent*
Gonorrhea	Neisseria gonorrhoeae
Non-gonococcal urethritis	Chlamydia trachomatis (D-K)
Syphilis	Treponema pallidum
Lymphogranuloma venereum	Chlamydia trachomatis (L)
Chancroid	Haemophilus vaginalis
Granuloma inguinale	Donovania granulomatis
Nonspecific vaginitis	Haemophilus vaginalis
Mycoplasma infection	Mycoplasma hominis(genitalium)

2. **Viral**

AIDS	• Human immunodeficiency virus • HIV 1 OR HIV 2
Genital herpes	Herpes simplex virus (HSV 2)
Condyloma acuminata	Human papilloma virus (HPV)
CIN	HPV-16, 18 OR 31
Molluscum contagiosum	Pox virus
Viral hepatitis	Hepatitis B & C virus

3. Protozoal

Bacterial vaginosis	Gardnerella vaginalis
Trichomonas vaginitis	Trichomonas vaginalis

4. Fungal

Monilial vaginitis	Candida albicans

5. Ectoparasite

Scabies	Sarcoptes scabiei
Pediculosis pubis	Crab louse (Pthirus pubis)

Gonorrhea

- Causative agent—Neisseria gonorrhea (G negative diplococcus)
- Incubation period-3-7 days
- Site of invasion—columnar and transitional epithelium of genitourinary tract
- Primary site—endocervix, urethra, Skene's gland & Bartholin's gland
- Other sites—oropharynx, anorectal region and conjunctiva

Q7. Mention the clinical features of gonorrhea?

Asymptomatic—50%
If symptoms present—nonspecific
Clinical features are as follows

Local:

Symptoms

- Dysuria (25%)
- Profuse, non-irritating, white to yellowish vaginal discharge (50%)
- Unilateral pain and labial swelling
- Rectal discomfort
- Others: Pharyngeal infection, inter menstrual bleeding

Signs

- Labia-swollen and inflamed
- Vaginal discharge—mucopurulent
- Bartholin's duct opening—congested
- External urethral meatus—congested
- Pressure on Bartholin's duct and external urethral meatus—purulent exudates
- Bartholin's gland—enlarged, tender
- Per speculum
  Ectocervix-congested
  Cervical secretion-mucopurulent

Distant or metastatic
Features of perihepatitis or septicemia

Q8. Diagnosis for gonorrhea

NAAT of urine or endocervical discharge is done
NAAT—sensitive and specific (95%)
Preferred 1st void morning urine sample

Q9. Mention the treatment protocol

Preventive

- Male partner should be treated simultaneously
- Avoid multiple sexual partner
- Barrier method should be used

According to CDC 2020
Injection Ceftriaxone—500 mg-IM-single dose
Tab Azithromycin—1 g-PO-once

Curative: Any one single dose regimen according to CDC 2020

Follow up:
- Cultures should be done 7 days after therapy
- Repeat cultures monthly following menses for 3 months

Syphilis
Causative organism: Treponema Pallidum (spirochete)
Incubation period: 9-90 days
Acquired by—direct contact with infected person
Transmission through—abraded skin or mucosal surface

Clinical features:
- **Primary lesion**—Chancre (single or multiple located in labia)-heals spontaneously
- Fourchette, anus, cervix and nipples other site of lesion
- Small papule—formed 2-3 weeks after exposure-erode to form ulcer
- Margin—raised, smooth shiny floor
- Ulcer—painless

Secondary syphilis
Time—within 6 weeks to 6 months of onset of primary chancre
Location—in vulva in the form of condyloma lata
Lesion—coarse, flat-topped, moist, necrotic lesion & teeming with treponemes
Transmission—hematogenous spread
Symptoms:
- Fever
- Headache
- Sore throat
- Maculopapular skin rashes in palm and sole
- Generalized lymphadenopathy
- Mucosal ulcer
- Alopecia

Primary and secondary stage can last up to two years

Latent syphilis
Quiescence phase after stage of secondary syphilis is resolved
Duration: 2-20 years
Serology—positive without sign and symptoms
Tertiary syphilis—characterized by gumma
About 1/3rd of untreated patients progress from late latent stage to tertiary syphilis
- Damages CNS, CVS and musculoskeletal system

Symptoms
- **Cranial nerve palsies (III, VI, VII and VIII)**
- Hemiplegia
- Tabes dorsalis
- Aortic aneurysm
- Gummas of skin and bone
- Endarteritis and periarteritis of small and medium sized vessels

Q10. How will you diagnose syphilis?

For the diagnosis of syphilis we should take detailed history and investigations:

- History: Exposure to infected person
- Organism identification
- Serological test:
  - Nonspecific nontreponemal test are-
    - VDRL: Positive after 6 weeks of initial infection
      - Pregnancy
      - SLE

Specific test

- TPHA
- FTA-Abs
- TPI
- RPR card test: Positive after 4-6 weeks after initial exposure
- PCR and immunoblotting: Are more sensitive and confirmatory test nowadays.

Q11. Write the treatment protocol for syphilis?

Early syphilis:

<1 year duration

Benzathine penicillin G 2.4 million units-IM-Single dose

If allergic to penicillin

Tab Tetracycline—500 mg-PO-QID

OR

Tab Doxycycline 100 mg-BID-PO for 14 days

Late syphilis:

>1 year duration

Benzathine penicillin G 2.4 million units-IM—for 3 weeks

Alternative regimen:

Tab doxycycline 100 mg bid

Or, Tab tetracycline 500 mg QID for 4 weeks

The sexual partner of infected women should be evaluated clinically and serologically and, should be treated.

Follow up:

Serological test to be performed 1, 3, 6, and 12 months after treatment of early syphilis.

Chlamydia infections:

Causative organism- Chlamydia trachomatis

Incubation period—6-14 days

Affected epithelium—columnar and transitional epithelium of genitourinary tract.

Lesion—limited superficially

Symptoms—localized to urethra, Bartholin's gland and cervix

20-40% associated with gonococcal infection

Clinical features:

Asymptomatic—75%

Presenting symptoms—Dysuria, dyspareunia, postcoital bleeding and intermenstrual bleeding

Discharge—mucopurulent cervical discharge

Complications:

Urethritis and bartholinitis

Chlamydia cervicitis spreads upwards to produce endometritis and salpingitis

Fitz-Hugh-Curtis syndrome—spread to liver from pelvic organs via lymphatics and peritoneal cavity

Diagnosis

Materials-to be collected from urethra by using cytobrush
Nucleic acid amplification testing (NAAT)
Tissue culture: 100% specific

Treatment

According to CDC-2015
Tab Azithromycin—1g-PO-single dose
OR
Tab Doxycycline 100 mg-BID-7 days
OR
Tab Ofloxacin 300 mg-BID-7 days
OR
Tab Erthromycin—500 mg-PO-QID-7 days

Q12. How will you treat chlamydia in pregnancy ?

Tab Erythromycin-500 mg-QID-7 days
OR
Tab Erythromycin-500 mg-BID-14 days
OR
Tab Amoxicillin 500 mg—TDS-7 days

Chancroid (Soft sore)
Causative organism-*Haemophilus ducreyi*
Incubation period—3-5 days
Lesion:
Multiple
Small vesicopustules over vulva, vagina, or cervix
Pain—painful lesion
Discharge—foul purulent and hemorrhagic
Buboes present
Presence of chancroid genital ulcer facilitate transmission of HIV

Diagnosis:
Syphilis must be ruled out first
Specialized culture media—confirmatory
Gram stain—Shoal of fish

Treatment:
According to CDC 2015
Ceftriaxone 250 mg-IM-single dose (sexual partner should also be treated)
Azithromycin-1g-PO-single dose
Erythromycin 500 mg-PO-8 hourly for 7 days

Bacterial vaginosis
It is sexually associated with infection
Cause—due to shift of vaginal flora
Organism—G. vaginalis, anaerobic organisms (Bacteroides species, *peptococcus* species, Mobiluncus, Prevotella, and Mycoplasma hominis
It is cause of symptomatic vaginitis (15-50%)

Clinical features

- Discharge—malodorous fishy discharge
- Color-grayish-white and adherent to vaginal wall

Risk factors

- Multiple or new sexual partners
- Early age of SI
- Absence of hydrogen peroxide producing lactobacilli
- IUCD
- Immunosuppression

Diagnosis

Amsel's four diagnostic criteria

1. Homogenous vaginal discharge
2. Vaginal pH >4.5
3. Positive whiff test
4. Presence of clue cells (>20% of cells)

   Three of four criteria are sufficient for the presumptive diagnosis.

Gram stained vaginal smear (Hay/Ison)

Presence of more Gardnerella or Mobiluncus morphotypes with few or absent lactobacilli

Presence of clue cells are diagnostic

Histology: Absence of inflammation in specimen of vagina

Complications

- Recurrent infection leading to PID
- Development of PID following abortion
- Vaginal cuff cellulitis following hysterectomy

Q13. How will you treatment bacterial vaginosis?

Treatment according to CDC 2015

- Metronidazole 500 mg-PO-BID-7 days
- Tinidazole 2g-PO-3 days

OR

- Clindamycin 300 mg—PO-BID-7 days

And

- Clindamycin ovules 100 mg-intravaginally, once at bed time for 3 days

HERPES GENITALIS

Causative organism—Herpes simplex virus (HSV)

Incubation period—2-14 days

Clinical features

Time—appear in less than 7 days after sexual contact

Lesion—initially red, painful, inflammatory area on

Location—clitoris, labia, vestibule, vagina, perineum, and cervix

Constitutional symptoms:

Fever, malaise, and headache

Vulvar burning, pruritus, dysuria or retention of urine

Diagnosis

- Clinical inspection
- PCR test—HSV DNA

- ELISA or immunofluorescent method
- Western blot

Risks

Adverse effects in primary infection during pregnancy

- Increased risk of miscarriage and PTL
- Transfer of infection from mother to neonate during NVD, if primary (50%) or recurrent (5%)
- Baby may suffer from damage to CNS
- Delivery by LUCS is indicated

Treatment

Treatment should be done according to

- Primary episode
- Recurrent episode
- Daily suppression

General

Rest and analgesics.

Specific

Initial therapy

- Acyclovir 200 mg—5 times daily for 7-10 days

OR

- Valacyclovir 1g—twice daily for 7-10 days

OR

- Famciclovir 250 mg—thrice daily for 7-10 days

Recurrent episode

- Acyclovir 400 mg—3 times daily for 5 days

OR

- Valacyclovir 1g—once daily for 5 days

OR

- Famciclovir 125 mg—BID for 5 days

Then 500 mg OD then 250 mg-twice daily for 2 days

Daily suppressive therapy

Acyclovir 400 mg twice daily

OR

Valacyclovir 1 g once daily

OR

Famciclovir 250 mg TID

Human Immunodeficiency Virus Infection and Acquired Immunodeficiency Syndrome

Causative agent: HIV1 AND HIV2

Retrovirus (double stranded RNA family)

Risk factors

- Multiple sex partners
- Prostitution
- Homosexual males
- IV drug abuser
- Multiple transfusion
- STD
- Mother to infant

Q14. What are the mode of transmission of HIV?

- Sexual intercourse:
  Women are more affected then men
  Transmission from male to female is high
  Both by heterosexual and homosexual contact
- IV users
- Transfusion from an infected person
- Use of contaminated needles
- Breastfeeding
- Perinatal transmission

Q15. What are the AIDS defining conditions?

- Candidiasis of bronchi, trachea or lungs
- Cervical carcinoma
- Cryptosporidiosis, chronic intestinal encephalopathy HIV related
- Kaposi's sarcoma
- Lymphoma (Burkitt's)
- Mycobacterium tuberculosis
- Salmonella septicemia (recurrent)
- Toxoplasmosis of brain
- Wasting syndrome due to HIV

Q16. What are the gynecological symptoms with HIV?

- Infection of genital tract
  - Vaginitis
  - PID
- Neoplasms of genital tract are increased
- Increased morbidity following gynecological surgery
- Menstrual abnormality

Q17. How a patient affected with HIV presents?

Following exposure patient develops antibodies in about 8-12 weeks
Flu like symptoms

Acute infection syndrome is characterized by:

Fever, skin rash, arthralgia, lymphadenopathy, and diarrhea (seroconversion illness)
Last for 2-3 weeks and resolves spontaneously

Q18. Mention the diagnostic test for HIV?

The screening test is the antigen/antibody combination immunoassay

- Detection of IgG antibody to Gp 120
- Viral P-24 antigen
- ELISA
- Western blot or immunoblot
- HIV RNA by PCR—Gold standard

Q19. How will you treat HIV patient?

1. Preventive
2. Definitive

Preventive measures:

- Safer sex: Barrier method

- LNG-IUS with condoms
- Male circumcision
- Used of blunt tipped needles
- HIV negative blood transfusion
- Postexposure prophylaxis
- Termination of pregnancy in HIV positive women
- Avoid breastfeeding
- Cervical cytology screening yearly
- Widespread integrated counselling and testing

Definitive

- **Antiretroviral therapy (ART)**
  - i. **Nucleoside reverse transcriptase inhibitors (NRTIs):** zidovudine, tenofovir, lamivudine, abacavir
  - ii. **Non-nucleoside reverse transcriptase inhibitors (NNRTIs):** Delavirdine, Nevirapine, Efavirenz
  - iii. **Protease inhibitors (PI):** Indinavir, Darunavir, Ritonavir
  - iv. **Entry inhibitor:** Enfuvirtide
  - v. **Integrase inhibitor:** Dolutegravir, Raltegravir

Q20. When to start therapy?

- Acute HIV infection syndrome
- Symptomatic HIV infection
- Asymptomatic but CD4 cell count <350 cells/mm^3 or viral load >50000 copies/ml
- Postexposure prophylaxis
- Opportunistic infections

Efavirenz is the first line therapy in all patient unless she is planning to conceive and has NRTI or NNRTI resistance

GENITAL TUBERCULOSIS

Genital tuberculosis is almost always secondary to primary infection. The fallopian tubes(100%) usually are the primary sites from where secondary spread occurs to other genital organs.

Q1. What is the causative organism?

Mycobacterium tuberculosis of human type.

Q2. Mention the mode of spread of genital tuberculosis.

1. **Hematogenous (90%):** From any primary site
2. **Lymphatic or direct:** From infected organs such as peritoneum, bowel or mesenteric nodes
3. **Ascending:** Sexual transmission from a male partner with urogenital tuberculosis is possible in vulvar, vaginal or cervical lesion.

Q3. Mention the affection rate of genital organs with tuberculosis.

- Fallopian tube—100%
- Endometrium—50-60%
- Cervix—5-15%
- Ovaries—30%
- Pelvic peritoneum—40-50%
- Vulva, vagina—1%

Q4. What are the clinical features of genital tuberculosis?

Patient profile:

- The infection is affected mostly (80%) in childbearing period (20-40 years)

- May have past history of tubercular affection of lungs or LN
- Positive family history
- Flare up may occur following HSG or D&C

Symptoms: Cases are called as silent tuberculosis

Vary according to severity and staging.

- Usually no symptoms but sometimes may have
  - Low grade fever
  - Anorexia
  - Anemia
  - Night sweats
- The lesion is incidentally diagnosed during investigation of infertility or AUB
- The patient may also present with **infertility**
  May be primary or secondary
  Present in about 70-80% of pelvic tuberculosis
- Menstrual abnormality: Suppression of ovarian function due to tubercular toxin:
  About 50 %
  Menorrhagia 20-30%
  Amenorrhea or oligomenorrhea
- Chronic pelvic pain:
  Dysmenorrhea 20-30%
  T-O mass
- Vaginal discharge
- Weight loss, malaise

Signs

General:

- Weakness
- Low grade fever
- Anemia
- Active or healed extragenital tubercular lesion

Perabdomen

- Rarely irregular tender mass present arising out of pelvis
- May feel doughy due to matted intestines
- Tubercular ascites when encysted mimics an ovarian cyst

Pervaginam

- Pelvic findings negative in 50%
- Vaginal or vulvar ulcer—undermined edges
- Thickening of tubes—felt in lateral fornices or nodules, felt through posterior fornix
- B/L pelvic mass—indistinguishable due to pyogenic infection

Q5. What are the investigations to be done?

Investigations should be done for

1. To identify the primary lesion
2. To confirm the genital lesion

- Complete blood count
  WBC & ESR raised
- Mantoux test
- Chest X-Ray: to see healed or active pulmonary lesion
- USG: to detect adnexal mass

- CT/MRI: to detect pelvic or abdominal masses, LN with better resolution
- Diagnostic uterine curettage:
  - Done during week preceding menstruation
  - Tubercles come to surface during this period
  - **Materials should be send to laboratory in two portions:**
    - One part in normal saline for histopathology
    - Another part for
      - Culture in Lowenstein-Jensen media
      - Identification of acid fast bacilli by Ziehl-Neelsen's stain
      - Nucleic acid amplification
      - Guinea pig inoculation-positive test is diagnostic
- First day menstrual discharge:
  Should be collected by a pipette and the material subjected to mycobacterial nucleic acid amplification, culture and guinea pig inoculation
- Biopsy from lesion in cervix, vagina or vulva
- Hysterosalpingography
  - Contraindicated for the risk of reactivation of the lesion.
  - Routinely done for work up of infertility
- Imaging: USG, IVU, CT OR MRI:
  - MRI is helpful where mass and/or ascites present
  - However, it cannot confirm the diagnosis.
- Laparoscopy: in absence of endometrial evidence used for identification of tubercles in pelvic organs
- Hysteroscopy:
  - Early cases: cavity and tubal ostia appear normal
  - Advance cases:
    - Cavity is reduced with intrauterine adhesion formation
    - Ostia is closed

Q6. What the suggestive features for pelvic tuberculosis on hysterosalpingography?

- Vascular or lymphatic extravasation of dye
- Lead pipe tubes with nodulation
- Tobacco pouch with blocked fimbrial end beaded appearance of tube
- Distal tube obstruction
- Coiling of tubes
- Bilateral cornual block
- Tubal diverticula and/or fluffiness of tubal outline
- Uterine cavity:
  - irregular outline
  - Honeycomb appearance
  - Presence of uterine synechiae

Q7. Mention the mode of treatment of genital tuberculosis?

- General
- Chemotherapy
- Surgery

General

- If active pulmonary tuberculosis: admission
- Good diet

- Anemia correction if present
- Until infection subside: barrier method should be used

Chemotherapy

Antitubercular therapy is the treatment of choice

- **Isoniazid (H):**
  Daily oral dose—maximum 300mg
  Nature—bactericidal
  Toxicity—hepatitis, peripheral neuropathy
- **Rifampicin (R)**
  Daily oral dose—maximum 600 mg
  Nature—bactericidal
  Toxicity—Hepatitis dysfunction, orange discoloration of urine
- **Pyrazinamide (Z)**
  Daily oral dose-1.5 g/day
  Nature—bactericidal
  Toxicity—Hepatitis, hyperuricemia, GI upset and arthralgia
- **Ethambutol (E)**
  Daily oral dose—1200 mg/day
  Nature—Bacteriostatic
  Toxicity—Visual disturbances, optic neuritis, loss of visual acuity

Surgery:

- If unresponsive to antitubercular chemotherapy
- Tubercular pyosalpinx, ovarian abscess or pyometra
- Persistent menorrhagia and/or chronic pelvic pai

Q8. What do you mean by multidrug resistant (MDR) tuberculosis and treatment protocol for it?

MDR is defined as infection with *M. tuberculosis* that is resistant to two or more agents including isoniazid.

MDR patient with HIV negative treatment protocol

6 drug regimen

Drug used—kanamycin (IM)
Ofloxacin (PO)
Ethionamide (PO)
Pyrazinamide (PO)
Ethambutol (PO)
Cycloserine (PO)

Initial phase:

For 6-9 months and 18 months in continuation phase

MDR patient with positive HIV treatment protocol

- Have high mortality and morbidity
  1. To complete TB drugs then to start ARV- therapy
  2. To treat TB (with rifampicin containing regimen) + efavirenz +2 NRTIs
  3. To treat TB (as above) + 2NRTIs then to start HAART (maximally suppressive) regimen

CHAPTER 11

Vaginal Discharge

- Vulvovaginitis in childhood
- Trichomoniasis
- Moniliasis
- Vaginitis due to *Chlamydia trachomatis*
- Atrophic vaginitis
- Nonspecific vaginitis
- Toxic shock syndrome

Vulvovaginitis in childhood

More common due to lack of estrogen, vaginal defense is lost

Etiology:

- Nonspecific vulvovaginitis
- Presence of foreign body
- Associated intestinal manifestation

Clinical features:

- Pruritus
- Vaginal discharge
- Dysuria

Inspection:

- vulva—soreness
- Labia minora—swollen and red
- Investigations
- Vaginal discharge collected—two smears collected one for direct examination and another for gram stain
- Vaginoscopy—to exclude foreign body
- Treatment
- Personal hygiene
- Estrogen cream local application
- Trichomonas vaginal infection

Most common:

- Causative organism
- Trichomonas vaginalis (flagellate anaerobic protozoa)

Mode of transmission:

- By sexual contact
- Incubation period
- 3–28 days
- Pathology
- 25% of women of reproductive period

Clinical features:
- Sudden profuse and offensive vaginal discharge
- Irritation and itching
- Urinary symptoms
- History of previous similar attacks

On examination:
Thin, grey, greenish yellow, frothy and offensive discharge
Vulva inflamed and evidence of pruritus.
Per speculum—strawberry appearance of upper vagina and cervix.

Diagnosis:
Hanging drop preparation.
NAATs—more sensitive.
Treatment: Metronidazole 500 mg per oral BD for 7 days
Or
200 mg TID for 7 days.

CANDIDA VAGINITIS (MONILIASIS)

Causative organism: Candida albicans (gram positive yeast like fungus)
Clinical feature: Intense vulvovaginal pruritus with discharge.
On examination— Discharge—thick, curdy white and inflakes (cottage cheese type)
Vulva—red, swollen with evidence of pruritus.
Vaginal examination—tender
If menopausal—atrophy of vulvovaginal structure.

Diagnosis:
- Wet smear (KOH 10% is added)
- Culture—positive in 24-72 hours.

Classification of vulvovaginal candidiasis (CDC 2015)

Uncomplicated:
- Sporadic or infrequent
- Mild to moderate in severity
- Non immune compromised women.

Complicated:
- Recurrent
- Severe
- Women with uncontrolled diabetes
- Immunosuppression

Treatment:
- Correction of predisposing factor
- Uncomplicated vulvovaginal candidiasis
- Topical antifungal agent for 1-3 days.
  Or
- Single dose of Fluconazole or Itraconazole.
- Complicated vulvovaginitis
- Topical azoles two doses for 7 to 14 days.
- Oral therapy—a second dose of fluconazole 150 mg 72 hours after 1st dose
- Vaginal boric capsules (600 mg in gelatin capsule)
- Acute vulvovaginal candidiasis (VVC)

Cap fluconazole 150 mg OD stat
OR
Clotrimazole pessary 500 mg single dose

- Severe VVC
  - Oral fluconazole 150 mg orally on day 1–4

  OR
  - Clotrimazole 500 mg pessary intravaginally on day 1–4
- Recurrent VVC
  - Oral fluconazole 150 mg every 72 hours * doses

  OR
  - Clotrimazole 500 mg pessary intravaginally 7–14 days

Chlamydia
Discharge—mucopurulent
Consistency—thick
Whiff test—negative
Diagnosis—NAAT
Treatment—Tab Azithromycin 1 gm—orally single dose

Bacterial vaginosis:
Color—grey, white to green yellow white
Consistency—thin, adherent homogenous
Whiff test—positive

Diagnosis:

- Clue cells
- Amine odor after adding KOH to wet mount

Treatment
Metronidazole 500 mg PO-BID for 7 days

CHAPTER 12

Infertility

Case Discussion 1

A 33-year-old para 0+0 woman presents to gynecology outdoor with complaints of inability to conceive. She has been married for 3 years and couple didn't use any contraceptive method. Her menstrual cycles is regular and have premenstrual symptoms. She has no dysmenorrhea or dyspareunia. She has no significant medical history, has never had a sexually transmitted disease, and has never had surgery. Her husband is 35 years old and has a history of hypertension controlled by β blockers.

Q1. Why do you label this couple infertile?
The woman has tried to conceive without contraception for 3 years.

Q2. Is history suggestive of ovulation?
Yes. The woman is <35 years, having regular menstrual cycle and having premenstrual symptoms.

Q3. What should be the first test to evaluate male partner?
Semen analysis.

Q4. What is the initial workup and basic investigations you advice to this couple?

- Medical history
- Physical examination
- Semen analysis
- Discussion about timing and frequency of intercourse
- Check for ovulation: BBT chart, ovulation prediction kits, and luteal phase serum progesterone

Q5. If semen analysis report shows abnormality what will be your next step?
Repeat semen analysis after 1 month from same laboratory.

Case Discussion 2

A 37-year-old para 1+1 woman has presented in the outpatient department (OPD) with complain of infertility. She is separated from her former husband and has now married again. She is keen to conceive, especially as her new partner has no children. She is trying for pregnancy for last 8 months and having regular sexual intercourse. She says that her periods are regular most of the times but occasionally she has missed a period for up to 2 months. The bleeding is moderate and lasts up to 5 days. There is no history of pelvic pain or dyspareunia and no irregular bleeding or discharge. She has no significant medical history. Her husband is 40 years old with no significant history of medical illness. Physical examination of both partners shows no abnormality. Her investigation reports during her next cycle are mentioned here:

		Normal range
Day 3 follicle-stimulating hormone	14.2 IU/L	Day 2-5.1-11 IU/L
Day 3 luteinizing hormone	8.2 IU/L	Day 2-5 0.5-14.5 IU/L
Prolactin	12 ng/mL	Up to 29 ng/mL
Testosterone	1.4 nmol/L	0.8-3.1 nmol/L
Day 21 progesterone	5.5 nmol/L	

Semen analysis report: Normal volume, count, normal forms and motility.
Hysterosalpingogram report: The uterine cavity is of normal shape with a smooth regular outline. There is spillage of contrast medium on either side of fallopian tubes.
Transvaginal ultrasound report: The uterus is normal size, anteverted, no polyp, fibroid, or uterine anomaly. Both ovaries are of normal morphology but without any follicle.

Q1. What is the cause of the infertility?
The woman is 37 years old and having irregular menstruation which means she is not ovulating. Anovulation in this case is confirmed by the low day 21 progesterone. The abnormality in this patient is high day 3 FSH level and the fact that no follicles are visualized at ultrasound scan. This is suggestive of anovulation due to premature failure of ovarian function.

Q2. What are the further investigations for her?
The FSH should be repeated, as it is possible that this could be a sporadic result or poorly timed sample, so confirmation is needed before continuing on to treatment.

Q3. What are the management options?
The woman is unlikely to conceive naturally or with in vitro fertilization (IVF) as her FSH level remains elevated. However, she may be counseled about the assisted reproduction using donor eggs. Donated oocytes are fertilized with the husband's sperm and then fertilized ova is implanted into the uterus.

Q4. Why has hysterosalpingogram done?
To determine tubal patency in a patient with infertility.

Q5. Among all tests for evaluation of tubal patency, which should be chosen first?
Hysterosalpingography (HSG) is usually considered the first test for suspected fallopian tube infertility. But if Hystero Contrast Sonography is available, it should be utilized instead. If there are any related comorbidities, like endometriosis or pelvic inflammatory disease, the patient may undergo laparoscopic chromopertubation first.

Q6. Which features are to be looked for HSG?
(i) Contour of the uterine cavity-size, shape, presence of any filling defect, any adhesion inside.
(ii) Contour of the cervix.
(iii) Tubal patency or obstruction, tubal dilatation, margin and appearance.

SHORT ANSWER TYPE QUESTIONS

Q1. Define infertility.
Infertility is defined as the failure to conceive after 1 year of regular unprotected intercourse.

Q2. What do you mean by primary and secondary infertility?
Primary infertility applies to those who have never conceived, whereas secondary infertility designates those who have conceived at some time in the past.

Q3. What is the definition of fecundability?
Fecundability is the probability of conception in each month of menstrual cycle.

Q4. What are sterility and fecundity?
Sterility implies an intrinsic inability to achieve pregnancy. The woman will be never able to conceive.
Fecundity is the probability of achieving a live birth in one menstrual cycle.

Q5. What is the incidence?
80% conceive in 1 year
10% by 2nd year
10% remain infertile

Q6. What are the causes of infertility?

Male: 30-40%

Female: 40-55%

Both: 10 to 20%

Unexplained: 10%

Q7. What are the essential factors needed for conception?

- Healthy spermatozoa deposited high in the vagina or near the cervix.
- Spermatozoa should undergo changes—capacitation, acrosome reaction and acquire motility.
- Motile spermatozoa should ascend through cervix into uterine cavity and fallopian tubes.
- There should be ovulation.
- Fallopian tube should be patent.
- Fimbria should pick the oocyte.
- Spermatozoa should fertilize the oocyte at the ampulla of the tube.
- Embryo should reach the uterine cavity after 3 to 4 days of fertilization.
- Endometrium should be receptive for implantation.
- Corpus luteum should function adequately.

Q8. When will you start investigations in infertile couples?

Infertile couples are usually advised to start their investigations after 12 months of trying to conceive or after 6 months if the female partner is >35 years old or immediately if there is an obvious cause for their infertility such as they have a history of male factor infertility, endometriosis, a tubal factor, pelvic inflammatory disease, or pelvic surgery.

Q9. How do you define male infertility?

The World Health Organization defines male factor infertility as the presence of ≥1 abnormalities in the semen analysis or the presence of inadequate sexual or ejaculatory function.

Q10. What is the first test to perform if history and physical examination of infertile couple offers no clue?

Semen analysis

Q11. What are the relevant characteristics of normal semen analysis?

Volume: ≥1.5 mL

Sperm concentration: ≥15 million sperms per mL

Motility: ≥32% progressively moving spermatozoa, ≥40% motile sperms (progressive + nonprogressive);

Morphology: >4% of normal shape).

Q12. Some common terms used in male infertility.

- **Normozoospermia:** All semen parameters are normal.
- **Aspermia:** Failure of emission of semen (no ejaculate).
- **Hypospermia:** Low semen volume (<2 mL).
- **Oligozoospermia:** Reduced sperm number. Mild to moderate: 5-20 million/mL , severe: <5 million/mL .
- **Polyzoospermia:** Count is more than 350 million/mL.
- **Azoospermia:** No spermatozoan in the semen.
- **Asthenozoospermia:** Reduced sperm motility.
- **Leukocytospermia:** Increased white cells in semen.
- **Necrozoospermia:** Spermatozoa are dead or motionless.
- **Teratozoospermia:** >70% spermatozoa with abnormal morphology.
- **Oligoasthenoteratozoospermia:** Disturbance of all 3 variables.

Q13. What are causes of male infertility?

Causes of male infertility are:

- Defective spermatogenesis
- Obstruction of efferent duct system
- Failure to deposit sperm high in the vagina
- Inadequate sexual and ejaculatory functions
- Error in the seminal fluid.
- Impaired sperm motility

Some common causes of male infertility:

Pre-testicular—(hypogonadotropic)

- Obesity
- Gonadotropin deficiency
- Thyroid dysfunction
- Hyperprolactinemia
- Erectile dysfunction, impotency
- Drug- antihypertensive, antipsychotic
- Klinefelter syndrome
- Y chromosome deletion

Single gene mutation

Testicular—(mainly hypogonadotropic)

- Undescended testes
- Infection—mumps, orchitis, chlamydia
- Toxins—drug, smoking and radiation
- Varicocele
- OATS (oligoasthenoteratozoospermia)
- Immunologic

Post-testicular—(mainly obstructive cause)

- Absence of vas deference
- Acquired infection—TB, Gonorrhea
- Surgical—herniorrhaphy, vasectomy

Others

- Ejaculatory failure
- Retrograde ejaculation
- Hypospadias
- Bladder neck surgery
- High or low volume of ejaculation
- Low fructose content

Q14. Name the basic and advanced investigations for male partner.

Basic investigation: Semen analysis (after 2-7 days of sexual abstinence): two analyses with 1 months apart at the same laboratory—WHO.

Advanced investigations:

- **Hormonal assay:**
  - FSH
  - LH
  - Testosterone
  - TSH
  - Prolactin.

- **Testicular biopsy:** To differentiate between obstructive and nonobstructive azoospermia.
- **Chromosomal karyotyping:** For suspected genetic disorders—sex chromosomal aneuploidy, cystic fibrosis, and deletion of Y-chromosome.
- **Anti-sperm antibodies**

Q15. What are the normal reference values of semen analysis (WHO):

	Normal reference values	
Semen analysis	**2010**	**2021**
Volume	1.5 mL	≥1.4 mL
pH	7.2-7.8	≥7.2
Sperm concentration	15-16 million/mL	≥15 million/mL
Total sperm number	39 million per ejaculate	≥39 million per ejaculate
Motility (%)	Total motility: 40% (Progressive motility = 32%)	Total motility: ≥42% (Non-progressive motility: ≥1%, Progressive motility: ≥30%, Immobile sperms: ≥20%)
Morphology (%)	4%	≥4%
Viability	58%	≥54% live spermatozoa
WBCs	Less than 1 million/mL	
Round cells	<5 million/mL	
Sperm agglutination	<10% spermatozoa with adherent particles	

Q16. What are the treatment options for male infertility?

The treatment options in male infertility include:

- Medical and surgical therapy
- ART-1UI/1CSI/ VF-ET

Q17. What are the causes of female infertility?

According to FIGO

- Ovulatory dysfunction: 30–40%
- Tubal disease: 25–35%
- Uterine factors: 10%
- Cervical factor: 5%
- Pelvic endometriosis: 1–10%

Q18. What are the causes of ovarian factor infertility?

- Anovulation or oligo—ovulation, hypothalamic.
- Luteal phase defect (LPD)
- Luteinized unruptured follicular syndrome (trapped ovum)
- Endocrine disorders (/pituitary amenorrhea, hyperprolactinemia, thyroid disorders, and adrenal disorders)
- Premature ovarian failure
- Aging and diminished ovarian reserve (DOR)

Q19. What do you mean by ovulation?

Ovulation the process whereby a secondary oocyte is released from the ovary following rupture of a mature graafian follicle and becomes available for conception.

Q20. How can you diagnose ovulation?

- Indirect
- Direct
- Conclusive

Indirect

From history:

- Menstrual history—cycle regular or not—irregular cycle indicate anovulation but 20% to 30% regular cycle may also have inovulation.
- Mid menstrual bleeding (spotting) or pain or excessive mucoid vaginal discharge (mittelschmerz syndrome) indicate ovulation
- Premenstrual syndrome or primary dysmenorrhea present in ovulation
- Biphasic temperature change

Investigation:

Serum progesterone:

D 21: >6 ng/mL suggest ovulation

Cervical mucous study:

- Disappearance of fern pattern beyond 22nd day of the cycle suggestive of ovulation

Sonography:

- Endometrial thickness >8 mm and trilaminar.
- Size of ovarian follicle attains max size 18-20 mm before ovulation.

Endometrial biopsy:

- Done on 21 - 23rd day of cycle (if cycle is irregular then done 24 hours of menstruation)
- Secretory activity of endometrial glands in the second half of the cycle - indicate ovulation.
- Subnuclear vacuolation is earliest sign of ovulation within 36 - 48 hour

(secretory changes are due to action of progesterone on the estrogen primed endometrium)

Direct

Laparoscopy:

- Visualization of corpus luteum or detection of ovum from aspirated peritoneal fluid from POD is direct evidence of ovulation.

Conclusive:

Pregnancy is the surest evidence of ovulation.

Q21. What is the procedure for BBI?

Body temperature is measured and recorded in each morning upon awakening, before arising, plotted on graph paper. Normal ovulation is reflected by a biphasic curve during ovulation, with a rise in temperature by 0.5-1 °F during the luteal phase (because of an increased level of progesterone).

Q22. What do you mean by biphasic temperature change?

Basal body temperature—by biphasic pattern of temperature variation in ovulatory cycle i.e., first half of the cycle is raised to 0.5–1 degree Fahrenheit following ovulation then the rise sustain throughout the second half of cycle and fall 2 days prior to next period called biphasic pattern.

Q23. Clinical importance of BBT.

- To determine ovulation
- Timing of postcoital test
- Timing of endometrial biopsy
- Timing for cervical mucus, all vaginal cytology study
- Helps to determine most fertile period for the couple who has irregular cycle

Q24. What are the limitation of BBT?

- BBT Indicate ovulation retrospectively
- Cannot predict ovulation precisely with time

- Rarely ovulation has been observed in monophasic temperature.
- Required continuous 3-4 months

Q25. Why fern pattern disappears after 22nd day?

- Fern pattern disappears after 22nd day because of presence of progesterone which causes dissolution of sodium chloride crystals.
- Loss of stretchability (spinnbarkeit) after ovulation.

Q26. Hormone estimation to diagnose ovulation.

1. **Serum progesterone:**
   - D8 —1 ng/mL
   - D 21—>6 ng/mL suggest ovulation
2. **S. LH:**
   - D3 -5 mIU/mL
   - After ovulation 60 mIU/mL
   - Ovulation occurs 34-36 hours after LH surge

   Urine LH:

   Ovulation usually occurs with 14-26 hours of detection of urine LH surge. (always within 48 hours).
3. **S. Estradiol:**
   - Normal value 300-600 pg/mL at ovulation and follicular phase but at luteal phase—100 pg/mL
   - Is maximum 24 to 36 hours after ovulation
4. **TSH—should be <2.5 for infertile couple**
5. **T4—0.8 - 1.8 ng/dL**
6. **S. Prolactin—**
   - Normal—1-20 ng/dL

Q27. How blood is collected for prolactin test?

- Morning sample
- No stimulus should be given
- Test done by ELISA method

Q28. What are the TVS features of ovulation?

- Collapsed follicle
- Fluid in POD
- Endometrial thickness >8 mm and trilaminar
- Size of ovarian follicle attains max size 18-20 mm before ovulation.

Q29. What is the next step in evaluation if semen analysis is normal?

Ovulatory function to be assessed.

Q30. What are causes of anovulation?

According to WHO, ovulatory disorders are grouped into:

Group 1 (Hypothalamic—Pituitary failure):

- Hypogonadotropic hypogonadism
- Low gonadotropin and low estradiol level, normal prolactin
- Progesterone challenge test (-ve)

Causes are:

Stress related amenorrhea

Sheehan's syndrome

Kallmann's syndrome

Anorexia nervosa

- Rx: hMG or GnRH with or without ARTs

Group 2 (Hypothalamic—pituitary dysfunction):

- Normogonadotropic, normoestrogenic, anovulatory, and oligomenorrheic
- Cause—PCOS
- Rx: Clomiphene citrate

Group 3 (Ovarian Failure):

- Hypergonadotropic and hypogonadal with low estrogen level

Causes:
Turner syndrome
Premature ovarian failure
Ovarian radiation or chemotherapy

- Rx: Ovum donation (ART)

Group 4 (Hypothyroidism and hyperprolactinemia)

Q31. What is clomiphene citrate (CC) and which patient is it used?

Clomiphene citrate is nonsteroidal anti estrogenic agent, which is recently reclassified as a selective estrogen receptor modulator. It competes for the estrogen receptor at the hypothalamus and normalizes the gonadotropin-releasing hormone (GnRH) release.

Indications:

- Anovulation or oligo-ovulation due to hypothalamic pituitary dysfunction
    - PCOS
    - Unexplained anovulation
    - Hyperprolactinemia
- Luteal phase defect (LPD)
- Unexplained infertility.

Q32. In which gynecological condition clomiphene citrate used?

- Anovulatory or oligo ovulatory infertility and unexplained infertility.
- To induce spermatogenesis in male infertility.

Less common:

- Secondary hypogonadism in males.
- Performance enhancement of healthy athletes.
- Primary ovarian hyperstimulation syndrome.
- short-lasting unilateral neuralgiform headache attacks.

Q33. How does clomiphene citrate act?

Clomiphene citrate is a selective estrogen receptor modulator (SERM), which selectively binds to estrogen receptor in the hypothalamus, ovary, endometrium and cervix and produces estrogenic and antiestrogenic effects. In the hypothalamus, it acts as a partial estrogen agonist, resulting a estrogen negative feedback inhibition. Thus, it increases compensatory pulsatile gonadotropin-releasing hormone GnRH) secretion and increases ovarian follicular activity: It increases the secretion of LH hormone as well as FSH hormone, thus increasing the secretion of testosterone.

Q34. How is clomiphene citrate used?

Ovulation induction: The standard dose of CC is 50 mg PO od for 5 days, starting on the menstrual cycle day 3-5 or after progestin-induced bleeding. The daily dose can be increased by up to 50 mg every 2 cycles to a maximum of 200 mg/dose as needed to induce ovulation.

Spermatogenesis induction: The regimen is 25 mg daily half of a tablet for 25 days, off for five days. Alternative administration is a 25 mg oral tablet every other day.

Q35. What are the side effects of clomiphene citrate?
Common side effects include headache, dizziness, exacerbation of psychiatric illnesses, nausea, vomiting, ovarian enlargement, blurred vision, scintillating scotoma, abnormal uterine bleeding, pelvic pain, hypertriglyceridemia, gynecomastia, testicular tumor, vasomotor flushing, gastro-intestinal disturbance, and mastalgia.

Q36. When is induction with gonadotropins indicated?
Gonadotropins are typically used as second-line treatment after CC has failed. However, they may be first-line options for patients with hypothalamic amenorrhea and for women with a nonfunctioning pituitary gland (e.g., Kallman's syndrome).

Q37. What agent should be used when a woman who has anovulation because of hyperprolactinemia?
Dopamine agonists such as bromocriptine or cabergoline.

Q38. What do you mean by ovarian reserve?
"Ovarian reserve" is the term used to describe the size and quality of the remaining supply of oocytes.

Q39. How will you assess ovarian reserve?
Diminished/poor ovarian reserve seen if:
- D3 S. FSH >10-15 IU/L
- D3 S. Estradiol > 60–80 pg/mL
- Clomiphene citrate challenge test +ve
- AMH 0.2–0.7 ng/mL
- AFC <10
- Ovarian volume measurement (OVM) decreases

Q40. What are the commonly used tests to assess ovarian reserve?
- FSH
- AMH
- AFC (antral follicle count)

Q41. Why AMH is better than other test?
AMH is better than other because:
- It is direct reflection of follicle.
- It is not influenced by any other hormones.
- It remains constant with menstrual cycle.

Normal level: 2-5 ng/mL

Poor ovarian reserve: <1 ng/mL

Q42. Why age is important in case of infertile female?
With increasing age ovarian reserve decreases.

Q43. What is IUI?
Intrauterine insemination is a technique by which a processed semen sample, washed to remove prostaglandins, leukocytes, and nonmotile sperm, is injected via catheter through cervix directly into the upper uterine cavity. The pregnancy rate is 4-6% per cycle when used alone, it is frequently used in combination with ovulation induction to achieve pregnancy rates of 10-18%.

Q44. What are the different modalities of assisted reproductive techniques (ARTs)?
- In vitro fertilization and embryo transfer (IVE-ET)

- Gamete intrafallopian transfer (GIFT)
- Zygote intrafallopian transfer (ZIFT)
- Intracytoplasmic sperm injection (1 CSI)
- Tubal embryo transfer
- Gamete and embryo cryopreservation
- Oocyte and embryo donation
- Gestational surrogacy.

Q45. How should a woman who presents with infertility and early stage endometriosis is treated for fertility?
Surgical resection of endometriosis lesions and other pelvic adhesions followed by a trial of clomiphene or gonadotropin plus intrauterine insemination (IUI).

Q46. What are tubo-peritoneal causes of female infertility?
Tubal causes are:
- Tubal infection – Chlamydia and Gonorrhea
- Tubal endometriosis
- Previous tubal surgery or sterilization
- Salpingitis isthmica nodosa
- Polyp or mucus debris within tubal lumen
- Tubal spasm

Peritoneal causes are: Peritubal adhesion due to PID or endometriosis

Q47. Which is the most common cause for secondary subfertility?
Tubo – peritoneal factor

Q48. What is the major cause of tubal factor infertility?
Pelvic inflammatory disease.

Q49. What are the other causes of tubal infertility?
- Lower abdominal surgery leading to pelvic adhesions
- Tubercular salpingitis
- Previous tubal surgery
- Use of an intrauterine device (rare)
- Any pelvic infection
- Endometriosis

Q50. How will you assess tubal factor?
Anatomical patency and functional integrity of tubes are needed to be assessed which may be done by following investigations:
- Hysterosalpingography
- Laparoscopy and chromopertubation (sensitivity is 65%, specificity is 83%)
- Sonohysterosalpingography
- Dilatation and Insufflation test (Rubin's test)
- Saline infusion sonography
- Falloposcopy: During hysteroscopy
- Salpingoscopy: During laparoscopy

Q51. What are uterine factors of infertility?
- Unfavorable endometrium for mediation and growth of fertilized ovum
- Chronic endometritis (TB)
- Fibroid

- Synechiae
- Uterine hyperplasia
- Inadequate secretory endometrium
- Congenital malformation

Q52. How will you assess uterine factor?

Uterine factor assessed by

- Hysteroscopy
- Ultrasonography
- Hysterosalpingogram
- Laparoscopy

Q53. What are cervical factors of infertility?

- Ineffective sperm penetration
- Chronic cervicitis
- Immunological factor (presence of anti-sperm antibody)
- Anatomic:
  - Congenital elongation of cervix
  - Second degree or more uterovaginal prolapse

Q54. What are the combined causes of infertility?

- Age >35 years
- Infrequent intercourse
- Lack of knowledge of coital technique and timing
- Apareunia
- Dyspareunia
- Use of lubricant during intercourse
- Immunological factors

Q55. What are the basic investigations should be done?

For male: Semen analysis, if the report of semen analysis is normal no need further investigations.

For female:

- Confirmation of ovulation (if the cycle is regular and age <35 years, no need for hormone analysis).
- Confirmation of tubal patency.

Some routine investigations for both partner

- Blood sugar
- Urine Examination
- Serology
- Thyroid function test

Q56. How will you manage a case of infertility?

For management of my case I need to evaluate tubal factor and male factor-semen analysis

Firstly I will counsel my patient about:

- Their condition
- Failure rate is more than success rate
- Advice for lifestyle modification:
  - Weight reduction in obese patient
  - Weight gain in underweight
  - Avoid smoking, alcohol
  - Avoid anxiety

- Correction of coital difficulty if any
- Folic acid, antioxidant and micronutrients supplementation
- Stabilizing preexisting medical condition like hypothyroid, HTN, epilepsy, SLE then I will go for treatment of the particular cause

If the cause is anovulation:

Basic management for anovulation is ovulation induction

- General management—weight reduction (5 to 10% of weight reduction cause correction of ovulation and normal menstruation).
- Medical management:
  - Oral—clomiphene citrate, letrozole
  - Injectable—GnRH, Gonadotrophin
  - Adjuvant—metformin, dexamethasone, conjugated estrogen
  - Substitute—metformin (DM patients), antithyroid (thyroid patients), bromocriptine (hyperprolactinemia)
  - Surgical—Ovarian drilling (PCO)

Q57. What are determinants of treatment options?

- Age of the patient
- Size and extent of lesions
- Severity of symptoms
- Location of disease
- Desire for fertility
- Results of previous therapy

Q58. For ovulation induction what do you prefer?

Letrozole is the first line drug for ovulation induction.

Q59. Why letrozole is better than clomiphene?

- It causes monofollicular development, so less chance of OHSS and less chance of multiple pregnancy (OHSS-Ovarian hyperstimulation syndrome).
- No effect on endometrium so endometrial thickness is not effective and implantation is more, less chance of miscarriage and more success rate.

Q60. How does letrozole work?

M/A of letrozole:

- Letrozole increases the release of gonadotropins from pituitary and stimulates development of ovarian follicle.
- Letrozole suppress ovarian estradiol secretion and reduces estrogen induced negative feedback. As a result, levels of FSH rises, intra-ovarian androgens are increased which increases FSH sensitivity.

Q61. How will you treat a patient with hypothyroidism?

Asymptomatic but TSH >4 start treatment with thyroxine supplement

It symptomatic but TSH >2.5 then do

- Antibody test if positive then treatment with thyroxine supplement
- If negative then only follow up 3 monthly

Thyroxine should be given 1/2 tab If TSH between 4-5

1 tab thyroxine if TSH 10 mIU/mL

Target level of TSH is 2.5

TSH (1.5–2.5) then same dose maintenance

Q62. If more dose of thyroxine is given what will happen?

Patient will develop hyperthyroidism

Mx:

- Drug should be stopped.
- Follow up
- When hormone level come back to normal then restart

Q63. What advice will you give after ovulation induction?

1. Timely intercourse daily or alternative days beginning 5 to 7 days after last dose of clomiphene/letrozole therapy.
2. If missed period then do BHCG and consult with report
3. If period start then come on D2 of next cycle
4. If abdominal distension then patient should come for consultation immediately

Q64. When to do laparoscopy in infertile female?

Diagnostic:

- Age >35 years
- Abnormal HSG
- Failure to conceive after reasonable period (6 months) with normal HSG
- Women with comorbid pelvic pathology (PID, endometriosis)
- Unexplained infertility
- Previously reconstructive tubal surgery was done

Operative:

- Adhesiolysis
- Fulguration of endometriotic implants
- GIFT and ZIFT
- Ovarian drilling in case of PCOS—when medical treatment is failed

Q65. What are the benefits of hysteroscopy?

Hysteroscopy is the gold standard for visualizing uterine cavity and tubal ostia. The benefits are

- Polypectomy for endometrial polyp
- Submucous resection of myoma
- Hysteroscopic adhesiolysis
- Resection of uterine septum

CHAPTER

13

Endometriosis

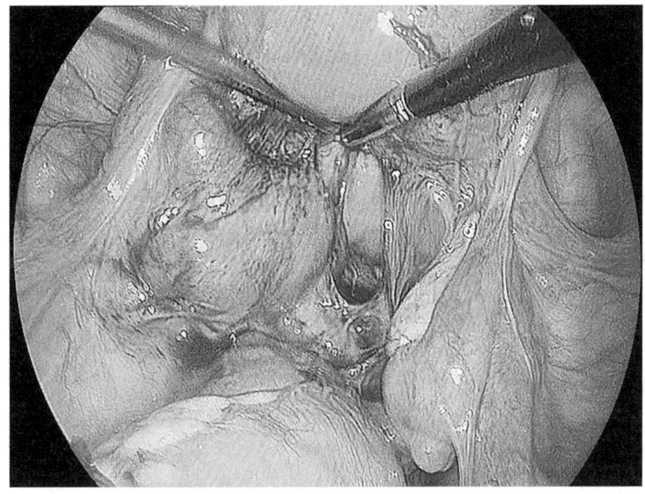

Courtesy: BMU Department of obstetrics and gynecology.

Case Discussion

A 35-year-old nulliparous woman presents with a history of progressively worsening menstrual pain for most of the period. She finds no relief from ibuprofen, and she misses 2-3 days of work each month. She has been married for 6 months and her relationship with husband is affected by associated stress and pain during intercourse. On vaginal examination, her uterus is of normal size and minimally tender. Rectovaginal examination reveals uterosacral nodularity and tenderness.

Q1. What is your diagnosis and why?

Endometriosis

The woman is 35 years nullipara presenting with dysmenorrhea and dyspareunia which are classic symptoms of endometriosis. She is having painful pelvic examination findings and uterosacral nodularity in rectovaginal examination which are features of endometriosis.

Q2. What is the risk factor of endometriosis present in this patient?

- Nulliparity.

Q3. What are the causes of pain in endometriosis?

The underlying cause of pain is not clearly known but following are possibilities:

- Peritoneal inflammation (PGF, cytokines)
- Tissue necrosis
- Adhesion
- Due to deep penetration irritation of nerve

- Local inflammatory mediators release
- Formation of endometrioma

Q4. Pain is related with severity of endometriosis how?
Degree of visible endometriosis has no correlation with the severity of pain. Pain is not related to the extent of tissue penetration.

Q5. What are the differential diagnoses?
- Pelvic inflammatory discase
- Adenomyosis
- Pelvic adhesion
- Uterine fibroids

Q6. Name the investigations you consider for the patient.
- Ultrasonography as it can diagnose chocolate cyst and excludes leiomyoma, and adenomyosis,
- Laparoscopy may be done to confirm the diagnosis.

SHORT ANSWER QUESTIONS

Q1. What is endometriosis?
The existence of active endometrium (glands and stroma) in locations outside the uterine lining is referred to as endometriosis.

Q2. What is the nature of endometriosis?
Endometriosis is an aggressive, progressive (31%), and invasive disease. Cyclic hormones promote growth, whereas continuous hormones inhibit it.

Q3. Prevalence of endometriosis?
The prevalence is about 10-15%. However, prevalence is high amongst the subfertile women (30-45%) as based on diagnostic laparoscopy and laparotomy.

Q4. What are the common sites of endometriosis?
- Ovaries (80%), bilateral (50%)
- Umbilicus
- Pelvic peritoneum
- Pouch of Douglas
- Uterosacral ligaments
- Rectovaginal septum
- Sigmoid colon
- Appendix
- Pelvic lymph nodes
- Fallopian tubes

Q5. What are the rarest sites of endometriosis?
- Scar-abdominal and episiotomy
- Lungs and pleura
- Kidney and ureter
- Arms Legs
- Nasal mucosa

Q6. What are the risk factors of endometriosis?

- Parity-low
- Elderly pregnant
- Family history-endometriosis
- Outflow tract obstruction
- Environmental toxins
- Peritoneal fluid abnormalities

Q7. How can you explain endometriosis in different sites?

Sites	*Theory*
Endometriosis-pelvic	Due to retrograde menstruation
Pelvic peritoneum	Due to coelomic metaplasia
Abdominal viscera and umbilicus Rectovaginal septum	Due to coelomic metaplasia
Scar-abdominal and Episiotomy Vagina, cervix	Directly implant on the scar
Lymph nodes	By lymphatic spread
Rare sites (lungs, pleura, skin, lymph nodes, nerves)	Can be due to vascular spread may be genetic or immunologic

Q8. What are the pathogenesis of endometriosis?

- Genetic mutations and immunological
- Molecular defects
- Mechanical (outflow tract obstruction)
- Environmental toxins (dioxins)
- Others: Neo angiogenesis, upregulation of aromatase, downregulation of 17-P HSD2 and decreased expression of PR-P (progesterone receptor-P) and development of progesterone resistance.

Q9. What are the pathology of endometriosis?

The endometrium (glands and stroma) at ectopic sites can experience changes because of the effects of ovarian hormones.

- Proliferative changes are regularly observed, whereas the secretory changes are strikingly absent. This may be due to an absence of steroid receptors in the ectopic endometrium.
- Cyclic growth and shedding persist until menopause. The blood that is released periodically might remain trapped in a cyst or, conversely, the cyst may enlarge and rupture.
- Blood is an irritant that activates a strong tissue reaction around the injury, resulting in fibrosis. When it happens on the pelvic peritoneum, it results in adhesions and wrinkling of the peritoneum.
- Deep lesions that penetrate beyond 5 mm are more advanced (DIE).
- Throughout , the cyst enlarges with occasional bleeding. The serum takes in during the gaps, and the substance changes to chocolate brown. Consequently, this cyst is known as a chocolate cyst and is usually located in the ovary.

Q10. What are the clinical features of pelvic endometriosis?

Patient Profile

- Age: 35-45
- Parity-nulliparous/para 1
- Infertility

- Higher social status
- Family history may be present

Symptoms

- Symptoms do not correlate with the size of the lesion.
  - Women with significant endometriosis can often be asymptomatic.
  - Women with slight endometriosis might experience debilitating chronic pelvic discomfort.
  - Women experiencing deep infiltrating endometriosis (DIE) endure intense pain. Lesions that extend beyond 5 mm cause pain, dysmenorrhea, and dyspareunia.
  - The clinical variability frequently relies on differences in cytokine production.
  - Symptoms are primarily associated with the location of the injury

Q11. What are the most common symptoms of endometriosis?

- Dysmenorrhea (70%)
- Dyspareunia (20-40%)
- Chronic pelvic pain
- Abdominal pain
- Abnormal uterine bleeding (AUB) (15-20%)
- Infertility (40-60%)
  - Endometriosis is found in 30-45% of infertile women
  - About 40-50% of patients with endometriosis suffer from infertility.

Other symptoms: Related to the organ involved.

- Urinary-frequency, dysuria, backpain, hydronephrosis or hematuria.
- Sigmoid colon and rectum-painful defecation (dyschezia), diarrhea, constipation, rectal bleeding or even melena.
- Chronic fatigue, perimenstrual symptoms (bowel, bladder).
- Hemoptysis (rarely), catamenial chest pain, hemothorax.
- Surgical scars-cyclical pain and bleeding.

Q12. What are the examinations performed in endometriosis?

Abdominal examination: Physical examination has poor sensitivity and specificity.

- May not reveal any abnormality.
- A mass may be felt in the lower abdomen arising from the pelvis which is tender with restricted mobility.

Pelvic examination:

- Bimanual examination may not reveal any pathology.
- Pelvic tenderness,
- Nodules in the pouch of Douglas
- Nodular feel of the uterosacral ligaments
- Fixed retroverted uterus
- Unilateral or bilateral adnexal mass of varying sizes

Speculum examination: Bluish spots in the posterior fornix or the cervix.

Rectal examination/for confirmation of the diagnosis

Q13. What are the classic symptoms of endometriosis?

- Progressively increasing secondary dysmenorrhea
- Dyspareunia
- Infertility

Q14. What are the criteria of dysmenorrhea in endometriosis?

- There is progressively increasing secondary dysmenorrhea. The pain starts a few days prior to menstruation, gets worsened during menstruation and takes time, even after cessation of period, to get relief of pain (co-menstrual dysmenorrhea).
- Pain usually begins after few years pain-free menses. The pain is usually deep seated and, on the back, or rectum.

Q15. What are the criteria of dyspareunia in endometriosis?

The dyspareunia is typically profound. It could be caused by the stretching of the structures in the pouch of Douglas or sensitivity from direct contact. Primarily located in endometriosis of the pouch of Douglas or rectovaginal septum and with a retroverted uterus that is fixed.

Q16. Types of abnormal uterine bleeding (AUB) in endometriosis?

- Menorrhagia: Predominant.
- Polymenorrhagia or epimenorrhagia.
- May be premenstrual spotting.

Q17. How endometriosis is related with infertility?

- 30-45% of infertile women have endometriosis
- Also, approximately 40-50% of patients with endometriosis suffer from infertility.

Q18. What is the role of Cancer antigen (CA) 125 in endometriosis?

Serum CA-125 is a serum marker which elevate moderately in severe endometriosis. It is not specific for endometriosis, as it is significantly raised in epithelial ovarian carcinoma. It is helpful to assess the therapeutic response and in follow-up also can detect any recurrence post therapy.

Q19. What are the serum markers in endometriosis?

- Serum CA-125
- Monocyte Chemotactic Protein (MCP-1)
- Glycodelin is elevated in endometriosis.
- Other predictive markers: Interleukin-1 (lL-1) and interferon gamma.

Q20. What are the imaging used in endometriosis?

- Ultrasonography
- Magnetic resonance imaging (MRI)
- Computed tomography (CT)
- Colonoscopy, rectosigmoidoscopy and cystoscopy when respective organs are involved.

Q21. What is the role of TVS in endometriosis?

TVS and ERUS are found to be useful for rectosigmoid endometriosis specially for diagnosis of deep infiltrating endometriosis (DIE).

Q22. What is the role of TVS in endometriosis?

Thick walled cyst with low level homogenous "ground glass" like internal echoes.

Q23. What is the role of MRI in endometriosis?

- It is the best diagnostic tool.
- Hyperintensity on Tl-weighted images and hypointensity on T2 weighted images
- Sensitivity and specificity of MRI is 91-95%.
- It is superior compared to TVS and CT with much better resolution and soft tissue interfaces.
- MRI is better to diagnose DIE and deep seated endometrioma.

Q24. What is the role of laparoscopy in endometriosis?

- Degree of the condition determined by a scoring method (ASRM-1996).
- Evaluation of the lesion regarding its location, dimensions, and severity
- A biopsy can be performed simultaneously.
- Staging is possible
- The degree of adhesions might be documented.
- Chance to perform laparoscopic surgery if necessary

Q25. What are the typical peroperative features of pelvic endometriosis?

- Fibrosis and thickening in the peritoneum
- Areas shaped like red flames
- Glistening red protruding regions.
- Brownish yellow spots
- Pale peritoneal regions
- Round peritoneal gaps
- Adhesions below the ovaries

Q26. What are the classic lesion of pelvic endometriosis peroperatively ?

The typical lesion of pelvic endometriosis can appear as 'powder burns' or 'matchstick' marks on the peritoneum in the pouch of Douglas. New lesions appear as bleb-like formations and are typically 1 cm or smaller.

Q27. What are the common characteristics of endometrioma?

- The ovaries are often affected, typically on both sides.
- Endometriomas (chocolate cysts) come in different sizes and appear as bluish spots

Q28. What are the microscopic appearance of endometriosis?

The cardinal histologic features are ectopic endometrial glands, stroma, hemorrhage in the tissues and hemosiderin-laden macrophages.

Biopsy confirmation of excised lesion is ideal but negative histology does not exclude it.

Q29. What is the role of IVU in endometriosis?

Useful in cases associated with deep infiltrating endometriosis (DIE) and suspected ureteric involvement.

Q30. What are the differential diagnosis of endometriosis?

- PID
- Adenomyosis
- Ovarian malignancy

Q31. How is ovarian endometrioma (chocolate cyst) formed?

The most common site for endometriosis (60-70%) is ovary. It starts with a superficial endometriotic implant over the ovarian surface. The endometriotic tissue gradually invades the ovarian stroma. Cyst formation is due to periodic shedding and bleeding from the implant.

Leakage of this altered blood along with inflammation leads to adhesion formation with the adjacent structures. If asymptomatic, may be confused with a benign ovarian tumor and in a symptomatic one, with a malignant ovarian. Presence of nodules in the pouch of Douglas confuses the diagnosis.

Q32. In which factors management depends?

a. Age
b. Desire of fertility
c. Severity of symptoms
d. Size

Q33. Can chocolate cyst rupture?

While separating the adhesions in the course of the procedure, the cyst consistently bursts, releasing blood that is chocolate colored. The cyst may rupture spontaneously, leading to acute abdominal pain with clinical signs indicative of acute ectopic. Acute abdomen can be mistaken for ovarian tumor torsion or rupture, ectopic pregnancy complications, appendicitis, or diverticulitis.

Q34. What are the causes of subfertility in endometriosis?

Pelvic region:

- Peritoneal fluid: Changes due to inflammation
- Increase in microphage numbers and secretion of proinflammatory substances
- Modifications in peritoneal fluid that affect sperm-oocyte interaction
- Altered pelvic structure (inability to capture ovum).

Ovaries:

- Absence of ovulation
- Oligomenorrhea
- Deficiency in the luteal phase
- Decreased ovarian reserve (damage caused by endometriosis and/or surgical intervention)
- Adhesions on ovaries and fallopian tubes
- Inadequate reaction to ovulation stimulation, COS and ART C.

Uterus:

- Decreased endometrial receptiveness
- Failure of implantation
- Progesterone resistance

Q35. What challenges arise from endometriosis?

Endocrinopathy—this might be a reason for infertility.

- Rupture of chocolate cyst
- Pollution of chocolate cyst
- Impeding traits
- Intestinal obstruction
- Blockage of the ureter → buildup of fluid → enlargement of the kidney → abrupt kidney infection.
- Women with endometriosis have a fourfold increased risk of ovarian cancer.

Q36. Significance of endometriosis staging.

The identified endometriosis must be accurately staged according to laparoscopic observations.

- To foresee outcomes
- To select therapy
- To assess the therapeutic approach

The assessment (updated) by the American Society of Reproductive Medicine (ASRM)

Q37. What are the constraints of ASRM Staging?

Either a laparoscopy or a laparotomy must be done.

- Differences among observers and within a single observer
- There is no connection between illness severity and symptom intensity.
- Staging has not been associated with fertility outcomes.
- Staging has not been connected to the most effective treatment approach

Q38. Importance of ENZIAN classification (2021).

A valid and useful tool for the classification of deep endometriosis (DE), as assessed by TVS, MRI or surgical methods. Enzian classification describes DE involving the retroperitoneal structures.

Q39. How is Endometriosis Fertility Index (EFI) calculated?

Calculated by addition of:

Total historical factors from history + Total surgical factors.

Q40. What are the factors on which Endometriosis Fertility Index (EFI) scoring is calculated?

Factors from the history include point scoring (0-2)

a. Age: ≤ 35 years = 2; 36-39 years = 1; ≥ 40 years = 0.
b. Years of infertility: ≤ 3 years = 2; >3 years = 0.
c. Prior pregnancy: History of (h/O) pregnancy = 1; no h/o pregnancy = 0.

Q41. What are the goals of treatment of endometriosis?

a. Pain relief
b. Improvement of fertility
c. To arrest the progression of the disease

Q42. What are the preventive measures should be taken to prevent endometriosis?

- To prevent a tubal patency test right after curettage or during the menstrual period.
- A forced pelvic examination should not occur during or right after menstruation.
- Married women who have a family history of endometriosis are advised to pursue their first conception without delay and to finish building their family

Q43. What are the objectives of curative treatment of endometriosis?

- To abolish or minimize the symptoms-pelvic pain and dyspareunia
- To improve the fertility
- To arrest the progress of the disease.
- To prevent recurrence.

Q44. What are the challenges to treat endometriosis?

- Assessing treatment outcomes is challenging due to the absence of consistent staging or grading.
- Many cases are asymptomatic.
- Personal symptoms do not correlate with observable signs.
- Commonly linked to infertility.
- Improvement during pregnancy and menopause

Q45. What are the treatment options for pelvic endometriosis?

- **Expectant management** (observation only)
- **Medical therapy:**
  - Hormones
- **Surgical**
  - Conservative
  - Definitive
- Both combined **therapy:**
  - Medical
  - Surgical

Q46. What are the determinants of treatment options of pelvic endometriosis?

- Age
- Location
- Size and extent
- Desire for fertility
- Severity of symptoms
- Results of previous therapy

Q47. How will you manage pain in pelvic endometriosis?

- *Minimal:* Expectant management
- *Mild:* NSAIDs, COCs, Progestogens, GnRH agonist (empirical)
- *Moderate to severe:* Laparoscopy (Diagnosis/staging)

Q48. Criteria of case selection for expectant treatment in pelvic endometriosis?

- Minimal endometriosis with no other abnormal pelvic finding
- Unmarried
- Young married who are ready to start family
- Approaching menopause

Q49. How will you manage infertility and moderate to severe pain in pelvic endometriosis?

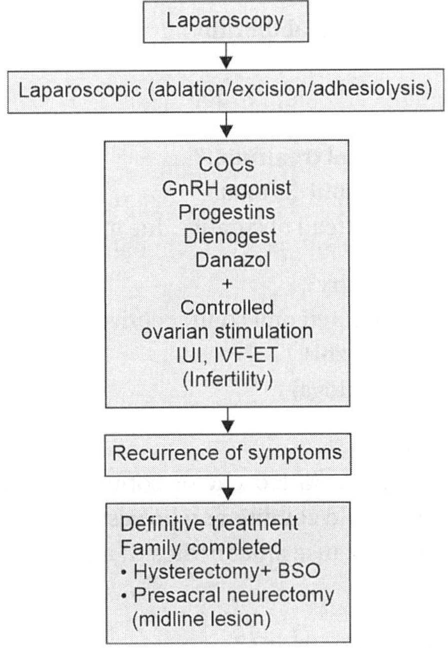

Q50. Name of NSAIDs used to relieve pain in endometriosis.

- Prostaglandin synthetase inhibiting (PSI) drugs
  - Ibuprofen 800-1200 mg can be given
  - Mefenamic acid 150-600 mg per day

Q51. How pregnancy is helpful for endometriosis?

The married women are advised to have conception. Pregnancy can improve the condition due to absence of shedding and decidual changes in the ectopic endometrium causing its necrosis and absorption.

Q52. Name of hormones used in endometriosis.

Oral

- Estrogen and progestogen together (daily for 6-12 months)
- Progestins
  - Medroxyprogesterone acetate (10 mg three times daily for 6-9 months)
  - Dydrogesterone 10-20 mg per day (for 6-9 months)
  - Norethisterone 10-30 mg each day (6-9 months)
  - Dienogest 2 mg orally once a day for 3 to 6 months

IM

- Depot medroxyprogesterone 150 mg 3 months interval (3-6 months)

IUCD

- Levonorgestrel-releasing- LNG-IUS having 52 mg with IUCD (LNG-IUS) 20 μg/day release of LNG (5 years).

GnRH analogs

- Goserelin 3.6 mg depot IM monthly (6 months)
- Triptorelin
- Leuprolide

Danazol: 400-600 mg given per oral in 4 divided doses in total 6–9 months

Gestrinone

Q53. What is the recurrence rate following medical therapy?

- 5 to 15% in the first year
- 40 to 50% in 5 years

Q54. What is the main purpose of the hormonal treatment?

- To promote shrinkage of the endometriotic lesions.
- It ought to be viewed as suppressive instead of curative due to a high recurrence rate.

Q55. What is the process of endometrial atrophy?

- By inducing 'pseudopregnancy' (combined oral contraceptives)
- By inducing 'pseudomenopause' (danazol)
- By 'medical oophorectomy' {GnRH analogs)

Q56. What is the role of OCP in endometriosis?

Low dose contraceptive pills can be given in a cyclic or continuous manner for a duration of 6-12 months. It offers benefits for young patients with mild conditions who wish to postpone pregnancy. It leads to endometrial decidualization and degeneration. It can cause amenorrhea. It alleviates menstrual pain. Symptoms improve in 80% of women.

Q57. What is the role of progestogens in endometriosis?

- It leads to the decidualization of the endometrium and subsequent atrophy.
- Elevated doses could inhibit ovulation and trigger amenorrhea

Q58. What is the role of dienogest in endometriosis?

- It is a 19-nortestosterone derivative.
- It is a selective progesterone that causes anovulation.
- It has antiproliferative effect on endometrial cells.
- It inhibits cytokine secretion.
- It decreases the nerve fiber density in endometriosis to relieve pain.

Q59. What is the role of LNG-IUS in endometriosis?

Levonorgestrel-releasing-IUCD: It reduce symptoms like dysmenorrhea, pelvic pain, dyspareunia, and menorrhagia significantly. It is useful for rectovaginal endometriosis.

Q60. What is the role of danazol in endometriosis?

Danazol causes atrophic alterations in the endometrium and the endometrial lesions. Danazol creates a state of low estrogen and high androgen levels. The patient should use barrier contraceptive methods to prevent virilization of a female fetus.

Q61. What is the role of GnRH agonists in endometriosis?

- It causes hypoestrinism and amenorrhea
- When used continuously act as medical oophorectomy.
- It causes down regulation and desensitization of the pituitary.
- GnRH agonist can be used in women >18 years if pain continues after NSAIDs and combined oral contraceptives (COCs) (ACOG).
- GnRH agonist can improve symptoms in 75 to 90%
- Ovarian function usually returns back to normal by 6 weeks or more, after using GnRH agonist for 6 months.

Q62. What are the drawback of GnRH agonists in endometriosis?

- The drugs are expensive.
- Therapy for more than 6 months should be avoided
- Add-on therapy may be needed to reduce the vasomotor symptoms, vaginal atrophy or the demineralization of bones.

Q63. What are the common side effective of GnRH agonists in endometriosis?

- Hot flushes
- Vaginal dryness
- Insomnia.
- Bone demineralization with prolonged use (≥6 months)
- Tolerable side effect than danazol.

Q64. What is the role of GnRH antagonist in endometriosis?

Oral (elagolix): Dose: 150-200 mg/day as effective as leuprolide acetate. Bone loss and other side effects are less.

Q65. What are the other drugs can be used in endometriosis?

- Progesterone antagonists (mifepristone)
- Selective progesterone-receptor modulators (SPRMs
- Aromatase inhibitors
- Pentoxifylline

Q66. What are the indications of surgical management in endometriosis?

Endometriosis with intense symptoms that do not respond to hormonal treatment.

- Profound and extensively invading endometriosis (DIE) to rectify the alteration of pelvic structure.
- Advanced endometriosis with pelvic adhesions.
- Endometriomas greater than 1 cm

Q67. What is the role of conservative surgery in endometriosis?

- To preserve the reproductive function.
- To restore the normal pelvic anatomy.
- The endometriotic tissues (endometriomas) are removed.
- Adhesiolysis.
- To destroy the endometriotic lesions.
- To preserve the reproductive function.

Q68. What are the conservative surgery done on endometriosis?

Laparoscopy

- Excision/cauterization
- Laser vaporization
- LUNA
- Adhesiolysis

Endometrioma

- Aspiration with irrigation
- Excision of cyst wall
- Cystectomy (size >3 cm)
- Peeling off the cyst wall

Q69. What will you do if small endometrioma (<3 cm)?

Small endometrioma (<3 cm) is aspirated laparoscopically. The cyst cavity is irrigated with normal saline. Cyst wall epithelium may be peeled off or destroyed by laser vaporization.

Q70. What will you do if large endometrioma (>3 cm)?

Large endometrioma is often associated with extensive adhesion to other pelvic structures. Laparoscopy is necessary for ovarian cyst drainage and adhesiolysis.

Q71. What are the advantages of conservative surgery?

- Laparoscopic cystectomy (if >3 cm) pain relief in about 74% cases of mild to moderate cases.
- Pregnancy rate about 60% cases with moderate and 35% cases with severe disease.

Q72. What are the disadvantages of conservative surgery?

Use of electrosurgery may cause decrease ovarian reserve. Surgical excision of endometriomas decrease the ovarian reserve.

Q73. What will you do in case of subfertile endometriosis patient?

After initial surgery, ART therapy is preferred as it is found to be more effective. Suppression of endometriosis with GnRH agonist for 3-6 months before IVF-ET improves outcomes.

Q74. What does definitive surgery mean?

Definitive surgery refers to a hysterectomy combined with bilateral salpingo-oophorectomy and thorough resection of the endometriotic tissues.

Symptom enhancement is observed in 91% of instances

Q75. What is the role of combined medical and surgical treatment in endometriosis?

- Preoperative hormonal therapy is given for the reduction of the size and vascularity of the lesion that can facilitate surgery.
- Post operative hormonal therapy given for the residual lesions left behind postsurgery and to pain control
- Duration of therapy is usually 3-6 months preoperatively and 3-6 months postoperatively.
- But it does not improve fertility.

Q76. When will you give empirical treatment and by which drug?

Empirical treatment of pelvic pain with the presumptive diagnosis of pelvic endometriosis may be given with combined oral contraceptives, if pain persists after NSAIDs.

Q77. What are the treatment options if infertility which is related to endometriosis?

If there is no improvement in infertility because of endometriosis with the ongoing treatment, couples should be counseled for ART. Controlled ovarian hyperstimulation with IUI, IVF, GIFT, and ICSI.

Q78. Mention the special sites where endometriosis can occur?

Scar-abdominal and episiotomy

- Bladder and ureter
- Cervix and vagina
- Lung

Q79. Short note on scar endometriosis.

- **When and how do you develop?**
  It occurs postabdominal hysterotomy, cesarean section, myomectomy or even after tubectomy.
- **Symptom** painful nodular swelling over or adjacent to the scar which increases in size and often bleeds during periods can be the main complaint
- **Examinations:** Variable, nodular mass, tenderness present with restricted mobility. It may not be associated with pelvic endometriosis. The same type of findings can be found over episiotomy scar.
- **Treatment:**
  - Excision.
  - Hormone therapy is ineffective.

CHAPTER 14 Adenomyosis

Case Discussion 1

Mrs, Bella, 42 years old, P 4+1(ab), presented with heavy menstrual blood loss and progressive painful menstruation for 2 years. She is moderately anemic. On pelvic examination, the uterus is about 14 weeks in size, pregnant uterus and the uterus is soft to firm in consistency, globular, and mildly tender; the fornices are free and nontender.

Q1. What is your provisional diagnosis?

Adenomyosis

Q2. What are the differential diagnoses?

- Submucous fibroid
- Endometriosis

Q3. What are the risk factors of adenomyosis in this case?

- Age 42 years
- Multiparous
- Patient has a history of 1 abortion.

Q4. How will you investigate her?

For diagnosis:

- TVS
- MRI (if diagnosis is uncertain)

For management purposes: Routine investigations for anesthetic fitness.

Q5. How will you treat her?

As the patient is 42 years old, multiparous, and has failed medical management, I will prefer hysterectomy with bilateral prophylactic salpingectomy with conservation of both ovaries if they are found normal.

SHORT ANSWER TYPE QUESTIONS

Q1. What is adenomyosis?

Adenomyosis is a condition characterized by the invasion of the endometrium, including both the glandular and stromal parts, directly into the myometrium. It can be either diffuse or focal. It is additionally referred to as endometriosis interna.

Q2. Causes of adenomyosis.

Growth of ectopic endometrial glands and stroma into the myometrium due to:

- Repeated childbirths
- Cesarean delivery
- Trauma to the endometrial-myometrial interface following induced abortion with curettage.

Q3. What are the co-existing pathologies of adenomyosis?

- Myoma
- Endometriosis: Pelvic endometriosis coexists in about 40%
- Endometrial hyperplasia
- Endometrial carcinoma.

Q4. What are the differences between adenomyosis and endometriosis?

In adenomyosis, endometrial glands and stroma are implanted within the myometrium, whereas in endometriosis, ectopic growth and proliferation of endometrial glands and stroma occur outside the uterus.

Q5. Pathogenesis of adenomyosis.

The endometrial glands and stroma expansion beyond the endometrial-myometrial boundary. Due to the absence of the submucosa, endometrial glands come into direct contact with the myometrium beneath. It creates nests, deep inside the myometrium. Thereafter, myometrial hyperplasia is present surrounding the endometriotic foci. The disruption of the normal junctional zone (JZ) is believed to make the inner myometrial zone more susceptible to secondary infiltration by endometrial glands and stroma.

Q6. Pathology of adenomyosis.

- The response of ectopic endometrial tissues to ovarian steroids influences the growth and tissue reaction in the endometrium. When only the basal layer exists, the tissue reaction is significantly reduced since it does not respond to hormones. However, if the functional zone exists that responds to hormones, the tissue response around the endometrium is significant.
- The myometrium exhibits hyperplasia, resulting in a generalized increase in the size of the uterus. The growth can be localized or can infiltrate a polyp (adenomyomatous).
- Appearance to the naked eye: Widespread symmetrical enlargement of the uterus, with the posterior wall typically thicker than the anterior wall. The size typically does not exceed that of a large orange (12–14 weeks pregnant uterus).
- The cut surface shows a darker coloration (myoma with a pale exterior), accompanied by thickening of the uterine wall. The sectioned surface displays distinct trabecular features. The growth lacks a surrounding capsule. Cystic dark areas and blood spots might be apparent in certain locations.

Q7. What are the types of adenomyosis?

- Based on the observations of MRI and 3D-ultrasonography, adenomyosis has been classified as:
  - Focal
  - Diffuse
  - Adenomyoma
  - Cystic
  - Noncystic varieties.
- Depending upon the extent of infiltration of endometrial glands and stroma within the layers of the uterus:
  - Type-1: Up to junctional zone
  - Type-2: Up to the middle myometrium and
  - Type-3: Up to the outer myometrium.
- Based upon the extent of the disease:
  - Mild (<25% affected)
  - Moderate (25–50% affected)
  - Severe (>50% affected)

Q8. Histological findings of adenomyosis.

Glandular tissue resembling the endometrium is surrounded by stromal cells in the myometrium.

Q9. What are the clinical features of adenomyosis?

- In about 50%, it remains asymptomatic.
- The patients are usually parous (90%), with age usually above 40 (80%).
- Menorrhagia (70%)
- Dysmenorrhea (30%)
- Dyspareunia or frequency of urination are due to an enlarged and tender uterus.
- Infertility
- A midline mass in the hypogastric region emerging from the pelvis may be detected during the abdominal examination. The size often does not go beyond a uterus of 14 weeks of gestation.
- Pelvic examination shows consistent swelling of the uterus

Q10. Why does heavy menstrual bleeding occur in adenomyosis?

The excessive bleeding results from an enlarged uterine cavity, endometrial hyperplasia, and insufficient uterine contractions. In typical menstruation, subendometrial contractions propagate forward from the fundus to the cervix. In adenomyosis with distortion of the junction zone, myometrial contractions are irregular and insufficient.

Q11. Why does dysmenorrhea occurs in adenomyosis?

Gradually intensifying colicky pain during menstruation results from the retrograde movement of uterine contractions. It also relies on the quantity and extent of adenomyotic foci present in the myometrium. When the penetration depth exceeds 80% of the myometrium, the pain becomes intense. Additional sources of discomfort include localized tissue swelling and prostaglandins.

Q12. Why does infertility occur in adenomyosis?

Women with adenomyosis experience a greater occurrence of infertility and miscarriage. The causes are:

- Irregular activity of the subendometrial myometrium.
- Contractions of the myometrium in a retrograde manner.
- Disruption of sperm movement and blastocyst attachment.
- Unusual endometrial immune reaction and nitric oxide concentration

Q13. What are the Ultrasound (3D) and color Doppler (TVS) features of adenomyosis?

- Heterogeneous echogenicity.
- Hypoechoicmyometrium featuring various small cysts in the myometrium (honeycomb-like appearance)
- Increased vascularity inside myometrium.
- Ill-defined endometrial echo.
- Striated projections from endometrium to myometrium.

Q14. What is MUSA criteria?

Morphological Uterus Sonographic Assessment (MUSA) criteria for diagnosis of adenomyosis has been currently used (2019).

Nine subdivisions have been made based on uterine involvement of the disease:

1. Globular
2. Asymmetric wall thickening
3. Cysts
4. Hyperechoic islands
5. Fan shaped shadowing
6. Echogenic subendometrial lines and buds
7. Translesional vascularity
8. Irregular junctional zones and
9. Interrupted junctional zones

Q15. What are the diagnostic criteria of adenomyosis (based on MRI)?

- Asymmetrical thickness of the uterine walls (posterior > anterior)
- Heterogeneous myometrial echotexture
- Small myometrial hypoechoic cysts (honeycomb appearance)
- Striated projections extending from endometrium to myometrium
- Endometrial echo poorly defined
- Uterus is globally enlarged
- J-Z thickening 2:12 mm.

Q16. What are the treatment options in adenomyosis?

Medical management: Medical treatment for adenomyosis is unsatisfactory.

Non-hormonal: NSAIDs can be used to control pain and bleeding.

Hormonal: Less useful hormone therapy.

Therapy involving progestins or a combination of cyclic estrogen and progestin offers minimal advantages.

- LNG-IUS is shown to enhance the symptoms of menorrhagia and dysmenorrhea.
- Intrauterine device (IUD) loaded with Danazol (300–400 mg)

Surgical management:

- Conservative surgery:
  - Adenomyomectomy
  - Uterine mass reduction (laparotomy or laparoscopy)
  - Uterine artery embolization
- Definitive surgery: Hysterectomy (parous and aged women).

CHAPTER 15

Chronic Pelvic Pain

Q1. Define PID and classify it clinically.

Infection and inflammation of upper genital tract involving fallopian tubes and ovaries.

Clinical syndrome	*Duration*
Acute	≤30 days
Sub-clinical	No symptoms and duration unknown
Chronic	≥30 days

Q2. What are the causes of PID?

The causes of PID are as follows:

i. Sexually transmitted disease
   - Chlamydial infection
   - Gonococcal infection

ii. Polymicrobial infection
   - Following abortion, MR, vaginal delivery

iii. Iatrogenic
   - IUCD insertion
   - Vaginal procedures
   - Hysteroscopy

iv. Special
   - Tuberculosis

Q3. What are the risk factors for PID?

- Sexually active teenagers
- Multiple sex partners
- Absence of contraceptive pills or barrier method use
- Previous history of PID
- IUD users
- Low socioeconomic status
- Partner with STD or urethritis
- Genetic predisposition

Q4. Mention the protective factors for PID.

1. Contraceptive practice
   - Barrier method, diaphragm with spermicides
   - Oral steroidal contraceptives
     - Produce thick mucus: Prevent ascent of sperm
     - Decrease in menstruation: Shorter interval of bacterial colonization of upper tract
   - Monogamy or partner with vasectomy

2. Others: Pregnancy, menopause, postcoital washing, and vaccines (Hep B and HPV)
3. Primary prevention: Reduction of STI
4. Secondary prevention: Universal screening of women at high risk for chlamydia and gonorrhea.

Q5. Name the organism responsible for PID.

Acute PID is usually polymicrobial infection caused by organism ascending upwards from downwards.

1. Primary organism:
   Sexually transmitted
   - *Neisseria gonorrhoeae* (30%)
   - Chlamydia trachomatis (30%)
   - Mycoplasma hominis (10%)
2. Secondary organism:
   - Aerobic: Nonhemolytic *Streptococcus, E. coli,* Group B *Streptococcus, Staphylococcus*
   - Anaerobic: *Bacteroid* species

Q6. Mention the clinical diagnostic criteria for acute PID.

According to CDC-2015

Minimum criteria:

- Lower abdominal tenderness
- Adnexal tenderness
- Cervical motion tenderness

Additional criteria for diagnosing PID:

- Oral temperature >38°C
- Mucopurulent cervical or vaginal discharge
- Abundant WBCs on saline microscopy of cervical secretions
- Raised CRP
- Elevated ESR
- Laboratory documentation of positive cervical infection with gonorrhea or *Chlamydia trachomatis*

Definitive criteria:

- Histopathologic evidence of endometriosis on biopsy
- Imaging study showing evidence of thickened fluid filled tubes +-free pelvic fluid or tuboovarian complex
- Laparoscopic evidence of PID
- Although initial treatment can be made before bacteriologic diagnosis of *C. trachomatis* or *N. gonorrhea* infection: Needs to treat the sex partner also.

Q7. What are the clinical features of PID?

Symptoms:

i. Lower abdominal and pelvic pain
   - Dull in nature
   - Onset of pain is more rapid and acute in gonococcal infection (3 days), chlamydia (5–7 days)

ii. Fever, lassitude and headache

iii. Irregular and excessive vaginal bleeding

iv. Abnormal vaginal discharge which becomes purulent and copious

v. Nausea and vomiting

vi. Dyspareunia

vii. Pain and discomfort in right hypochondrium (Fitz-Hugh-Curtis syndrome)

Signs

i. Temperature ≥38.3°C
ii. Abdominal palpation reveals tenderness on both the quadrants of lower abdomen. liver may be enlarged and tender (perihepatitis)
iii. Vaginal examination reveals:
   a. Abnormal vaginal discharge
   b. Congested external urethral meatus or opening of Bartholin's duct (pus may be seen)
   c. Speculum examination shows congested cervix with purulent discharge
   d. Bimanual examination reveals B/L tenderness on fornix palpation, cervical motion tenderness, thickening or a definite mass felt through the fornices.

Q8. What are the investigations done for diagnosis of PID?

1. Identification of organisms
   Materials collected from:
   - Urethra or Bartholin's gland
   - Cervical canal
   - Collected pus from fallopian tube during laparoscopy or laparotomy
2. Blood:
   CBC
   - Leukocytosis >10,000 per cu mm
   - ESR >15 mm per hour

Serological test for syphilis for both partners

3. Laparoscopy:
   Gold standard
   Useful for grading of PID
4. Sonography
   - limited value
   - fluid filled tubes
   - fluid in POD or adnexal mass S/O PID
5. Culdocentesis

Aspiration of peritoneal fluid (WBC >30,000/mL)
Extended investigations to be done for male partner.

Q9. What are the laparoscopic findings in patients with PID?

1. **Mild:**
   Tubes: Edema erythema, no spontaneous purulent exudates and tubes are freely mobile
2. **Moderate:**
   Material: Gross purulent
   Erythema and edema present
   Tubes: Not freely movable
   Fimbria stroma: Not patent
3. **Severe:** Pyosalpinx or abscess

Q10. What are the indications for hospitalization of PID patient?

According to CDC 2015

- Suspected tuboovarian abscess
- Severe illness, vomiting, temp. >38°C
- Uncertain diagnosis—where surgical emergencies cannot be excluded
- Unresponsive to outpatient therapy for 48 hours

- Intolerance to outpatient antibiotics
- Co-existing pregnancy
- Patients with HIV infection

Q11. How will you treat the patient with PID?

In outpatient:

1. Ceftriaxone 250 mg IM single dose
   OR
   Cefoxitin 2 g IM single dose and probenecid 1 g-PO-single dose
   OR
   Injection Cefotaxime IV
   Plus
2. Doxycycline 100 mg-PO-BID for 14 days with/out
   Metronidazole 500 mg-PO-BID for 14 days
3. Minimum criteria empirical treatment of PID should be initiated

Inpatient therapy:

Parenteral regimen

a. Cefoxitin 2 g IV every 6 hours for 7 days
   Plus
   Doxycycline 100 mg -PO-BID for 14 days
b. Clindamycin 900 mg -8 hourly
   Plus
   Gentamicin 2 mg/kg (loading dose) followed by 1.5 mg/kg IV (maintenance dose every 8 hours)
   Aztreonam 2 g-IV slowly is similar to aminoglycoside and can be used
   - No renal toxicity
   - Expensive
c. **Alternative parenteral regimen**
   Ampicillin- sulbactam 3 g-IV-6 hourly for 3–5 days
   Plus
   Doxycycline 100 mg-PO-BID for 14 days

Q12. What are the complications of PID?

Immediate:

- Pelvic peritonitis/generalized peritonitis
- Septicemia

Late complications:

- Dyspareunia
- Infertility
  - 1st episode: 12%
  - 2nd episode: 25%
  - 3rd episode: 50%
- Chronic pelvic inflammation (25%)
- Adhesion formation or hydro/pyosalpinx and T-O abscess
- Chronic pelvic pain and ill health
- Increased risk of ectopic pregnancy (6–10-fold)

Q13. What are the late sequels of PID?

- Infertility:
  - Due to cornual block
  - Damage to the wall of tube

- Chronic infection
- Chronic pelvic pain, dysmenorrhea
- Pelvic adhesive disease
- Ectopic pregnancy
- Residual inflection with periodic acute exacerbation
- Intestinal obstruction
- Chronic ill health
- Dyspareunia and marital disharmony
- Endometriosis
- May end in hysterectomy

Q14. Define chronic pelvic pain and mention its causes.

Chronic pelvic pain is defined as pain lasting for at least 6 months and localized at pelvis, the anterior wall at or below the umbilicus, lumbosacral back or buttocks that is of sufficient severity to cause functional disability or lead to medical care.

The causes are the following:
- Following acute pelvic infection—if initial treatment was inadequate
- Following low grade recurrent infection
- Tubercular infection

Q15. What are the clinical features of chronic pelvic infection.

Symptoms:
- Usually asymptomatic
- Has history of acute pelvic infection following childbirth or abortion
- Recurrent episodes of re infections
- IF patients are present with symptoms:
  Chronic pelvic pain: Varying magnitude
  Pain aggravates prior to menstruation

Dyspareunia: Deep and may be located unilaterally or bilaterally
Congestive dysmenorrhea
Lower abdominal pain
Menorrhagia or poly menorrhea
Vaginal discharge: Mucoid or mucopurulent
Infertility

Signs

On examination

Per abdomen-
- Iliac fossa—tenderness on one or both sides
- Pelvic mass—irregular and tender

Q16. Mention the investigations to be done for chronic pelvic infection?

The investigations depend on the diagnosis and causes:
1. Complete blood count
2. Urine R/ME
3. Endocervical swab—chlamydia, gonorrhea and culture sensitivity
4. USG of whole abdomen and pelvis: Doppler study may be needed
5. Laparoscopy: When pelvic abnormality is detected and to diagnose and treat the contributory condition.
6. MRI: Helpful in the diagnosis of deep endometriosis, adenomyosis and endometriomas
7. Intraserous phyclogim (IVP): Accordance to history and examination

Q17. What is the management protocol for chronic pelvic infection?

The goal of management includes self-managerial and improve quality of life.

1. General:
   - Health improvement
   - Anemia correction if present
   - Analgesics if required
2. Specific:
   - If IUCD in situ -to be removed
   - Long-term broad-spectrum antibiotics as per treatment protocol
3. Surgery:
   May be required in few cases with adhesions, endometriosis of tuboovarian mass.

Q18. How does PID causes infertility in a young lady?

- Cornual block
- Loss of cilia
- Loss of peristalsis due to thickening of tubal wall
- Closure of abdominal ostium and distortion of tube due to peritubal adhesion

Q19. How does PID causes ectopic pregnancy?

- Loss of cilia lining and impairment of mucosal peristalsis
- Narrowing of the tubal lumen
- Formation of the pockets due to adhesion between mucosal fold
- Peritubal adhesion resulting in kinking and angulation of the tube

CHAPTER 16

Uterine Leiomyoma (Fibroids) and Leiomyosarcoma

Case Discussion

A 40-year-old woman, para 2+0, complains of an abdominal mass with excessive menstrual blood loss. She had two normals deliveries. On general examination, she was moderately anemic. A firm nodular mass is palpable mass in lower abdomen and is about 20 weeks size of pregnant uterus. The mass is mobile side to side, but mobility is restricted above downwards. On pelvic examination, cervix moves along with movement of the mass.

Q1. What is your diagnosis and why?

Uterine leiomyoma (uterine fibroid). This 40-year-old woman with irregular, heavy menstrual bleeding (HMB) with anemia and a lump in lower abdomen which moves side to side, but up and down mobility is restricted, and mass is continuous with uterus.

Provisional diagnosis → Uterine leiomyoma

Positive findings:

1. Heavy menstrual bleeding
2. Anemia
3. Lump → mobility

Q2. What are the differential diagnoses?

- Pregnancy
- Adenomyosis
- Ovarian tumor

Q3. Why is this not a case of adenomyosis?

- Adenomyosis is more common in women of advanced reproductive age group (>40 years).
- And among multiparous women.
- This patient has no history of repeated curettage, MR, D&C.
- The patient has menorrhagia but no dysmenorrhea and dyspareunia.

From examination:

- In adenomyosis:
  - Uterus is uniformly enlarged and usually not more than 14 weeks size
  - Surface is smooth
  - Well-defined margin
  - Soft to firm in consistency
  - Tenderness may be present

Q4. Why is this not an ovarian tumor?

In ovarian tumor,

- No age is immune
- Usually there is not associated with menstrual symptoms
- Patient may have history of dyspepsia dull aching pain.
- If ovarian origin on examination: The lump is felt in lower abdomen, may be cystic in nature

- Lump is mobile in all direction, lower pole could be reached
- Bimanual examination reveals a normal sized uterus separate from the mass. A cleft can be felt between the mass and uterus. There is no movement of the cervix along with movement of the mass. The mass could be felt through all fornices.

Q5. Why HMB (menorrhagia) occurs in leiomyoma?

a. Increase endometrial surface area
b. Increased vascularity of uterus
c. Defective uterine contractions
d. Associated endometrial hyperplasia
e. Endometrial ulceration over a submucous leiomyoma,
f. Uterine congestion due to compression of venous plexus within myometrium.

Q6. How do you confirm your diagnosis?

By pelvic ultrasonography/TVS.

Q7. What other investigations will you do for her?

- A complete blood count to assess the degree of anemia
- An ultrasonography of kidneys, ureters, bladder, and renal function tests as a large leiomyoma may cause ureter obstruction and hydronephrosis.

Q8. How will you treat her?

After confirmation of fibroid at first I will counsel with the patient about her disease, treatment options, suitable treatment according to her age, parity and desire, complications that may arise if treatment is not taken or during treatment, availability of treatment and cost of treatment.

As my patient is 40 years old with 2 living children and already treated medically, with no improving response, I will prefer surgical management for her.

If patient desires for further child - myomectomy can be an option.

But if patient not desire of further childbirth I will go for definitive treatment i.e. Total abdominal hysterectomy with conservation of both ovaries (if they are found apparently healthy).

Before operation I will counsel with the patient that after total abdominal hysterectomy she will not menstruate or able to be pregnant but she will have no problem in her conjugal life.

Related information: If facilities available - If expert surgeon, availability of laparoscopic instrument and patient ability permits then Total laparoscopic Hysterectomy, (TLH) Laparoscopic assisted Vaginal Hysterectomy (LAVH) non descent vaginal hysterectomy (NDVH).

SHORT ANSWER QUESTIONS

Q1. What is leiomyoma?

Leiomyomas are the most common benign solid tumors of the uterus in female. Histologically, this tumor is composed of smooth muscle and fibrous connective tissue and also named as uterine myoma or fibromyoma.

Q2. Features on cut surface.

- Smooth whitish feature of whorled appearance
- Trabeculation due to intermingling of fibrous tissue with muscle bundles.
- False capsule: It is formed by compressed adjacent myometrium.
- The periphery of tumor is more vascular and center is least vascular.

Q3. What is the incidence and prevalence of leiomyomas?

- About 20-40% of women at the age of 30 years or older.
- The patients are usually between 30 and 50 years old

- About 50% remain asymptomatic.
- In outpatient department is about 3%.
- About 70% in white women.
- In African-American women, it is about 80%.
- Common in nulliparous or low parity.

Q4. What are the origin of fibroids?

- Still uncertain
- Monoclonal
- Arise from somatic mutation in a progenitor myocyte
- 40% chromosomal abnormality
- Role of polypeptide growth factor
- Positive family history

Q5. Is there any genetic correlation of fibroid?

Yes, there is genetic correlation in fibroid. About 40% of cases, there is a varying type of chromosomal abnormality, particularly the chromosome 6,7, 12,14 (rearrangements, deletions).

- Somatic mutations in myometrial cells.
- Genetic factors
- Myometrial cellular hypoxia

Q6. Is there any role of polypeptide growth factors?

- Epidermal growth factor (EGF),
- Insulin-like growth factor-I (IGF-1)
- Transforming growth factor-TGF, stimulate the growth of leiomyoma either directly or via estrogen.

Q7. What are the risk factors of leiomyoma?

- Increasing age
- Early menarche
- Nulliparity
- Obesity, body mass index (BMI)
- Polycystic ovary syndrome (PCOS)
- Hyperestrogenic state
- Black women
- High fat diet
- Family history

Q8. What are the protective factors of leiomyoma?

- Late menarche
- Multiparity
- Menopause
- Combined oral contraceptives (COCs)

Q9. Why is leiomyoma called predominantly an estrogen-dependent tumor?

- Both estrogen and progesterone receptors are found in higher concentrations in myomas.
- Myomas cells have higher levels of the enzyme aromatase. This increases the high local levels of estrogen.
- Myomas are rare before menarche and majority decreases in size following menopause.
- They often enlarge during pregnancy.
- Hypoestrogenic conditions (GnRH agonist use), menopause reduces the size of myomas.

Q10. Effect of progesterone and estrogen on myoma.

Progesterone:

- Increase the mitotic activity in the myoma of young woman
- Help in growth of myoma by down regulation of apoptosis in the tumor

Estrogen: Contribute to tumor enlargement by increasing the production of extracellular matrix.

Q11. What are causes of uterine enlargement?

- Pregnancy
- Fibroid
- Adenomyosis
- Myohyperplasia
- Pyometra
- Hematometra
- Lochiometra
- Malignancy of uterus:
  - Uterine sarcoma
  - Endometrial carcinoma
- Sarcomatous changes of pre-existing fibroid

Q12. When does rapid growth occur in fibroid uterus?

- During pregnancy.
- Degeneration
- Use of high dose OCP
- Malignant change.

Q13. What are the types of fibroid uterus? (Classification by Anatomic Location)

- Body (corporeal)
  - Interstitial (75%) (intramural)
  - Subserous (10%)
  - Submucous (5%)
  - Sessile Pedunculated
- Cervical
- Broad ligament (pseudo)
- Wandering (parasitic)

LASMAR'S classification

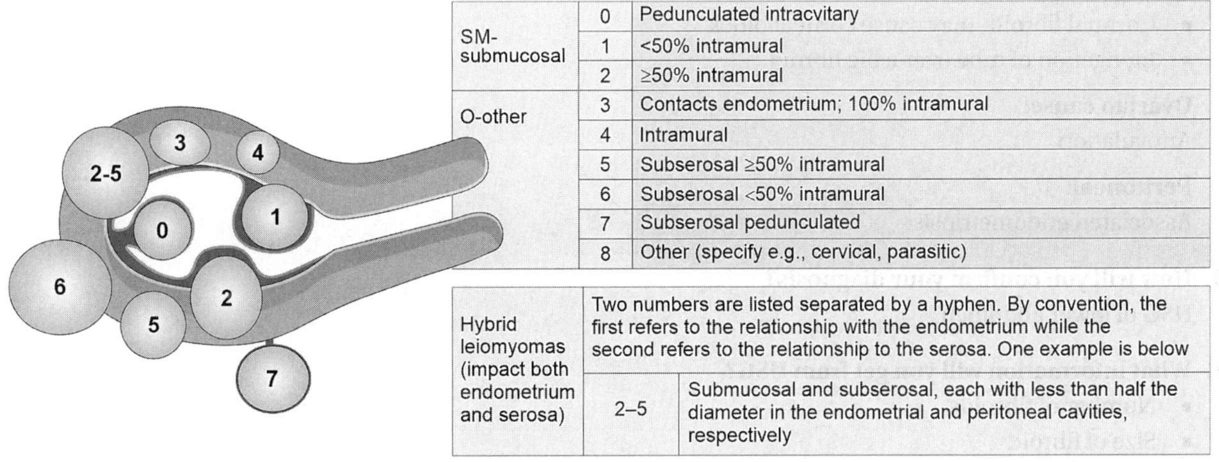

SM-submucosal	0	Pedunculated intracvitary
	1	<50% intramural
	2	≥50% intramural
O-other	3	Contacts endometrium; 100% intramural
	4	Intramural
	5	Subserosal ≥50% intramural
	6	Subserosal <50% intramural
	7	Subserosal pedunculated
	8	Other (specify e.g., cervical, parasitic)

Hybrid leiomyomas (impact both endometrium and serosa)	Two numbers are listed separated by a hyphen. By convention, the first refers to the relationship with the endometrium while the second refers to the relationship to the serosa. One example is below	
	2–5	Submucosal and subserosal, each with less than half the diameter in the endometrial and peritoneal cavities, respectively

Q14. What is intraligamentary leiomyoma?

When leiomyoma extends into the broad ligament, they are known as intraligamentary leiomyoma.

Q15. What is parasitic leiomyoma?

Pedunculated subserous leiomyoma may rarely get attached with omentum or intestines and may develop a secondary blood supply. The leiomyoma may be detached from uterus and loss primary blood supply and the resulting structure known as parasitic leiomyoma.

Q16. What are the causes of dysmenorrhea in fibroid uterus?

a. *Congestive dysmenorrhea:* It occurs due to pelvic congestion or associated endometriosis or PID.
b. *Spasmodic dysmenorrhea:* During passage of clot or when a submucous fibroid attempts to expel.

Q17. Is abdominal pain common in fibroid?

Pain is an uncommon feature of fibroid. If present it may be due to complications of fibroid—e.g.,

- Degeneration
- Torsion of pedunculated subserous fibroid
- Extrusion of submucous fibroid
- Sarcomatous change
- Adhesion with other organs
- Associated other pathology, e.g., PID, endometriosis

Q18. Can metrorrhagia occur in fibroids?

Yes, it can occur when there is:

- Ulceration of submucous fibroid
- Torn vessels from sloughing base of a polyp
- Associated endometrial carcinoma

Q19. Can infertility occur in fibroid uterus and why?

About 30% of the cases, majority unknown.

Uterine cause:

- Distortion and or elongation of the uterine cavity- difficult in sperm ascent.
- Prevention of rhythmic uterine contraction- impair sperm transport
- Congestion of endometrial venous plexus- defective implantation.
- Menorrhagia and dyspareunia

Tubal cause:

- Cornual fibroid- may cause corneal block
- Elongation of tube over a big fibroid

Ovarian cause:

Anovulation

Peritoneal:

Associated endometriosis

Q20. How will you confirm your diagnosis?

USG of lower abdomen

Q21. What information will you get from USG?

- Number of fibroids
- Size of fibroid

- Endometrial thickness
- Distortion of endometrium
- Endometrial polyp
- Echogenicity

Any central vascularization (which indicates degenerative changes).

- Any adnexal pathology - as because fibroid is associated with follicular cyst of ovary and endometriosis.

Q22. Why not TVS or when TVS is preferable?

- TVS better delineates the pelvic organs and it gives better delineation of endometrial thickness and endometrial pathology.
- As in my case the lump is palpable from abdomen, so USG of lower abdomen is better.

Q23. What are the typical features of leiomyoma on ultrasound?

- Leiomyomas can be hypoechoic (gray on screen), isoechoic, anechoic (black on screen), hyperechoic (white on screen) or mixed echoic
- Linear stripy fan shaped internal shadowing (rain in the forest appearance)
- Significant shadowing from the edge of the lesion beyond the serosa of the uterus
- Calcification: Posterior acoustic shadowing
- Peripheral calcification: Eggshell appearance and cavitation.

Q24. What is leiomyoma mapping?

Leiomyomas mapping is the term used to understand the relationship between the leiomyoma from serosa and endometrium by noting the exact distance between there. Leiomyomas mapping is important for the surgical management of leiomyomas and assessing the complications.

Q25. What other investigations do you want to do?

1. **Saline infusion sonography**—to detect submucous fibroid.
   - It is noninvasive
   - No anesthesia is required
   - Can be done as an alternative to hysteroscopy
   - No special preparation is required
2. **Hysteroscopy**
   Diagnostic: Preferable to detect submucous fibroid by direct visualization and along with endometrial sampling can be taken.
   Therapeutic: Hysteroscopic resection of fibroid can be done at same setting.
3. MRI
4. Pap's smear → for cervical screening
5. IVU

Q26. What is the role of MRI?

- **Diagnostic:** MRI is more accurate compared to USG. It is not routinely done. It is done when there is diagnostic dilemma between fibroid and adenomyosis. It can also be done for infertility workup in fibroid uterus and also to see endometrial thickness.
- **Therapeutic:** MRI guided focused Ultrasound.

Q27. Why MRI not done routinely?

- MRI is expensive
- Not widely available

Q28. What other investigations do you need to do?

For management purpose I want to do some baseline investigations. Those are mainly for anesthetic fitness.

- Blood grouping and Rh typing
- CBC - Hb% for degree of anemia
- S. Creatinine
- S.electrolytes
- HBsAg
- Anti-HCV
- Urine - R/M/E
- Chest X-ray
- ECG
- Echo if age >30 years

Q29. What is the role of endometrial curettage in case of fibroid?

Endometrial curettage is mandatory in patients with fibroid with irregular per vaginal bleeding to exclude endometrial pathology.

Q30. What is the role of Pap's smear?

Pap's smear can be done as routine screening procedure if it has not been done before.

Q31. What is the role of IVU?

IVU is recommended in case of:

- Large subserous fibroid
- Cervical fibroid
- Broad ligament fibroid to see relation of ureter and any sign of compression.

Q32. What complications can be anticipated in a patient with fibroid?

Following Complications are anticipated:

1. **Degeneration:**
   - Hyaline degeneration (most common)
   - Cystic
   - Fatty
   - Atrophic
   - Calcific
   - Red-common in pregnancy and puerperium.
2. **Necrosis** (common in submucous fibroid).
3. **Infection** (common in submucous fibroid).
4. **Torsion** of subserous pedunculated fibroid.
5. **Hemorrhage:** It can be intracapsular or intraperitoneal due to rupture of surface veins of a subserous fibroid.
7. **Sarcomatous change** (rare) <0.1% of all fibroids. Sarcomatous change is suspected when there is sudden enlargement of fibroid and pain. Sometimes associated with postmenopausal bleeding.
8. Polycythemia

Q33. What is red degeneration?

In red degeneration, the peripheral vessels become thrombosed and there is extravasation of blood which is responsible of red color of the tumor. The extravasated blood stretches the pseudocapsule resulting in severe abdominal pain. The cut section of tumor has a raw beef appearance with a fishy odor from fatty acids.

Q34. What is the clinical presentation of red degeneration?

The patient is pregnant or in puerperium and complains of sudden onset pain. She may have fever, vomiting, and tachycardia. The tumor may be enlarged and tender.

Blood examination reveals peripheral leukocytosis and raised ESR.

Q35. How do you treat red degeneration?

The condition is conservatively treated with bed rest, analgesics, sedatives and IV fluids. There is no place of surgery. Pregnancy usually proceeds uneventfully.

Q36. Why polycythemia occurs in fibroid?

Polycythemia occurs in fibroid

- Due to erythropoietic function by the tumor
- Altered erythropoietic function of the kidney due to ureteric pressure.

Q37. What are life threatening complications of fibroid?

- Persistent menorrhagia, metrorrhagia—may cause severe anemia—anemic heart failure
- Severe intraperitoneal hemorrhage due to rupture of veins over subserous fibroid.
- Severe infection leading to peritonitigs or septicemia
- Sarcoma

Q38. What are the diseases commonly associated with myoma?

- Follicular cyst of ovary
- Endometrial hyperplasia
- Endometrial carcinoma
- Endometriosis

Q39. What are the pregnancy related complications?

Effects on pregnancy:

- May be none
- Pressure symptoms due to impaction -
  - Bladder- retention of urine
  - Rectum - constipation
- Abortion
- Malpresentation
- Preterm labor and prematurity
- Red degeneration
- Placental abruption

Effects on Labor:

- May be unaffected
- Non-engagement of presenting part
- Uterine inertia
- Cervical dystocia due to cervical or broad ligament fibroid
- Obstructed labor
- Difficulty during cesarean section.

Effects on puerperium:

- PPH (due to atonicity or due to morbid adherent placenta)
- Subinvolution
- Sepsis
- Lochiometra and pyometra
- Secondary PPH
- Inversion of uterus

Effects of pregnancy on fibroid:

- Red degeneration
- Infection
- Torsion

Q40. Why do you want to preserve ovary in your case?

- Less incidence of vasomotor symptoms, osteoporosis, atherosclerotic change.
- Ovarian function continues up to 60-65 years of age, so menopausal symptoms appear late and severity will be less.

Q41. What are the risks of preservation of ovary?

- Risk of development of ovarian neoplasm.
- Residual ovarian syndrome within 1-3 years.
- Chronic pelvic pain and dyspareunia.
- Risk of re-laparotomy (1-3%).

Q42. When do leiomyomas need not to be treated?

If the leiomyoma is asymptomatic and the patient not anemic, no treatment is necessary. In asymptomatic leiomyoma, observation with periodic examination and investigation every 3-6 months.

Q43. What are treatment options for fibroid uterus?

a. Treatment option for asymptomatic fibroid:

Expectant management -

Indications

- Size <12 weeks of pregnant uterine size
- Diagnosis is certain.
- Follow up possible (6 monthly with history, clinical examination, USG evaluation)

b. Treatment options for symptomatic fibroid:

1. Medical management
   - Non-hormonal
     - Tranexamic acid
     - Prostaglandin synthetase inhibitors (PSI)
   - Hormonal
2. Conservative surgical treatment
3. Definitive surgical treatment

Medical management

- For temporary palliation
- An alternative to surgery.
- It can also be given preoperatively
- During waiting for surgery at least for 3 months.

Q44. Different treatment options of leiomyoma in different patients.

Patient characteristics	*Treatment options*
Asymptomatic women	Observation
Symptomatic women who desire fertility preservation	Nonsurgical treatment or myomectomy
Symptomatic women who do not desire future fertility but wish to preserve the uterus	Nonsurgical treatment or myomectomy or myolysis or uterine artery embolization
Women who desire fertility preservation and have had a pregnancy complicated by uterine leiomyoma	Myomectomy
Infertile women with distortion of uterine cavity	Myomectomy
Women with severe symptoms who desire definitive treatment	Hysterectomy

Q45. Whom to give medical treatment?

Medical treatment can be given to -

- Young woman desires of pregnancy
- To improve menorrhagia and to correct anemia before surgery
- To minimize the size and vascularity of the tumor in order to facilitate surgery
- To facilitate hysteroscopic and laparoscopic surgery
- Where postponement of surgery is planned temporarily.

Q46. What are the names of hormonal drugs used for symptomatic fibroid?

- OCP—It decreases mean blood loss but not size
- Selective progesterone receptor modulators (SPRM)—Ulipristal acetate given 5 mg once for 3-6 months.
- Progesterone if endometrial hyperplasia
- LNG - IUS
- *GnRH analogue:*
  - Agonist - Goserelin, Buserelin
  - Antagonist - Cetrorelix or Ganirelix
- Anti-progesterone (Mifepristone)
- *Anti-gonadotrophin:* Danazol, gestrinone

Q47. How does GnRH analogue, LNG-IUS, SPRM, mifepristone, antigonadotropin work?

- **GnRH against:** Initially causing surge in LH+ FSH (Have effect), followed by prolonged stimulation that leads to down regulation of GnRH receptors of dememorization of pituitary
- **GnRH antagonist:** Work by directly blocking GnRH receptors in pituitary gland. Preventing release of LH of FSH.
- **GnRH analogue:**

  Advantages:
  - Improvement of menorrhagia and may produce amenorrhea
  - Improvement of anemia
  - Relief of pressure symptoms
  - Reduction in size by 50% when used for a period of 6 months
  - Reduction in vascularity of the tumor
  - Reduction in blood loss during myomectomy
  - May facilitate laparoscopic or hysteroscopic surgery
  - May facilitate non descent vaginal hysterectomy

  Disadvantages:
  - Need add- back therapy due to hypo estrogenic side effects (vasomotor symptoms, trabecular bone loss)
  - Regrowth of myoma on cessation of therapy
  - Degeneration (Some leiomyoma) causing difficulty in myoma enucleation
  - Costly
- **LNG-IUS:** It reduces blood loss, produce amenorrhea and reduce size
- **SPRM:** Induce apoptosis of tumor
- **Mifepristone:** It reduces fibroid size and blood loss
- **Anti-gonadotropin:** It reduces blood loss, produce amenorrhea, and reduce size

Q48. Contraindication of LNG-IUS.

- If uterus is >12 weeks size
- Distortion of uterine cavities

Q49. What is the role of prostaglandin synthetase inhibitor?

These are used to relieve pain; they cannot improve menorrhagia.

Q50. What are the surgical options in case of fibroid?

a. Conservative surgery:

Traditional: myomectomy

Endoscopic:

- Laparoscopic myomectomy
- Hysteroscopic resection of myoma

Recent updates:

- Embolotherapy (UAE)
- Laparoscopic uterine artery ligation
- Magnetic resonance guided focused ultrasound
- High intensity focused ultrasound
- Myolysis
- Electrocautery
- Laser
- Cryotherapy

b. Definitive surgery:

- TAH (Total abdominal hysterectomy)
- TLH (Total laparoscopic hysterectomy)
- LAVH (Laparoscopic-guided vaginal hysterectomy)
- VH (Vaginal hysterectomy)

Q51. If your patient does not want to go for surgery then what will you do?

At first, I want to know whether she has taken medical treatment properly, if not then I will offer her 3-6 cycle of medical treatment, if size of uterus is <12 weeks. If size of uterus is >12 weeks, I will offer her conservative surgery.

Q52. What is myomectomy?

Myomectomy is the enucleation of myoma from the uterus leaving behind a potentially functioning organ capable of future reproduction.

Q53. What are indications of myomectomy?

- Persistent uterine bleeding despite medical therapy
- Excessive pain or pressure symptoms
- Size more than 12 weeks of pregnant uterus
- Recurrent pregnancy loss
- Rapidly growing myoma
- Subserous pedunculated fibroid
- Distortion of uterine cavity due to submucous fibroid

Q54. What are the important considerations prior to myomectomy?

- It should be done mainly to preserve the reproductive function.
- Wish to preserve the menstrual function in parous women.
- Myomectomy is a riskier operation when the fibroid is too big and too many in number.
- At least 2-unit blood should be kept in ready
- Counselling with the patient:
  - Risk of recurrence and persistence of fibroid is about 30 to 50%
  - Risk of persistence of menorrhagia is about 1 to 5%
  - Risk of re-laparotomy is about 20 to 25%
  - Pregnancy rate following myomectomy is about 40 to 60%
  - Pregnancy following myomectomy should have a mandatory hospital delivery, although the chance of scar rupture is rare, little more when the cavity is open.

Q55. What are the pre-requisites for myomectomy?

- Urine pregnancy test- to exclude pregnancy
- Hb% should be at least 11 g/dL
- Ultrasonography—confirmation and location of leiomyoma
- Hysteroscopy or hysterosalpingography—to exclude any submucous fibroid or a polyp or any tubal block.
- Hysteroscopy/endometrial biopsy—in cases of irregular cycle to exclude endometrial carcinoma, 25% chance having endometrial carcinoma.
- Pap's smear to exclude cervical carcinoma
- Ovarian reserve (if subfertile)
- Semen analysis

Q56. What are the different routes of myomectomy?

Myomectomy can be performed via laparoscopy, robotic surgery and hysteroscopy, mini laparotomy and laparotomy.

Q57. What are the contraindications of myomectomy?

- Infected fibroid
- Growth of myoma after menopause
- Suspected malignant change (sarcoma).
- Women with no desire fertility or uterine preservation
- Parous women where hysterectomy is safe and a definitive treatment
- Functionless fallopian tube
- Pelvic or endometrial tuberculosis
- During pregnancy or during C/S (relative)

Q58. What are the complications of myomectomy?

Preoperative:

- Hemorrhage
    - Injury to surrounding structures, e.g., bladder, ureter, fallopian tube, bowel
    - Anesthetic hazard

Postoperative:

- Immediate:
    - Abdominal distension
    - Low grade pyrexia
- Late:
    - Persistence of menorrhagia
    - Recurrence of menorrhagia
    - Adhesion formation to bowel

Q59. How to reduce the adhesion formation following myomectomy?

Adhesion formation can be reduced by careful operative techniques such as:

- Limited number of incisions
- Anterior incision
- Application of absorbable barrier like intercede, Gore-Tex, and seprafilm to reduce contact between damage tissue
- Medical approaches using dextran 40, factor 13 with fibrinogen
- Plication of round ligament to maintain version
- Bony's hood
- Proper hemostasis

- Baseball suture
- To keep a drain tube
- Peritoneal toileting

Q60. How can you reduce hemorrhage during myomectomy?

Before operation: GnRH analogue—It reduces the vascularity of the tumor and decrease blood loss.

During operation:

- Inj. Vasopressin—1 ample (1 mL = 20 unit) dilute with 100 mL normal saline injected into myometrium and surface of the myoma for vasoconstriction.
- Intramyometrial bupivacaine plus epinephrine
- Inj. Tranexamic acid—1g IV
- Vaginal misoprostol
- Incision—preferably midline on the anterior wall of uterus
- Bonney's myomectomy clamp should be applied around the uterine vessels and the round ligament to decrease uterine artery blood flow.
- *Oxytocin:* Cause vasoconstriction and myometrial contraction—20-unit IV bolus dose then 10 to 20 unit in 1000 mL of normal saline or dextrose.
- *Tourniquet:* An avascular part of broad ligament at the level of uterine isthmus.

Q61. What is the role of preoperative GnRH administration prior myomectomy?

Adantages:

- Increased preoperative hemoglobin level
- Decreased uterine size
- Lower incidence of vertical |incisions
- Decrease estimated blood loss
- Decrease in number of blood transfusion

Limitation:

- No shortening of duration of surgery or complications
- Loss of histologic cleavage plain during surgery making surgical removal of leiomyoma limited.

Q62. How does vasopressin act?

Vasopressin causes vasoconstriction due to its effect on V1 receptors. Uterine contractions are also stimulated by vasopressin through myometrial V1a receptors. Vasopressin receptors are present in the myometrium of both pregnant and nonpregnant uterus. Vasopressin causes antidiuresis in the kidneys through its effect on V2 receptors.

Q63. What is the procedure for using vasopressin to reduce hemorrhage during myomectomy?

- Vasopressin should be diluted in the range of 0.1-0.2 U/mL using 100-200 mL of normal saline.
- A total dose of 5 units should not be exceeded for a one-time injection.
- Before injecting vasopressin, the entire surgical team, including the anesthetist, should be informed.
- Injecting into blood vessels should be avoided, and double-checking should be done prior to injecting vasopressin.
- The injection needle is inserted between the uterus and the myoma. The whole of the normal saline is injected.
- Usually, a single insertion is sufficient, but the position of the needle may be changed if needed.
- Injections can be repeated after 45-60 minutes if the first is uneventful.

Q64. What are the complications of vasopressin injection?

Vasopressin induced increase in blood pressure may cause vagal-mediated bradycardia, and the vasoconstrictive effect of vasopressin may cause coronary artery vasospasm, thus leading to cardiac ischemia and cardiac arrest. Other complications include hypotension, hypertension and pulmonary edema.

Q65. When patient will try for pregnancy after myomectomy?

Chance of pregnancy is more within 2 years, so when she think she is fit for herself she should try to conceive as early as possible. If age is more, then we can give ovulation inducing drugs. If failed, after 3 months hysterosalpingogram should be done.

Q66. Mode of delivery after myomectomy.

NVD can be done even vertical incision can be given because chance of rupture of myomectomy scar is less and better healing.

Q67. Is there any effect on ovary after myomectomy?

Early menopause may occur in 10% due to decrease in blood supply to ovary when large myoma is removed.

Q68. What advice will you give your patient after hysterectomy?

- Resected uterus should be sent for histopathology and check histopathology report
- Avoid heavy work for three months which is required to gain normal strength otherwise they develop hernia.
- Avoid sexual intercourse for six weeks
- Counsel the patient that she will never menstruate nor be pregnant but she will not have any problem in her conjugal life.

Q69. What are indications of emergency surgery in fibroid?

- Torsion of a subserous pedunculated fibroid
- Massive intraperitoneal hemorrhage following rupture of veins over subserous fibroid
- Uncontrolled infected fibroid
- Uncontrolled bleeding fibroids

Q70. What is Bonney's hood operation?

It is done to remove a large fundal fibroid. A low transverse incision is made on the myoma over the anterior uterine surface. After removal of the fibroid the capsule is trimmed and is sewn over the anterior uterine wall. This procedure is done to minimize adhesion formation.

Q71. How myomectomy is performed for central cervical fibroid?

After incising the peritoneum of the uterovesical pouch and dissecting the bladder down hemisection of the uterus is done from above downward to reach the fibroid which is then enucleated. The Dead Space is obliterated without closing the cervical canal followed by repair of the bisected uterus.

Q72. What precautions are mostly taken during hysterectomy of cervical fibroid?

There are greater chances of inadvertent injury to the ureter, bladder and uterine vessels.

In this case the principle is enucleation followed by hysterectomy to minimize injury to the ureter. Alternatively one can also give preoperative GnRH analogue 3 months prior to facilitate surgery.

Q73. What are the advantages and disadvantages of laparoscopic myomectomy?

Advantages:

- Shorter hospital stay
- Lower morbidity
- Cosmetically better

Disadvantages:

- Require expertise
- Laparoscopic myomectomy is limited to patients with fibroid size <8 cm or <4 fibroids
- Recurrence rate (35%) is more
- More adhesion formation
- There is chances of rupture in pregnancy

CHAPTER 17

Benign Ovarian Lesions

Q1. What are the causes of enlargement of ovaries?

Causes of enlargement of ovary

- Hypertrophy (congenital and acquired)
- Corpus luteum hematoma
- Ovarian pregnancy
- Oophoritis (Acute or chronic)
- Endometriosis
- Lutein cysts and luteoma of pregnancy
- Distension or retention cysts
- Primary ovarian neoplasms (Benign or malignant)
- Secondary (metastatic) neoplasms

Q2. What are the functional cysts of ovary?

Classification of ovarian cyst

a. Functional cyst/cystic ovary
   - Follicular
   - Corpus luteum
   - Theca lutein and granulosa lutein
   - PCOS
b. Non functional cyst
   Endometrial cyst (chocolate cyst)

Physiological cysts of ovary

- Atretic cysts
- Germinal inclusion cysts
- Follicular and theca lutein cysts

Q3. How can you diagnose?

Symptoms and signs of follicular cyst of ovary

- Asymptomatic (majority)
- And polymenorrhagia
- Amenorrhea
- Infertility
- Pain in the iliac fossa
- Usually multiple and small
- Unilocular
- Contains clear fluid inside unless hemorrhage occurs.

Q4. How can you differentiate between cystic ovary and ovarian cyst?

Differences between cystic ovary and ovarian cyst.

Cystic ovary	*Ovarian cyst*
Non-neoplastic cyst	Neoplastic cyst (Benign or malignant)
Usually, 6–8 cm in diameter	May be of any (Mucinous cyst adenoma is the largest benign ovarian tumor)
Usually, asymptomatic	Symptomatic
Regression occurs spontaneously usually after correction of the related functional disturbances	Spontaneous regression does not occur
Contains clear fluid inside unless hemorrhage occurs	May contain serous or mucinous fluid
The lining epithelium reflects the functional epithelium of the unit from which it originates	Emerges from the totipotent surface epithelium of the ovary and is covered by columnar or cuboidal epithelium

Q5. How will you treat a case of functional cyst of ovary?

Treatment of functional ovarian cysts

- *Follicular cysts:*
  - Follicular cyst ≤8 cm: no evaluation needed
  - Follow up along with repeated ultrasound in 3 to 6 months if Simple cyst, 8 cm, unilocular, echo free without solid areas or papillary projections, with normal serum CA 125
  - Persisting/growing cyst:laparoscopy/laparotomy
- *Corpus luteum cysts:*
  - In uncomplicated cases: Spontaneous regression is expected
  - In complicated cases: Laparotomy with enucleation of the cyst along with resuscitation (if features of acute abdomen occur)
- *Lutein cysts:* Spontaneous regression is anticipated within weeks after successful tumor therapy, with gonadotrophin levels returning to normal
- *PCOS:* Laparoscopic ovarian drilling (when medical methods such as clomiphene citrate fails)

Q6. Classify ovarian tumor.

Classification of ovarian tumor

- Epithelial tumor (60–70%)
  These tumors usually are benign, borderline malignant or malignant
  - Serous
  - Mucinous
  - Endometrioid tumors
  - Clear cell tumors
  - Brenner tumors
  - Mixed epithelial tumors
  - Undifferentiated carcinoma
  - Unclassified epithelial tumors
- Sex cord stromal tumors (6-10%)
  - Granulosa cell tumor
  - Tumors of thecoma and fibroma group
    - Thecoma
    - Fibroma
    - Unclassified

  - Androblastoma
    - Sertoli cell tumor
    - Sertoli Leydig cell tumor
    - Hilus cell tumor
  - Gynandroblastoma
  - Unclassified
- Germ cell tumors
  - Dysgerminoma
  - Endodermal carcinoma
  - Embryonal carcinoma
  - Polyembryoma
  - Choriocarcinoma
  - Teratoma
    - Immature
    - Mature (Dermoid cyst)
    - Monodermal (Struma ovarii and carcinoid)
  - Mixed forms
- Lipid cell tumors
- Gonadoblastoma
- Soft tissue tumors not specific to the ovary
- Unclassified tumors
- Secondary (metastatic) tumors

Q7. How will you differentiate between serous and mucinous tumors of the ovary?

Differences between serous and mucinous tumors of the ovary

Serous ovarian tumor	*Mucinous ovarian*
Benign form: Serous cyst adenoma Malignant form: Serous cyst adenocarcinoma	Benign form: Mucinous cyst adenoma Malignant form: Mucinous cyst adenocarcinoma
More common	Less common that serous tumor
Chance of malignancy in case of serous cyst adenoma is more (40%)	Chance of malignancy in case of mucinous cyst adenoma is less (5-10%)
The cysts are usually smaller than mucinous type	Mucinous cyst adenoma accounts to be the largest benign ovarian tumor
The wall is smooth, shiny and greyish white	The wall is smooth, lobulated with whitish on bluish white hue
The content of the fluid is clear, rich in serum proteins—albumin and globulin	The content of the fluid is thick, viscid and mucin
Lined by single layer of cubical epithelium	Lining is single layer of tall columnar epithelium

Q8. Name 4 common types of benign ovarian tumor.

Common benign ovarian tumor

- Mucinous cyst adenoma
- Serous cyst adenoma
- Dermoid cyst
- Brenner tumor
- Endometrioid tumors
- Clear cell tumors

Q9. What are the solid tumors of the ovary?

Solid tumors of the ovary

- Krukenberg tumor
- Granulosa cell tumor
- Thecoma
- Malignant teratoma
- Fibroma

Q10. Name the hormone producing tumors of the ovary.

Hormone producing ovarian tumor

- Granulosa cell and theca cell tumor
- Sertoli- Leydig and Hilus cell tumor
- Struma ovarii (thyroid hormones)
- Choriocarcinoma

Nice to know

- Conditions where we get follicular cysts of ovary
    - Metropathia hemorrhagica
    - Polycystic ovary disease
    - Associated fibroid
- Conditions where we get Lutein cysts of ovary
    - Hydatidiform mole
    - Choriocarcinoma
    - Multiple pregnancy
    - Patients receiving chorionic gonadotrophin

Nice to know

- Etiological factors for ovarian malignancy
    - Family history of two or more affected first-degree relatives
    - Nulliparity
    - Infertility
    - Late menopause
    - Early menarche
    - Ovulation inducing drug users
    - Streak gonad in Turner's syndrome
    - Unknown

Q11. How will you manage a case of benign ovarian tumor?

Management of benign ovarian tumor

- **Diagnosis**
    - Clinical features
        - Patients profile
            - Mainly in late childbearing period. But, dermoid (90%) specially with mucinous cyst adenoma is more common in reproductive period
            - Not related with parity of the patient
        - Symptoms

          Most tumors are asymptomatic. Presenting symptoms may be
            - Lower abdominal heaviness
            - Mass gradually increasing in size
            - Lower abdominal pain dull aching in nature

- In neglected cases, the size of tumor is not large to produce any cardiorespiratory symptoms or GI symptoms like nausea or indigestion
- Menstrual pattern remains unaffected

- Signs
  General examination
  - General condition remains unaffected
  - The patients may be cachectic (in huge mucinous cystadenoma)
  - Pitting oedema of legs may be present (when a huge tumor presses on the great veins)
- Abdominal examination
  - Inspection
    - Bulging of the lower abdomen
    - The mass may be placed centrally or in one side
    - The flanks remain flat
- Palpation
  The mass may be
    - Size : Variable
    - Consistency : Cystic or tense cystic
    - Surface : Smooth
    - Margin : Well-defined
    - Mobility : Mobile in all directions
    - Tenderness : Non-tender

- *Percussion:* The lump will be dull on percussion and the flanks will be resonant (In ascites-just the opposite)
- *Auscultation:* A friction rub may be present over the tumor
- *Pelvic examination:* Bimanual examination
  - The uterus is separated from the mass.
  - A groove is felt between the uterus and the mass.
  - Movement of the mass per abdomen fails to move the cervix.
  - On elevation of the mass per abdomen, the cervix remains in stationary position.
  - The lower pole of the cyst can be felt through the fornix.
  - Absence of pulsation uterine vessels from fornices.

Investigations

- For diagnosis
  - Ultrasonography
  - Tumor marker: CA 125 (for exclusion of malignancy)
  - CT scan
  - MRI (not routinely done but it can be helpful for determining whether the cyst is benign or malignant)
  - Laparoscopy (for differentiation of a painful cystic mass and a disturbed ectopic pregnancy)
  - Plain X-ray of whole abdomen over the tumor
  - Laparotomy (if inconclusive clinical diagnosis)
  - Cytology (if ascites or pleural effusion)
- Routine investigations
  Done pre-operatively to make the patient fit for anesthesia
  - Blood for Hb%, TC, DC, ESR
  - Blood grouping and Rh typing
  - Urine R/M/E
  - X-ray chest P/A view
  - ECG
  - Random creatinine

Treatment

Laparotomy and planning of surgery which depends on age, parity and nature of the tumor. Surgery-definitive

- In young patients
  - Ovarian cystectomy leaving behind the healthy ovarian tissue is the operation of choice.
  - Ovariotomy (salpingo-oophorectomy) is reserved for a big tumor that has destroyed almost all the ovarian tissues or for a gangrenous cyst.
  - If both the ovaries are involves, ovarian cystectomy should be done at least in one ovary.
- In parous women around 40 years
  Total abdominal hysterectomy with bilateral salpingo-oophorectomy

Q12. Write a short note on dermoid cyst.

Dermoid cyst

- *Origin:* Arises from the germ cells arrested after the first meiotic division.
- *Pathology:*
  - Constitutes about 97% of teratoma
  - Incidence is about 30-40% amongst ovarian tumor and constitutes about 20-40% of all ovarian tumors in pregnancy.
  - Torsion is the most common (15-20%) and rupture is an uncommon (1%) complication
  - Chance of malignancy is about 1-2%. Squamous cell carcinoma is the commonest
- *Characteristics:*
  - Commonly occurs at relatively early and may complicate pregnancy
  - This tumor is usually uniocular but may contain a few locules
  - The capsule is thick, smooth and greyish yellow in color (yellow is due to the presence of sebaceous material within it)
  - The tumor has a long pedicle and so there is more chance of torsion
  - This tumor is usually felt through the anterior fornix.

Q13. Write down the macroscopic and microscopic findings of dermoid cyst.

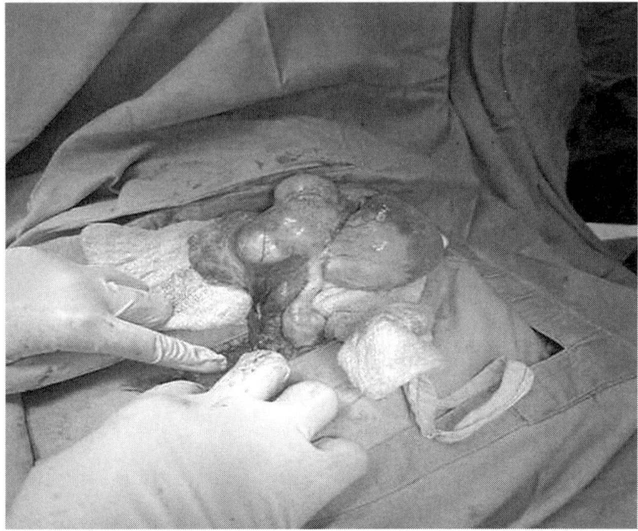

Macroscopic findings of dermoid cyst

- *Size:* Moderate
- The capsule is thick, smooth greenish yellow in color
- On cut section, the content is a predominantly sebaceous material with hair.

- There may be clear fluid (cerebrospinal fluid) derived from the neural tissues (choroid plexus)
- There is one area of solid projection called 'Rokitansky's protuberance' which is covered by skin with sweat and sebaceous glands. It is here teeth and bones are found.

Microscopic findings of dermoid cyst

- The wall is lined by stratified squamous epithelium; and at places by granulation tissue. The epithelium may be transitional or columnar
- The most common tissue elements are ectodermal.

Q14. What is risk malignancy index (RMI)?

The RMI is a scoring system which is used to predict whether an ovarian mass is benign or malignant. There are two scoring systems RMI 2, each of which calculates scores using ultrasound features, menopausal status, and preoperative CA-125 level according to the equation:
RMI score = Ultrasound score × menopausal sore × CA-125 level U/mL.

Q15. Which RMI should be used?

A systematic review of diagnostic studies concluded that the RMI I is the most effective and should be used for women with suspected ovarian cancer (RCOG 2011).

CHAPTER 18

Precancerous Lesions of Cervix: Cervical Intraepithelial Neoplasia

Q1. Enumerate the benign lesions of the cervix.

Benign lesions of the cervix:

1. Cervical ectopy (erosion)
2. Eversion (ectropion)
3. Cervical tear
4. Cervical cysts:
   a. Nabothian cysts
   b. Endometriotic cysts
   c. Mesonephric cysts
5. Elongation of the cervix (congenital and supravaginal)

Q2. Write down some pathological conditions of cervix:

Pathological conditions of the cervix:

1. Inflammation
   - Chronic cervicitis
   - Acute cervicitis
2. Benign lesions
   - Cervical ectopy (erosion)
   - Eversion (ectropion)
   - Cervical tear
   - Cervical cysts
   - Elongation of the cervix
3. Premalignant lesion
   a. Squamous cell metaplasia
   b. Basal cell hyperplasia
   c. Cervical intraepithelial neoplasia (CIN)
4. Cervical polyp
5. Neoplasms (benign)
   a. Leiomyoma of uterus
   b. Others papilloma
6. Neoplasms (malignant)
   a. Sq cell carcinoma
   b. Adenocarcinoma
   c. Sarcoma
   d. Melanoma

Q3. Enumerate the common cervical pathology encountered in gynae OPD.

Common cervical pathology encountered in gyne OPD:

1. Cervical erosion/ectopy
2. Chronic cervicitis
3. Cervical polyp
4. Cervical malignancy
5. Incompetence of cervix in pregnancy
6. Elongated cervix

Cervical Ectopy

Q1. Define cervical ectopy.

Cervical ectopy, known as cervical erosion, refers to a condition in which the squamous epithelium of the ectocervix is substituted by columnar epithelium that is continuous with the endocervix. It is not a sore.

Q2. What are the causes of cervical erosion?

Causes of cervical erosion:

1. Congenital
2. Acquired
   a. Use of hormone such as pills
   b. Pregnancy
   c. Infection

Q3. Describe the pathology of cervical erosion.

Pathological aspects of cervical erosion:

1. In cervical erosion, the squamous layer on the vaginal side of the cervix is substituted by columnar epithelium that is continuous with the lining of the endocervix.
2. It is not a region stripped of epithelium as the term suggests (misnomer). Microscopically observed small ulceration areas can sometimes result from secondary infections, local trauma, or may be artifacts.
3. An ectopy appears bright red with a distinctly defined border.

   The columnar epithelium can be structured in a regular formation, but it can also proliferate and group together to form a villous outgrowth – a papillary ectopy

   The columnar epithelium can be structured in a uniform pattern, but it may also proliferate and group together to form a villous outgrowth – a papillary ectopy.
4. Below the epithelium, the tissue frequently displays round cell infiltration and glandular growth.
5. Ectopy is a dynamic condition, and the boundary between the two types of epithelium shifts toward and away from the external os.

Q4. What are the clinical features of a case of cervical erosion and how will you manage it?

Management of cervical erosion:

- Diagnosis:
  - Symptoms
    1. Asymptomatic nearly all cases
    2. Vaginal discharge
    3. Post-coital bleeding
    4. Associated cervicitis may produce
       a. Backache
       b. Pelvic pain
       c. Infertility

- Signs

  Internal examination reveals

  a. Inspection: Bright red region that continuous with the endocervix and featuring a distinctly outlined outer boundary

  b. Palpation
- Non-tender—if no signs of infection: Multiple pinpoint areas may bleed if touched or rubbing with a swab
- Soft, granular feel and gives rise to a grating sensation when touched with finger tip

Treatment:

1. Asymptomatic caşes need no treatment.
2. In pregnancy and early puerperium treatment is not required. Reassessment is necessary after 12 weeks of puerperium.
3. Those who take pills, should be stopped and advised barrier method and reassessment after 3 months.
4. If erosion still persists, treatment should be given.

Treatment options are:

a. Electrocautery (mostly used)
b. Cryosurgery
c. Laser vaporization

Q5. Write a short note on cervical erosion.

Cervical erosion, or ectopy, is a benign condition in which the glandular epithelium from the cervical canal is present on the outer surface of the cervix. It commonly occurs under the influence of estrogen and may present with discharge or contact bleeding, though many cases remain asymptomatic.

Etiology/causes:

- High estrogen states (puberty, pregnancy)
- Use of oral contraceptive pills
- Chronic cervicitis
- Hormonal imbalance

Clinical features:

- Often asymptomatic
- Excessive mucoid vaginal discharge
- Postcoital bleeding
- Contact bleeding on examination

Examination findings:

- Red, velvety area around the external os
- May bleed on touch

Diagnosis:

- Clinical examination (per speculum)
- Pap smear (to exclude malignancy)
- Colposcopy if needed

Management:

- Usually no treatment if asymptomatic
- Treat underlying infection if present
- Ablative methods if symptomatic:
  - Cryotherapy
  - Cauterization (diathermy)
  - Laser therapy

Q6. Write a short note on ectropion.

Ectropion (outward turning).

In chronic cervicitis, substantial thickening of the cervical lining occurs alongside swelling in the underlying tissue. These condensed tissues frequently bulge through the external os along the route of minimal resistance.

The entity is most visible in areas where the cervix has been torn.

In these conditions, the longitudinal muscle fibers can operate without resistance. As a result, the cervix's edges curl upward and outward, exposing the red-tinged endocervix, resulting in ectropion/eversion.

Treatment: Trachelorrhaphy.

Cervical Intraepithelial Neoplasia

Q1. What is CIN?

Cervical intraepithelial neoplasia: CIN is a histological condition, where part or whole of the thickness of the thickness of the cervical squamous epithelium is replaced by varying degrees of atypical cells.

Q2. What are the types of CIN?

Types/grading of CIN:

- CIN-I in the basal third or less of the epithelium is filled with undifferentiated cells.
- CIN-II (Dysplasia of moderate severity): If the undifferentiated cells make up between one-third and two-thirds of the epithelium
- CIN-III (Severe dysplastic changes or carcinoma in situ): If over two-thirds of the thickness of the epithelium is filled with undifferentiated cells

Q3. What are the risk factors of CIN?

Risk factors of CIN:

1. Infection with HPV (16, 18, 31, 33 high risk HPV) HIV, chlamydia
2. STDs
3. First pregnancy at young age
4. Frequent births
5. Socioeconomic status-low
6. sexual partners-multiple
7. Immunosuppressed
8. Oral contraceptive users
9. smoking

Q4. What is Pre-invasive carcinoma of the cervix?

Carcinoma in situ of the cervix (CIS)/Pre-invasive cervical carcinoma.

Pre-invasive carcinoma of the cervix refers to the situation where neoplastic, abnormal cells are limited to the epithelial layers of the cervix and do not penetrate the basement membrane.

Q5. Give a pathological picture of carcinoma cervix in situ.

Pathological picture of carcinoma in situ of cervix:

a. Epithelial layer-affected
b. Loss of stratification
c. Cells vary in size and shape
d. The nuclei exhibit intense staining with frequent mitosis and an unusual chromatin arrangement.
e. The nuclei are oversized and hyperchromatic with minimal cytoplasm.
f. The basement membrane stays permeable

Q6. How will you manage a case of CIN?

Management of CIN/carcinoma in situ of cervix

- Diagnosis
  - Clinical features
    - CIN are symptomless conditions which may show no naked-eye signs of their presence
    - Incidentally diagnosed during routine screening by cervical cytology (pap smear) or colposcopy
    - The affected cervix usually looks remarkably healthy
  - Investigation:
    a. Cervical smear for cytology
    b. Colposcopy
    c. Cervical biopsy
       - Cone biopsy
       - Punch biopsy
    d. Schiller's test

Treatment

Treatment option depend on:

- Patient age
- CIN-nature
- Future fertility desired

Treatment of CIN according to grading.

- CIN I: Pap's smear should be done and follow up at 6 months or should do HPV DNA test at every 12 months
- CIN II: Commonly treated with Large loop (electrosurgical) excision of transformation zone (LLLETZ)
- CIN III: Treated by local ablative methods
  - Cryotherapy
  - Electrodiathermy
  - Cold coagulation
  - Laser vaporization

Q7. How CIN can be prevented?

Prevention of CIN:

1. The bivalent HPV vaccine (Cervarix) protects against 90% of cervical cancer cases caused by types 16 and 18.
2. To delay sexual activity until the cervical epithelium, especially in the transformation zone, has attained physiological maturity.
3. Proper hygiene to avoid vaginal infections
4. Barrier method should be used in early sexual life

CHAPTER 19

Cervical Cancer

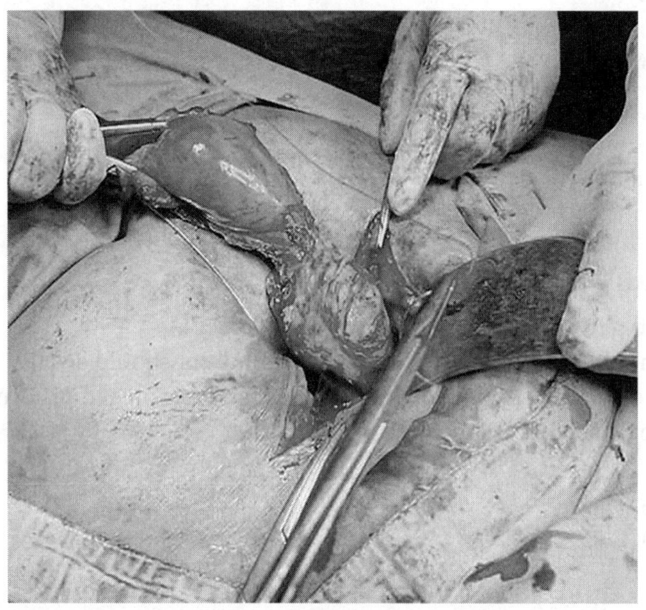

Courtesy: BMU Department of obstetrics and gynecology.

Q1. Which of the female genital tract cancer is common in Bangladesh?

Carcinoma cervix.

Q2. What are the common gynecological malignancy?

Common gynecological malignancy

i. Carcinoma cervix
ii. Malignancy ovarian tumor
iii. Choriocarcinoma

Q3. What are the types of carcinoma cervix?

Types/Pathological types/Histopathological types of Ca cervix

i. Squamous cell carcinoma (90%)
ii. Adenocarcinoma (5%)
iii. Mixed (5%) such as adeno-squamous variety

Q4. What are the risk factors for Ca cervix?

Risk factors/predisposing factors of carcinoma cervix

i. Early marriage and early sexual intercourse
ii. Early age of first pregnancy

iii. Too many and too frequent child birth
iv. Low socio-economic condition
v. Multiple sexual partners
vi. Sexually transmitted disease (STD) like HPV (16, 18, 31, 33), HIV and chlamydia infection
vii. Immunosuppressed (HIV positive) individuals
viii. Husband, whose previous wife died of cervical carcinoma
ix. Oral pill user
x. Smoking habits

Etiological factors of carcinoma cervix

i. Unknown
ii. HPV infection (16, 18, 31, 33)
iii. HIV and chlamydia infection
iv. Long term OCP use
v. Race: More in Hindus
vi. Low socio-economic condition

Q5. How carcinoma cervix spread?

Mode of spread of carcinoma cervix

a. By direct extension
    - The growth spread directly to the adjacent structures, to the vagina and to the body of the uterus.
    - It extends laterally to the parametrium, paracervical and paravaginal tissues
    - It may spread backwards along the uterosacral ligament, to involve the rectum or forwards to involve the base of the bladder
b. By lymphatics
    - The primary group involved are
        i. Parametrial nodes
        ii. Internal iliac nodes
        iii. Obturator nodes
        iv. External iliac nodes
        v. Sacral nodes
    - The secondary group involved are
        i. Common iliac group
        ii. Inguinal nodes para-aortic nodes
c. By blood stream
    - Blood borne metastasis is late and usually by veins rather than the arteries,
    - Lungs, liver or bone are usually involved
d. By direct implantation

    Direct implantation of the cancer cells at operation on the vault of the vagina or abdominal or perineal wound is very rare.

Q6. What are the stages of carcinoma cervix?

0	Tumor confined to the surface layer (the cell lining) of the cervix; also called carcinoma in situ.
I	Extension deeper into the cervix with no spread beyond (extension to the corpus is disregarded)
IA	Invasive carcinoma; may only be diagnosed at microscopy
IA1	Stromal invasion ≤3
IA2	Stromal invasion >3.0 mm and ≤5 mm
IB	Clinically visible lesions limited to the cervix uteri or preclinical cancers higher than stage IA
IB1	Stromal invasion >5 mm and ≤2 cm
IB2	Stromal invasion >2 cm and ≤4 cm
IB3	Stromal invasion >4 cm

II	Cervical carcinoma extends beyond the uterus but not to the pelvic wall or the lower one-third of the vagina
IIA	Upper 2/3rd of vagina
IIA1	Invasive carcinoma ≤4 cm in greatest dimension
IIA2	Invasive carcinoma >4 cm in greatest dimension
IIB	With obvious parametrial invasion
III	Extension to the pelvic wall, involvement of lower one-third of the vagina, or hydronephrosis or nonfunctioning kidney
IIIA	Involvement of lower one-third of the vagina with no extension to the pelvic wall
IIIB	Extension to the pelvic wall, hydronephrosis, or nonfunctioning
IIIC	Kidney
IIIC1	Pelvic lymph nodes metastasis
IIIC2	Para aortic lymph node metastasis.
IV	Extension beyond the true pelvis or involvement of the bladder or rectal Mucosa (biopsy proved); bullous edema does not convey stage IV disease
IVA	Spread to adjacent organs
IVB	Spread to distant organs

Q7. How can you diagnose early carcinoma cervix?

Diagnosis of early carcinoma cervix

- Patient profile
  Mean age is 38-42 years
- Symptoms
  a. Asymptomatic (majority)
  b. Blood stained vaginal discharge
  c. Intermenstrual bleeding
  d. Post coital or postmenopausal bleeding
- Sings
  - General examination
    a. Anemia may be present
    b. Cachexia may be present
  - Per abdominal examination
    Usually normal findings
  - Per vaginal examination
    a. Cervix may look unhealthy
    b. Cervical erosion or cervicitis may be present
- Investigation:
  Colposcopy guided biopsy and histopathology

Q8. How will you manage a case of carcinoma cervix?

Management of Ca Cervix

- Diagnosis
- Patient profile
  a. Usually multiparous, in premenopausal age group
  b. Previous H/O postcoital or intermenstrual bleeding
- Symptoms
  a. Irregular vaginal bleeding
  b. Watery vaginal discharge (may be blood stained, having foul smell)
  c. Post coital bleeding

d. Urinary symptoms
    - Dysuria
    - Frequency of micturition
    - Urinary incontinence
e. Rectal pain
f. Backache
g. Oedema of the legs
h. Loss of weight

- Signs
  A. General examination
     a. Anemia
     b. Cachexia
     c. Oedema
  B. Abdominal examination
     This may reveal enlarged uterus in case of
     - Pyometra
     - Hematometra
     - Associated fibroid
     - Associated pregnancy
     - Associated pregnancy
  C. Vaginal examination
     a. Speculum examination
        May reveal the cervix to be
        - Enlarged and irregular b
        - Ulcerated and excavated
        - Completely destroyed
        - Replaced by hypertrophic mass
        - Bleeding on touch
     b. Bimanual examination
        May reveal
        - Cervix
          - Enlarged
          - Fixed, hard, friable and bleeds on touch (Cardinal signs of Ca Cervix)
        - Vagina
          - Involvement of fornices, upper parts or lower parts of the walls
          - The parametrical tissue and lateral pelvic wall may be involved
     c. Rectal examination
        - To excluded rectal mucosal involvement
        - To see the extent of the disease in the pelvis

- Investigations
  a. Pap's smear
  b. Colposcopy
  c. Cervical biopsy (confirmatory)
  d. To see the extent of the disease
     i. Chest X-ray (lung involvement)
     ii. IVU (Ureteric involvement)
     iii. Cystoscopy (bladder involvement)
     iv. Sigmoidoscopy (rectal involvement)

Treatment modalities

1. Surgery (Radical/ Wertheim's hysterectomy) : Up to stage IIA
2. Radiotherapy: All stages
3. Surgery followed by radiotherapy
4. Radiotherapy followed by surgery
5. Combined radiotherapy and chemotherapy: Advanced stage
6. Palliative treatment: Advanced stage

Treatment of carcinoma cervix according to staging

1. Stage IA
   a. Stage IA_1 without LVSI (lymphovascular space invasion):
      - Cone biopsy if fertility is desirable
      - Extrafascial hysterectomy if family is complete
   b. Stage IA_1 with LVSI and stage IA_2 :
      - Modified radical hysterectomy and pelvic lymphadenectomy.
      - Intracavity radiation in a medically unfit patient.
   i. Stage IB_1 & IIA
   Radical hysterectomy with pelvic lymphadenectomy followed by adjuvant radiotherapy with or without chemotherapy.
   ii. Stage IIB and beyond (stage IIB – stage IV)
      a. Primary external beam radiation plus brachytherapy is the gold standard.
      b. Neoadjuvant chemotherapy before radiation.
      c. Concurrent chemoradiation.

Q9. Name the types of surgery which are done in early-stage disease?
Stage IA1: Conization (when fertility desired) or total-hysterectomy.
Stage 1A2-IIA: Radical hysterectomy with bilateral pelvic lymphadenectomy.
Stage 1A2-1B1 (when fertility desired): Radical trachelectomy.

Q10. When will you consider radiotherapy following surgery?
If surgical pathology reveals positive lymph nodes, involvement of parametrium, or positive margins, postoperative chemoradiation is required. Postoperative radiation therapy is also recommended in patients who have at least two intermediate risk factors [including tumor size >2 cm, deep stromal invasion, or lymphovascular space invasion (LVSI)].
For patients with IB2 or IIA cancer and selected in most cases. Many of these patients will meet either intermediate- or high-risk criteria after radical hysterectomy and therefore are strong candidates for this approach.

Q11. If she is unfit for surgery, how do you treat her?
Combined external beam radiation with brachytherapy and/or chemotherapy.

Q12. If she is having advanced stage disease (say stage IIIB), how do you treat her?
By chemoradiotherapy, external bean radiation therapy shrinks the central tumor and treats regional lymph nodes. This therapy is followed by brachytherapy. Chemotherapy is usually given with radiation therapy, to sensitize the tumor to radiation.

Q13. Why chemoradiation is better than radiotherapy alone?
National Cancer Institute (NCI) in US in 1999 identified a large survival advantage for the administration of concurrent chemotherapy with radiotherapy. The benefits of chemoradiotherapy over radiotherapy alone were further confirmed in a Cochrane meta-analysis. Weekly cisplatin during radiotherapy has been studied in more advanced stage.

Q14. What are the cardinal signs of carcinoma cervix?

Cardinal signs of Ca Cervix

a. Fixed
b. Hard
c. Friable
d. Bleeds on touch

Q15. What are the complications of carcinoma cervix?

Complications of CA Cervix

a. Pyometra
b. Vesicovaginal and vesicocervical fistulas
c. Rectovaginal fistula
d. Hydronephrosis and pyonephrosis
e. Uremia

Q16. What are the causes of death in carcinoma cervix?

Causes of death in Ca Cervix

a. Uremia
b. Hemorrhage
c. Sepsis
d. Cachexia
e. Metastases to the distant organs:
   - Lung (36%)
   - Lymph nodes (30%)
   - Bone (16%)
   - Abdominal cavity (7%)

Q17. What are the differential diagnosis of carcinoma cervix?

Differential diagnosis of Ca Cervix

a. Cervical tuberculosis
b. Syphilitic ulcer
c. Cervical ectopy
d. Chronic cervicitis
e. Fibroid polyp
f. Products of conception in incomplete abortion

Q18. What are the complications of radiotherapy in the treatment of carcinoma cervix?

Radiotherapy treatment of Ca Cervix

- Treatment of choice in majority cases and applicable for all stages of the disease.
- It aims at giving a cancericidal dose of gamma-rays to all areas where there is growth or there is likely to be growth.
- Radiation Techniques
  a. Teletherapy (external bean radiation)
  b. Brachytherapy (Intracavity therapy)
- Pre-requisites of radiotherapy
  a. From examination
     Anemia and PID are to be excluded
  b. Investigations
     Should confirm:
     a. Hemoglobin level more than 10 gm%

b. Total WBC count more than 3000/cu mm
c. Platelet count more than 1,00000/cu mm

- Complications of radiotherapy
  - Early effects
    1. Enteritis
    2. Proctosigmoiditis
    3. Cystitis
    4. Vulvitis
    5. Bone marrow depression
    6. Diarrhea
  - Delayed effects
    1. Chronic proctosigmoiditis
    2. Hemorrhagic cystitis
    3. Small and large bowel strictures
    4. RVF and VVF
    5. Pelvic fibrosis
    6. Loss of ovarian function

Q19. How can you prevent carcinoma cervix?

Prevention of carcinoma cervix

A. Primary Prevention
   i. Health education
   ii. Identification of the high risk group
   iii. Prophylactic HPV vaccine (Cervarix)
   iv. Use of condom during early intercourse
      - Raising the age of marriage and of first birth
      - Limitation of family
      - Maintenance of local hygiene and effective therapy of STD

B. Secondary prevention: By screening procedures

Q20. What is the recent advance in prevention of carcinoma cervix?

Recent advance in prevention of carcinoma cervix

Prophylactic recombinant HPV vaccine (cervarix) is the recent advancer in prevention of carcinoma cervix.

- Cervarix is a bivalent vaccine against HPV 16, 18 in Bangladesh used in girls and women in 10-45 years of age.
- It should be used ideally before potential exposure to HPV through sexual contact or who have not vaccinated. This vaccine reduce the incidence of HPV related cervical and genital cancer
- Intramuscular injection of 0.5 mL vaccine is given at 0, 1 and 6 months

Q21. What are the screening tests available for carcinoma cervix?

Screening procedures of carcinoma cervix

a. Pap's smear (cytodiagnosis)
b. Visual inspection of the cervix
   i. Unaided: Down staging
   ii. Aided:
      - With Acetic acid (VIA)
      - With Lugol's iodine (Schiller's test)
   iii. Colposcopy
   iv. HPV DNA testing

Importance of cervical cancer screening

a. Prevention if Ca cervix
b. Early diagnosis of Ca cervix and CIN
c. Formulation of line of treatment in case of CIN

Q22. What is the treatment of carcinoma cervix with pregnancy?

Treatment of carcinoma cervix with pregnancy

1. Role of radiotherapy
   - During the first half of pregnancy: Application of radium will kill the fetus resulting in spontaneous abortion. Thereafter full dose of radiotherapy can be applied.
   - During the second half of pregnancy: Pregnancy is to be terminated by abdominal hysterectomy. Then it is flowed by radiotherapy.
   - If the pregnancy is advanced: Radiotherapy can be deferred till fetus becomes mature. Thereafter case section can be followed by radiotherapy.
2. Role of surgery
   During early weeks of gestation, Wertheim's hysterectomy can be performed with pregnancy in situ.

Q23. What do you mean by stump carcinoma?

Stump carcinoma

Carcinoma developed in the cervical stump after subtotal hysterectomy is called carcinoma.

Treatment

Radiotherapy is the treatment of choice.

CHAPTER 20

Ovarian Malignancy

Q1. What are the causes of enlargement of ovaries?

Causes of enlargement of ovary

1. Hypertrophy (congenital and acquired)
2. Corpus luteum hematoma
3. Ovarian pregnancy
4. Oophoritis (Acute or chronic)
5. Endometriosis
6. Lutein cysts and luteoma of pregnancy
7. Distension or retention cyst
8. Primary ovarian neoplasms (Benign or malignant)
9. Secondary (metastatic) neoplasms

Q2. What are the functional cysts of ovary?

Classification of ovarian cyst

1. Functional cyst/cystic ovary
   a. Follicular cysts
   b. Corpus luteum cyst
   c. Theca lutein and granulosa lutein cysts
   d. Polycystic ovarian syndrome
2. Non-functional cyst
   Endometrial cyst (chocolate cyst)

Q3. How can you diagnose a functional cyst in ovary?

Symptoms and signs of follicular cyst of ovary

1. Asymptomatic (majority)
2. Polymenorrhea and polymenorrhagia
3. Amenorrhea
4. Infertility
5. Pain in the iliac fossa
6. Usually, multiple and small
7. Unilocular
8. Contains clear fluid inside unless hemorrhage occurs.

Q4. How can you differentiate between cystic ovary and ovarian cysts?

Differences between cystic ovary and ovarian cyst

Cystic ovary	*Ovarian cyst*
1. Non-neoplastic cyst. (Also called functional cysts of the ovary)	Neoplastic cyst (Benign or malignant)
2. Usually 6–8 m in diameter	May be of any size (Mucinous cyst adenoma is the largest benign ovarian tumor)
3. Usually asymptomatic	Symptomatic/asymptomatic
4. Spontaneous regression occurs usually following correction of the functional disturbances to which it is related	Spontaneous regression does not occur
5. Contains clear fluid inside unless hemorrhage occurs	May contain serous or mucinous fluid
6. Lining epithelium corresponds to the functional epithelium of the unit from which it arises	Arises from the totipotent surface epithelium of the ovary and lined by columnar or cubical epithelium

Q5. How will you treat a case of functional cyst of ovary?

Treatment of functional ovarian cysts

1. Follicular cysts
   a. Follicular cyst ≤5 cm: Requires no further investigations
   b. Simple cyst 8 cm, unilocular, echo free without solid areas or papillary projections, with normal serum CA 125: Follow up with repeat ultrasound in 3 to 6 months time
   c. Persisting or growing cyst: Removal of cyst by laparoscopy/laparotomy
2. Corpus luteum cysts
   a. In uncomplicated cases
      Spontaneous cases regression is expected
   b. In complicated cases
      Laparotomy with enucleation of the cyst along with resuscitation (if features of acute abdomen occur)
3. Lutein cysts
   Spontaneous regression is expected within few weeks following effective therapy of the tumors with the gonadotrophin level returning back to normal.
4. Polycystic ovarian syndrome
   Laparoscopic ovarian drilling (when medical methods such as clomiphene citrate fails)

Q6. Classify ovarian tumor.

Classification of ovarian tumor

1. Epithelial tumor (60–70%)
   Theses tumors may be benign, borderline malignant or malignant
   a. Serous tumor
   b. Mucinous tumor
   c. Endometrioid tumors
   d. Clear cell tumors
   e. Brenner tumors
   f. Mixed epithelial tumors
   g. Undifferentiated carcinoma
   h. Unclassified epithelial tumors
2. Sex cord stromal tumors (6–10%)
   a. Granulosa cell tumors
   b. Tumors of thecoma-fibroma group
      - Thecoma
      - Fibroma
      - Unclassified

c. Androblastoma
- Sertoli cell tumor
- Sertoli Leydig cell tumor
- Hilus cell tumor

d. Gynandroblastoma
e. Unclassified

3. Germ cell tumors
a. Dysgerminoma
b. Endodermal sinus tumor
c. Embryonal carcinoma
d. Polyembryoma
e. Choriocarcinoma
f. Teratoma
- Immature
- Mature (dermoid cyst)
- Monodermal (Struma ovarii and carcinoma)

g. Mixed forms

4. Lipid cell tumors
5. Gonadoblastoma
6. Soft tissue tumors not specific to the ovary
7. Unclassified tumors
8. Secondary (metastatic) tumors

Q7. How will you differentiate between serous and mucinous tumors of the ovary?

Differences between serous and mucinous tumors of the ovary

Serous ovarian tumor	*Mucinous ovarian tumor*
1. Benign form: Serous cyst adenoma Malignant: Serous cyst adenocarcinoma	Benign from: Mucinous cyst Adenoma Malignant: Mucinous cyst adenocarcinoma
2. More common	Less common than serous tumor
3. Chance of malignancy in case of serous cyst adenoma is more (40%)	Chance of malignancy in case of mucinous cyst adenoma is less (5-10%)
4. The cysts are not so big as that of mucinous type	Mucinous cyst adenoma is the largest benign ovarian tumor
5. The wall is smooth, shiny and greyish white	The wall is smooth, lobulated with whitish on bluish white hue
6. The content of the fluid is clear, rich in serum proteins-albumin and globulin	The content of the fluid is thick, viscid and mucin
7. Lined by single layer of cubical epithelium	Lined by single layer of tall columnar epithelium

Q8. Name 4 common types of benign ovarian tumor.

Common benign ovarian tumor

1. Mucinous cyst adenoma
2. Serous cyst adenoma
3. Dermoid cyst
4. Brenner tumor
5. Endometrioid tumor
6. Clear cell tumors

Q9. What are the solid tumors of the ovary?

Solid tumors of the ovary

1. Krukenberg tumor
2. Granulosa cell tumor
3. Thecoma
4. Malignant teratoma
5. Fibroma

Q10. Name the hormone producing tumors of the ovary.

Hormone producing ovarian tumor

1. Granulosa cell and theca cell tumor
2. Sertoli–Leydig and Hilus cell tumor
3. Struma ovarii (thyroid hormones)
4. Choriocarcinoma

- Conditions where we get follicular cysts ovary
  1. Metropathia hemorrhagica
  2. Polycystic ovary disease
  3. Associated fibroid
- Conditions where we get Lutein cysts of ovary
  1. Hydatidiform mole
  2. Choriocarcinoma
  3. Multiple pregnancy
  4. Patients receiving chorionic gonadotrophin
- Etiological factors for ovarian malignancy
  1. Family history of two or more affected first-degree relatives
  2. Nulliparity
  3. Infertility
  4. Late menopause
  5. Early menarche
  6. Ovulation inducing drug users
  7. Streak gonad in Turner's syndrome
  8. Unknown

Q11. How will you manage a case of benign ovarian tumor?

Management of benign ovarian tumor

- Diagnosis
  1. Clinical features
     a. Patient profile
        1. Mainly observed during the later stages of childbearing. Nonetheless, dermoid (90%), particularly with mucinous cyst adenoma, frequently occurs during the reproductive stage
        2. Not related with parity of the patient

Symptoms

Most tumors are asymptomatic. The patient may present with:

i. Feeling of heaviness in lower abdomen
ii. A mass of increasing in size in lower abdomen
iii. Dull aching pain
iv. If not treated in time the tumor may be big enough to fill whole abdomen producing cardiorespiratory symptoms or gastrointestinal symptoms like nausea or indigestion
v. No menstrual abnormality

Signs

General examination

i. The patient's overall condition is unaffected.
ii. Cachexia may be observed in cases of large mucinous cystadenoma.
iii. Pitting oedema of the legs may be present if a large tumor is compressing the great veins.

Abdominal examination

- Inspection
  i. The lower abdomen may appear swollen.
  ii. The mass may be positioned in the center or on one side.
  iii. The flanks remain flat.
- Palpation
  The mass may have the following characteristics:
  i. Size: Variable
  ii. Consistency: Cystic or tense cystic
  iii. Surface: Smooth
  iv. Margin: Well-defined
  v. Mobility: Mobile in all directions
  vi. Tenderness: Non-tender
- Percussion
  The lump is dull on percussion, while the flanks are resonant.
  (In cases of ascites, this is the opposite.)
- Auscultation
  A friction rub may be heard over the tumor.
- Pelvic examination
  Bimanual examination
  i. The uterus is separated from the mass.
  ii. A groove is felt between the uterus and the mass.
  iii. Movement of the mass from the abdomen does not move the cervix.
  iv. When the mass is elevated from the abdomen, the cervix remains stationary.
  v. The lower pole of the cyst can be felt through the fornix.
  vi. There is no pulsation of the uterine vessels through the fornices.
- Investigations
  - For diagnosis
    i. Ultrasonography
    ii. Tumor marker: CA 125 (to rule out malignancy)
    iii. CT scan
    iv. MRI (not routinely done, but helpful in determining whether the cyst is likely to be benign or malignant)
    v. Laparoscopy (to differentiate a painful cystic mass from an ectopic pregnancy)
    vi. Plain X-ray of the abdomen over the tumor
    vii. Laparotomy (if clinical and ancillary investigations fail to diagnose the mass)
    viii. Cytology (when the patient presents with ascites or pleural effusion)
- Routine investigations
  These are carried out pre-operatively to ensure the patient is fit for anesthesia
  i. Blood tests for hemoglobin percentage, total count, differential count, ESR
  ii. Blood grouping and Rh typing
  iii. Urine routine and microscopy
  iv. Chest X-ray (posteroanterior view)
  v. ECG
  vi. Random blood sugar
  vii. Serum creatinine

- Treatment
  Laparotomy is performed along with planning of surgery, which depends on the patient's age, parity, and the nature of the tumor.

Definitive surgery

1. In young patients
   - Ovarian cystectomy, preserving healthy ovarian tissue, is the preferred operation.
   - Ovariotomy (salpingo-oophorectomy) is reserved for large tumors that have destroyed most of the ovarian tissue or for gangrenous cysts.
   - If both ovaries are involved, ovarian cystectomy should be performed at least in one ovary.
2. In parous women around 40 years
   Total abdominal hysterectomy with bilateral salpingo-oophorectomy.

Q12. Write a short note on dermoid cyst.

Dermoid cyst

- Origin: These cysts develop from germ cells that stop developing after the first meiotic division.
- Pathology:
  - They make up approximately 97% of teratomas.
  - They occur in about 30–40% of ovarian tumors and account for about 20–40% of all ovarian tumors.
  - They are also responsible for about 20–40% of all ovarian tumors during pregnancy.
  - Torsion is the most common complication, occurring in 15–20% of cases, while rupture is a less common complication, affecting about 1% of cases.
  - The risk of malignancy is low, at around 1–2%.

Squamous cell carcinoma.

Q13. Write down the macroscopic and microscopic findings of dermoid cyst.

Macroscopic and microscopic findings of dermoid cyst

1. Size: Moderate
2. The capsule is thick, smooth greenish yellow color
3. On cut section, the content consist of sebaceous material with hair
4. There may be clear fluid which is derived from the neural tissue (choroid plexus)
5. Area of solid projection called 'Rokitansky's protuberance' that is covered by skin with sweat and sebaceous glands also teeth and bones are found.

Microscopic findings of dermoid cyst

1. The wall is covered by stratified squamous epithelium; and in some areas by granulation tissue. The epithelium can be columnar or transitional
2. The most common tissue elements—ectodermal

Q14. How will you manage a case of malignant ovarian tumor?

Management a case of malignant ovarian tumor?

Diagnosis

1. Patient profile
   a. Postmenopausal (60%) and premenopausal (20%)
   b. Nulliparous (Mostly)
   c. Family history may be present
2. Symptoms
   i. Asymptomatic in initial phases
   ii. Swift growth of the lower abdominal mass
   iii. Abdominal discomfort and distention

iv. Rapid weight loss
v. Respiratory difficulty (could be mechanical due to pleural effusion or ascites)

3. Signs
   a. General examination
      i. Patient is cachexic and anemic
      ii. Jaundice in late stage
      iii. Left supraclavicular lymph gland (Virchow's) may be palpable
      iv. Oedema of leg or vulva (characteristic of malignant tumor)
   b. Abdominal examination
      - Inspection
        The abdomen may be hugely enlarged or distended with shiny skin.
      - Palpation
        A mass is detected in the hypogastrium and may frequently occur bilaterally. It includes the following features:
        i. Consistency: Partly cystic, partly solid
        ii. Surface: Irregular
        iii. Margins: Well-defined margin
        iv. Fixity: Fixed to the surrounding structures
        v. Tenderness: Usually present
      - Liver may be enlarged, firm and nodular
      - Percussion examination dull over the tumor, and may be resonant due to overlying intestinal adhesions
   c. Vaginal examination
      - Yterus may be separated from the mass
      - Nodules may be felt through the posterior fornix.
      - POD—Nodule felt

Investigations

a. To confirm malignancy
   i. Cytological examination of pleural or ascitic fluid or cul-de-sac aspiration (to detect malignant cells)
   ii. Tumor markers
      - CA - 125 (>65 U/mL with a pelvic mass suggests malignancy)
      - CA - 19 - 9
      - CA - 15 - 3
      - OVXI
      - HE4
b. To identify the extent of lesion
   i. Chest X-ray (to exclude pleural effusion and chest metastasis)
   ii. Barium enema (to detect any lower bowel malignancy)
   iii. Cytological examination of thoracocentesis fluid.
   iv. Ultrasonography (to detect involvement of the omentum or contralateral)
   v. CT scan and MRI
   vi. Examination under anesthesia
   vii. uterine curettage for diagnosis
c. To detect the primary site
   i. X-ray Barium meal
   ii. Colonoscopy
   iii. Mammography
d. Routine investigations

Done pre-operatively to make the patient fit for anesthesia

i. Blood for Hb% TC < DC, ESR
ii. Blood grouping and Rh typing
iii. Random blood sugar
iv. Serum creatinine
v. Urine R/M/E
vi. Chest X-ray P/A view
vii. ECG

Treatment

- Definitive treatment: Irrespective of age and parity
  TAH with BLSO with infracolic omentectomy followed by chemotherapy
- If not operable:
  - Debulking (reduce the size of the tumor) followed by chemotherapy
  - If debulking not possible: Chemotherapy

Q15. How will you differentiate between benign and malignant ovarian tumor?

Differentiation between benign and malignant ovarian tumor

- From clinical examination

Points	***Benign***	***Malignant***
Patient profile 1. Age	Usually reproductive age	Extreme age (more young and more old)
Symptoms 2. Rapidity of growth	Slow	Rapid
Signs: G/ E 3. Pallor	Absent	Present
Signs: P/A 4. Consistency	Cystic	Solid or partly solid and partly cystic
5. Surface	Smooth	Irregular
6. Mobility	Mobile in all directions	Fixed to the surrounding structures
7. Tenderness	Non-tender	Usually tender
8. Ascites	Absent	Present
Distribution	Unilateral	Bilateral
Secondary deposits in pouch of Douglas	Absent	Present

- From laparotomy findings

Points	***Benign***	***Malignant***
1. Engorged blood vessels over the surface of ovary	Absent	Present
2. Abdominal Ascites	Absent	Present (often hemorrhagic)
3. On surface Exophytic growth	Absent	Present
4. Adhesions	Absent	Present
5. Cut section	Cystic	Solid and hemorrhagic areas
6. Peritoneal nodules	Absent	Present

Q16. Write down the findings of a case of malignant ovarian tumor.

From the following points malignancy can be suspected

1. Extreme age, i.e., more young and more old

2. Rapidly growing tumors
3. Solid, nodular and irregular tumors
4. Tumor associated with pain and tenderness
5. Bilateral distribution
6. Fixity of the tumor
7. Associated ascites
8. Oedema of the feet and vulva
9. Secondary deposits in pouch of Douglas

Q17. Write down the per operative findings of malignant ovarian tumor.

Signs of malignancy at laparotomy

1. At opening of the abdomen there may be presence of hemorrhage peritoneal fluid
2. Broken capsule
3. Engorged blood vessels over the surface of the ovary
4. Distribution-bilateral
5. Solidity of the tumor
6. Multiple secondary deposits over the peritoneum and pelvic structures
7. Adhesion with surrounding structures

Q18. What are the chemotherapeutic drugs used in the treatment of malignant ovarian tumor?

Chemotherapeutic drugs used in the treatment of malignant ovarian tumor

1. Cyclophosphamide
2. Cisplatin
3. Carboplatin
4. Adriamycin
5. Paclitaxel
6. Etoposide
7. Bleomycin
8. Doxorubicin
9. Vicristine

Q19. What do you mean by second look operation?

Second look operation

Second look operation either by laparoscopy or laparotomy done in patient with no evidence of persistent tumor after an interval of chemotherapy.

A second look procedure performed through laparoscopy or laparotomy in a patient showing no signs of remaining tumor after a course of chemotherapy.

- *Objectives/Significance*
  1. To verify "healing" and to cease chemotherapy
  2. To evaluate the reaction to chemotherapy
  3. To modify the medications when resistance is detected.
- *The results of a second look surgery could be:*
  1. Negative (both clinically and microscopically)
  2. Microscopically positive but clinically negative
  3. Positive (both clinically and microscopically)
     - **When to be done?**

     Second look operation either by laparoscopy or laparotomy done in patient with no evidence of persistent tumor after an interval of chemotherapy.

Q20. Write down the tumor markers used in investigating malignant ovarian tumor?

Tumor markers used in investigating malignant ovarian tumor

1. CA - 125
2. CA - 19 - 9
3. CA - 15 - 3
4. Carcinoembryonic antigen (CEA)
5. α-fetoprotein
6. Human chorionic gonadotrophin (hCG)
7. Lactic dehydrogenase (LDH)

Q21. What are the tumor markers of germ cell tumor?

Tumor markers of germ cell tumor

1. α-fetoprotein
2. hCG
3. lactic dehydrogenase (LDH)
4. CA - 125

A-fetoprotein and hCG are more commonly used.

PCOS

Q22. Define PCOS.

Polycystic ovary disease (PCOD)

Polycystic ovarian disease is manifested by amenorrhea, hirsutism, obesity and enlarged ovaries with multiple cyst which is associated with

- Androgen production is excessive
- Impaired ovarian follicular growth leading to anovulation

Stein Leventhal first described it in 1935. So it is also called Stein-Leventhal syndrome

Diagnostic criteria

Diagnosis according to the presence of any two of the following three criteria:

1. Oligo and/or anovulation
2. Hyperandrogenism (clinical and/or biochemical)
3. Polycystic ovaries, with the exclusion of the other etiologies

Clinical features

1. Menstrual abnormality: Oligomenorrhoea, amenorrhea
2. Infertility
3. Obesity
4. Hirsutism
5. Acanthosis nigricans
6. HAIR - AN syndrome
7. Vaginal examination usually

Investigations

1. Transvaginal sonography
   - Enlarged ovary with volume (≥ 10 cm^3)
   - No of follicle (>12) of peripherally arranged cysts (2-9 mm)
   - Transvaginal sonography in obese patient.
2. Serum LH elevated and LH:FSH is >3:1
3. Serum Androstenedione: Increased

4. Serum testosterone and DHEA-S: May be marginally elevate
5. Serum insulin level is raised (Fasting insulin may be >20 IU/mL)
6. Laparoscopy: Bilateral polycystic ovaries will be seen

Diagnostic criteria of PCOS according to Rotter dam (2003) 2 out of 3 required
1. Menstrual irregularity
2. Hyper androgens
3. USG polycystic ovary of exclusion of other etiology.

Management of PCOS
1. Lifestyle modifications.
2. Hormonal contraceptives
3. Spironolactone
4. Immediate: Correction
   - Hirsutism
   - Regulation of menses
   - Fertility issue
5. Long-term issue:
   - IR
   - CVS risk
   - Obstructive sleep
   - Malignancy

Pharmacological treatment for non-fertility indication:
1st line therapy
- COCS

2nd line therapy
- COC_1 with metformin
- COC_s with anti-androgen drugs
- Metformin alone.

Q23. What is krukenberg tumor?

Krukenberg tumor

Krukenberg tumor may be defined as a metastatic adenocarcinoma of the ovary.
- Primary sites
  1. Stomach
  2. Colon
  3. Gall bladder
  4. Breast
- Mode of spread lymphatic retrogression or through implantation from metastatic sites in the peritoneal cavity.
- Naked eye appearance
  1. Bilateral, solid with smooth surfaces and usually with shape of the ovary
  2. They usually create firm white masses that are rounded or kidney-shaped
  3. No tendency of adhesion (i.e., intact capsule)
  4. Cut surfaces show yellow or white in color cystic spaces at places because of degeneration.
- Histological appearance
  1. The stroma is highly cellular
  2. The mucin within epithelial cells compresses the nuclei to one pole, producing 'signet ring' appearance
  3. The scattered 'signet ring' looking cells are characteristic of krukenberg tumor.

Treatment

Oophorectomy followed by chemotherapy and treatment of the primary site.

Nice to Know

Meig's syndrome

It is a triad of findings including ascites, pleural effusion and benign ovarian fibroma

The causes is unknown

The ascites and pleural effusion resolve spontaneously when the ovarian tumor is removed.

CHAPTER 21

Endometrial Carcinoma and Endometrial Hyperplasia

ENDOMETRIAL CARCINOMA

Q1. What are the risk factors for development of endometrial carcinoma?

Risk factors related to endometrial carcinoma:

1. Delayed menopause
2. Parity—nulliparity
3. Only estrogen therapy
4. PCOS
5. Infrequent menstruation and excessive premenopausal bleeding
6. Obesity, and comorbidities like DM, HTN
7. Family history of breast, ovary, colon or endometrial cancer
8. Endometrial hyperplasia
9. Post-tamoxifen therapy
10. Menopause followed by radiation

Q2. What are the types of endometrial carcinoma?

Types/varieties of endometrial carcinoma (reference from doctor slide):

1. Adenocarcinoma (endometrioid 80%)
2. Adenocarcinoma with squamous elements
3. Papillary serous carcinoma (5–10%)
4. Mucinous adenocarcinoma (5%)
5. Clear cell adenocarcinoma (5%)
6. Secretory carcinoma (1%)
7. Squamous cell carcinoma
8. Mixed carcinoma

Nice to know:

Mode of spread of endometrial carcinoma

1. Direct: Infiltrate the myometrium and spread to the parametrium or into the peritoneal cavity. It could spread downward and involve the cervix in about 15% cases.
2. Lymphatic: Usually late stage involving pelvic, para-aortic and rarely inguinal and femoral nodes.
3. Hematogenous: Common sites of metastases are lungs, liver, bones and brain.

Q3. How will you manage a case of endometrial carcinoma?

Management of endometrial carcinoma

- Diagnosis
  1. Patient profile
     - Typically a nulliparous woman, probably postmenopausal
     - There might be a history of postponed menopause.
     - The patient could be overweight; probably suffering from hypertension or diabetes
  2. Symptoms
     - Bleeding after menopause (75%) that can be minimal, sporadic, or constant.
     - In women before menopause, there can be abnormal and heavy bleeding.
     - Sometimes, there is a discharge that is watery and foul-smelling because of pyometra.
     - Experiencing pain is fairly common
       - Few patients (<5%) remain asymptomatic
  3. Signs
     - General examination
       - Pallor of varying degree
       - Obesity
       - Hypertension
     - Pelvic examination
       a. Speculum examination
          - Cervix looking healthy
          - Blood or purulent offensive discharge from external os
       b. Bimanual examination
          The uterus can be atrophic, normal, or possibly enlarged due to tumor spread, associated fibroids, or pyometra.
          The uterus is typically movable, but becomes stationary in the later stages.
       c. Rectal examination: Supports the findings from the bimanual assessment

Investigations
1. Endometrial biopsy
2. Papanicolaou smear
3. Ultrasound and color Doppler (TVS)
4. Hysteroscopy
5. Fractional curettage
6. CT scan of pelvic and abdomen
7. MRI
8. Positron emission tomography (PET)

Treatment
Modalities of treatment
1. Surgery
2. Radiotherapy
3. Chemotherapy
4. Combined therapy (surgery and radiotherapy)

Stage I: Total abdominal hysterectomy (extrafascial) along with bilateral salpingo-oophorectomy

Stage II:
a. Radical hysterectomy and pelvic lymph node dissection
b. Primary radiation (intrauterine and vaginal implants, and external radiotherapy) followed by extrafascial hysterectomy
c. Simple hysterectomy followed by external beam radiation

Radiotherapy: Given to patients with advanced disease for symptom relief.
Chemotherapy advanced and recurrent cases or in cases where cancer has spread to other parts of the body.

Combined therapy: Extrafascial hysterectomy followed by adjuvant radiotherapy 4–6 weeks after surgery. This is done to prevent the cancer from recurring in the local area.
Nice to know: Indications for radiotherapy in endometrial carcinoma:
1. Women who are not fit for surgery
2. Women with significant other health conditions
3. Women with disease that cannot be surgically removed
4. Women at high risk of cancer returning
5. Patients with advanced disease for symptom relief

Chemotherapeutic agents used in endometrial carcinoma:
1. Progestogens
2. Tamoxifen
3. *Cytotoxic drugs:* Commonly used drugs include Adriamycin, cisplatin, carboplatin, paclitaxel, and cyclophosphamide

Chemotherapeutic agents used in endometrial carcinoma:
1. Progestogens
2. Tamoxifen
3. *Cytotoxic drugs:* Commonly used drugs are Adriamycin, cisplatin, carboplatin, paclitaxel, and cyclophosphamide

Q4. How endometrial carcinoma can be prevented?

Primary prevention
a. Maintain a healthy weight from an early age
b. Limit the use of estrogen in women who have not had a hysterectomy after menopause
c. Educate women about the importance of irregular vaginal bleeding during the perimenopausal and postmenopausal periods

Secondary prevention: Screening high-risk women during menopause to detect precancerous changes or early-stage cancer is an important step

Endometrial Carcinoma Stage

Stage I	Confined to uterus IA2 → Nonagreement a. Limited to endometrium on <50% myometrium b. >50% myometrium	72% survival
Stage II	Cervix stroma	50% survival
Stage III	Pelvic: a. Senora, adnexa (SA) b. Vagina and parametrium c. LN	31% Pelvic
Stage IV	a. Bladder on bowel b. Distal including c. Abdominal on inguinal LN	10% sy Survival

ENDOMETRIAL HYPERPLASIA

Q1. Define endometrial hyperplasia.

Endometrial hyperplasia may be defined as a premalignant endometrial lesion in which there is abnormal proliferation of both glandular and stromal elements showing altered histologic architecture.

Q2. What are the types of endometrial hyperplasia?

Types of endometrial hyperplasia (WHO classification)

1. Simple/cystic hyperplasia
2. Complex/adenomatous hyperplasia
3. Atypical endometrial hyperplasia
   a. Atypical simple hyperplasia
   b. Atypical complex hyperplasia

Q3. What are the risk factors of endometrial hyperplasia?

1. Unhindered estrogen stimulation (primary factor)
2. Delayed menopause
3. PCOS
4. Diabetes
5. Obesity
6. Hypertension
7. Nulliparity
8. Previous exposure to radiation therapy
9. Family history—endometrial carcinoma, carcinoma of breast, ovary or colon
10. Post-tamoxifen therapy

Q4. What are the protective factors of endometrial hyperplasia?

1. Multiparity
2. Average weight
3. COCs
4. Progestogen
5. If menopause ≤49 years

Q5. How will you manage a case of endometrial hyperplasia?

Management of endometrial hyperplasia

Diagnosis

1. No classic symptom
2. Abnormal perimenopausal uterine bleeding (constant feature)
   An incidental diagnosis occurs while examining infertility, DUB, PCOS, or an excised sample from a removed uterus
3. Procedure for screening
   a. Vaginal pool smear
   b. Endometrial aspiration
   c. Endometrial biopsy (curettage) and transvaginal ultrasound (thickened endometrium; 13 mm in premenopause and >4 mm in postmenopause)
4. Ultimate diagnosis is by uterine curettage and histology

Treatment protocol

Related to age of the patient and histologic type of hyperplasia

1. Young-age patient with cystic or hyperplasia (adenomatous)
   a. Cyclical progesterone therapy for about 6–9 months and should follow-up at 6 months' interval by evaluation with endometrial sampling
   b. Ovulation induction (in cases of PCOS to improve fertility in young women)
2. Perimenopausal and postmenopausal women
   a. Hyperplasia without atypia
      - Continuous progesterone therapy
      - Hysterectomy with bilateral salpingo-oophorectomy
   b. Moderate-to-severe atypical hyperplasia
      Hysterectomy with bilateral salpingo-oophorectomy

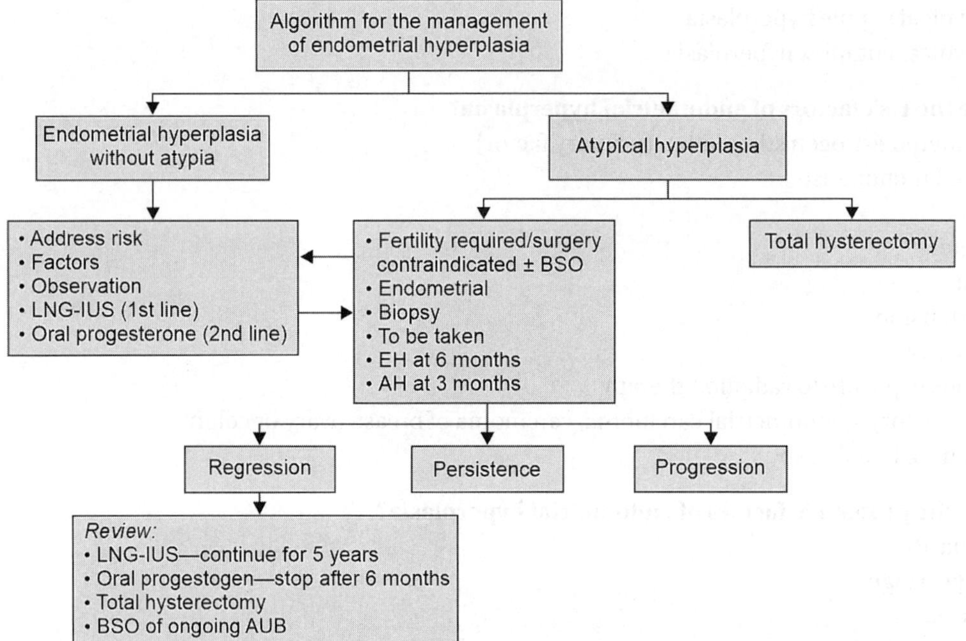

CHAPTER 22

Gestational Trophoblastic Disease

Q1. Define gestational trophoblastic disease.

Gestational trophoblastic disease (GTD)

Abnormal growth and proliferation of the trophoblast that continue even after the end of pregnancy.

Gestational trophoblastic neoplasia encompasses persistent hydatidiform mole, invasive mole, choriocarcinoma and a rare entity of placental site trophoblastic tumor.

Q2. Define trophoblastic tumor.

Trophoblastic tumor: The neoplasm which arise from the fetal tissue within the maternal host and are composed of both syncytiotrophoblastic and cytotrophoblastic cells is called trophoblastic tumor.

Q3. Classify gestational trophoblastic disease.

Classification of gestational trophoblastic disease:

1. Hydatidiform mole (complete and partial)
2. Gestational trophoblastic neoplasia:
   a. Persistent hydatidiform mole
   b. Invasive mole
   c. Choriocarcinoma
   d. Placental site trophoblastic tumor

Q4. What do you mean by persistent gestational trophoblastic disease?

Persistence of trophoblastic activity following evacuation of molar pregnancy.

Clinical features:

1. Irregular vaginal bleeding
2. Subinvolution of the uterus
3. Persistence of theca lutein cysts
4. Level of hCG either plateaus or reelevates after an initial fall

CHAPTER 23

Hydatidiform Mole

Q1. What is hydatidiform mole?

Hydatidiform mole

It is an abnormal condition of the placenta where there are partly degenerative and partly proliferative changes in the young chorionic villi.

Hydatidiform mole may be defined as a benign neoplasia of the chorion with malignant potential.

Q2. What is molar pregnancy?

Molar pregnancy

Molar pregnancy is an abnormal pregnancy characterized grossly by multiple grape like vesicles filling and distending the uterus, usually in the absence of an intact fetus

Invasive mole/chorioadenoma destruens.

It is a locally malignant growth, which invades the myometrium even the perimetrium, giving rise to intraperitoneal hemorrhage.

Q3. What are the types of hydatidiform mole?

Types hydatidiform mole

1. Complete mole
    - All the chorionic villi are changed to hydropic villi, a small amniotic sac may present which is difficult to find out
    - Usually arises in the ovary early weeks of pregnancy so the fetus is absorbed.
2. Partial mole
    - Hydropic villi will be present along with the normal villi and a fetus
    - It is usually associated with chromosomal abnormality, which is triploid (69 XXX, 69 XXY) in majority of cases.
    - Malignant change is very rare

Differences between complete and partial mole:

Features	***Complete mole***	***Partial mole***
Embryo/fetus	Absent	Present
Hydropic degenerations of villi	Pronounced and diffused	Variable
Trophoblast hyperplasia	Diffuse	Focal
Uterine size	More than the date (30–60%)	Less than the due
Theca lutein cysts	Common (25–50%)	Uncommon
Karyotype	46XX (85%), paternal origin	Triploid (90%), diploid (10%)
β-hCG	High (>50,000)	Slight elevation (<50,000)
Classic clinical symptoms	Common	Rare
Risk of persistent GTD	20%	<5%

Q4. What are the pathological changes in hydatidiform mole?

Pathological changes in hydatidiform mole

- Naked eye appearance: A mass of varying size filling the uterus each attached by a fine stalk
- Microscopic appearance:
  1. Marked proliferation of the syncytial and cytotrophoblastic epithelium
  2. Marked thinning of the stromal tissue due to hydropic degeneration
  3. There is absence of blood vessels in the villi
  4. The villus pattern is distinctly maintained

Q5. How will you manage a case of molar pregnancy?

Management of hydatidiform mole.

Diagnosis

From history

1. Short period of amenorrhea (8–12 weeks)
2. Exaggerated early pregnancy symptoms
3. Irregular vaginal bleeding which may be heavy
4. Expulsion of grape like vesicles per vagina (diagnosis of vesicular mole)
5. No fetal movement

- General examination
  1. Ill looking
  2. Anemia
  3. Features of preeclampsia (hypertension, edema and/or proteinuria): Present in about 50% cases
- Abdominal examination
  1. Size of the uterus is more than the period of amenorrhea (70% cases)
  2. Doughy feeling of the uterus
  3. Absence of fetal parts and fetal sounds
- Vaginal examination
  1. Bilateral cystic enlargement of the ovaries may be felt through fornices
  2. Findings of vesicles in the vaginal discharge (pathognomonic of hydatidiform mole)
  3. If the cervical os is open, instead of the membranes, blood clot or the vesicles may be felt
- Investigation
  1. USG of the uterus and adnexa: "Snow storm" appearance of the mole which is diagnostic
  2. Serum hCG: Markedly elevated
  3. X-ray chest: May show cannon ball opacities due to metastatic deposits
  4. Complete blood count, ABO and Rh grouping.

Treatment:

1. Suction evacuation and curettage of the mole
   a. It is to be done both during the process of expulsion or even when no mole has been expelled out
   b. If bleeding is severe prior to complete evacuation, a single dose ergometrine may be used (inj. oxytocin is not used prior or during evacuation due to risk of embolization but in case of severe bleeding it can be used during the time of evacuation)
   c. Following evacuation, curettage is to be done to remove the residual mole
   d. Blood transfusion is to given simultaneously
   e. This is to be followed by check D and C if necessary after one week.
2. Evacuation and curettage: If there is spontaneous expulsion of the mole, evacuation and curettage is to be done to remove the residual mole
3. Hysterectomy: It is the choice of treatment with the mole in situ or after evacuation, for women who are more than 40 years and/or have three or more children

4. There is no need to treat the lutein cysts in the ovaries even if they are large. They will disappear with the cessation of chorionic activity
5. Rh(–) women should receive Rh immunoglobulin as trophoblast cell express the RhD factor (in case of partial mole but it is given in both molar pregnancy)

Q6. What are the complications of hydatidiform mole?

Complications of hydatidiform mole
1. Hemorrhage and shock
2. Perforation of uterus
3. Infection
4. Choriocarcinoma
5. Coagulation failure
6. Acute pulmonary insufficiency

Q7. What are differential diagnosis of hydatidiform mole?

Differential diagnosis of hydatidiform mole
1. Threatened abortion
2. Multiple pregnancy
3. Fibroid or ovarian tumor pregnancy

Q8. A patient is evacuated for molar pregnancy. How will you follow up the patient?

Follow-up schedule after evacuation of mole

After evacuation of the mole, observation of the patient is essential for at least 2 years to detect the first sign of remaining or reawakening of chorionic activity.

History:

The patient should be enquired about:
1. Vaginal bleeding
2. Persistence of amenorrhea for a longer period
3. Hemoptysis, dyspnea, chest pain, etc.
4. Paresis and paralysis, headache, visual disturbance, etc.
5. Nodules in the vulva
6. Hematemesis
7. Hematuria

Examination:
1. General examination
   a. Anemia
   b. Cachexia
2. Abdominal examination: Presence of any lump
3. Vaginal examination
   a. Speculum examination: To see any deposits over the vulva, vagina, cervix and urethra.
   b. Bimanual examination: To see:
      - The size of the uterus
      - Lutein cysts of the ovaries

- Investigation
  1. Serum β-hCG estimation
     - Weekly until 3 consecutive level becomes negative
     - Monthly interval for next 1 year

     The average time to achieve the first normal hCG level after evacuation of mole is about 9 weeks.

2. Chest X-ray
   - 1st prior to evacuation of mole
   - 2nd after 4 weeks

   In a patient with falling hCG level, not more than one or two X-rays are necessary

- Advices
  1. Not to become pregnant during the period of follow-up
  2. Contraceptive advices
     a. Combined oral pill is actually preferred because they provide reliable contraception
     b. Progesterone only pill and IUCD should not be used because they cause irregular bleeding
     c. Barrier contraceptives can be used

At a glance
- IUCD use will create problem in diagnosing persisting molar activity
- Insertion of IUCD before normalization of hCG level also carries the risk of perforation.

Q9. Why not to become pregnant during the period of follow-up?

Because positive pregnancy test during this period will give rise to difficulty in differentiating persisting chorionic activity from occurrence of a new conception.

- Indications of chemotherapy following evacuation of a mole or hysterectomy:

Methotrexate and folic acid is commonly used.
1. Raised β-hCG level 6 month level 6 months after evacuation even if falling
2. β-hCG plateau in three consecutive serum samples
3. β-hCG > 20,000 mIU/mL more than 4 weeks after evacuation
4. Rising β-hCG in two consecutive serum samples
5. Pulmonary, vulval or vaginal metastasis unless the β-hCG level is falling
6. Heavy P/V bleeding or GI/intraperitoneal bleeding
7. Histological evidence of choriocarcinoma
8. Brain, liver or lung metastases >2 cm

CHORIOCARCINOMA

Q1. What is choriocarcinoma?

Choriocarcinoma is a highly malignant tumor arising from the chorionic epithelium.

Q2. How will you manage a case of choriocarcinoma?

Management of choriocarcinoma
- Diagnosis
  - Clinical features
    A. Symptoms
       1. Persistence of irregular vaginal bleeding following expulsion of mole (50%), abortion (25%) and term pregnancy (25%)
       2. Metastatic symptoms
          - Lung: Cough, breathlessness, hemoptysis
          - Vaginal: Irregular and at times brisk hemorrhage
          - Cerebral: Headache, convulsion, paralysis or coma
          - Liver: Epigastric pain, jaundice
- Signs
  - General examination
    a. Ill looking
    b. Severe anemia

- Abdominal examination
  a. Tenderness in abdomen may be present (due to intraperitoneal hemorrhage)
  b. Palpable lump in lower abdomen may be present (due to enlarged uterus and/or large theca lutein cyst)
- Vaginal examination
  a. Enlarged and tender uterus
  b. Unilateral or bilateral theca lutein cyst
- Speculum examination: Sometime show metastatic nodule
- Investigation:
  1. Serum β-hCG assay: Remarkably increased
  2. USG
     It can detect:
     a. Uterine enlargement
     b. Theca lutein cyst in ovaries and hepatic metastasis
  3. Chest X-ray: It can detect pulmonary metastasis.
  4. CT scan: for brain metastasis
  5. Diagnostic uterine curettage

Treatment

1. Chemotherapy
   Choice of treatment for choriocarcinoma
   a. Low-risk group: (FIGO score up to 7) best treated with single drug therapy mostly with methotrexate and folinic acid

Methotrexate	1–1.5 mg/kg	I/V, I/M	Days 1,3,5,7
Folinic acid		I/V	Days 2,4,6,8

   b. High-risk group: Best treated with multi agent chemotherapy (EMA-CO therapy)

E = Etoposide, M = Methotrexate, A = Actinomycin D
C = Cyclophosphamide, O = Oncovin (vincristine)

2. Surgery:
   a. Total abdominal hysterectomy with preservation of both ovaries
   b. Lung resection (thoracotomy) in pulmonary metastasis
3. Radiation: In patients with brain metastasis

Follow-up

- Mandatory for all patients at least for 2 years
- Serum β-hCG is measured:
  - Weekly until it is negative for 3 consecutive weeks
  - Monthly for 6 months
  - 6 monthly for lifelong

Nice to know

Indication of surgery (hysterectomy) in choriocarcinoma

1. Lesions confined to the uterus in women aged >35 years, not desirous of fertility
2. Placental site trophoblastic tumor
3. Intractable vaginal bleeding
4. Localized uterine lesion resistant to chemotherapy
5. Accidental uterine perforation during uterine curettage.

Q3. Who are the high-risk patient for treatment of choriocarcinoma?

High-risk group

1. Metastatic disease with poor prognosis
2. FIGO prognostic score 7 or above

Low-risk group

1. Nonmetastatic disease
2. Metastatic disease with good prognosis
3. FIGO prognostic score is 6 or less

Prognosis of choriocarcinoma

- Cure rate is almost 100% in low-risk cases and 70% in high-risk case
- Brain and liver metastases have the worst prognosis

When to stop chemotherapy

- WBC <3,000/cu.mm
- Polymorphonuclear leukocyte <1,500/cu.mm
- Platelet count: <1,00,000/cu.mm
- Significant elevation of serum creatinine, serum bilirubin, SGPT, and SGOT

Q4. How choriocarcinoma can be prevented?

Prevention of choriocarcinoma

1. Prophylactic chemotherapy in "at risk" women following evacuation of molar pregnancy may be considered.
2. Meticulous follow up following evacuation of hydatidiform mole is essential for at least 6 months to detect early evidences of trophoblastic reactivation
3. Selective hysterectomy in hydatidiform mole over 35 years
4. Diagnostic uterine curettage in unexplained abnormal bleeding, 8 weeks following term delivery or abortion
5. In suspected cases, serum β-hCG is to be determine.

Q5. Write a short note on methotrexate.

Methotrexate is a chemotherapeutic drug (anti-metabolites/folic acid antagonist) which prevents reduction of folic acid to folinic acid used by inhibiting the enzyme dihydrofolate reductase.

- Route of administration
  1. Oral (weekly)
  2. Parenteral (IM/IV)
  3. Subcutaneous
  4. Intrathecal
- Indication/use:
  1. Autoimmune diseases (rheumatoid arthritis, psoriasis, psoriatic arthritis, SLE, etc.)
  2. As chemotherapeutics in the treatment of a number of cancer (breast, leukemia, lymphoma, trophoblastic neoplasms, Lung bladder and osteosarcoma)
  3. First trimester termination of pregnancy (as abortifacient)
  4. Medical treatment of ectopic pregnancy
- Adverse effects
  1. Ulcerative stomatitis
  2. Predisposition to infection (lowers WBC count)
  3. Nausea
  4. Abdominal pain
  5. Fatigue
  6. Fever
  7. Headache and dizziness
  8. Dry cough and shortness of breath
  9. Diarrhea
  10. Sore throat

CHAPTER 24

Pelvic Organ Prolapse

CASE TAKING

Salient Points

Age: Common in perimenopausal and postmenopausal age

Occupation: Manual labor and lifting of heavy weights

Parity: Common in multipara

Symptoms: Feeling of something coming out vagina, heaviness or pressure in pelvis, urinary symptoms, bowel symptoms, sexual symptoms and local symptoms

Menstrual history: Menopause or not

Obstetric history: Number of pregnancies, number of vaginal delivery, duration of second stage, instrumental delivery and weight of baby

Medical history: Chronic cough, constipation, muscular dystrophy, multiple sclerosis and spinal cord injury

Surgical history: Vaginal or abdominal hysterectomy, previous prolapsed surgery.

General and systemic examination: Body mass index, chronic obstructive pulmonary disease (COPD), and neuropathy

Abdominal examination: Abdominal lump/ascites

Pelvic examination: Open genital hiatus (GH), smooth bulging mass, decubitus ulceration, and stress incontinence. Measurement of extent of prolapse in relation to hymen and introitus, measurement of GH, perineal body (PB), vaginal length, tone of perineal muscles, size, position, and mobility of uterus, and palpation of adnexa.

Per rectal examination: Tone of external anal sphincter, differentiate rectocele, and enterocele.

Rectovaginal examination: Palpation of enterocele, rectovaginal septum, and PB.

Case Discussion 1

A 60-year-old multiparous woman presents with sensation of something coming out of vagina. Symptom worsens with prolonged physical exertions such as heavy weight lifting, straining and standing. On occasion, she can see and feel something bulging from vaginal opening. Increasingly, she is experiencing difficult in emptying bladder and she needs to reduce the bulge with her fingers in order to empty her bladder. She does not have any urinary leakage during physical exercise and coughing. She gives history of chronic cough and constipation.

Q1. What is your diagnosis?

A stage III uterovaginal prolapse with cystocele, rectocele and enterocele diagnosed.

Q2. Identify the risk factors of pelvic organ prolapse (POP) that are present in this patient.

- Elderly patient
- Multiparity

- Chronic cough
- Constipation

Q3. Apart from the symptoms of POP mentioned here which other symptoms she might have?

Urinary symptoms: Poor stream, positional changes to complete micturition, urinary tract infection.

Bowel issues: Trouble with bowel movements, loss of control over gas, loose stools or firm stools, urgency to defecate, using fingers or support to aid defecation, sensation of not fully emptying, rectal bulging during or postdefecation (rectal prolapse).

Sexual issues: Difficulty with infrequent intercourse, pain during sex, absence of pleasure or climax, involuntary urination during sexual encounters.

Additional local symptoms include perineal pain, discomfort in the lower back that improves with lying down, abdominal pressure or pain, and vaginal discharge that is blood-stained and/or unusual

Q4. What do you mean by stage III uterovaginal prolapse?

- The most distal prolapse is >1 cm below the hymen but no further than 2 cm less than the total vaginal length (TVL).
- What is the role of vaginal estrogen in patients with

Q5. How do you demonstrate the findings of anterior vaginal wall prolapse?

- Fulfill the prerequisites of examination
- Use a Sims speculum to pull back the posterior vaginal wall and instruct the patient to cough

Q6. How do you demonstrate findings of uterine prolapse?

- Fulfill the prerequisites of examination
- Cusco's speculum is placed in the vaginal vault slowly, the speculum is withdrawn, and the patient is asked to cough or strain, and observe for descent of the cervix.

Q7. Name the operation that should be performed in this patient.

As the woman is 50 years of age, she can be treated with vaginal hysterectomy, pelvic floor repair and repair of enterocele.

Q8. How the support of vaginal apex is to be restored?

Support of vaginal apex can be restored by any of the following operation:

i. Uterosacral ligament suspension
ii. Sacrospinous ligament fixation
iii. Iliococcygeal vaginal suspension

Case Discussion 2

A 70-year-old woman P5 + 0 with onset of menopause for 20 years presents with sensation of something coming out through vagina. The symptom is more noticeable when she is standing for a long period of time. She does not complain of urinary or bowel symptoms. Her medical history is well controlled hypertension and chronic bronchitis. She has never had surgery. Pelvic examination reveals normal appearing external genitalia except generalized atrophic changes. A cystocele and rectocele are noted. The cervix descends to the introitus with the patient in an upright position. Uterus is small, atrophied and fornices are free. Rectal sphincter tone is slightly decreased. The patient prefers nonsurgical treatment. A pessary is placed and vaginal estrogen prescribed to address atrophic changes.

Q1. What are the risk factors in this case for development of POP?

- Aging and menopause
- Multiparity
- Chronic cough and bronchitis

Q2. What is the role of vaginal estrogen?

Pessaries may cause vaginal irritation and ulceration. They are better tolerated when the vaginal epithelium is well estrogenized. In hypoestrogenic patient like this woman, exogenous estrogen is prescribed but not oral estrogen.

Q3. What are other nonsurgical treatments apart from pessary treatment?

a. Observation
b. Medical treatment for symptoms
c. Pelvic floor exercises

Q4. When is surgery indicated in this patient?

a. When she is desirous of surgical treatment
b. Recurrent vaginal ulceration with pessary treatment.

Case Discussion 3

A 65-year-old woman with parity 6+0 complains of a sensation of something coming out of vagina and lower back pain when standing or walking. It has been present for last 15 years, but she can now only stand for a short time. It is not noticeable at night. All her deliveries were through vaginal route. She had her menopause at 52 years. She is generally constipated and sometimes finds that she can only defecate by placing her fingers into the vagina and. She has mild frequency of micturition. There is no dysuria or hematuria.

Examination: On examination, she is of average build. The abdomen is soft and nontender. There is atrophic changes of the vulva. On examination, in the supine position, there is a mild prolapse. There is a large posterior wall prolapse reaching up to introitus and a minimal posterior wall prolapse.

Q1. What is your diagnosis?

The diagnosis is second-degree uterine prolapse with rectocele. According to POP-Q Staging system, stage II middle and posterior compartment prolapse.

Q2. What increases this patient's risk for POP?

a. Aging and menopause
b. Multiparity

Q3. How would you manage this patient?

Her initial treatment involves treatment of constipation with dietary changes and laxatives. This may resolve some of the symptoms. If surgical treatment is chosen, treatment of constipation will prevent recurrence as well.

SHORT ANSWER TYPE QUESTIONS

Q1. What is POP?

Pelvic organ prolapse describes the unusual displacement or protrusion of pelvic organs from their normal location in the pelvis.

Q2. Support of the urogenital system.

Upper tier

- Round ligament
- Broad ligament
- Endopelvic fascia

Middle tier

- Uterosacral ligament
- Mackenrodt's ligament
- Pubocervical ligament

Lower tier

- Urogenital diaphragm
- Perineal body
- Levator ani muscle

Deficiencies in biomechanical support

Level-1:

- Uterosacral ligament
- Mackenrodt's ligament

Level-2:

- Pubocervical ligament
- Rectovaginal fascia
- Arcus tendinous

Level-3:

- Urogenital diaphragm
- Perineal body
- Levator ani muscle plate

Q3. Which anomalies are frequently linked to POP?

Typical POP anomalies include:

Cystocele is a condition in which the pubocervical ligament weakens and the bladder lowers into the vagina from its normal anatomical position, creating a bulge in the upper two-thirds of the anterior vaginal wall.

Urethrocele: Due to the triangle ligament's weakening, the urethra moves from its anatomical location downhill toward the vagina, creating a bulge in the lower third of the anterior vaginal wall.

Rectocele: The weakening of the rectovaginal fascia (Denonvilliers' fascia) results in a bulge in the middle third of the posterior vaginal wall as the rectum protrudes into the vagina. A protrusion in the upper portion of the body is known as an enterocele or pouch of Douglas hernia.

Q4. How can uterovaginal prolapse be categorized?

Uterovaginal prolapse can be classified based on:

- Compartment
- Degree—Shaw's classification
- Baden and Walker's system of grading
- POP-Q system.

Q5. What are the compartment-based classifications of prolapse?

i. Anterior compartment defect: urethrocele, cystocele, cystourethrocele
ii. Middle compartment defect: uterine prolapse, vault prolapse
iii. Posterior compartment defect: enterocele, rectocele, and relaxed perineum.

Q6. What does Shaw's classification of prolapse entail?

According to Shaw, descent is categorized into four degrees:

1st degree—Descent of the uterus while the cervix remains within the introitus
2nd degree—Cervix descends to the level of the introitus
3rd degree—When the cervix projects out through the vulva
4th degree—Complete procidentia

Q7. What is procidentia?

Complete prolapse of the uterus outside the introitus

Q8. What is the Baden and Walker's system for grading prolapse?

In the Baden system, the hymen serves as a reference point:
Grade 0—No prolapse
1st degree—Descent halfway to the hymen
2nd degree—Descent of the cervix up to the hymen
3rd degree—When the cervix projects through the vulva
4th degree—Complete procidentia

Q9. What is POP-Q System?

The pelvic organ prolapse quantification (POP-Q) system was developed by the standardization subcommittee of the International Continence Society in 2002. It provides a method for quantifying pelvic organ prolapse stages by measuring, in centimeters, the positions of nine locations on the vagina and perineal body in relation to the hymen. The pelvic organ prolapse quantification (POP-Q) assessment:

The stages are determined by the furthest extent of the prolapse in relation to the hymen. Stage 0: No signs of prolapse.

Stage I: The most distal point of the prolapse is more than 1 cm above the hymen.

Stage II: The most distal point of the prolapse is between 1 cm above and 1 cm below the hymen.

Stage III: The most distal point of the prolapse is more than 1 cm below the hymen but not exceeding 2 cm less than the total vaginal length (TVL).

Stage IV: Signifies procidentia or complete prolapse.

Q10. Picture of POP-Q grid.

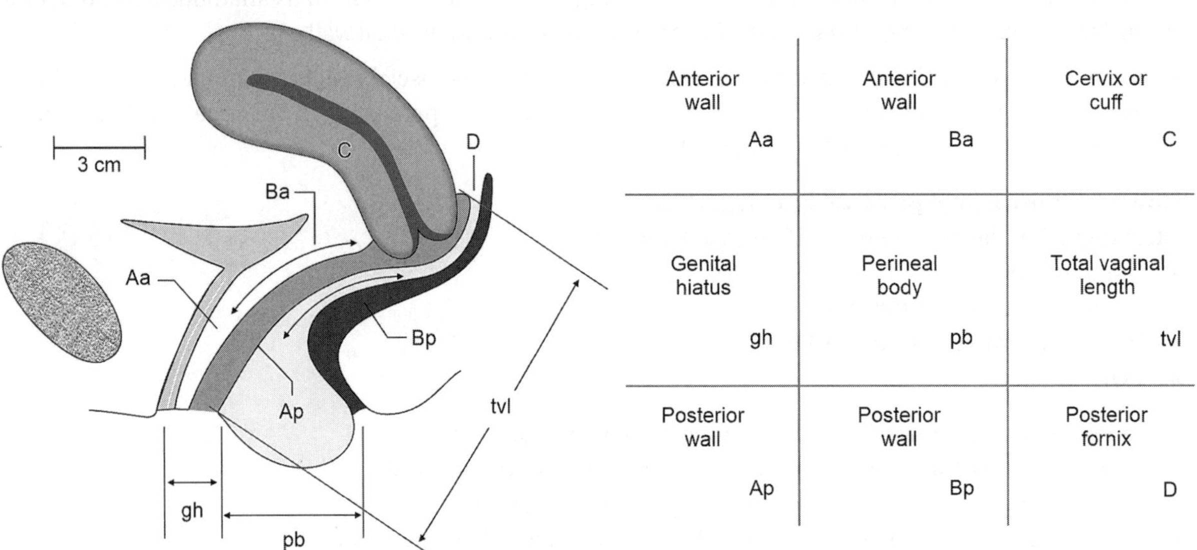

POP- Q grid.
Courtesy: VA Duddalwar, A Bhalerao et al. 2021

Q11. What are the advantages and disadvantages of POP Q system?

Advantages:

- More objective
- Site-specific
- Anatomical
- The system relies on specific measurements in the midline of the vaginal wall

- Less risk of mismanagement
- Can compare outcome of surgical repair
- Interindividual reliability
- Standard in written publication and scientific presentation

Disadvantages:

- Every gynecologist is not aware about the method.
- Measurements are changed according to position of the patient.
- It needs more training.

Q12. What are the risk factors of POP?

- Multiparity
- Advancing age
- Menopause
- Increased intra-abdominal pressure
- Large fibroid or tumor
- Obesity
- Heavy lifting
- Previous pelvic surgery
- Spinal cord injury
- Muscular atrophy

Q13. What are the predisposing factors and what are the aggravating factors in your case?

Predisposing factors include:

a. Congenital weakness of support
b. Poor management of the second stage of labor; and
c. Bearing down effort prior to full cervical dilation
d. Intense instrumental delivery; prolonged second stage of labor; and downward pressure to deliver the placenta
e. Shortly spaced repeat vaginal deliveries
f. Early activity resume history following each birth
g. Genetic collagen deficiency (Ehlers–Danlos syndrome, Marfan syndrome)

Among the aggravating causes include menopause, persistent coughing, and persistent constipation.

Q14. How childbirth is responsible for development of POP staging?

The pudendal nerve, connective tissue, and muscular structure are all harmed during vaginal birth. The strength and suppleness of some of the injured muscles and ligaments will never entirely return. The pelvic muscles and ligaments can be strained by a variety of reasons, including the baby's weight, protracted second stage of labor, episiotomy, forceps delivery, anal sphincter lacerations, and birth stressors.

Q15. What is most common symptom of POP?

A feeling of something coming out of vagina and heaviness or pressure in the pelvis.

Q16. How does one evaluate POP?

To determine the type and severity of prolapse:

1. Examination must be made with the patient straining (cough or Valsalva) forcefully enough that the prolapse is at its maximum.
2. The examiner must examine each element of support independently.

Q17. What are the morbid changes occur in case of uterine prolapse?

Morbid changes can occur in vaginal mucosa, cervix and urinary system.

Vaginal mucosa:

- Hyperpigmentation and hyperkeratinization: When exposed to air, it thickens and dries, resulting in a rough surface.
- Decubitus ulcer: It is a trophic ulcer located at the lower part of the prolapsed mass that is positioned outside the introitus.

Cervix:

- Vaginal part of the cervix- hyperplasia and hypertrophy of the fibromuscular glandular components which causes congested, bulky cervix.
- Supravaginal part of cervix
  - Stretching occurs because the tension of the cardinal ligament holds the cervix in place, while the uterus's weight causes it to descend through the vaginal axis.
  - Ongoing obstruction of venous and lymphatic drainage promotes elongation

Uetrus:

- Edema
- Incarceration: Infection of the perivaginal and cervical tissues causes the entire prolapsed mass to become swollen and congested, resulting in irreducibility

Urinary system:

Urinary bladder: During straining a incomplete emptying of the bladder is visible due to sharp angulation of the urethra against the pubourethral ligament. As a result there is hypertrophy of the bladder wall and trabeculation. Incomplete evacuation favors cystitis.

Ureters:

- Hydroureteric and hydronephrolic changes may occur due to ureters are mechanically obstructed and may be compressed.
- Pyelitis, pyelonephritis due to infection of the urinary bladder can ascend up.
- Uremia due to long standing cases of procidentia (rare).

Q18. What is acute emergency in case of prolapse?

When prolapsed part become incarcerated it is an acute emergency.

Q19. How decubitus ulcer is formed?

Decubitus ulcer occurs as a result of ischemic necrosis of tissue. There is downward displacement of the uterus. The anatomy becomes distorted. As a result, there is impaired blood supply. So ischemic necrosis occurs which leads to infections, cracks and ulceration.

Q20. How will you treat decubitus ulcer?

The aim of treatment is to restore the blood supply which can be achieved by reposition of the prolapsed part. Vaginal pack is to be given with roller bandage soaked with antiseptic lotion, glycerin and acriflavine. It takes about 7–14 days to heal the ulcer.

Q21. If there is decubitus ulcer why it is important to treat it prior to surgery?

The tissues around the ulcer remain unhealthy due to ischemia and associated infection. So, there will be difficulty in dissection leading to more bleeding as well as spreading of infection which impairs tissue healing.

Q22. How do you differentiate rectocele and enterocele?

Enterocele is present in upper one-third of posterior vaginal wall, whereas a rectocele typically is in the middle one-third of the vagina. A rectocele is best diagnosed by a finger in the rectum, demonstrating the defect, as the palpated between the rectum and vagina during rectovaginal examination, confirming enterocele.

Q23. How do you differentiate second and third-degree uterine prolapse?

Second- and third-degree uterine prolapse cannot be differentiated by inspection alone, palpation is essential. In second degree uterine prolapse get over test is found negative. During palpation of the prolapse mass, the thumb is placed anteriorly and four fingers are placed behind the mass. If the anterior and posterior fingers can be apposed above the mass outside the introitus, then the uterine prolapse is of the 3rd degree.

Q24. What may be the differential diagnosis of uterine prolapse?

- Elongated cervix
- Myomatous polyp
- Uterine inversion
- Gartner duct cyst

Q25. How do you differentiate Gartner duct cyst, elongated cervix, fibroid polyp, uterine prolapse and cystocele?

Gartner duct cyst

- Well-defined, nonreducible cystic lump on anterior or anterolateral vaginal wall
- Vaginal mucosa overlying lump is tense with loss of rugosities
- No impulse on cough
- The metallic catheter is introduced per urethra fails to come below the vaginal mucosa
- Vaginal ultrasound can detect a cystic mass
- Treatment: Excision

Elongated cervix

- Vaginal fornices are deep and narrow
- Vaginal part of cervix is elongated lying below the level of ischial spine
- Bimanual examination shows a normal size and position of the body of uterus

Fibroid polyp

- Often presents with menstrual abnormality-menorrhagia, metrorrhagia, and dysmenorrhea
- Polypoid mass coming out of cervix without any visible opening on leading part
- The mass is shaggy with broad leading part
- Bimanual examination reveals pedicle coming out through cervical canal or arising from cervix
- Rectal examination reveals normal shape and position of the uterus
- Treated by polypectomy

Uterine inversion

- Irregular bleeding per vagina
- It looks shaggy
- External os is not visible. Broad mass protrudes through cervix like a rim
- During bimanual examination and per rectal examination cup-shaped depression may be felt at fundus
- Body of uterus is not felt on per rectal examination
- USG: Absent body of uterus
- Treated by Haultain or Spinelli operation

Cystocele:

- Ill-defined, reducible bulge in upper two-thirds of anterior vaginal wall vaginal mucosa overlying bulge is not tensed and rugosities present.
- Tip of female metal catheter can be felt below the bulge.

Q26. Name some measures that may be helpful to prevent POP.

Proper management of labor, pelvic floor exercise following childbirth, treatment of constipation, cough, and precipitating factors, concomitant procedures to prevent vault prolapse during hysterectomy. Pelvic floor exercises after childbirth may help to prevent prolapse in future.

Q27. What are the concomitant procedures at the time of hysterectomy to prevent POP?

Concomitant procedures at the time of hysterectomy, different sling operations, closure of the pouch of Douglas with a Moschcowitz's procedure or uterosacral plication, may reduce the incidence of prolapse.

Q28. What investigations you want to do POP case?

History and clinical examination findings are enough for confirmation of the diagnosis of uterine prolapse. Routine investigations with USG of whole abdomen are to be done for management purpose.

Q29. Why you want to do USG of whole abdomen?

- To see any adnexal mass or pelvic pathology
- Hydroureter and hydronephrosis can be seen

Q30. Before going to operation what are the points you want to consider?

Before going for operation I must exclude stress incontinence, if present then can be treated at the same sitting and I want to exclude complete perineal tear because I need gut preparation before operation.

Q31. Why stress incontinence may present along with prolapse? How will you treat stress Incontinence in that case?

Uterovaginal prolapse may be associated with stress incontinence due to loss of urethrovesical angle. Stress incontinence should be corrected along with pelvic floor repair by Kelly's suture.

Q32. How Kelly's suture is given?

Following careful exposure of the bladder neck and urethra through the vaginal approach, a Kelly's suture is placed around the proximal urethra and bladder neck using a vertical mattress technique to plicate the pubocervical fascia.

Q33. What type of surgery you want to do in POP case?

Vaginal hysterectomy with pelvic floor repair—anterior colporrhaphy, posterior colpoperineorrhaphy and correction of enterocele.

Q34. Why vaginal hysterectomy performed in POP case?

Pelvic floor repair is the actual corrective surgery for utero vaginal prolapse, vaginal hysterectomy is not the surgery for prolapse. But before pelvic floor repair vaginal hysterectomy is to be done for better exposure. Uterus is removed as because is a potential site of malignancy in postmenopausal lady.

Q35. What is the management of asymptomatic POP?

Observation or watchful waiting is appropriate. Pelvic floor muscle rehabilitation may be offered despite the lack of data supporting its use to prevent progression.

Q36. What is the traditional procedure for anterior colporrhaphy?

The vaginal epithelium is dissected from the underlying fibromuscular connective tissue and bladder, then plicating the vaginal muscularis across the midline. Excess vaginal epithelium is excised and the wound is closed.

Q37. What are the different surgical options for treatment of vault (apical) prolapse?

a. Transvaginal repairs:
   - Sacrospinous ligament
   - Uterosacral ligament suspension

b. Abdominal repairs: Abdominal sacrocolpopexy (laparoscopy/laparotomy)

Q38. What is the traditional procedure for posterior vaginal wall prolapse (rectocele)?

Colpoperineorrhaphy:

The vaginal epithelium is separated off the underlying fibromuscular layer and endopelvic fascia. Repair often includes plication of the levator ani muscles and bulk lateral plication of tissue oversewing the rectovaginal fascia. Excess vaginal epithelium is excised and the wound closed.

Q39. When is a hysterectomy warranted?

For treatment of uterine prolapse or if concomitant uterine pathology is present at the time of prolapse surgery.

Q40. How enterocele can be corrected?

Upon locating the neck of the enterocele sac, a purse-string suture is placed as high as feasible. Excess part of the peritoneum is removed and the edges of the peritoneum are brought together with interrupted sutures. While suturing, I need to be cautious to prevent bowel damage since the bowel is part of the enterocele contents.

Q41. What are the complications of vaginal hysterectomy?

Early complications:

During surgery

- Hemorrhage
- bladder and rectum injury

After surgery

- Reactionary hemorrhage
- Secondary hemorrhage
- Retention of urine
- Cystitis
- Infection

Late complications: Dyspareunia

Q42. Why vaginal pack is given after vaginal hysterectomy?

Vaginal pack is given after vaginal hysterectomy to prevent reactionary hemorrhage.

Q43. If vaginal bleeding occurs within 24 hours following vaginal hysterectomy then what will you do?

Vaginal bleeding that happens within 24 hours after a vaginal hysterectomy results from inadequate hemostasis during the procedure caused by slippage of the ligature. The patient must be taken to the operating room for exploration to identify the source of the bleeding.

Q44. What is secondary hemorrhage? Why it occurs following vaginal hysterectomy and what will you do if secondary hemorrhage occurs?

Secondary hemorrhage:

Secondary hemorrhage usually occurs 24 hours after operation. But it commonly occur between 5th and 10th day due to sepsis.

Management:

- In cases of rapid secondary hemorrhage, the patient must be taken to the operating room for exploration under general anesthesia in addition to resuscitative measures
- If there is any visible bleeding point, hemostatic suture should be given followed by tight vaginal packing.
- High vaginal swab should be taken and send for culture and sensitivity and antibiotics should be started.

Q45. Following vaginal hysterectomy for how many days you will keep catheter in situ?

Usually catheter should be kept for 3–5 days

Q46. During vaginal hysterectomy nothing is done to bladder then why catheterization is to be done for so long time?

1. For giving rest to the bladder as more dissection of bladder is done.
2. If during operation bladder is injured it helps healing.

Q47. Why vaginal pack is given after vaginal hysterectomy and for how long it should be kept?

Following vaginal hysterectomy vaginal pack is to be given to prevent reactionary hemorrhage and it should be removed 24 hours following operation.

LONG ANSWER TYPE QUESTIONS

Q1. Write short note on rubber ring pessary.

Rubber ring pessary: If surgery is not wanted, she can be treated with ring pessary. Pelvic floor exercise is unlikely to benefit her prolapse.

Types of pessaries:

There are two types of main pessaries: Support pessaries and space occupying pessaries.

M/A:

It reduces the prolapse by lateral stretching with elevation of the vaginal sidewalls.

Indications:

i. Elderly patients with severe prolapse, unfit for surgery
ii. Women with symptomatic POP who decline surgery
iii. Who need temporary relief of pregnancy-related prolapse or incontinence
iv. Women who may yet bear children.

Choice of exact size of pessary:

At first bimanual examination should be done and use the forefinger to measure the distance between the posterior vaginal fornix and external urethral orifice. The measurement of the pessary would be given after deducting 1.5 cm from the former measurement. Sometimes trial and error may be only way to determine which size of pessary should be used and clinicians should keep a variety of sizes.

Procedure:

i. Ensure that the patient's bladder and bowel are empty.
ii. Depress the perineum and posterior vaginal wall with left index finger
iii. Introduce the pessary being lubricated vertically inside vagina and then rotate to place it properly
iv. The pessary fits well if a finger can be swept between the pessary and the walls of the vagina.
v. The goal is to fit the largest pessary that does not cause discomfort.

Sterilization:

By boiling.

Complications:

- Spontaneous expulsion
- Irritation of the vaginal wall
- Ulceration
- Bleeding
- Pain
- Odor

Time of pessary change:

If there are no adverse symptoms, the pessary can be changed every 9-12 months.

Contraindication:

i. Untreated vaginal infection
ii. Pelvic inflammatory disease
iii. Follow-up is not possible

Q2. Steps of anterior colporrhaphy.

Principles:

- To remove a segment of the loosened front vaginal wall.
- To elevate the bladder and move it upwards after severing the vesicocervical ligament. The bladder is subsequently supported permanently by folding the endopelvic fascia and the pubocervical fascia beneath the bladder neck at the midline

Steps:

Following the administration of adequate anesthesia, the patient is positioned in lithotomy. Antiseptic solution should be applied to swab the vulva and vagina. The perineum is to be covered with a sterile towel and the legs with leggings. Metal catheter will be used to drain the bladder. A vaginal exam is performed to evaluate the type and extent of prolapse. Sim's posterior vaginal speculum is inserted, and the anterior lip of the cervix is grasped by the vulsellum and lowered by the assistant. A metal catheter is inserted to determine the bladder's lower boundary. A T-shaped incision is created on the front wall of the vagina. The horizontal cut is performed under the bladder, and the vertical cut initiates from the center of the horizontal incision extending down to approximately 1.5 cm below the external urethral meatus. The triangular vaginal flaps along with the fascia on both sides are divided from the endopelvic fascia that encases the bladder by gauze. The cleavage line is the vesicovaginal area. The bladder, along with the surrounding endopelvic fascia, is now revealed. When the vaginal wall edges are pulled laterally, the vesicocervical ligament is grasped with an Allis tissue forceps and cut. The bladder is subsequently elevated by fingers wrapped in gauze until the peritoneum of the uterovesical pouch becomes apparent. The vesicocervical area is revealed, and the pubocervical fascia is folded using interrupted stitches. The excess part of the vaginal mucosa is trimmed on both sides. The edges of the vagina are brought together with interrupted stitches. The catheter is inserted again. The vagina is densely filled with roller gauze. A self-retaining catheter is inserted.

Q3. What are the operative steps of vaginal hysterectomy?

Following the administration of adequate anesthesia, the patient is positioned in lithotomy position. The antiseptic solution should be used to swab the vulva and vagina. The perineum should be covered with a sterile towel, and the legs with leggings. Metal catheter is to empty the bladder. Vaginal examination serves to evaluate the type and severity of prolapse.

Sim's posterior vaginal speculum is inserted, and the anterior lip of the cervix is grasped by a vulsellum and lowered by the assistant. A metal catheter is inserted to determine the bladder's lower limit. An inverted T incision is performed on the front vaginal wall. A horizontal cut is created beneath the bladder, and a vertical cut begins at the midpoint of the transverse incision, extending to a point approximately 1.5 cm below the external urethral opening. The triangular vaginal flaps, along with the fascia on both sides, are detached from the endopelvic fascia covering the bladder using gauze. The cleavage line is the vesicovaginal space. The bladder along with the surrounding endopelvic fascia is now visible. As the vaginal wall edges are pulled back laterally, the vesicocervical ligament is grasped with Alli's tissue forceps and then cut. The bladder is subsequently elevated by fingers wrapped in gauze until the peritoneum of the uterovesical pouch becomes evident. The peritoneum between the uterus and bladder is incised. Landon's retractor is inserted and will be held by an assistant. The posterior vaginal wall at the cervicovaginal junction is incised. The vaginal wall is opened until the pouch of Douglas is accessed. The peritoneum is surgically incised. The initial clamp is positioned, which encompasses the uterosacral ligament, Mackenrodt's ligament, and the descending cervical artery. The tissues are trimmed near the cervix and secured with sutures. The same process is carried out on the opposite side. The second clamp is now applied, which encompasses the uterine artery and the base of the broad ligament. The structures are trimmed near the uterus and substituted with ligature. The fundus is now extracted through the anterior pouch using a pair of Allis tissue forceps.

The bladder is then pushed up by gauze covered fingers till the peritoneum of the uterovesical The pouch can be seen. Uterovesical peritoneum is incised. Landon's retractor is placed and will be held by an assistant. The posterior vaginal wall at the cervicovaginal junction is incised. The vaginal wall is carefully cut until the pouch of Douglas is accessed. The peritoneum is incised. The first clamp is then positioned, encompassing the uterosacral ligament, Mackenrodt's ligament, and the descending cervical artery. The tissues are trimmed near the cervix and secured with sutures. The identical process is carried out on the opposite side. The second clamp is now applied, encompassing the uterine artery and the base of the broad ligament. The structures are trimmed near the uterus and substituted with ligature. The fundus is now extracted from the anterior pouch using a pair of Allis tissue forceps. The third clamp is now applied, encompassing the round ligament, fallopian tube, mesosalpinx, and ovarian ligament. The structures are severed and substituted with transfixing suture.

Q4. How does posterior colpoperineorrhaphy proceed?

In posterior colpoperineorrhaphy, a third pair of Allis tissue forceps is applied to the midline of the posterior vaginal wall, high above the rectocele bulge, while another pair is placed on each side at the lower end of the labia minora. A horizontal incision is then made at the mucocutaneous junction to connect the two lateral Allis forceps. Using perineorrhaphy scissors, the posterior vaginal wall is dissected from the rectum and perineal body up to the level of the third Allis forceps. From the apex down to the midpoint of the horizontal incision, a vertical incision is made. Dissection of the resulting triangular flaps laterally exposes the rectum along with the underlying musculofascial structures.

Vault Prolapse

Case Discussion

Mrs X, 50 years old, para 3 + 2, a housewife of low socioeconomic condition complains something coming down per vagina for 3 years and difficulty in micturition for 6 months. She has a history of abdominal hysterectomy 7 years back. Regarding her obstetrical history, she has four living children, all of them delivered vaginally at home by untrained birth attendant. She gave no history of chronic cough or constipation. On inspection-there is a bulge protruding through the introitus which is increased when the patent in asked to strain, on per speculum examination - a transverse scar and two dimples one on each end of the scar. On straining it descent further to the level of 1 cm above the introitus. There is a large bulging at the upper two-thirds of the anterior vaginal wall. Posterior vaginal wall has two bulgings, one at the upper part and another at the middle part, separated by a transverse sulcus. On bimanual examination -Vault scar is felt as a transverse band of tissue which is firm than the adjacent vaginal wall and dimple is felt on each end of the scar. Uterus is absent with no pelvic mass.

On per rectal examination the examining index finger could be hooked into the lower bulged but it could not reach the upper swelling.

Q1. What is your diagnosis?

Vault prolapse with cystocele and rectocele.

Q2. During operation what prophylactic measures can you take to prevent for vault prolapse?

During vaginal hysterectomy:

- Attachment of the uterosacral ligament and cardinal ligament to the vaginal vault.
- Prophylactic McCall culdoplasty

During abdominal hysterectomy:

- Modified McCall culdoplasty: the uterus is to be pulled up to make the uterosacral ligament taut and then permanent tag sutures are employed on each uterosacral ligament at a point 2 cm distal to pelvic wall. These are subsequently fixed to the vaginal vault.
- Moschcowitz's suture: Obliteration of the pouch of Douglas can be done by circumferential sutures.

Q3. What are the conservative measures you can take to treat vault prolapse?

- Pelvic floor muscle training.
- Pessaries are suitable for women who are not sexually active.

Q4. What operation you can do to repair vault prolapse?

Repair of vault prolapse can be done by different approaches

- Abdominally: Sacrocolpopexy
- Vaginally: Sacrospinous fixation
- Laparoscopically: Sacrocolpopexy

Abdominal sacrocolpopexy:

Prolene mesh or tissue graft is required to pull the vaginal vault and fixed into ligament in front of the S3 vertebrae.

Sacrospinous fixation:

During sacrospinous fixation dissection into the para vaginal space and ischial spine is identified. Two nonabsorbable sutures are placed. One end of the suture is attached to the undersurface of the poster vaginal wall of the apical area. A longitudinal incision is made over the posterior vaginal wall and extend it to the apex of the vaginal wall. The vaginal mucosa is dissected from the recto vaginal fascia until the puborectal muscle is identified. The sacrospinous ligament is then identified. Two stitches are inserted through the sacrospinous ligament and secured to the apex of the vagina.

CHAPTER 25

Urinary Incontinence

Case Discussion-1

A 55-year-old female presents with 6 years history of urinary leakage with coughing or sneezing. It also occurs during physical exertion and sexual intercourse. She is greatly embarrassed with her problem and limited her social activities. A medical history and medication review are noncontributory.

Q1. What kind of incontinence this patient might have?

Suggestive of stress urinary incontinence (SU1).

Q2. What elements of the physical examination are important to obtain?

Physical examination should include pelvic, rectal, and neurologic examination.

Pelvic examination:

- Urinary stress test should be done with full bladder
- Evaluation for pelvic organ prolapse
- Evaluate for urethral hypermobility
- Bimanual examination

Rectal examination: To identify fecal impaction, rectal masses, and sphincter tone.

Neurological examination:

- Perineal sensation, voluntary anal sphincter contraction (S2-S4).
- The anal wink reflex (S4-S5), which is anal sphincter contraction triggered by lightly stroking perianal skin.
- The bulbocavernosus reflex (S2-S4), which is anal sphincter contraction triggered by pressure on clitoris.

Q3. What investigations can be performed to this patient?

- Urine analysis and/or urine culture
- Ultrasonography—postvoid residual (PVR) urine
- Blood urea nitrogen
- Serum creatinine
- Urodynamic testing (UDT)—if surgery is planned.

Q4. How she should be treated?

Because the clinical history is noncontributory, conservative management includes pelvic floor exercise and surgical treatment includes transvaginal or transobturator vaginal tap or colposuspension.

Case Discussion-2

A 70-year-old woman has presented with involuntary loss of urine for 10 years. Initially, it was infrequent, but it has progressed over years and now it has become troublesome. Leaking of urine is small in amount, because of frequent occurrence she wears a pad all the time. She never leaks urine on sneezing or coughing, urgency, and frequency. She used to pass urine every hour during daytime and wakes up 2-3 times every night. Her obstetric history reveals she has two uncomplicated vaginal deliveries. She has been menopausal for 20 years.

Examination: There is no prolapse found in anterior, apical, or posterior vaginal compartment.

Routine urine examination: No abnormality detected.

Urodynamics: The first urge to void 50 mL bladder urge, involuntary detrusor contractions were noted while attempting to inhibit micturition. There was no loss of urine with coughing.

Q1. What is your diagnosis?

The diagnosis is of overactive bladder (OAB) syndrome. This was formerly referred to as detrusor instability. Patient has urgency, frequency, nocturia, and urine routine examination reveals no infection. She has no neurological illness. Urodynamic study confirms involuntary detrusor contraction during filling phase of bladder.

Q2. How would you manage this patient?

Lifestyle changes

- Should avoid intake of caffeine.
- Take normal fluid per day and avoid taking fluid after 7 PM to avoid nocturia.
- Bladder retraining for 6 weeks.

Medical treatment

If above measures fail: Anticholinergic drugs such as oxybutynin or tolterodine.
The side effects include dry mouth, dry eyes, and constipation.

SHORT ANSWER TYPE QUESTIONS

Q1. What is urinary incontinence?

Urinary incontinence refers to the involuntary loss of urine that can be clearly observed, leading to difficulties in maintaining proper hygiene or participating in daily activities due to social or practical challenges.

Q2. What is the incidence of urinary incontinence?

About 5-7% in 15-44 years age group and range between 8-12% after 45 years of age.

Q3. Pathophysiology of urinary incontinence.

The fundamental pathology of incontinence involves the increase of intravesical pressure beyond the maximum urethral pressure. It could result from mechanical damage to the bladder neck supports after childbirth, trauma (surgery), or as a consequence of aging. Heightened activity of the detrusor muscles may also be linked.

Q4. Name and describe major types of incontinence.

Stress incontinence: SUI is defined as involuntary escape of urine from the external urethral meatus due to sudden rise in intra-abdominal pressure (IAP).

Occult stress incontinence is a type of stress urinary incontinence that is only recognized after the underlying pelvic organ prolapse has been corrected.

- Urgency incontinence involves uncontrollable urine leakage that occurs due to a sudden and strong urge to urinate, making it difficult to delay.
- Mixed incontinence occurs when urine leakage is caused by both urgency and increased pressure within the abdomen.
- Overflow incontinence happens when the bladder fills with urine to an excessive level and is unable to empty properly.
- This leads to a large bladder and may result in urine leakage that happens continuously or when coughing or straining.
- Functional incontinence refers to urine leakage that results from conditions affecting cognitive or physical abilities, such as dementia or stroke, or from environmental barriers that prevent the person from reaching the bathroom in time.

Q5. What is meant by following symptoms?

- Urgency: A sudden, strong urge to urinate.
- Enuresis: The involuntary loss of urine, typically during sleep.
- Nocturnal enuresis: The loss of urine that happens while sleeping.
- Continuous urinary incontinence: A constant leakage of small amounts of urine.
- Nocturia: Waking up more than once during the night to urinate.
- Overactive bladder: A condition that includes a strong, sudden urge to urinate, often along with frequent urination and waking up at night to urinate.

It may also involve unintentional leakage of urine, but it is not caused by a urinary tract infection or other clear medical issues.

- Continuous urinary incontinence: A steady, small amount of urine leaks out continuously.
- Urinary frequency: Urinating eight or more times in a 24-hour period

Q6. What are the known risk factors for urinary incontinence?

Childbearing, advanced age, obesity, family history, chronic cough, ascites, and pelvic masses.

Q7. Definition of Genuine Stress Incontinence.

Genuine stress incontinence (GSI) is defined as involuntary urethral loss of urine when the intravesical pressure exceeds the maximum urethral pressure in the absence of detrusor activity. (According to the International Continence Society)

Q8. Incidence of Genuine Stress Incontinence.

40% associated with pelvic organ prolapse.

Q9. Etiopathogenesis of Genuine Stress Incontinence.

- Urethral hypermobility due to alteration of the typical urethrovesical structure.
- The lowering of the bladder neck and proximal urethra, which typically rests above the urogenital diaphragm, obstructs the increase of intraurethral pressure when straining.
- Reduced urethral pressure at rest beneath the intravesical pressure

Q10. What are the risk factors of Genuine Stress Incontinence?

- Developmental weakness of the supporting structures
- Genetic variations in collagen and other connective tissues
- Childbirth trauma
- Gestation:
  - Because of elevated progesterone levels.
  - Challenging vaginal birth, forceps or ventouse assistance, or even higher parity.
- Postmenopausal: Lack of estrogen results in the degeneration of the supporting structures.
- After the operation
  - Anterior colporrhaphy,
  - Local treatment of vesicovaginal fistula (VVF)
  - Surgery on the bladder neck may result in fibrosis of the urethra and the muscles of the urethra.
- Advancing in age.
- Overweight (BMI: >30).
- Medications: Diuretics, benzodiazepines.
- Coexisting conditions: Diabetes, parkinsonism, and cerebrovascular accident

Q11. What are the modifiable factors of Genuine Stress Incontinence?

- Gynecologic: Cystocele, uterine prolapse.
- Medications
- Smoking, obesity, high intake of caffeine.

Q12. What are the morbid anatomic changes of Genuine Stress Incontinence?

- Intrinsic sphincter deficiency (ISD)—20%.
- The base of the bladder flattens and aligns with the back wall of the proximal urethra.
- Funneling of the proximal urethra.

Q13. How will you diagnose Genuine Stress Incontinence?

Clinical Features

The patients are usually parous, may be obese, postmenopausal.

Symptoms

Escape of urine with coughing, sneezing, or laughing.

The loss of urine has got the following features:

- Brief and coincides precisely to the period of raised IAP.
- Unassociated with a desire to pass urine.
- Rarely, occurs in supine position or during sleep.
- Patients are fully aware of it.
- The amount of loss is small

Examination

- Clinical stress test-positive
- Pad test-positive
- Midstream urine analysis-normal
- Bladder diary (volume frequency chart)
- Uroflowmetry—normal
- Cystometry—normal
- Significant lowering of urethral closure pressure during strain
- Leak—point pressure (Valsalva) test—positive
- Cystourethroscopy—negative finding
- Video cystourethrography (VCU)—bladder neck funneling
- Transvaginal endosonography—altered anatomical relationship (descent) of urethrovesical junction and bladder base.

Q14. Differences in clinical presentation of different types of incontinence.

Stress incontinence	***Urge incontinence (sensory)***	***Overactive bladder***
Leakage of urine with stress No prior urge to void	Unable to control the escape of urine, once there is an urge to void	The incontinence may occur abruptly even without a full bladder or a clinical cause
Amount-small	Amount-large	Amount-large
Patient-fully aware of	Patient-aware of the urge	Patient-not aware of it
Micturition-normal	Urgency and frequency	Frequency and nocturia
Leakage with running water—No	Yes	No
Midstream urine examination Not informative	Evidences of infection	Usually, non-informative
Uroflowmetry: Normal	Normal	High in idiopathic group
Cystometry: During strain, there is significant lowering of the urethral pressure. (urethral pressure profile)	Normal	Urge to pass urine is provoked at much lower bladder filling Detrusor pressure is increased during filling
Cystourethroscopy: Normal	Offending factor present	Diminished bladder capacity
Lateral cystourethrography: Funneling of the proximal urethra	Normal	Normal

Q15. What is frequency volume chart/urinary diary?

Patient is asked to record her fluid intake, voiding habit, voided volume, episodes of leakage in relation to time and activity. It should be recorded at least for 3 days. This diary gives an idea about daily urine output, number of voids per day and functional bladder capacity.

Q16. Normal findings of cystometry.

- Residual volume: 0-50 mL
- First sensation of urination: 150-200 mL
- Capacity: 400-600 mL
- Intravesical pressure on filling and standing: 0-15 cmH_2O
- Absence of systolic detrusor contraction
- No leakage on coughing
- Able to interrupt the urine flow on command
- Maximum detrusor pressure during voiding: <50 cmH_2O
- Peak urinary flow rate: >15 mL/sec

Q17. How will you prevent stress urinary incontinence?

- Avoidance of repeated childbirth trauma and delay in second stage of labor.
- Management of obesity, diabetes, chronic pulmonary, and neurological diseases.

Q18. What are the aims of treatment of stress urinary incontinence?

- Restoration of the function of the muscles of the urethrovesical junction.
- Strengthening the support of the urethra.

Q19. What are the indications of surgery?

1. Various forms of SUI especially ISD.
2. SUI with concomitant pelvic organ prolapse.

Q20. How will you treat stress urinary incontinence?

Stress urinary incontinence (SUI) refers to the involuntary leakage of urine during physical activities that increase intra-abdominal pressure, such as coughing, sneezing, laughing, or exercise. Treatment for stress urinary incontinence is tailored to the severity of symptoms and the patient's specific needs, and can involve conservative measures, pharmacologic treatments, or surgical interventions.

1. Conservative Management:
   - Pelvic Floor Muscle Training (PFMT): Often the first line of treatment, PFMT, including Kegel exercises, strengthens the pelvic floor muscles, helping prevent urine leakage.
   - Bladder Training: Involves scheduling regular trips to the bathroom to train the bladder to hold urine longer.
   - Lifestyle Modifications: Weight management, fluid management, and avoiding bladder irritants (e.g., caffeine and alcohol) can be helpful.
2. Pharmacologic Treatment:
   - Topical Estrogen: For postmenopausal women with vaginal atrophy, local estrogen treatment can help improve the tone of the urethral and pelvic floor muscles.
   - Duloxetine: This serotonin-norepinephrine reuptake inhibitor is sometimes prescribed as an off-label treatment for stress urinary incontinence, as it can improve the function of the urethral sphincter.
3. Surgical Treatment:
   - Midurethral Sling Surgery: The most common surgical procedure for SUI, where a sling (often made from synthetic mesh or autologous tissue) is placed around the urethra to provide support.
   - Colposuspension (Burch procedure): Surgical elevation and fixation of the bladder neck to the pelvic sidewall to restore continence.

- Artificial Urinary Sphincter (AUS): This is often reserved for more severe cases of SUI, particularly in men or women with intrinsic sphincter deficiency.

4. Minimally Invasive Options:
   - Injectable Bulking Agents: Agents such as collagen or carbon-coated beads are injected into the tissue around the urethra to improve its closure during times of increased pressure.
   - Percutaneous Tibial Nerve Stimulation (PTNS): A form of neuromodulation where a small needle is inserted near the ankle to stimulate the tibial nerve, which then affects the bladder function.
5. Psychological and Supportive Therapies:
   - Cognitive behavioral therapy (CBT) and other psychological support measures can help patients manage any emotional or social stress associated with the condition.

Q21. What are the conservative treatment of stress urinary incontinence?

To improve the tone of the pelvic floor muscles:

- Pelvic floor muscle training (supervised)
- Biofeedback therapy: During PFMT visual, auditory, and/or verbal feedback are given to the patient with GSI of minor degree.
- Kegel exercises: Patient is taught to contract and hold the levator ani muscles voluntarily for 50-60 times a day.
- Vaginal devices: Pessary with a knob.
  - It stabilizes the urethra to reduce urethral hypermobility and to increase urethral pressure.
- Vaginal cone with weight ranging from 20-100g.
- Weight reduction in obese patients.
- Electrical stimulation of pelvic floor muscles by stimulation of pudendal nerves.

Drugs management:

- Sympathomimetic
  - Duloxetine (SNRI), 400 mg, twice daily
  - Imipramine, 10-25 mg orally twice daily
  - Ephedrine, 15-30 mg orally twice daily
- Estrogen
- Paraurethral implant—Calcium hydroxyapatite, Teflon (↑ functional length of urethra)
- Periurethral injection of GAX collagen, Bovine Collagen

Q22. How is pelvic floor muscle training (supervised) given?

To strengthen the muscular part of rhabdosphincter and pelvic floor muscle. The pelvic floor muscle training (PFMT) is in the form of drawing up the anus and tightening the vagina for stopping micturition. This squeeze and release is repeated 10 to 15 times with a total of 8 contractions 3 times a day. This should be done for minimum 3 months.

Q23. What are the surgical management of stress urinary incontinence?

1. **Kelly's cystourethroplasty:**
   - Common procedure
   - Plication of pubocervical fascia is done to strengthen the urethral pressure.
2. **Retropubic cystourethropexy**
   a. Burch colposuspension:
      - Gold standard procedure
      - Endopelvic fascia lateral vaginal fornix is sutured to the ipsilateral iliopectineal ligament
      - Success rate 80-90%—5 years

   b. Marshall Marchetti-Krantz—paravaginal and paravesical fascia are fixed with periosteum of pubic bones.

   c. Laparoscopic bladder neck suspension

3. **Tension free midurethral tape procedure**
   - TVT (Tension free vaginal tape)
     - Success rate (80-90%) in 3 years.
     - Gortex tape is passed vaginally U shaped manner and kept tension free.
     - Improves the midurethral support.
   - Trans obturator tape
     - Support the urethral as a hammock
     - Success rate 80%
     - A tape is passed through the obturator foramen
   - Bladder sling procedure
     - Mini sling/micro sling
     - Pubovaginal sling
4. **Urethral bulking agent**
   - Intrinsic sphincter deficiency.
   - Bovine collagen. Teflon
5. **Salvage procedures:** where all other procedures have failed.
   - Implantation of artificial sphincter
   - Urinary diversion

Q24. What are the advantages of surgery of stress urinary incontinence?

- Restoration of normal anatomy to maintain bladder neck and proximal urethra.
- Strengthening the support of bladder neck and proximal urethra.
- To increase the functional urethral length.

Q25. What are the complications of surgery?

- Hemorrhage.
- Urinary tract and visceral injury.
- UTI.
- Wound infection.
- Voiding dysfunction.
- OAB.
- Pelvic organ prolapse.
- Nerve injuries.
- Osteitis pubis.
- Other's:
  - Dyspareunia
  - Chronic suprapubic pain
  - Sinus tract formation.

Q26. What is Tension free vaginal tape?

Tension free vaginal tape (TVT) is a surgical procedure for correction of stress urinary incontinence. It is one of the latest method of surgical treatment (SUI) which is recommended as "Grade- A" evidence-based level.

Q27. How much effective Tension free vaginal tape?

Success rate: 80-90%.

Q28. What is the aim of TVT?

1. To strengthen pubourethral ligament.
2. To prevent proximal relaxation.

Q29. In which patient Tension free vaginal tape is effective?

- When PFMT failed
- Severe stress urinary incontinence
- Associated with pelvic organ prolapse

Q30. What are the prerequisite of TVT procedure?

- Advise counsel the women that is a permanent implant and complete removal might not be possible.
- Give the women written information about the implant
    - Including its name.
    - Manufacturer.
    - Date of insertion.
    - Implanting surgeons name and contact details

Q31. What are the steps of TVT procedure?

- Anesthesia: Local Anesthesia (LA)
- A Marlex or Gortex, length (40 cm) and breath (10 mm) is passed vaginally in a U shaped manner under the midurethral to the either side with especially designed needles.
- The needles are passed along the back of the pubic bone to the skin incision on either side of midline. Cystoscopy is done at the end of procedure.
- Tape is not suture to any structure.

Q32. Mechanism of action of TVT procedure?

TVT increase the urethral coaptation by kinking the urethra during IAP.

Q33. What are the advantages of TVT procedure?

- Less invasive
- Short hospital stay
- Operative time is short
- Patient compliance good
- Success rate 80-90% for 3 years
- Can be done under LA.

Q34. What are the limitations of TVT procedure?

- Injury to:
    - UB
    - Intestine
    - Blood vessels
- Bladder perforation (3-9% common)
- Retropubic hematoma.
- Overactive bladder.
- Mesh erosion
- Voiding difficulty
- Tape rejection

Q35. Postoperative management of TVT procedure?

- Catheterization for 5 days
- Prophylactic Antibiotics
- Kegels exercise and Biofeedback method.

Q36. Before discharge what precautions should be taken?

USG to see the:

- Retropubic hematoma
- Residual volume.

Q37. When follow-up should be given after procedure?

Within 6 months of surgical procedure of SUI.

Q38. Definition of overactive bladder (Detrusor Overactivity)

An overactive bladder (OAB) is defined by the International Continence Society as 'one that is shown objectively to contract spontaneously or on provocation during the filling phase while the patient is attempting to inhibit micturition'.

Q39. Incidence and prevalence of overactive bladder.

Among the elderly women, OAB is the most common cause. Overall prevalence is 12-15% in women aged 40 years or more.

Q40. What are the common etiology of overactive bladder?

Gynecological

- Genitourinary prolapse
- Genuine stress incontinence
- Menopause (tissue atrophy due to estrogen deficiency)
- Pelvic mass
- Pregnancy

Urological

- Urinary tract infection
- Detrusor overactivity (DO)
- Urethral syndrome
- Interstitial cystitis
- Diabetes

Medical

- Neurological lesions (multiple sclerosis, Alzheimer's disease)
- Diuretic therapy

Others

Psychological and idiopathic

Q41. What is the pathophysiology of overactive bladder?

The pathophysiology is obscure. There may be increased in a-adrenergic activities causing increased detrusor contraction. It is thought that inappropriate detrusor contraction results when there is passage of urine into the proximal urethra due to incompetence of the bladder neck. Incompetent bladder neck → urine in proximal urethra → OAB/DO → incontinence. This occurs despite the effort of the individual to inhibit them. Other explanation is change in the detrusor smooth muscle property (due to atherosclerosis or neuropathy) that leads to inappropriate DO.

Q42. What are the symptoms of overactive bladder?

- Involuntary loss of urine without any prior urge to urinate.
- Urgency, frequency (>8 times/day), nocturia (>once/night) and bed wetting.
- Associated with GSI too often.

Q43. How will you diagnose overactive bladder?

- Maintenance of urinary diary for 4 days.
- Detailed neurological examination.
- Midstream urine examination for culture and sensitivity test.
- Post-void residual (PVR) urine measurement.
- Urodynamics done in selected cases.

Q44. How will you manage overactive bladder?

General

- Psychosomatic problems: Psychotherapy.
- Other medical problems (neurological, diabetes) should be properly attended.

Behavioral therapy

- Limit the intake of fluid to l liter/day
- Drugs-diuretics may be stopped if possible
- Avoidance of bladder irritants: caffeine, alcohol, carbonated beverages
- Weight loss
- Cessation of smoking
- Bladder training including PFMT
- Bladder retraining

Drugs:

- **Antimuscarinic drugs**
  - If patient compliance good
    - Oxybutynin tab 5 mg daily
  - If patient complain dry mouth, change in to
    - Oxybutynin patch
  - If patient compliance not good
    - *Tolterodine*: 1-2 mg daily, BD
    - *Darifenacin*: 7.5-15 mg daily
    - *Solifenacin*: 5-10 mg daily
- **Selective B3 agonist:**
  - Mirabegron 25-50 mg daily
    If no response:
  - MDT needed
  - No need urodynamic, should not give to cardiac patient.
- **If patient have nocturia:**
  - Ist-line management: Desmopressin should not give for CVD/HTN
  - 2nd-line management:
    - Imipramine
    - Trospium (elderly frail women) 40-60 mg daily

Surgical intervention

- Neuromodulation and pelvic floor elective stimulation
- Botulinum toxin
- Percutaneous tibial nerve stimulation
- Augmentation cystoplasty
- Urinary diversion

CHAPTER 26

Vesicovaginal Fistula and Rectovaginal Fistula

Q1. Define genitourinary fistula.

Genitourinary fistula

Genitourinary fistula is an abnormal communication between the urinary and genital tract either acquired or congenital with involuntary escape of urine into the vagina.

Fistula

A fistula is an abnormal communication between two or more epithelial surfaces.

Q2. What are the types of genitourinary fistula?

Types of genitourinary fistula

The communication may occur between the bladder, urethra or ureter and genital tract.

1. Bladder
   - Vesicovaginal (commonest)
   - Vesicourethrovaginal
   - Vesicouterine
   - Vesicocervical
2. Urethra
   - Urethrovaginal
3. Ureter
   - Ureterovaginal
   - Ureterouterine
   - Uterocervical

VESICOVAGINAL FISTULA (VVF)

Q1. What is VVF?

Vesicovaginal: Abnormal communication between the bladder and the vagina and the urine escapes into the vagina causing true incontinence.

Q2. What are the causes of VVF?

Causes of Vesicovaginal fistula

1. Obstetrical causes (80-90%)
   a. Ischemic: In obstructed labor, prolonged compression effect on the bladder base between head and symphysis pubis—ischemic necrosis-Infection-sloughing-Fistula
   b. Traumatic:
      - Following instrumental vaginal delivery (such as destructive operations or forceps specially with Kielland)
      - Following abdominal operations (such as hysterectomy for rupture uterus or caesarean section)

2. Gynecological causes:
   a. Operative injury: Anterior colporrhaphy, abdominal hysterectomy etc.
   b. Traumatic: Following fall on a pointed object or by a stick used for criminal abortion.
   c. Malignancy: Advanced carcinoma of the cervix, vagina, or bladder
   d. Radiation
   e. Infection: Vaginal tuberculosis, Lymphogranuloma venereum, schistosomiasis etc.
   f. Congenital malformation: Aberrant ureter, persisting urogenital sinus.

Q3. What is the mechanism of development of VVF in obstructed labor?

Mechanism of formation of obstetrical fistula

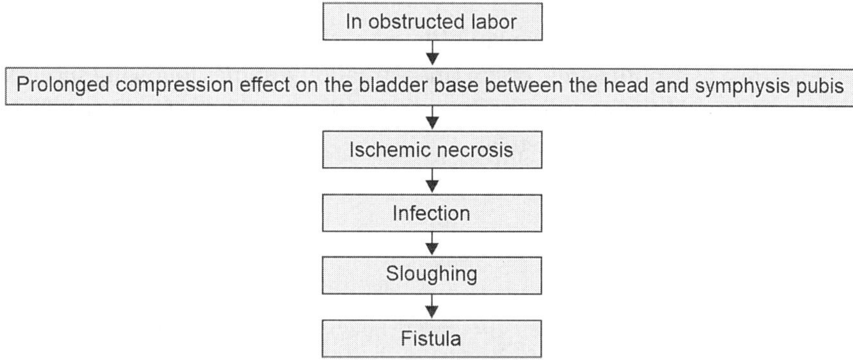

It takes few days (3-5) following delivery to produce obstetric of fistula.

Types of VVF

Depending upon the site of fistula, it may be:

1. *Juxtacervical (close to cervix):* The communication is between the supratrigonal region of the bladder and the vagina.
2. *Midvaginal*: The communication is between the base (trigone) of the bladder and vagina.
3. *Juxtaurethral*: The communication is between the neck of the bladder and vagina (may involve upper urethra)
4. *Subsymphysial*: Circumferential loss of tissue in the region of bladder neck and urethra. The fistula margin is fixed to the bone.

Q4. How will you manage a case?

Management of VVF

- Diagnosis
  - Clinical features
    - Patient profile
      - Usually, young primiparous
      - History of difficult labor or instrument delivery in recent past.
- Symptoms
  - Continuous escape of urine per vagina (true incontinence) - classic symptom
  - No urge to pass urine
  - There is associated pruritus vulvae
- Signs
  - General examination
    - Usually short statured
    - Uriniferous smell from the patient
    - Wetting of clothes

- Vulval inspection
  - Escape of watery discharge per vaginam of ammoniacal smell is characteristic.
  - Evidences of sodden and excoriation of the vulval skin
  - Varying degrees of perineal tear may be present.
- Internal examination
  - Its fistula is big enough, its position, size and tissue at the margins are to be noted.
- Speculum examination
  - Size, site, and number of fistula
  - The bladder mucosa may be visibly prolapsed through a big fistula.
  - A tiny fistula is evidenced by a puckered area of vaginal mucosa.

Associated clinical features that may be present in VVF.
1. Secondary amenorrhea of hypothalamic origin (menstruation resumes following successful repair)
2. Foot-drop (due to prolonged compression of the sacral nerve roots by the fetal head during labor)
3. Complete perineal tear or rectovaginal fistula

Investigation: To confirm the diagnosis
1. EUA (examination Under Anesthesia)
2. Dye test
3. Three swab test
4. Cystoscopy
5. IVU (for diagnosis of ureterovaginal fistula)

Treatment: Operative treatment

Definitive surgery: Local repair of vesico-vaginal fistula by flap splitting method with or without graft.

Different tissue may be used for grafting
1. Vulval fat pad graft (Martius graft)
2. Gracilis muscle graft
3. Omentum graft

Other types of operation can be done in different routes:
1. *Vaginal route*:
   a. *Saucerization*: Closure of a small fistula using interrupted stitches without dissection of bladder from the vagina.
   b. *Colpocleisis*: Partial or total
2. Abdominal route
   a. Transvesical
   b. Transperitoneal
   c. Combined

Q5. What is three swab test?

Three Swab Test

The three-swab test not only confirms the VVF but also differentiates it from ureterovaginal and urethrovaginal fistula.

Procedure
- Three cotton swabs are placed in the vagina:
  - One at the vault
  - One at the middle
  - One just above the introitus

- The methylene blue/1% gentian violet is instilled into the bladder through a rubber catheter, and the patient is asked to walk about for about 5 minutes.
- She is then asked to lie down, and the swabs are removed for inspection.

Interpretation

Observation	***Inference***
1. Upper most swab soaked with dye. The lower two fistula swabs remain dry.	Ureterovagina fistula
2. Upper and lower swabs remain dry, but the middle swab stained with dye	Vesicovaginal fistula
3. The upper two swabs remain dry, but the lower swab stained with dye.	Urethrovaginal fistula

Q6. Write down Pre-operative management before VVF repair?

Pre-operative assessment

1. Fistula status (site, size, number, mobility, and status of the margins of the fistula)
2. Urethral involvement (assessed by introducing a metal catheter through external urethral meatus into the bladder)
3. Cystoscopy
4. To exclude associated rectovaginal fistula or complete perineal tear.
5. Routine investigation
   - CBC with ESR
   - Blood grouping & Rh typing
   - Random blood sugar level
   - Blood urea and serum creatinine
   - Urine R/ME
   - Chest X-ray
   - ECG

- Pre-operative preparations
  - Improvement of general condition
  - Treatment of local infection in the vulva
  - Urinary infection, if any, should be corrected beforehand.

Principles of local repair by flap splitting method

1. Perfect asepsis and good exposure of the fistula
2. Excision (minimal) of the scar tissue round the margins
3. Mobilization of the bladder wall from the vagina
4. Suturing the bladder wall without tension in two layers

Q7. What is the ideal time to repair VVF after delivery and why?

Timing of VVF repair after delivery

The ideal time to repair VVF is between 3-6 months following delivery. This time is necessary for:

1. Improvement of general condition
2. Local tissue reaction to subside
3. Tissue are free from infection.

Q8. How will you prevent obstetric fistula in our country?

Prevention of VVF/Reduction of incidence of VVF in Bangladesh

1. Adequate antenatal care (to rule out at risk mothers likely to develop obstructed labor)
2. Proper utilization of partograph to curtail prolonged labor
3. Continuous bladder drainage for about 14 days following delivery either vaginally or abdominally in case of long standing obstructed labor
4. Meticulous care during obstetrical and gynecological surgery to avoid injury to the bladder

5. Training of doctors and paramedics for anticipation, early detection, and proper management of obstructed labor.
6. Community awareness to arrange transport for sending the patient to the proper place for safe delivery.

Q9. What are the criteria for successful repair of VVF?

Criteria for successful repair of VVF

1. Number of fistula : Single
2. Site : Vesicovaginal fistula (VVF)
3. Size : <4 cm
4. Urethral involvement : Absent
5. Vaginal scarring : Absent
6. Tissue loss : Minimal
7. Ureter involvement : Absent
8. Circumferential defect : Absent

Q10. What is the postoperative management of local repair of VVF?

Postoperative management of local repair of VVF

1. Nothing by mouth till bowel sound returns
2. Antibiotic should be given preferably ampicillin.
3. Continuous catheter drainage for 2–3 weeks
4. Urinary output should be measured meticulously and should be balanced against the fluid intake (to detect early catheter blockage)
5. Patient should be advised to take plenty of water by mouth.
6. The patient should be asked about the soiling of bed.
7. Before removal of the catheter, it should be clamped periodically (to regain the tone of the bladder and to see any leakage of urine)

Advice during discharge

1. To pass urine more frequently
2. To check up after 6 weeks
3. Avoid intercourse for 3 months
4. To defer pregnancy for 1 year
5. Antenatal checkup is mandatory in subsequent pregnancies. The baby must be delivered by caesarean section.

Q11. What is the treatment of failed local repair of VVF?

Treatment of failed local repair of VVF

- Local repair should again be attempted after 3 months. The Fistula may become smaller when the second attempt may be successful.
- In case of repeated failures, Urinary diversion operation is preferred.

How many times repair can be attempted in case of failure?

Repair can be tried several times as far as healthy and adequate tissue around the fistula is an available.

Q12. How will you manage a case of recently formed fistula?

Management of recently formed VVF

1. If injury to the bladder is recognized while performing destructive vaginal delivery or during caesarean section: Injury is to repaired at once followed by continuous bladder drainage for 3 weeks under urinary antiseptic such as nitrofurantoin or any other antibiotics.
2. If history of recent fistula of about 1–2 weeks old
   Conservative management by continuous bladder drainage for about 2–3 weeks. With this treatment small fistula may heal spontaneously and big fistula may become smaller in size.

RECTOVAGINAL FISTULA (RVF)

Q1. Define Rectovaginal fistula.

Rectovaginal fistula (RVF)

Abnormal communication between the rectum and vagina with involuntary escape of flatus and/or feces into the vagina is called rectovaginal fistula (RVF).

Q2. What are the causes of RVF?

Causes of RVF

- Acquired
  a. Obstetrical:
    i. Incomplete healing or unrepaired recent complete perineal tear (commonest)
    ii. Obstructed labor
    iii. Instrumental injury inflicted during destructive operation.
  b. Gynecological
    i. Following incomplete healing of old complete perineal tear (commonest)
    ii. Trauma inflicted inadvertently and remains unrecognized in operations like:
      - Perineorrhaphy
      - Repair of enterocele
      - Vaginal tubectomy
      - Posterior colpotomy (to drain pelvic abscess)
      - Reconstruction of vagina
    iii. Fall on a sharp pointed object
    iv. Malignancy of vagina (common), cervix, or bowel
    v. Radiation
    vi. Lymphogranuloma venereum or TB of the vagina
    vii. Diverticulitis of the sigmoid colon → abscess → bursts into the vagina.
    viii. Crohn's disease involving the canal or lower rectum
- Congenital: The anal canal may open into the vestibule or in the vagina

Q3. How will you manage a case of RVF?

Management of VVF

Diagnosis:

1. Involuntary escape of flatus and or feces into the vagina
   If the fistula is small, there is incontinence of flatus and loose stool only but not of hard stool.
2. Rectovaginal examination reveals the site and size of the fistula
3. Confirmation of diagnosis
   a. By passing a probe through the vagina into the rectum
   b. Dye test: Methylene blue is introduced into the rectum which is seen escaping out through the fistula into the vagina
   c. Examination under anesthesia (EUA)
4. Investigations:
   1. Barium enema
   2. Barium meal and follow through
   3. Sigmoidoscopy
   4. Proctoscopy

Treatment:

1. Definitive treatment

   Definitive surgery includes:

   a. Situated low down: To make it a complete perineal tear
   b. Situated in the middle-third: Repair by flap method
2. Preventive treatment:
   a. Good intranatal care
   b. Identification of complete perineal tear and its effective repair
   c. Consciousness about the possible injury of the rectum in gynecologic surgery

URETERO-VAGINAL FISTULA

Q1. How will you manage a case of uretero-vaginal fistula?

Management of urtero-vaginal fistula

Diagnosis:

1. Escape of urine through vagina.
2. Patient has urge to pass urine and can Pass urine normally

Investigations:

1. Three swab test
2. IVU
3. Cystoscopy
4. Renal ultrasound
5. CT scan

Treatment: Ureteroileonecystostomy

Q2. How will you differentiate between vesicovaginal, uretero-vaginal and urethra-vaginal fistula?

Differences between three types of fistula

Traits	*Vesico-vagina fistula (VVF)*	*Uretero-vaginal fistula*	*Urethro-vaginal fistula*
1. Form history	• Continuous dribbling of urine • No desire to pass urine	• Continuous dribbling of urine • Desire to pass urine	No incontinence unless the internal urethral sphincter is damaged
2. From examination a. Inspection b. Palpation	• Can be seen by speculum examination. • Can be palpated by fingers.	• Can not be seen by speculum examination • Can be palpated by fingers	• Can be seen by speculum examination • Can be palpated by fingers.
3. Three swab test	Upper and lower swabs remain dry but the middle swab stained with dye	Upper most swab soaked with urine but unstained with dye. The lower two fistula swabs remain dry	The upper two swabs remain dry, but the lower swab stained with dye

CHAPTER 27

Anal Incontinence: Old Complete Perineal Tear

Q1. Write down the name of genital tract injuries.

Genital tract injuries

1. Foreign bodies in the genital tract
2. Vaginal burns
3. Direct trauma to vulva and vagina
4. Defective or deficient perineum
5. Complete perineal tear
6. Laceration of the cervix
7. Rupture and perforation of the uterus
8. Broad ligament hematoma
9. Genital tract fistulas
10. Acquired atresia and stenosis of the genital tract

Perineal Tear

Q1. Define complete perineal tear.

Complete perineal tear: Complete perineal tear or third-degree perineal tear is one, which involves perineal skin, perineal body, vaginal mucosa, and the sphincter ani externus with or without involvement of the anorectal mucosa.

Q2. What are types of perineal tear?

Ans. Classification/types/Degree of perineal tear

First degree	: Laceration of vaginal epithelium or perineal skin
Second degree	: Involvement of the perineal body but not the anal sphincter
Third degree	: Disruption of the anal sphincter complex (both external and internal)
Fourth degree	: Injury to the anal sphincter complex with tear of the anal epithelium.

Q3. What are the causes of complete perineal tear?

Causes of complete perineal tear:

1. Obstetrical
   a. Mismanaged second stage of labor
   b. During delivery of a large baby
   c. Face-to-pubis delivery
   d. Face delivery
   e. Forceps delivery
   f. Uncontrolled delivery of the fetal head at the height of uterine contraction.
   g. Precipitate labor
   h. Liberal episiotomy is not given in case of a rigid perineum or having previous perineorrhaphy done.
   i. Extension of a midline episiotomy

Q4. How will you manage a case of complete perineal tear?

Management of complete tear

- Diagnosis
  - Clinical feature
- Patient profile
  1. Usually primiparous
  2. History suggestive of inadequate care during childbirth
- Symptoms
  1. Inability to hold the flatus and feces
  2. Soreness over the perianal region (due to constant irritation by the stool)
- Signs
  - Inspection
    1. Absence of perineum
    2. Vaginal and rectal mucous membranes are found to be continuous, only separated by a bridge of fibrous tissue
       Rectal mucosa is reddish and vaginal mucosa is pinkish in color
    3. Visible dimple on the skin on either side of the fused mucosa may be present.
- Palpation
  1. Absence of the sphincteric grip evidence when a finger is introduced into the rectum.
  2. The anal canal is separated from the vagina only by a septum.

Treatment

- *Definitive surgery:* Repair of the perineal tear with restoration of the perineal body (perineorrhaphy) immediately after injury or within first 24 hours under G/A.

Q5. When a patient of complete perineal tear will come for definitive treatment?

Timing of repair of complete perineal tear

- Complete perineal tear should be repaired immediately after injury or within first 24 hours under G/A because during that period infection has not yet established.
- If there is a delay, repair should be postponed for at least 3–6 months following the injury. This will help as following:
  1. Local infection to subside
  2. Return of an adequate blood supply to the margins of the tear
  3. Return of optimum viability of the perineal tissue
- Deferment beyond 6 months should be avoided as there will be more fibrosis at the margins which will hinder adequate dissection and healing process.

Q6. How will you prepare a patient for repair of complete perineal tear?

Pre-operative preparation of complete perineal tear

1. The patient is to be admitted at least 5 days prior to surgery
2. Diet
   a. Low residual diet (milk, biscuits, etc.) for days following admission
   b. Liquid diet only for 48 hours prior to surgery
   c. Nothing by mouth from the morning on the day of operation
3. Bowel preparation
   a. Laxatives twice daily following admission.
   b. Enema should be given for 2 days prior to surgery and should be repeated until the rectum is clear
   c. Enema should be avoided in the morning of the day of operation.

4. Intestinal antiseptics
   Started 5 days prior to surgery. Ampicillin 2501 mg four times daily and metronidazole 400 mg twice daily has to be given for 5 days.

- Now a days this long bowel preparation procedure is replaced by following preparation:
  1. Oral intake of mannitol (5 mL/kg) solution 12 hours before operation (mannitol causes mechanical bowel clearance by strong purgation)
  2. Parenteral antibiotics and metronidazole are to be given.
  3. Normal saline or Hartsol solution is to be started I/V for correction of dehydration.

Q7. What is the postoperative management of complete perineal tear?

Postoperative management of Complete Perineal tear

1. Diet:
   a. Nothing by mouth for the first 48 hours following surgery and intravenous fluid is maintained
   b. She is allowed to have liquid diet from 48 hours
   c. Low residual diet for next 3 days.
   d. Normal diet may be given from the 5th post-operative day
2. Milk of magnesia 10–15 mL twice daily from the 3rd day to soft the stool
3. *Parental antibiotic:* Ampicillin, gentamicin, and metronidazole regimen for 7 days

Q8. Write down the steps of complete perineal tear repair operation.

Steps of complete perineal tear repair operation

1. This operation is done under general or spinal anesthesia in lithotomy position.
2. Vulva and vagina are to be swabbed with antiseptic solution.
3. The perineum is to be draped with sterile sheet.
4. Mobilization of the rectum and anal sphincter
5. **Repair**
   a. Rectal wall is closed by a series of interrupted sutures with no. 2.0 or 3.0 vicryl with a round body atraumatic needle staring from the apex.
   b. The pararectal fascia is approximated over the first layer by interrupted sutures using the same suture material.
   c. Th torn one end of the external anal sphincter is stretched across the other end and then sutured with either vicryl "2.0" or 3.0 PDS (NICE guidelines)
   d. Two to three interrupted sutures are placed through the perineal muscles.
   e. The vaginal wall and the perineal skin are then approximated by 2-0 vicryl.

Q9. How can you prevent complete perineal tear?

Prevention of complete perineal tear

1. Controlled delivery of the head
2. Delivery by early extension is to be avoided.
3. Spontaneous forcible delivery of the head is to be avoided by assuring the patient not to bear down during contractions.
4. To deliver the head in between contractions
5. To perform timely episiotomy (when needed)
6. To take care during delivery of the shoulders

Q10. What are the complications of complete perineal tear repair operation?

Complications of complete perineal tear repair

- Immediate
  1. Difficulty in dissection due to scarring

2. Difficulty in identifying the torn ends of the sphincter
3. Injury to the rectum

- Late
1. Wound infection and defecation
2. Recto-vaginal fistula (RVF)
3. Painful or difficult defecation
4. Dyspareunia
5. Anal incontinence

Q11. What are the advices given during discharge following repair of complete perineal tear?

Advice on discharge following complete perineal tear repair

1. Stool should be kept soft using laxatives for at least 2 weeks
2. Avoidance of coitus for 6 weeks
3. Maintenance of perineal hygiene
4. Postoperative checkup after 6 weeks to see the condition of the wound
5. Mandatory hospital delivery and liberal episiotomy during subsequent pregnancies.

CHAPTER 28

Menopausal and Hormone Therapy

Q1. What do you mean by menopause?

It is defined as permanent cessation of menstruation resulting from the loss of ovarian follicular activity. The duration of cessation should be at least 12 months from last cycle.

Q2. What is the age of menopause?

- Age of menopause is genetically predetermined. It is not related to age of menarche or age of last pregnancy but related to lactation, pill use, race, height.
- Age of menopause ranges between 45-55 years.

Q3. Who has chances to get late or early menopause?

- Late menopause—high parity or higher BMI
- Early menopause—chemotherapy, ovarian resection, or women with smoking habit.

Q4. What are the other phases of menopause?

- **Menopause transition:** Period of time during which a woman passes from reproductive to non-reproductive stage. Covers 4-5 years of either side of menstruation. Associated with elevated FSH and length of cycle.
- **Perimenopause:** Starting from few years before continuing after the period of onset of menopause
- **Climacteric:** Time after the cessation of reproductive function
- **Post menopause:** Phase of life after menopause.

Q5. What are the common symptoms of menopause?

Common symptoms include hot flashes, night sweats, vaginal dryness, mood changes, and sleep disturbances. These symptoms can vary in intensity and duration among individuals.

Q6. What are the organ changes during menopause?

Ovary:

- Size shrink, wrinkled and white
- Thinning of cortex

Fallopian tubes: Features of atrophy, cilia disappear, plicae less prominent

Uterus:

- Becomes smaller, ratio of body and cervix—1:1
- Endometrium—thin and atrophied

Menstrual changes: Abnormal uterine bleeding due to anovulation and unopposed estrogen effects

Vagina:

- Narrower due to loss of elasticity
- Epithelium—thin
- Rugae—flatten

- pH alkaline
- Maturation index—10/85/5

Vulva:
- Atrophy
- Labia—flattened
- Pubic hair—scanty

Breast fat:
- Reabsorbed, gland atrophy
- Flat and pendulous breast
- Bladder and urethra
- Epithelium—thin
- More prone to infection
- Dysuria, frequency or even stress incontinence

Loss of muscle tone: Pelvic relaxation, uterine descent and anatomical changes in urethra and neck of bladder

Adrenal: Decline DHEAS

Q7. What are the symptoms of menopause transition?

a. Menstrual changes
   Shorter cycle, irregular bleeding
b. Vasomotor symptoms
   - Hot flashes
   - Upper body sweating
   - Anxiety and lack of sleep
c. Psychological
   - Irritability
   - Mood swings
   - Poor memory
   - Depression
d. Sexual dysfunction
   - Vaginal dryness
   - Decreased libido
   - Dyspareunia
   - Itching vulva
e. Urinary
   - Incontinence
   - Urgency
   - Frequency
   - Dysuria
   - Recurrent UTI
f. Others
   - Back ache
   - Joint aches
   - Weight gain
   - Palpitation

Q8. What are the risk factors for vasomotor symptoms?

- Early menopause
- Surgical menopause

- Use of SERMs
- Sedentary lifestyle
- Smoking

Q9. How do you diagnose menopause?

1. Cessation of menstruation for consecutive 12 months during climacteric
2. Average age 51.3 years
3. Appearance of menopause symptoms: Hot flashes and night sweats
4. Vaginal cytology: 10/85/5 (features of low estrogen)
5. Low level of AMH
6. Increasing symptoms of urogenital atrophy
7. Serum estradiol <20 pg/mL
8. Serum FSH and LH >40 mIU/mL (3 values at weeks interval needed)

Q10. Mention abnormal menopause.

Abnormal menopause refers to menopause that occurs earlier or later than the normal physiological age or is associated with abnormal symptoms or pathological causes affecting ovarian function.

Q11. What are some lifestyle changes to ease menopausal symptoms?

- Maintain a healthy weight through diet and exercise.
- Practice stress-reduction techniques such as yoga or meditation.
- Stay hydrated and limit alcohol and caffeine intake.

Q12. What is postmenopause?

Postmenopause refers to the period after menopause has occurred, marking the end of the menopausal transition. During this phase, women may experience a reduction in menopause symptoms but may still face long-term health considerations related to hormone changes.

Q13. Where does the menopause osteoporosis begin?

In the spine.

Q14. Write down the treatment ways.

1. **Nonhormonal**
    - Lifestyle modification
    - Nutritious diet
    - Supplementary calcium
    - Exercise
    - Vitamin D
    - Cessation of smoking and alcohol
    - Biphosphonates to prevent bone resorption
    - Calcitonin inhibits bone resorption by inhibiting osteoclasts
    - Selective estrogen receptor modulators (SERMs)
    - Bazedoxifene controls vasomotor symptoms
    - Clonidine—reduce severity and duration of hot flashes
    - Antidepressants
    - Parathyroid hormone
    - Phytoestrogens
    - Soy protein
    - Vitamin E
2. **Hormonal**

    To overcome short term and long-term consequences of estrogen therapy

Q15. What are the indications for hormone therapy?
- Relief of menopausal symptoms
- Relief of vasomotor symptoms
- Prevention of osteoporosis
- Maintain quality of life after menopause

Q16. Mention the special group who are prescribed for hormonal therapy.
- Premature ovarian failure
- Gonadal dysgenesis
- Surgical or radiation menopause

Q17. What are the benefits of hormonal therapy?
- Improvement of vasomotor symptoms (70-80%)
- Improvement of urogenital atrophy
- Increase in BMD (2-5%)
- Decreased risk in vertebral and hip joint (25-50%)
- Reduction in colorectal cancer
- Possibly cardioprotection

Q18. What are the contraindications of HRT?
1. Known or suspected breast cancer
2. Undiagnosed genital tract bleeding
3. Estrogen-dependent neoplasm in body
4. History of DVT
5. Untreated HTN
6. Acute liver disease, prior cholestatic jaundice
7. Gallbladder disease
8. Prior endometriosis
9. Prior stroke, MI

Q19. What are the available preparations for hormone therapy?
The principal hormone used is estrogen in women following hysterectomy but women with intact uterus estrogen and progestin used.

Q20. What happens if only estrogen used in women with intact uterus?
Causes endometrial hyperplasia and even endometrial carcinoma

Q21. What is the commonly used HT?
Estrogens: Conjugated equine estrogen (CEE)—0.3,0.45 OR 0.625 mg/day or micronized estradiol 1-2 mg/day

Oral:
- CEE 0.3 mg + MPA 2.5 mg or 5 mg
- CEE 0.3 mg+MPA 1.5 mg

Progestins:
- Medroxyprogesterone acetate 1.5-5 mg/day
- Micronized progesterone 100-200 mg/day
- Dydrogesterone 5-10 mg/day

Subdermal implants:
- 17 β-estradiol implants 25 mg/50 mg or 100 mg
- Inserted subcutaneously over the anterior abdominal wall using local anesthesia for 6 months

Percutaneous estrogen gel: 1 g applicator of gel = 1mg estradiol daily

Transdermal patch: 17 β estradiol (0.025, 0.05, 0.75 or 0.1 mg/day) applied over buttock twice weekly

Vaginal cream: 1.25 mg daily effective for atrophic vaginitis

LNG-IUS: Protects endometrium from hyperplasia and cancer

Tibolone (19-nortestosterone derivative)

Q22. How will you monitor patient prior and during HRT?

A base level parameter of the following and their subsequent checkup at least annually are mandatory.

- Physical examination and pelvic examination
- Breast examination and mammography
- Cervical cytology
- Pelvic USG (TVS) for endometrial thickness (<5 mm)
- AUB should be investigated by endometrial biopsy or hysteroscopy.
- Serum level of estradiol and FSH.

Q23. Are there long-term health risks associated with menopause?

Yes, postmenopausal women may be at increased risk for osteoporosis, heart disease, and certain cancers. Regular check-ups and preventive health strategies are important for managing these risks.

CHAPTER 29

Postmenopausal Bleeding

Q1. A 60 years old lady presented with 2 episodes of postmenopausal bleeding.

a. How will you evaluate her?

b. How will you treat her?

Bleeding per vaginum following established menopause is called as postmenopausal bleeding. 75% of malignancy patient present with postmenopausal bleeding.

For evaluation of the above case a thorough history, clinical examination and investigations.

The most possible causes are:

1. **Gynecological:**
   a. Benign lesion:
      - Senile vaginitis and senile endometritis—60-80%
      - Endometrial hyperplasia 5-15%
      - Endometrial polyp 2-12%
      - HRT 15-25%
      - Cervical polyp

   b. Malignant:
      - Endometrial carcinoma 10%
      - Carcinoma cervix
      - Estrogen producing tumor

   c. Idiopathic 25%
2. **Non-gynecological:**
   - Urethral caruncle
   - Bladder carcinoma
   - Rectum carcinoma

For evaluation

History

- Age:
  - 50-55 years—carcinoma cervix
  - 60 years—endometrial carcinoma
- Parity:
  - Nulliparous—increased risk of endometrial carcinoma
  - Multiparous—carcinoma cervix
- Symptom analysis
  i. Amount of bleeding: Significant amount—carcinoma cervix, endometrial carcinoma, polyp
  ii. Number of episodes: 2 or more episode is significant
  iii. Any preceding cause: Postcoital bleeding—carcinoma cervix, polyp

- Associated symptoms:
  i. Foul smelling discharge:
    - Ca cervix
    - Endometrial carcinoma
    - Senile vaginitis
    - Foreign body
  ii. Discharge with itching: Trichomoniasis
  iii. Discomfort/fullness of vagina: Vaginitis
  iv. Any bowel/bladder symptom
  v. History of something coming down per vagina
    - Uterovaginal prolapse
    - Pessary
- Postmenstrual history: Early menarche or late menopause: endometrial carcinoma
- Medical history: Increased risk of endometrial carcinoma if DM, HTN, obesity
- Family history:
  - Ca breast
  - Ca ovary
  - Ca colon
  - Ca endometrium
- Contraceptive history: Use of ocp for >10 years increases risk of cervical carcinoma
- Drug history: Irregular intake of estrogen, HRT increases the risk of endometrial carcinoma

Clinical Examination

General

- BMI
  - High in endometrial carcinoma
  - Low in carcinoma cervix
- Anemia—depends on blood loss
- Blood pressure—increased in endometrial carcinoma
- Edema—carcinoma cervix
- Abdominal examination:
  - Any mass/ovarian tumor
  - Any organomegaly
  - Ascites
- Vaginal examination

Inspection:

- Vulva, vagina atrophic-senile vaginitis
- Vulva red, congested, itchy-diabetic vulvitis
- Prolapse

Per speculum

- Senile vaginitis—patchy redness in vagina, blood stained discharge
- Any pessary
- Cauliflower like growth
- Polyp

Bimanual examination

i. Carcinoma cervix: Cervix hard, fixed, friable bleeds on touch
ii. Endometrial carcinoma: Uterus is bulky and soft

iii. Endometrial polyp
   - Uterus-bulky
   - Cervix-patulous

iv. Unilateral/bilateral: Ovarian tumor

Investigations: Aim of investigation is to

Confirm diagnosis:

a. USG of pelvic organ/TVS
   Endometrial carcinoma
   - Endometrial thickness ≥4 mm
   - Hyperechoic irregular outline

   Tubo-ovarian region adnexal mass
b. Saline infusion sonography
   Endometrial polyp
   - Homogenous, hyperechoic
   - Intracavitary mass
c. Hysteroscopy: For biopsy
d. Fractional curettage: For endometrial carcinoma
e. Colposcopy and pap smear

For diagnosis of extension of disease:

i. MRI
ii. CT scan
iii. Chest X-ray
iv. Sigmoidoscopy
v. Colonoscopy
vi. Routine investigations for anesthesia check-up

Management will be done according to the cause

General

- Patient should be counselled about
  - Diagnosis
  - Treatment option
  - Risk and benefit
  - Outcome
- Reassurance
- Follow-up
- Correction of anemia if present
- Control of HTN, DM

Specific

If no cancer detected—careful observation

1. Endometrial carcinoma
   Stage I:
   - Low risk—TAH with BLSO with LN sampling
   - High risk—TAH with BLSO with pelvic lymphadenectomy followed by adjuvant radiotherapy

   Stage II: TAH with BLSO with pelvic lymphadenectomy followed by adjuvant radiotherapy
   Stage III: Hysterectomy with BLSO with selective lymphadenectomy, omentectomy followed by radiotherapy (debulking surgery)

2. Carcinoma cervix
   Stage IA1—Extrafacial hysterectomy
   Stage IA2—Modified Radical hysterectomy with pelvic lymphadenectomy
   Stage IB-IB2—radical hysterectomy with pelvic lymphadenectomy
   Stage IB3-IIA2—CCRT/Surgery
   Stage IIB-IVA—Primary CCRT
   Stage IVB—Systemic CT+RT
3. Cervical polyp: Polypectomy, D & C and histopathological examination
4. Endometrial hyperplasia: Hysterectomy (>65 years)
5. Senile vaginitis: Improve general condition and antibiotics, local estrogen cream
6. Estrogen producing ovarian tumor: Surgical staging with TAH with BLSO
7. Pessary (forgotten): Removal with antibiotics
8. If estrogen therapy
   - Stop therapy
   - Malignancy evaluation

Nongynecological:

1. Urethral caruncle:
   - Estrogen therapy locally by pessaries
   - Local antiseptic
   - Long standing-excision and biopsy
2. Hemorrhoids:
   - Stool softener
   - Refer to colorectal surgery
3. Ca bladder/rectum:
   - Observation and assurance
   - Follow up after 6 months

Hormone therapy is indicated in menopausal women to overcome the short-term and long-term consequences of estrogen therapy.

Indication

- Relief of menopausal symptoms
- Relief of vasomotor symptoms
- Prevention of osteoporosis
- To maintain quality of life in menopausal years

Special group

- Premature ovarian failure
- Gonadal dysgenesis
- Surgical or radiation menopause

Complications

1. **Endometrial carcinoma:** If estrogen given to women with intact uterus causes endometrial proliferation, hyperplasia and carcinoma
2. **Breast cancer:** Combined estrogen and progestin replacement therapy for a long term (5 years) increases the risk of breast cancer
3. **Venous thromboembolic disease:** Increased risk due to combined estrogen and progestin
4. **Coronary artery disease:** There is increased risk of total cholesterol and LDL. Coagulation parameter altered with rise in factor VII and fibrinogen
5. **Stroke:** Oral estrogen is associated with a small increase in the risk of stroke
6. **Lipid metabolism:** Increased risk of gallbladder disease has been observed following ERT due to rise in cholesterol.

CHAPTER 30

Contraception

Q1. What do you mean by contraception?

Contraception means all measures taken temporary or permanent to prevent pregnancy due to coital act. Ideal contraception method should be highly effective acceptive safe, reversible, cheap, having non contraceptive benefit, simple to use and requiring minimal motivation, maintenance and supervision.

Q2. What are the methods of contraception?

Method of Contraception

Temporary methods:

- *Barrier methods:*
  - Mechanical:
    - Male: Condom
    - Female:
      - Female condom
      - Vaginal diaphragm
      - Cervical occlusion cap
  - Chemical (vaginal contraceptives)
    - Cream
    - Jelly
    - Foam
    - Sponge
  - Combination: E.g., condom along with a spermicidal
- *Natural contraception:*
  - Rhythm method
  - Coitus interruptus.
  - Lactational amenorrhea method
  - Basal body temperature method
- *Intrauterine contraceptive devices (IUCDs):*
  - Non-medicated: E.g., Lippies loop
  - Medicated:
    - Copper devices: Cu-T
    - LNG-IUS
- *Steroidal/Hormonal contraceptives:*
  - Oral contraceptives:
    - Combined pills
    - Sequential pill
    - Progesterone only pill (mini pill)
    - Post coital pill (emergency pill)
  - Parenteral preparations (progestogens)

    - Injections: E.g., DMPA, NET-EN
    - Sub dermal implants e.g., Norplant

Permanent methods:
- Female:
  - Tubal ligation
  - Tubal occlusion
- Male: Vasectomy

Intrauterine Contraceptive Device

IUCD: Intrauterine contraceptive device are the devices with small plastic carrier placed in the uterus for the purpose of contraception.

Types of IUCD:
- Non medicated or inert IUCDs: E.g., Lippies loop
- Medicated IUCDs:
  - Cu releasing IUCDs:
    - Cu-7
    - Cu T 200
    - Multiload Cu 250
    - Multiload Cu 375
    - Cu T 380 A
    - Cu T 380Ag
  - Hormone releasing IUCDs:
    - Progestasert
    - Levonorgestrel IUCD

Mechanism of action of 1st and 2nd generation IUCDs:
- IUCD causes a foreign body reaction in the uterus causing cellular and biochemical changes in the endometrium and uterine fluid. These changes impair the viability of the gamete and thus reduce its changes of fertilization rather than its implantation.
- 2nd generation medicated IUCD affects the enzyme in the uterus by altering the biochemical composition of cervical mucus.
- Copper ion may affect sperm motility, capacitation and survival.

Mechanism of action of 3rd generation IUCDs:
- Progesterone of 3rd generation IUCDs increases the thickness of cervical mucus and prevents sperm from entering the cervix.
- It decreases the thickness of endometrial mucosa and thereby prevents implantation.

Timing of IUCD insertion:
- *At the end of menstruation:* It is preferable to insert 2-3 days after the period is over.
- *Postabortal:* Following termination of pregnancy by evacuation or D&C, or following spontaneous abortion.
- *Postpartum:* Following delivery insertion is usually done after 6 weeks.
- *Postplacental delivery:* Following the delivery of the placenta.

Advantages of IUCD/Cu-T:
- Less expensive.
- Simplicity in techniques of insertion.
- Prolong contraceptive protection after insertion and suitable for the rural population of developing countries.
- Systemic side effects are nil.

- Suitable for hypertensive, breastfeeding women.
- Reversibility to fertility is prompt after removal.

Disadvantages of IUCD:
- Require motivation.
- Limitation in its use.
- Adverse local reactions manifested by menstrual abnormalities, PID, pelvic pain and heavy periods.
- Risk of ectopic pregnancy.

Complications of IUCD/Cu-T:
Immediate:
- Cramp like pain.
- Syncopal attack.
- Partial or complete perforation.

Delayed:
- pain.
- Abnormal menstrual bleeding.
- PID
- Spontaneous expulsion.

Contraindications of IUCD:
- Pregnancy or suspected pregnancy.
- Undiagnosed per vaginal bleeding.
- Acute pelvic infection.
- Distortion of the shape of the uterus or uterine cavity as fibroid.
- Severe dysmenorrhea.
- Known or suspected uterine or cervical neoplasia.
- Sexually transmitted diseases (STDs)
- Gestational trophoblastic diseases.
- Immunosuppressive disorders.
- Breast cancer

Indications of removal of IUCD:
- Persistent excessive regular or irregular uterine bleeding.
- Flaring up of salpingitis.
- Uterine perforation.
- Partial expulsion of the device.
- Suspected pregnancy.
- Missing thread.
- One year after menopause.

Management of missing Cu-T:
History: Questions about:
- When did she feel the thread last?
- Is the tread torn out?
- Is there any pain?
- Is there any missed period?

Examination:
- Breast examination: Is there any signs of pregnancy
- Abdominal and pelvic examination: Signs of pregnancy, any tenderness?

Investigation:

USG of lower abdomen and pelvis

- Hysteroscopy
- X-ray pelvis

Treatment:

- If device inside the uterine cavity—uterine curette or hysteroscopic removal
- If the device is outside the uterine cavity but inside the abdominal cavity—laparoscopy or laparotomy.

Levonorgestrel-IUS (Mirena):

Mechanism of action:

- It induces strong and uniform suppression of endometrium.
- Cervical mucus becomes very thick and scanty. It impedes sperm motility and access to the upper genital tract.
- Anovulation and insufficient literal phase activity has also altered.
- Decreases tubal motility.

Advantages of LNG-IUS:

- Higher efficacy with lowest pregnancy rate.
- Can be used for longer duration of action (for 5-10 years)
- Lower expulsion rate and fewer indications for medical removal.
- Used as reduction in the risk endometrial and cervical carcinoma.
- Can be used as fertility sparing treatment of early stage endometrial carcinoma.
- Safe and effective as an alternative to sterilization method.
- It can provide the benefits of hormone replacement therapy.

Disadvantages of LNG-IUS:

- Expensive.
- Not available everywhere
- Can cause amenorrhea.
- Long duration of use can cause infertility or abortion.

Steroidal Contraceptions

Types of Hormonal or steroidal contraceptives:

- Oral contraceptives (oral pills)
    - Combined oral pills:
        - Monophasic
        - Biphasic
        - Triphasic.
        - Emergency/post-coital pill.
    - Single preparation:
        - Estrogen only pill.
        - Progesterone only pill.
        - Sequential pill.
- Parenteral preparations:
    - Injectable:
        - DMPA
        - NET-EN
    - Implants:
        - Implanon
        - Norplant-||
        - LNG Rod.

- Device:
  - IUD: LNG-IUS
  - Vaginal ring
- Transdermal patches: Nesterone.

Mechanism of actions of oral pill:

- Inhibition of ovulation by suppression of LH surge.
- Alteration in the composition of cervical mucus. The cervical mucus becomes thick, viscid, and scanty and prevents sperm penetration.
- Atrophy of the endometrium that prevents implantation of the fertilized ovum.
- Interference with the mobility and secretion of the fallopian tubes.

Selection criteria of a client for OCP:

Thorough history, examination and some investigations may be needed to exclude contraindications.

From history and examination:

- Age: If the patient is more than 35years OCP should be prescribed with caution and regular check-up.
- History of smoking
- Menstrual history should be taken to exclude pregnancy.
- Obstetrical history including breast feeding.
- Family history of cerebrovascular disease including hypertension or breast carcinoma.
- Medical history regarding thromboembolic episodes, jaundice, epilepsy, hypertension, diabetes, migraine etc should be excluded.
- Weight and blood pressure should be noted.

Investigations:

- Lipid profile
- Serum bilirubin
- Cervical smear

Choice of pill—should be one, containing the lowest effective dose of estrogen and progesterone.

Instructions:

- OCP should be started on the first day of menstruation.
- Patient should be instructed to take pill at the same time everyday, preferably at night.
- Patient should starts with the white pill and after completing one strip, new strip should be started without any interval.
- If one tablet is missed, it must be taken immediately as soon as she remembers, in addition to the scheduled one.
- If two consecutive tablets are missed additional contraceptive protection such as barrier method should be taken along with the rest of the tablets.
- For lactating mothers, OCP should be commenced 6months after delivery because estrogen-progesterone preparations affect the quality and quantity of the milk.

Indications of combined oral contraceptives:

According to WHO category:

Category-1: (No restriction of use)

- Age: Menarche to 40years.
- Postabortion.
- Anemia (iron deficiency, malaria)
- HIV or AIDS (additional to condom use)
- GTN following normal hCG level.

- History of ectopic pregnancy.
- Endometriosis, uterine fibroid, ovarian or endometrial carcinoma.
- Dysmenorrhea, DUB.
- Pelvic inflammatory disease
- Epilepsy
- Thyroid disease
- Varicose vein
- Tuberculosis
- Benign breast disease.

Contraindications of COC's

Relative contraindications:

WHO category-2:

- Age >40 years.
- Smoker <35 years
- History of jaundice
- Mild hypertension
- Gallbladder disease
- Diabetes
- Sickle cell disease
- Headache
- Cancer cervix or CIN

WHO category-3:

- Unexplained vaginal bleeding.
- Hyperlipidemia.
- Liver tumors (benign)
- Breastfeeding (postpartum 6weeks to 6months)
- Heavy smoker (>20 cigarettes/day)
- Past breast cancer.

Absolute contraindications:

WHO category-4:

- Circulatory disease:
    - Arterial or venous thrombosis
    - Severe hypertension
    - History of stroke
    - Valvular heart disease
    - Ischemic heart disease
    - Diabetes with vascular complications
    - Migraine with focal neurological symptoms.
- Disease of liver:
    - Active liver disease.
    - Liver adenoma, carcinoma.
- Others:
    - Pregnancy
    - Breast feeding (postpartum 6 weeks)
    - Major surgery or prolong immobilization.
    - Estrogen dependent neoplasm e.g., breast cancer.

Disadvantages or complications of COC's:

- *Minor complications:*
- Nausea, vomiting, headache and leg cramps.
- Mastalgia
- Weight gain
- Cloasma and acne
- Menstrual abnormalities
  - Breakthrough bleeding or spotting.
  - Hypomenorrhea.
  - Menorrhagia.
  - Amenorrhea.
- Loss of libido.
- Leukorrhea.

Major complications:

- Depression
- Hypertension
- Vascular complications:
  - Venous thromboembolism
  - Arterial thrombosis
- Cholestatic jaundice
- Neoplasia
  - Breast cancer
  - Cervical cancer

Progesterone only pill

Mini pill/Progesterone only pill: Mini pill contains only very low dose of progesterone and devoid of estrogen. The commonly used forms are:

- Levonorgestrel 75 microgram
- Norethisterone 350 microgram
- Desogestrel 75 microgram
- Norgestrel 30 microgram
- Lynestrenol 500 microgram

Mechanism of action:

- Thickening of cervical mucous hinders sperm penetration.
- Endometrial atrophy prevents blastocyst implantation.
- Ovulation inhibition in 2% cases.
- Abnormal luteal function.
- Decrease tubal motility.

Timing of starting mini pill: The pill should be started from the first day of the cycle, one pill per day, throughout the cycle, without break in between the packs.

Indications:

- Patients aging more than 35 years.
- Patients whom estrogen is contraindicated.
- Lactating mother.

Complications:

- Acne, mastalgia, headache.
- Breakthrough bleeding or at times amenorrhea.

- Simple ovarian cyst may be seen.
- Failure rate about 0.5 to 2 per 100 women per year.

Contraindications:
- Pregnancy
- Unexplained vaginal bleeding.
- Breast carcinoma.
- Arterial disease.
- Thromboembolic disorders.
- Epilepsy patients.

Injectable contraceptives

Types of injectable contraceptives:
- Depot medroxy progesterone acetate (DMPA) 150 mg 3 monthly.
- Norethisterone oenanthate (NET-EN) 200 mg 2 monthly.

Mode of action:
- Inhibition of ovulation by suppressing the mid cycle LH peak.
- Making cervical mucus thick, thus prevent implantation of sperm.
- Endometrium is atrophic that prevents blastocyst implantation.

Advantages of injectable contraceptives:
- Does not required regular medication.
- Can be used safely during lactation. It can increases the milk secretion without altering its composition.
- No estrogen like side effects.
- Menstrual symptoms e.g, menorrhagia, dysmenorrhea are reduced.
- Protective against endometrial cancer.
- Reduce PID, endometriosis, ectopic pregnancy and ovarian cancer.
- DMPA reduces the risk of:
  - Salpingitis.
  - Endometrial cancer.
  - Iron deficiency anemia.
  - Sickle cell problems.
  - Endometriosis.

Timing of injection:
- In menstruating women, the first injection should be given within 5 days of the menstrual period.
- Incase of post-abortion or termination of pregnancy, injection should be given on the same day of procedure.
- Postpartum: 5-6 weeks after delivery.

Side effects of injectable contraceptives:
- Irregular bleeding.
- Amenorrhea.
- Weight gain.
- Delayed return of fertility.
- Galactorrhea.
- Mild androgenic effect.
- Enuresis.
- Others, like depression, loss of libido, vaginal dryness, headache, leg cramps, etc.

Contraindications:
- Suspected pregnancy.
- Patients wants to conceive
- Acute or chronic liver disease.
- Undiagnosed abnormal genital tract bleeding.
- Thromboembolic disease.
- Recent trophoblastic disease.
- Obesity
- HTN

Norplant/Implanon

Norplant is a single implant containing 68 mg etonogestrel, the metabolite of Desogestrel and releasing about 60 microgram/day initially later 30 microgram/day over 3 years.

Mechanism:
- It inhibits ovulation in 90% of the cycles for the 1st year.
- Atrophy changes in the endometrium, thus prevents implantation.
- Making cervical mucus thick, thus prevent penetration of the sperm.

Time of insertion:
- During menstruation or the 1st day of menstruation.
- Immediately after abortion.
- 3 weeks after postpartum.

Site of insertion: The implants are placed in a fan shaped manner subdermally in the medial aspect of the non-dominant upper arm, 6-8 cm above the elbow fold.

Advantages:
- Highly effective for long term use and rapidly reversible.
- Suitable for women who have completed their family but do not desire permanent sterilization.
- Efficacy of Norplant is extremely high. This safe and effective method is considered as 'reversible sterilization'
- It eliminates regular medication as imposed by oral pill.
- It can be used safely during lactation.
- Menstrual symptoms e.g., menorrhagia, dysmenorrhea are reduced.
- Productive against endometrial.
- Reduction in PID, endometriosis, ectopic pregnancy and ovarian cancer.

Disadvantages:
- May disturb menstrual cycle.
- Irregular and prolong bleeding in most common compliant.
- Heavy bleeding and amenorrhea seldom occurs.

Emergency contraceptives

Emergency contraception is any drug or device used after unprotected intercourse to prevent pregnancy. The dose should be taken within 72 hours.

Available preparations:
- Levonorgestrel *(E. pills)*: 0.75 mg, 2 doses given at 12 hours interval.
- Ethinyl estradiol: 2.5 mg 12 hourly for 5 days
- Conjugated estrogen: 15 mg 12 hourly for 5 days.
- Ethinyl estradiol: 2.5 mg 12 hourly.
- Mifepristone: 100 mg single.

Complications:
- Nausea and vomiting.
- Failure leading to pregnancy.
- Ectopic pregnancy.

Sterilization

Sterilization/Permanent contraception: Sterilization is a surgical method where the reproductive function of an individual (male/female) is purposefully and permanently damaged.

Methods:
- For female: Tubal ligation/Tubectomy.
- For male: Vasectomy.

Tubal ligation/Tubectomy: It is an operation where resection of a segment of both fallopian tubes is done to achieve permanent sterilization.

Selection criteria of a patient for Tubectomy:
- Family must be completed.
- Age of the last child must above 3 years
- Written consent of husband.

Indications:
- For the purpose of family planning.
- To limit the size of the family.
- Socioeconomic purpose.
- In some medical conditions like diabetes, renal disease, heart disease where further pregnancy can be hazardous for the maternal health.

Time for sterilization:
- Intrapartum: During cesarian section.
- During puerperium: 24-48 hours following delivery.
- Random: following the menstrual period in the proliferative phase.
- Combined with MTP.

Methods of Tubectomy:
- Abdominal:
  - Laparotomy/Conventional:
    - Pomeroy method (A loop of the fallopian tube is tied with absorbable suture and the cut)
    - Parkland method (A segment of the fallopian tubes are excised and then the ends are ligated separately).
    - Irving's method (The cut end is buried in the myometrium and the distal end is tied and left free).
    - Uchida technique (A segment is cut and the proximal end is buried in the mesosalpinx).
    - Madlener's technique/fimbriectomy.
  - Minilaparotomy:
    - Small abdominal incision (2-3 cm) is made just above the pubic hairline.
    - Common in post-partum and interval sterilization.
    - Often done under local or regional anesthesia.
- Laparoscopic sterilization:
  - Performed using laparoscopy through a small abdominal port.
  - Tubes are occluded using: falope rings, Filshie clips, electrocautery.

Vasectomy: It is a permanent sterilization procedure done in the male where a segment of vas deferens of both side is resected and cut ends are ligated.

Methods:
- Conventional vasectomy
- Non scalpel technique
- Open ended vasectomy
- Chemical occlusion.

Post-operative care:
- In 1st 3 months the couple must use other methods like condoms
- Follow up semen analysis reports must confirm sterility.

Complications:
- Immediate:
  - Wound sepsis.
  - Cellulitis.
  - Scrotal hematoma.
- Delayed:
  - Frigidity or impotency.
  - Sperm granuloma.
  - Antisperm antibody formation.
  - Spontaneous recanalization leading to pregnancy.

Barrier methods of contraception

Types of barrier methods:
- *Mechanical barrier:*
  - Male: Condom
  - Female:
    - Female condom
    - Vaginal diaphragm
    - Cervical occlusion cap
- *Chemical barriers:*
  - Vaginal cream e.g., Delfen
  - Jelly e.g., koromex
  - Foam e.g., aerosol foam
  - Sponge

Advantages of condom:
- Easily available
- Cheaper with no contraindications
- Non-hormonal, no systemic side effects.
- Easy to carry, simple to use and easily disposable.
- Protection against sexually transmitted diseases.
- Protection against pelvic inflammatory disease.
- Fertility returns immediately after discontinuation.
- No need of medical supervision.

Disadvantages:
- Risk of accidentally break or slip off during coitus, so failure rate is high.
- Inadequate sexual pleasure.
- Latex allergy.
- Have to discard after one time use.

Natural Contraception

Natural contraceptives: These methods are based on the recognition of fertility and infertile phases of a menstrual cycle from the symptoms and signs of ovulation and to remain abstain from sexual intercourse during the fertile period.

Fertility awareness methods are:

- *Safe period/calendar method:* Avoid intercourse during the fertile period (typically day 10-18 in a 28 days cycle)
- *Basal body temperature method:* A women's body temp slightly raises after ovulation (0.3-0.5°C), avoid intercourse until 3 days after the temp raise.
- *Cervical mucus method:* Observes changes in vaginal discharge and avoid intercourse during fertile mucus.
- *Symptothermal method:* It combines BBT, cervical mucus and calendar methods.
- Lactational amenorrhea method (LAM).
- Coitus interruptus/withdrawal method.

Lactational Amenorrhea Method (LAM)

Lactational amenorrhea:

The Lactational amenorrhea method is based on the fact that breastfeeding provides 98% protection during the first six months postpartum if the baby is exclusively breastfeeding and the mother has not yet had a menstrual period.

Failure rate is 0.5-0.6%

Mechanism:

- During breastfeeding, high level of prolactin thus inhibits ovarian response to FSH.
- Hypo-estrogenic state cause no menstruation.
- If the patient does not breastfeed the baby, her menstruation would return by 6th week following delivery in about 40% and 80% by 12th week.

Limitations:

- It is temporary, only works for first 6 months postpartum.
- Requires exclusive breastfeeding.
- Not effective once menstruation returns or feeding is reduced.
- May not be reliable if feeding patterns are inconsistent.

CHAPTER 31

Minor Gynecological Operation

Q1. What are the different minor gynecological operations?

- Dilatation of cervix
- Dilatation and curettage
- Hysterosalpingography
- Dilatation and insufflation
- Cervical biopsy
- Thermal cauterization
- Cryosurgery
- Perineoplasty
- Amputation of cervix

Q2. What are the indication of dilatation of cervix?

The indications are:

- Before cervical amputation
  - Before hysteroscopy
  - Uterine infection or blood accumulation in the uterus
  - Before the introduction of a uterine curette and the insertion of an intrauterine device, radium or laminaria tents.
  - Dysmenorrhea-spasmodic

Q3. What should be done if dilatation is difficult?

Dilatation difficulties may be overcome by:

- Using a metallic probe-lacrimal duct probe
- Simultaneous use of USG to guide the probe/uterine sound
- Prior use of misoprostol to soften the cervix

Q4. What are the indication of dilatation and curettage (D&C)?

- Diagnostic criteria for D&C
  - Infertility
  - AUB amenorrhea
  - Tuberculosis of endometrium
  - carcinoma of endometrium
  - PMB
- Therapeutic
  - AUB
  - Polyp
  - Removal of Intrauterine device

- Combined
    - AUB
    - Polyp

Q5. What are the contraindications of D&C?

- Pregnancy
- Acute PID
- Clotting disorder
- Acute cervical or vaginal infection
- Cervical stenosis
- Cervical obstructive lesion

Q6. How much dilatation should be done during the procedure?

Usually 8-10 mm

Q7. What are the steps of D&C?

- Bladder evacuation
- Anesthesia-GA/diazepam sedation with/out paracervical block
- Lithotomy position
- Painting and drapping
- B/M/E to be done
- Vaginal speculum introduced posteriorly
- Anterior cervical lipis grasped by Allis forceps
- Uterine sound used to confirm position and length of uterocervical canal
- Cervical canal dilated
- Cervix made steady using traction
- After adequate dilatation uterine cavity is curetted by using curette either in clockwise or anticlockwise starting from fundus to internal os
- Speculum removed
- Curette material sent for histopathology

Q8. How is Hawkin Ambler dilator used?

The dilator knob needs to be positioned within the palm.

- Index finger should be placed on the instrument's body
- Finger tip positioned approximately 3 cm away from the instrument's tip
- The instrument's tip should go through the internal os
- Tip of dilator oriented anteriorly or posteriorly based on uterus position

Q9. What are the complication of D&C?

- Immediate
    - Cervical injury
    - Perforation
    - Hemorrhage
    - Injury to bowels
    - Infection
- Remote
    - Incompetence of cervix
    - Uterine synechiae

Q10. How can uterine perforation be identified?

- Abrupt loss of resistance
- Instrument travels deeper
- Instrument freely mobile

Q11. How will you manage uterine perforation?

- Operation should be stopped once perforation occurs
- Vital and peritoneal signs observed for several hours
- Abdominal injury should be excluded by laparoscopy
- Resuscitative measure
- If active bleeding—laparotomy

Q12. How Asherman's syndrome develops following D&C and how will you diagnose it?

- Due to vigorous curettage-basal layer of endometrium destroyed
- Healing result in synechiae between walls of uterus
- Diagnosis-by HSG, hysteroscopy
- Treatment-hysteroscopic lysis of adhesion and postoperative estrogen therapy.

Q13. What are the indication and complication of dilatation and insufflation?

Indication of dilatation and insufflation:

- To note the tubal patency in:
  - Investigation for infertility
  - Following tuboplasty operation

It should be done in first half cycle and should not be done in pelvic infection

Complications:

- Immediate
  - Air embolism
  - Rupture of tube
  - Recurrence of prior pelvic infection
- Remote
  - Pelvic endometrial tissue growth
  - Formation of granulomas

Q14. What do you mean by hysterosalpingography?

It is a radiographic procedure with contrast material employed to evaluate the internal structure of the uterus and tubes, including the patency of the tubes.

Q15. What are the indication of HSG?

- Evaluation of tubal patency in infertility after tuboplasty
- Identification of uterine anomalies
- Assessment of cervical insufficiency
- Identification of displaced IUD—within or beyond the cavity

Diagnosis of uterine adhesions

- After placing essure, validate the blockage of the fallopian tubes

Q16. What are the contraindication of HSG?

- Pelvic infection
- Patient with hydrosalpinges

- Presence of adnexal mass
- PID
- Pregnancy
- Suspected pelvic TB
- AUB

Q17. What advantages can you see in between HSG over D&I?

- Reduced number of false negatives reported
- Accurate determination of location and area of blockage
- Detection of uterine cavity irregularity

Q18. When HSG should be done?

D6-D10 of cycle

Q19. Which contrast media or dye is used for HSG?

- Oil based media
  - Ethiodized oil
- Water based media
  - Meglumine diatrizoate

Q20. What are the steps of HSG?

- Bladder evacuation
- Position-dorsal
- PV examination done
- Speculum inserted in posterior wall
- Anterior lip of cervix grasped
- HSG cannula fitted with syringe containing radio-opaque dye
- Dye slowly introduced
- 5-10 mL introduced

The entry of dye into the interior can be detected utilizing an X-ray image intensifier paired with a video display unit

- Speculum and allis removed
- Two radiographic views taken
  - To show filling of uterine cavity
  - Completion of procedure showing tubal findings

Q21. What are the types of cervical biopsy?

- Surface biopsy
- Punch biopsy
- Wedge biopsy
- Ring biopsy
- Cone biopsy

Q22. What are different methods of conization of cervix?

Conization can be done with a scalpel, laser and electrosurgical wire loop (LEEP)

Q23. What are the indication and complication cone biopsy?

It entails excising the cone of the cervix that encompasses the complete squamocolumnar junction, stroma with glands, and endocervical mucous membrane.

Indication: Diagnostic and therapeutic purpose
- Diagnosis/confirmation of CIN, microinvasion or invasive carcinoma
- Treatment of CIN
- CIS
- Unsatisfactory colposcopy finding
- Positive endocervical curettage

Complication of cone biopsy:
- Hemorrhage
- Cervical stenosis may cause hematometra
- Infertility can occur
- Decreases cervical mucus
- Cervical incompetence leading to recurrent miscarriage
- Midtrimester abortion or preterm labor.

Q24. What is thermal cauterization?
It is performed by damaging the eroded section of the cervix through thermoregulation or red-hot cauterization.

Q25. Indication of thermal cauterization.
Cervical ectopy accompanied by bothersome discharge
- Before cervical smear or biopsy

Q26. What is colposcopy?
It is a diagnostic procedure in which lighted and magnifying instrument (colposcope) used to examine cervix, vagina and vulva.

Q27. What are the indications of colposcopy?
- Women with abnormal pap test
- Positive HPV DNA test
- VIA positive
- Suspicious cervix
- Postcoital or postmenopausal bleeding even pap smear is normal
- Persistent inflammatory cervical cytology
- Abnormal vaginal discharge
- History of utero DES exposure
- Conservative management of intraepithelial neoplasia
- Posttreatment follow-up

Q28. How TZ is classified during colposcopy?
- *Type 1:* The entire transformation zone, including its upper limit, is ectocervical.
- *Type 2:* The upper limit of the transformation zone is either partially or fully visible within the canal and can be seen completely around 360 degrees.
- *Type 3:* A portion or the entire upper limit of the transformation zone is not visible within the canal.

Q29. What is the usual magnification of colposcope?
The colposcope typically offers interchangeable magnifications of 10x and 18x, utilizing both a normal light filter and a green filter. The green light is specifically employed to help identify vascular patterns.

Q30. What is cryosurgery?
This is a method in which tissue destruction is achieved through freezing.

Q31. What are indication of cryosurgery?

- Cervical ectopy
- CIN, condyloma acuminata, leukoplakia
- VaIN, vault granulation tissue following hysterectomy.

Q32. What are the advantage of cryosurgery then thermal cautery?

- No requirement of anesthesia
- Restruction of tissue
- No hemorrhage
- Cervical stenosis can occur

Q33. What are the drawback?

Excessive discharge for about 2-3 weeks.

CHAPTER 32

Major Operation in Gynecology

Q1. What are the major gynecological operation?

1. Hysterectomy
   a. Abdominal
   b. Vaginal
   c. Laparoscopy
2. Ovarian cystectomy
3. Ovariotomy
4. Wedge resection
5. Salpingectomy
6. Salpingo-oophorectomy
7. For inversion of uterus
   a. Haultians operation
   b. Kustner operation
   c. Ventrosuspension operation
8. Myomectomy
9. Vulvectomy

Q2. What are the types of hysterotomy?

1. Total hysterectomy
2. Subtotal
3. Panhysterectomy
4. Extended hysterectomy
5. Radical hysterectomy

Q3. What are the indication of abdominal hysterectomy?

Benign lesion	• Heavy menstrual bleeding • Fibroid uterus • Tubo-ovarian mass • Endometriosis • Adenomyosis • CIN • Endometrial hyperplasia • Benign ovarian tumor in perimenopausal age
Malignancy	• Carcinoma cervix • Carcinoma ovary • Carcinoma endometrium • Uterine sarcoma • Choriocarcinoma

Contd...

Contd...

Traumatic	• Uterine perforation • Cervical tear • Rupture uterus
Obstetrical	• Atonic postpartum hemorrhage (PPH) • Placenta accrete spectrum (adherent placenta) • Hydatidiform mole >35 years • Septic abortion

Q4. What are types of radical hysterectomy?

1. Simple extrafascial hysterectomy
2. Modified radical hysterectomy
3. Radical hysterectomy
4. European organization for research and treatment for cancer
   I. Type I: Simple hysterectomy
   II. Type II: Modified radical hysterectomy (same as above) + Uterine arteries are ligated at the site of crossing ureters.
   III. Type III: Radical hysterectomy (same as above) and uterine arteries are ligated at the origin
   IV. Type IV: Extended radical hysterectomy, removal of upper ¾ of vagina + paravaginal tissues.
   V. Type V: Partial exenteration
   VI. Type II-V: Completed with bilateral pelvic lymphadenectomy and with or without paraaortic node dissection.

Q5. What are the complications of Hysterectomy?

1. Intraoperative
   - Hemorrhage
   - Anesthetic hazard: Atelectasis, pulmonary edema, embolism
   - Visceral injury: Bladder or ureter
2. Postoperative

Immediate

- Hypovolemia (hemorrhagic)—shock
- Urinary
  - Retention due to pain and spasm
  - Cystitis
- Anuria may be due to inadequate fluid replacement (parenteral) or ureteric obstruction (postrenal)

Late

- Retention of urine
- Incontinence
  - Stress
  - True incontinence
  - Complication due to anesthesia
- Pyrexia
- Hemorrhage
- Hematomas
- Paralytic ileus and intestinal obstruction
- Necrotizing fascitis
- DVT
- Pulmonary embolism

Remote
- Vault granulation
- Vault prolapse
- Incisional hernia
- Prolapse of fallopian tube through the vault
- Depression, sexual dysfunction

Q6. What are the types of hemorrhage that occur postoperatively?
1. *Primary:* Slipping due to ligature
2. *Secondary:* Occurs between 7–14 days after operation is due to sepsis

Q7. What are the advantages of abdominal hysterectomy?
- Scope of wide exploration of the abdominal and pelvic organ
- Tubo-ovarian pathology can be tackled effectively and simultaneously
- Concurrent surgical procedure can be performed if needed
- Done by surgeon with average surgical skill

Q8. What are the disadvantages of abdominal hysterectomy?
- Longer recovery time and hospital stay
- Increased pain
- Increased need of analgesia
- Difficult in obese patients
- Delayed resumption in day to day life
- Leave a scar

Q9. What are the advantages of vaginal hysterectomy?
- Can be done in obese patient
- Less postoperative complications
- Less postoperatively pain
- Less hospital stay
- No incisional scar

Q10. What are the disadvantages of vaginal hysterectomy?
- More skilled and experience surgeon needed
- Exploration of abdominal organ cannot be done
- Less space—difficulty in cases with restricted mobility and associated adnexal pathology
- Difficult if uterus >12 weeks size, pelvic adhesion or previous history of laparotomy with adhesion

Q11. Mention the steps of abdominal hysterectomy?
- Position: Trendelenburg
- Painting and draping done
- Incision: Low transverse, intraumbilical, paramedian or midline
- Uterus: Drawn out
- Bowels and omentum—packed off from operative area
- Pelvic organ examined—preservation of adnexa decision is made
- Myoma screw used
- Paired clamp placed around round ligament—cut, clamp, ligate
- If ovaries to be removed—paired clamps in infundibulopelvic ligament a window is created in broad ligament before the clamp placed—tissue are cut and replaced by transfixation

- If ovaries to be preserved—clamps near the cornu including fallopian tube, mesosalpinx with uterine vessels and ovarian ligament—cut clamp and transfix
- Loose peritoneum of uterovesical fold
- Bladder is pushed down and out
- Posterior leaf of broad ligament is dissected down at the level of uterosacral ligament
- Uterus pulled forward to make uterosacral ligament prominent
- Clamps are placed over the uterosacral ligament as close as to cervix
- Ligaments are cut, peritoneum in between ligaments is dissected clamps replaced by suture
- Clamps on the Mackenrodts ligament cut and replaced by ligature
- Vault is open
- Edges of the vaginal vault is grasped
- Lateral vaginal angles closed by transfixation
- Vault closed by interrupted suture
- Pelvic peritonization done
- Peritoneal toileting done
- Abdomen closed in layers

Q12. What is ovariotomy?

Ovariotomy is the removal of the tumor along with healthy ovarian tissue, also known as oophorectomy.

Q13. Mention the steps for myomectomy?

- Incision-linear or elliptical incision in the midline or anterior wall of uterus
- Incision is deepened through myometrium and the capsule till myoma is reached
- Myoma enucleation—myoma is grasped, dissected continuing in the plane between myoma and capsule.
- Myoma is enucleated (intracapsular) from its bed
- Myoma bed is obliterated by interrupted mattress or figure of eight suture
- Endometrial cavity is opened up and repaired
- Exploration of other pelvic organ
- Abdomen closed in layers

Q14. What are the complication of myomectomy?

- Hemorrhage
- May need hysterectomy if excessive bleeding
- Postoperative pyrexia due to hematoma formation in myomectomy bed
- Risk of adhesion
- Recurrence of myoma
- Injury to bladder and ureter, fallopian tube and bowel

Q15. Measures taken to control bleeding during myomectomy?

- Preoperative treatment with GnRH analogue reduces vascularity of tumor
- Use of vasoconstrictive agent: Commonly used vasopressin (20 mL in 50 mL of normal saline)
- Oral or vaginal misoprostol and tranexamic acid
- Use of tourniquets to occlude uterine vessels and also ovarian vessels

Index

D

K

L

M

N

O

P

R

S

T

NCERT BIOLOGY

REVISION WORK BOOK

Most Effective Revision
& Concept Zipper for >>>>

NEET & CUET

Vol. 2 CLASS XII

Authors
Dr. Parul Goel
Juhi Bhatia

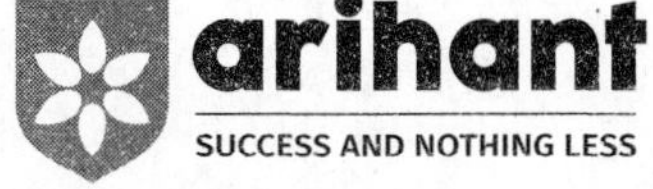

Super 6

ADVANTAGES OF REVISION WORK BOOKS

1. Learn with fun while practicing with Self Assessment.
2. Different question types are helpful in increasing the learning and understanding about **Core Concepts** and **Conceptual Applications**.
3. Figure based small methodical questions also help in increasing **figure visualisation**.
4. Innovative style of practice in Workbook manner helps in breaking the **monotonicity** of subject.
5. Complete sync with NCERT along with **Competition Connect** and **Competition Edge Up** helps in building the foundation for the preparation of competitions like NEET and CUET.
6. Questions with one word or maximum one sentence long answers are very helpful in **Faster Revision** and **Confidence Boost Up**.

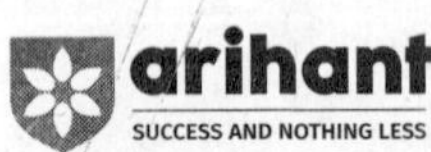

ARIHANT PRAKASHAN (SERIES), MEERUT

卐 **Administrative & Production Offices**

Regd. Office

'Ramchhaya' 4577/15, Agarwal Road, Darya Ganj, New Delhi -110002
Tele: 011- 47630600, 43518550

卐 **Head Office**

Kalindi, TP Nagar, Meerut (UP) - 250002
Tel: 0121-7156203, 7156204

卐 **Sales & Support Offices**

Agra, Ahmedabad, Bengaluru, Bareilly, Chennai, Delhi, Guwahati, Hyderabad, Jaipur, Jhansi, Kolkata, Lucknow, Nagpur & Pune.

卐 **PRICE** ₹310.00

卐 **PO No :** TXT-59-T061770-11-24

Published by Arihant Publications (India) Ltd.

For further information about the books published by Arihant, log on to www.arihantbooks.com or e-mail at info@arihantbooks.com

Follow us on    

FAB 4 Features

TOPIC 1

Flower and Pre-Fertilisation : Structures and Events NCERT Pg. 3-11

NCERT Tracker
Every topic is tagged with NCERT page numbers for better syncing with NCERT.

1. All flowering plants show sexual reproduction.
True ☐ False ☐
2. Identify the parts labelled as *A* to *G* in following figure.

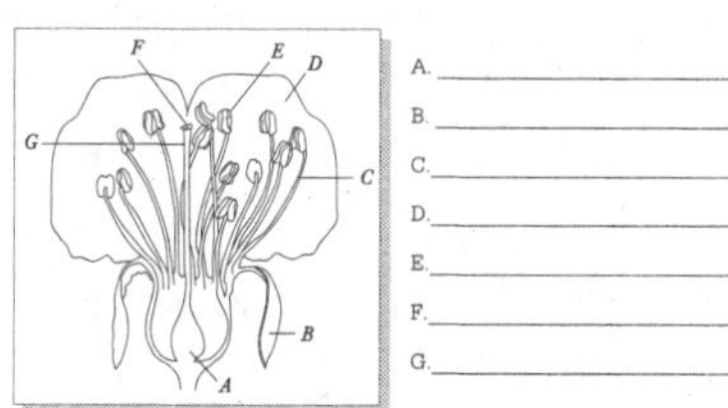

A. __________
B. __________
C. __________
D. __________
E. __________
F. __________
G. __________

***101.** Which of the following is not a correct match?
(a) Proliferative phase–Rupture of Graafian follicle in ovary ☐
(b) Secretory phase–Development of corpus luteum and increased secretion of progesterone ☐
(c) Menstruation–Breakdown of endometrium ☐
(d) Ovulation–LH and FSH attain peak level and cause rupture of Graafian follicle ☐

Important Concept Tagging
Every question which is based on the important concept from NEET & CUET point of view is marked with *.

Competition Connect
Supplement containing related portions of old NCERT which are present in NEET & CUET syllabus but removed from latest NCERT.

COMPETITION CONNECT

Topic 1. Organism and Its Environment [NCERT (Old) Pg. 220-226]

***1.** __________ is a subject which studies the interactions among organisms and between the organism and its environment.

2. Write the four levels of biological organisation.

____

3. The variations in the intensity and duration of temperature and precipitation account for the formation of biomes.
True ☐ False ☐

COMPETITION EDGE UP

1. Identify the set of correct statements. **[NCERT Pg. 13, NEET 2024]**
A. The flowers of Vallisneria are colourful and produce nectar.
B. The flowers of water lily are not pollinated by water.
C. In most of water-pollinated species, the pollen grains are protected from wetting.
D. Pollen grains of some hydrophytes are long and ribbon like.
E. In some hydrophytes, the pollen grains are carried passively inside water.
Choose the correct answer from the options given below.
(a) C, D and E only ☐
(b) A, B, C and D only ☐
(c) A, C, D and E only ☐
(d) B, C, D and E only ☐

(a) Wind pollinated plant inflorescence showing flowers with well exposed stamens. ☐
(b) Water pollinated flowers showing stamens with mucilaginous covering. ☐
(c) Cleistogamous flowers showing autogamy. ☐
(d) Compact inflorescence showing complete autogamy ☐

3. What is the function of tassels in the corn cob? **[NEET 2023]**
(a) To trap pollen grains ☐
(b) To disperse pollen grains ☐
(c) To protect seeds ☐
(d) To attract insects ☐

4. In angiosperm, the haploid, diploid and triploid structures of a fertilised embryo sac sequentially are **[NCERT Pg. 18, NEET 2023]**
(a) Antipodals, synergids and primary endosperm nucleus ☐

Competition Edge Up
Selected PYQs in Sync with NCERT Chapter.

CONTENTS

Chapter 01

Sexual Reproduction in Flowering Plants

Scan and take Chapter Test

TOPIC 1

Flower and Pre-Fertilisation Structures and Events

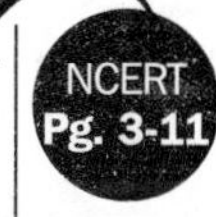

1. All flowering plants show sexual reproduction.

True ☐ False ☐

2. Identify the parts labelled as *A* to *G* in following figure.

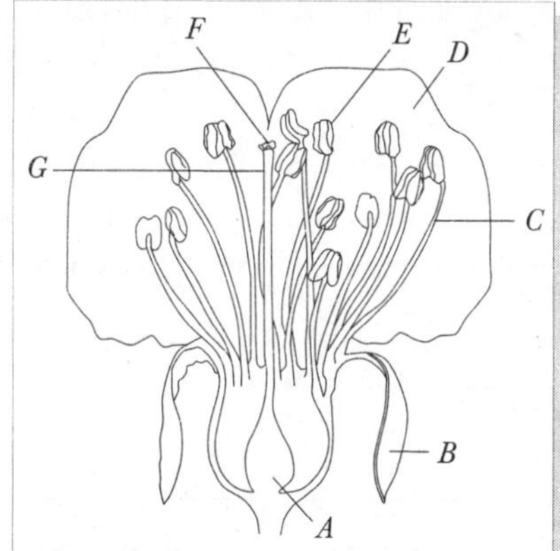

A. ____________________

B. ____________________

C. ____________________

D. ____________________

E. ____________________

F. ____________________

G. ____________________

3. Gynoecium represents the ____________________ (male/female) reproductive organ.

4. Arrange the following floral whorls on the thalamus from outermost to innermost.

Corolla, Androecium, Calyx, Gynoecium

____

5. Name the long, slender stalk of a typical stamen.____________________

6. The usually bilobed terminal structure of a typical angiospermic stamen is ____________

*Concepts of all questions bearing * are important for NEET & CUET*

7. The distal end of the filament is attached to the thalamus or petal of the flower.
(*Rewrite the statement after correcting the underlined word.)*

____

8. Each lobe in a typical angiospermic anther is monothecous.

True ☐ False ☐

9. There are ________________ (two/three/four) microsporangia in an anther.

10. After maturation, microsporangia develop into ________________ .

11. Identify the parts labelled as *A* to *D* in the following diagram.

A. ________________

B. ________________

C. ________________

D. ________________

12. Arrange the following layers of microsporangia in the order of outermost to innermost.

Tapetum, Endothecium, Epidermis, Middle layer

____

13. Name the layer of microsporangium which performs the following functions.

(i) Layers which perform the function of protection and help in dehiscence of anther to release the pollen.

____

(ii) Layer that nourishes the developing pollen grains.

____

14. Tapetum cells are ________________ (mononucleate/multinucleate).

15. Select the correct words from the box given below to fill in the blanks.

Centre, Corner, Endogenous, Sporogenous, Homogeneous, Heterogeneous

A group of compactly arranged ________________ cells called the ________________ tissue occupies the ________________ of each microsporangium in a young anther.

16. The sporogenous tissue undergoes mitotic division to form microspore tetrads.

True ☐ False ☐

17. Identify the parts labelled as *A* to *F* in the following diagram.

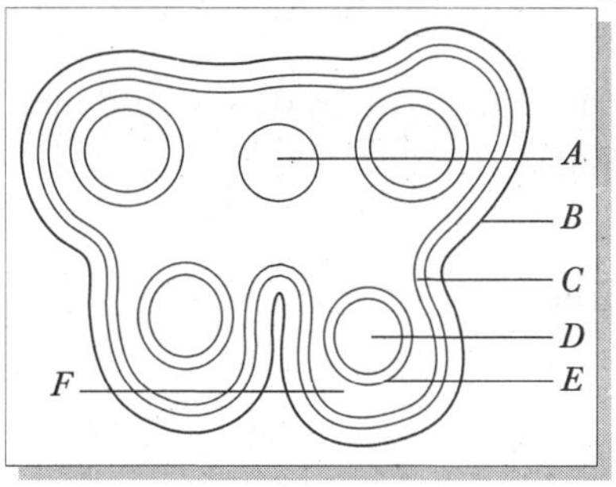

A. ____________
B. ____________
C. ____________
D. ____________
E. ____________
F. ____________

18. Identify the parts labelled as *A* to *E* in the following diagram.

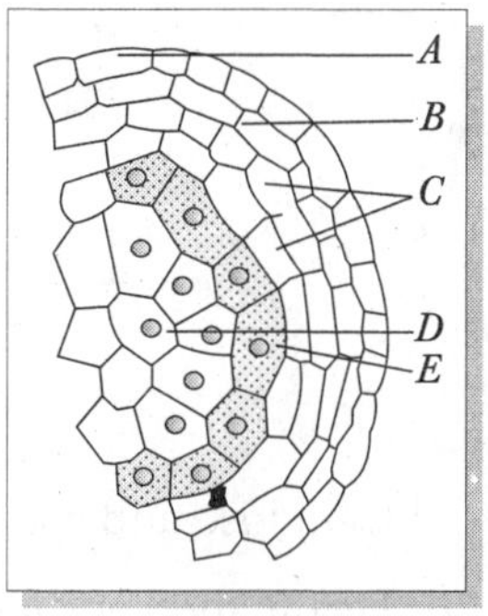

A. ____________
B. ____________
C. ____________
D. ____________
E. ____________

19. Write the expanded form of PMC.____________

20. Name the process of formation of microspores from a PMC.____________

21. Microspores are arranged in ____________ . As the anthers mature and dehydrate, microspores develop into the ____________ .

22. Which of the following combination is correct for ploidy of PMC and microspores?

(a) PMC - N, Microspore - 2N ☐ (b) PMC - N, Microspore - N ☐

(c) PMC - 2N, Microspore - 2N ☐ (d) PMC - 2N, Microspore - N ☐

23. Match the following columns.

Column I (Parts of microsporangia)	Column II (Structural/Functional details)
A. Tapetum	1. Potential pollen
B. Anther	2. Released when anther dehisce
C. Pollen grains	3. Innermost layer
D. Sporogenous tissue	4. Bilobed

A.____________ B.____________ C.____________ D. ____________

24. Pollens have two prominent walls which are ____________ and ____________ .

25. Exine is made up of ____________ .

26. Germ pores lack sporopollenin.

True ☐ False ☐

27. Consider the following statements.

Statement I Pollen grains are generally spherical in shape, measuring roughly about 25-50 micrometers in diameter.

Statement II Sporopollenin is resistant to enzymatic degradation and action of acids.

Choose the correct option from the following.

(a) Statement I is true, but statement II is false ☐

(b) Statement I is false, but statement II is true ☐

(c) Both statements I and II are true ☐

(c) Both statements I and II are false ☐

28. Consider the given image and mark the option that best represents the composition of structure labelled *X*.

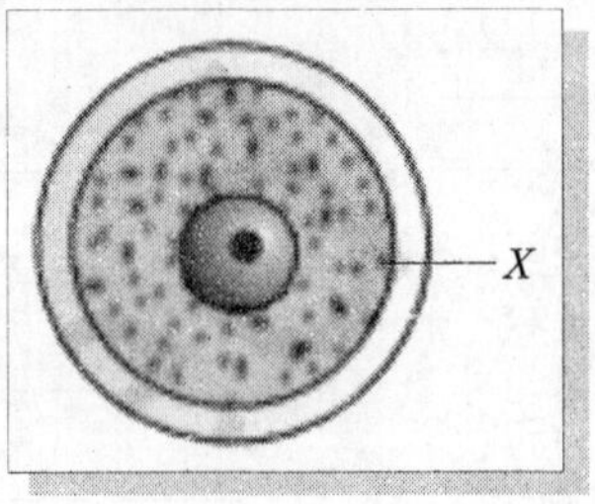

X

(a) Cellulose and hemicellulose ☐ (b) Cellulose and sporopollenin ☐

(c) Cellulose and pectin ☐ (d) Pectin and sporopollenin ☐

29. Find odd one out related to pollen grain structure.

Cellulose, Pectin, Hemicellulose, Sporopollenin

____

30. When the pollen grain is mature, it contains two cells, the ________________ and ________________.

31. Abundant food reserve is found in ________________ (vegetative/generative) cells.

32. Identify the structures marked *A* to *F* in the given diagram.

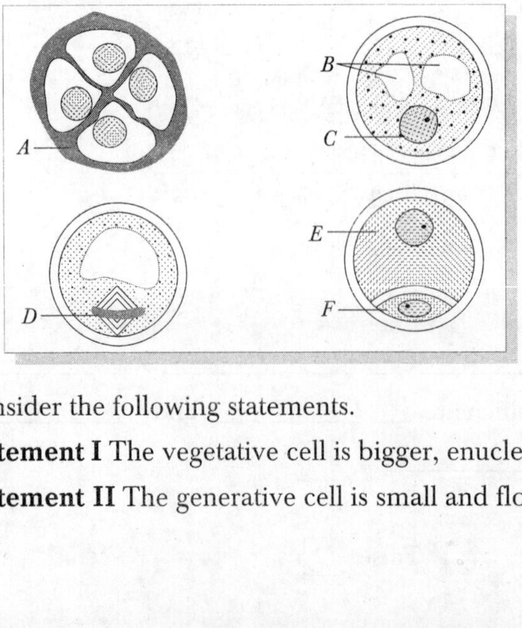

A B C D E F

A. ________________

B. ________________

C. ________________

D. ________________

E. ________________

F. ________________

33. Consider the following statements.

Statement I The vegetative cell is bigger, enucleate and has abundant food reserve.

Statement II The generative cell is small and floats in the cytoplasm of the vegetative cell.

Choose the correct option from the following.

(a) Statement I is true, but statement II is false ☐

(b) Statement I is false, but statement II is true ☐

(c) Both statements I and II are true ☐

(d) Both statements I and II are false ☐

34. Male gametes in angiosperms are formed by the division of________________ .

35. 60% of the angiosperms shed their pollens at the ____________________.

36. Pollen grains cause allergies and chronic respiratory disorders in some people.

True ☐ False ☐

37. Write scientific name of carrot grass that came to India as contaminant causing pollen allergy ________ .

38. Filament consumption increases the performance of athletes.
(*Rewrite the statement after correcting the underlined word.*)

____

39. Find odd one out with respect to pollen viability in following members of family.

Rosaceae, Leguminosae, Solanaceae, Poaceae

____

40. The pollen grains of a plant 'A' lose viability 30 minutes post their release. The plant is supposed to be

(a) potato ☐ (b) wheat ☐

(c) tomato ☐ (d) cucumber ☐

41. Pollen grains can be stored for years in liquid nitrogen at 196°C.

True ☐ False ☐

42. Match the following columns.

Column I (Male gametophytes)	Column II (Structures)
A. Pollen	1. Irregular shaped nucleus
B. Pollen viability	2. Race horses
C. Generative cell	3. Depends upon temperature and humidity
D. Vegetative cell	4. Spindle-shaped, floating in cytoplasm

A.________ B.________ C. ________ D. ________

43. Fill in the blanks using words given in the box below.

Multicarpellary, Monocarpellary, Androecium, Gynoecium

The __________ representing female reproductive parts of flower, may consist of single pistil, called __________ or more than one pistil, called __________ .

44. Identify whether the following diagrams are multicarpellary/monocarpellary and syncarpous/apocarpous.

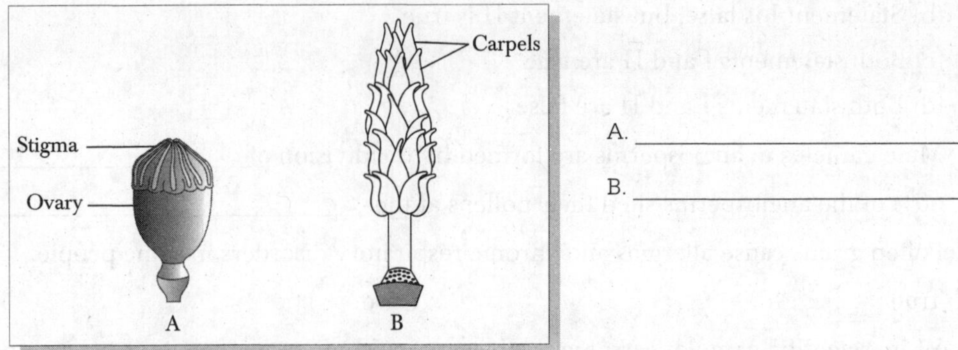

A. ____________________

B. ____________________

45. ____________________ is the landing platform for pollen grains.

46. Name the following.

(i) Basal bulged part of pistil ____________________

(ii) Elongated slender part beneath stigma ____________________

***47.** Considering the given diagram, identify the part where fertilisation takes place.

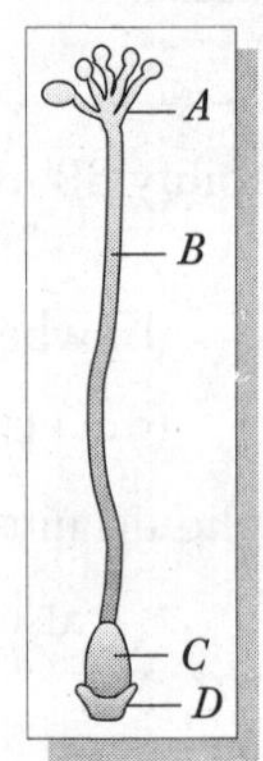

____

48. Find the odd one out.

Stamen, Stigma, Style, Ovary

____

49. The placenta is located inside the ovarian cavity.

True ☐ False ☐

50. Write the other name of megasporangia. ____________________

51. Complete the following analogy with respect to number of ovules.

Wheat : ____________ : : Papaya : Many

***52.** Identify the parts labelled as *A* to *I* in the given diagram.

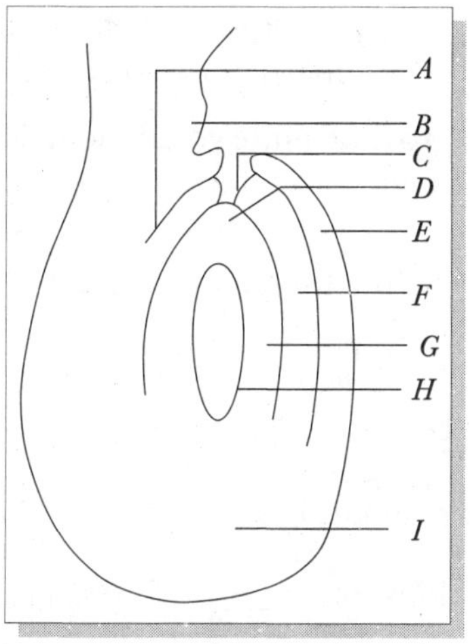

A. ________________

B. ________________

C. ________________

D. ________________

E. ________________

F. ________________

G. ________________

H. ________________

I. ________________

53. The mass of cells enclosed within the integument is called the nucellus.

True ☐ False ☐

***54.** Match Column I with Column II.

	Column I		Column II
A.	Funicle	1.	Stalk connecting to placenta
B.	Chalaza	2.	Abundant reserve food
C.	Integuments	3.	Protective envelope
D.	Nucellus	4.	Basal part of ovule

	A	B	C	D			A	B	C	D	
(a)	1	4	3	2	☐	(b)	1	2	3	4	☐
(c)	1	4	2	3	☐	(d)	1	2	4	3	☐

55. Female gametophyte present inside nucellus is also known as ________________

56. Arrange the following structures in the order they appear from innerside to outerside of a typical ovule.

Nucellus, Outer integument, Inner integument, Embryo sac

____

***57.** Consider the following statements.

Statement I Integuments are the protective covering of the ovule, encircling the nucellus except for the tip where micropyle is present.

Statement II Nucellus enclosed within integuments, provide nourishment to the developing embryo after fertilisation.

Choose the correct option from the following.

(a) Statement I is true, but statement II is false ☐

(b) Statement I is false, but statement II is true ☐

(c) Both statements I and II are true ☐

(d) Both statements I and II are false ☐

58. Write the full form of MMC.______________________________

59. The MMC undergoes ________________ division, which results in the production of ____________ megaspores. The formation of megaspore is termed as ______________ .

60. If nucellus provides nourishment to the growing embryo and female gametophyte represents embryo sac, the ploidy of the nucellus and female gametophyte, respectively will be

(a) Diploid and haploid ☐ (b) Diploid and diploid ☐
(c) Haploid and diploid ☐ (d) Haploid and haploid ☐

61. Fill in the blanks with words provided in the box given below.

Monosporic, Megaspore, Functional, Female, Embryo sac, Male, Disporic, Pollen tube

Only one __________ megaspore develops into _________ gametophyte and other three degenerate. This method of ________ formation from a single ______________ is termed as ___________ development.

62. Identify the parts labelled as (A-C) in the given diagrams.

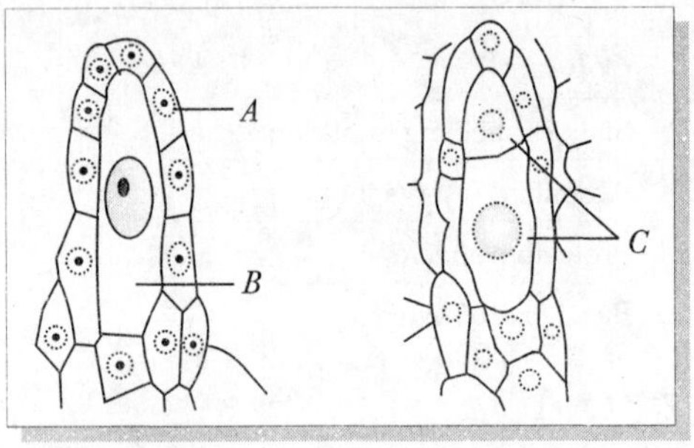

A. ______________________
B. ______________________
C. ______________________

63. Write the types of cell division (meiosis-I /meiosis-II/mitosis) involved in the following.

(i) Megaspore mother cell to megaspore dyad. ______________________
(ii) Megaspore dyad to megaspore tetrad. ______________________

***64.** Identify the parts labelled as *A* to *F* in the diagram given below.

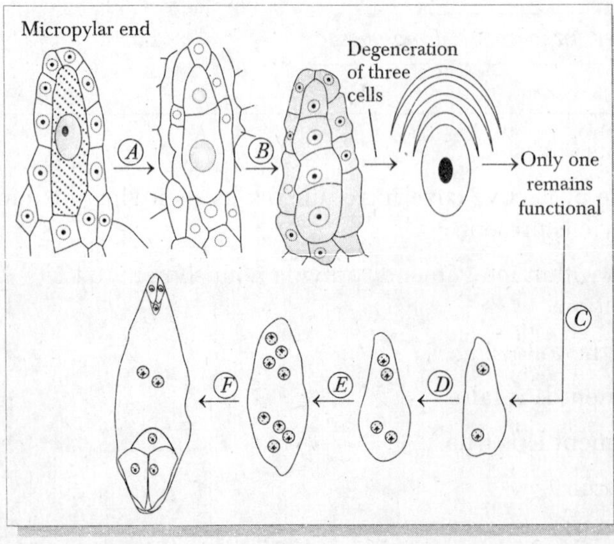

Micropylar end
Degeneration of three cells
Only one remains functional

A. ______________________
B. ______________________
C. ______________________
D. ______________________
E. ______________________
F. ______________________

65. Consider the given image and choose the incorrect statement regarding the same.

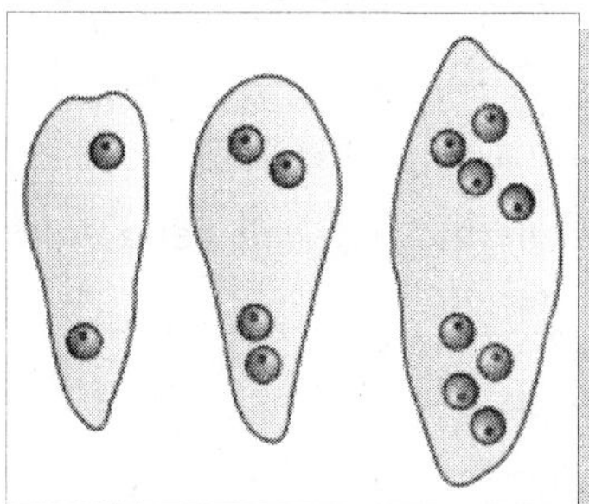

(a) Functional megaspore divides mitotically to form the 2,4 and 8 nuclear stage ☐
(b) Nuclear divisions are not followed immediately by cell wall formation ☐
(c) Two of the eight nuclei are arranged at the centre in a large central cell ☐
(d) Cell wall formation occurs only after the 16 nuclear stage. ☐

66. Identify the parts labelled as *A* to *E* in the diagram given below.

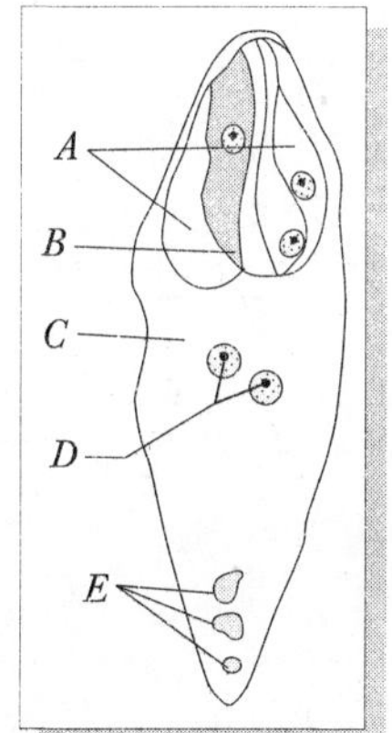

A. ____________________
B. ____________________
C. ____________________
D. ____________________
E. ____________________

67. The two nuclei that are not surrounded by the cell wall in embryo sac are called ______ ________________ nuclei.

68. Consider the following statements.

I. Ovules generally differentiate one MMC in the chalazal region of nucellus.
II. Ovarian cavity that lies inside the ovary, consists of a single embryo sac.
III. The nucleus of the functional megaspore after meiotic division, form two nuclei that move to the opposite poles, forming 2-nucleate, embryo sac.
IV. Orchids and watermelon have several number of ovules.
V. Polar nuclei that are two in number, occupy the central cell.

Choose the set of incorrect statements.

(a) II, IV and V ☐ (b) I, II and III ☐
(c) II and III ☐ (d) III and V ☐

69. The egg apparatus consists of two ____________ and one ______________ .

70. Name the structure that is found at the micropylar tip, which guides the pollen tubes into the synergid. ____________________

71. Antipodals are the three cells present at the ____________ end.

72. In embryo sac, the number of synergid, egg cell, central cell, antipodal cell follows the order ____________________

***73.** Consider the following statements.

Statement I A typical angiospermic embryo sac is 7-nucleate and 8-celled with a large central cell containing two polar nuclei.

Statement II The egg apparatus constituted by a group of three cells is situated at the chalazal end.

Choose the correct option from the following.

(a) Statement I is true, but statement II is false ☐

(b) Statement I is false, but statement II is true ☐

(c) Both statements I and II are true ☐

(d) Both statements I and II are false ☐

74. Complete the sequence.

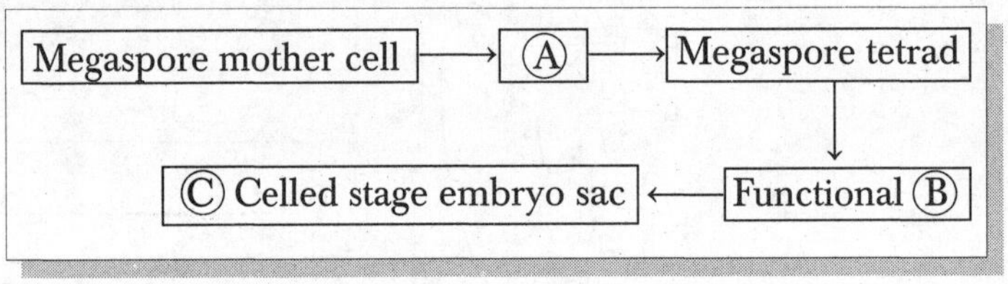

Megaspore mother cell → (A) → Megaspore tetrad → Functional (B) → (C) Celled stage embryo sac

A.____________ B.____________ C.____________

***75.** Identify the parts labelled as *A* to *F* in the diagram given below.

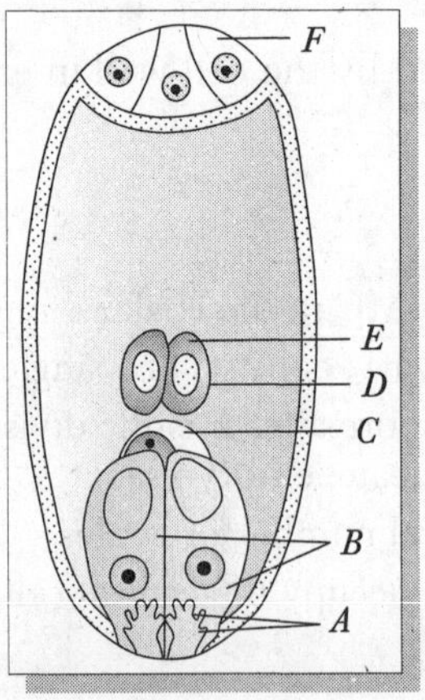

A. ____________

B. ____________

C. ____________

D. ____________

E. ____________

F. ____________

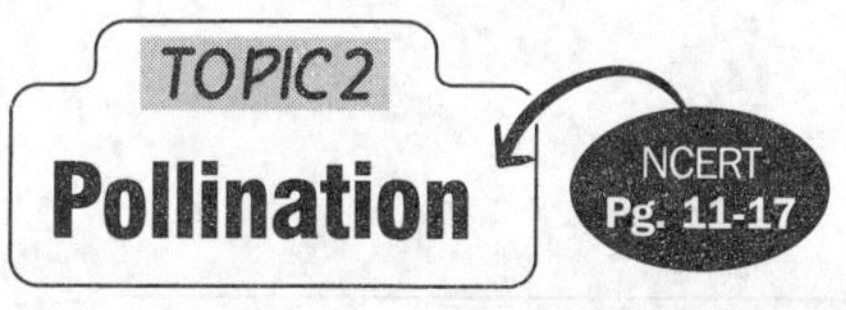

76. Mechanism of transfer of pollen grains to the ovule of a pistil is termed as pollination. (*Rewrite the statement after correcting the underlined word.*)

____

77. Identify the incorrect statement out of the following.

(a) Male and the female gametes produced in flower are non-motile ☐

(b) Angiosperms have a unique array to achieve pollination with the aid of external agents. ☐

(c) Windstorm and rain pour are natural phenomenon, not considered as external pollinating agents. ☐

(d) Plants like *Viola* possess two types of flowers chasmogamous and cleistogamous. ☐

***78.** Identify the structures *A* and *B* shown in the figure of *Commelina* plant given below.

A. ____________________

B. ____________________

***79.** Cleistogamous flowers are strictly autogamous because they remain __________

***80.** In chasmogamy, pollination takes place in ____________________

***81.** Cleistogamous flowers produce assured seed set even in the absence of pollinators.

True ☐ False ☐

82. Geitonogamy is genetically similar to xenogamy.

True ☐ False ☐

83. Which of the following can be an advantage of xenogamy over other types of pollination?

(a) Assured seed set ☐ (b) Genetic variability ☐

(c) Involvement of pollinating agent ☐ (d) Obtaining pure line variety ☐

***84.** Write the biological terms for the following.

(i) Transfer of pollen from anther to stigma of same flower. __________

(ii) Transfer of pollen from anther to stigma of different plant. __________

(iii) Transfer of pollen from anther to stigma of different flower on same plant.__________

***85.** Find odd one out regarding pollination.

Wind, Light, Water, Insects

____

86. Which type of pollen grains consist of the following characteristics?

(i) Non-sticky (ii) Light

(iii) Produced in large number

____

***87.** Study the diagram given below about its structural details and write two characteristics of flowers which get pollinated by wind.

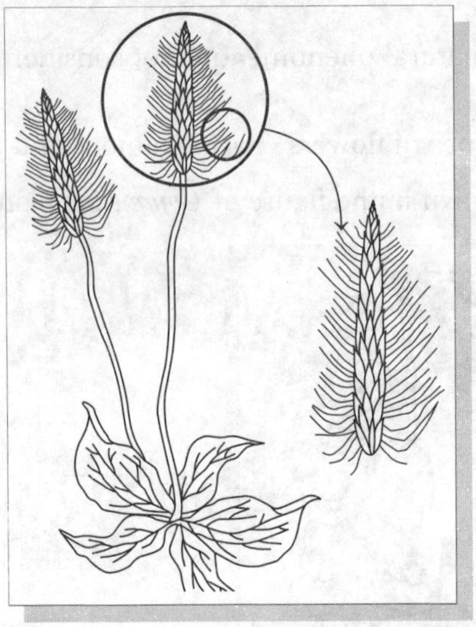

(i) ____________ (ii) ____________

***88.** Write any two examples of wind pollinated plants. ____________

89. Complete the following analogy.

Hydrilla : Maize : : ____________ : Wind pollinated

90. Long, ribbon-like pollens are commonly seen in water pollinated plants.

True ☐ False ☐

***91.** Consider the following statements.

Statement I Female flowers of *Vallisneria* are provided with long stalks to reach water surface.

Statement II All aquatic plants are not necessarily pollinated by water currents.

Choose the correct option from the following.

(a) Statement I is true, but statement II is false ☐

(b) Statement I is false, but statement II is true ☐

(c) Both statements I and II are true ☐

(d) Both statements I and II are false ☐

92. In some water pollinated plants, pollens are protected from getting wet by a ____________ covering.

93. ____________________________ are the dominant biotic pollinating agents.

94. Identify the pollinators of the following flowers.

(i) Colourful, fragrant flowers ____________

(ii) Foul odour flowers ____________

95. Write the two floral rewards for the animal pollinators. ____________

96. Write the name of plants which provide following floral rewards.

(i) Safe place to lay eggs. ____________

(ii) Deposition of eggs in the locule of ovary by a moth. ____________

***97.** Match Column I with Column II.

	Column I		Column II
A.	Water lily	1.	Light non-sticky pollens
B.	*Zostera*	2.	Safe place for laying eggs
C.	Grass	3.	Insect pollination
D.	*Amorphophallous*	4.	Water pollination

	A	B	C	D			A	B	C	D
(a)	3	4	1	2	☐	(b)	4	3	1	2
(c)	3	4	2	1	☐	(d)	4	3	2	1

98. Which one of the following plants shows a very close relationship with a species of moth, where none of the two can complete its life cycle without the other?

Banana, Yucca, Hydrilla, Viola

____

***99.** Write the common terms used for insects consuming pollen or nectar without bringing about pollination. ____________

***100.** Continued self-pollination results in ____________

101. Write any two ways by which flowering plants prevent self-pollination.

____

102. Which of the following can prevent inbreeding depression?

(a) Geitonogamy ☐ (b) Hermaphrodite flowers ☐

(c) Anther pollen synchrony ☐ (d) Self-incompatibility ☐

103. Identify the incorrect pair.

(a) Castor, maize - Monoecious ☐

(b) Maize, papaya - Dioecious ☐

(c) Papaya, date palm - Dioecious ☐

(d) Coconut, Maize ☐

104. In which of the following, both autogamy and geitonogamy are prevented?

Wheat, Papaya, Castor, Maize

____

***105.** Monoecious plants prevent <u>geitonogamy</u>, but not <u>autogamy</u>.
(*Rewrite the statement after correcting the underlined words.*)

____

106. Acceptance or rejection of a pollen is a result of continuous dialogue between pollen grain and the pistil.

True ☐ False ☐

107. Arrange the following events of pollen grain germination in a sequence.

(i) Pollen tube growth through stigma tissues.

(ii) Shedding of pollen grains at 2/3 celled condition.

(iii) Entry of pollen into the ovule through micropyle.

(iv) Pollen grain germination on the stigma.

____

108. Consider the following statements.

Statement I Pollen tube after reaching ovary, enters the embryo sac *via* chalazal end.

Statement II Filiform apparatus present at the micropylar end guides the entry of pollen tube.

Choose the correct option from the following.

(a) Statement I is true, but statement II is false ☐

(b) Statement I is false, but statement II is true ☐

(c) Both statements I and II are true ☐

(d) Both statements I and II are false ☐

***109.** Identify the parts labelled as *A* to *F* in the given diagram.

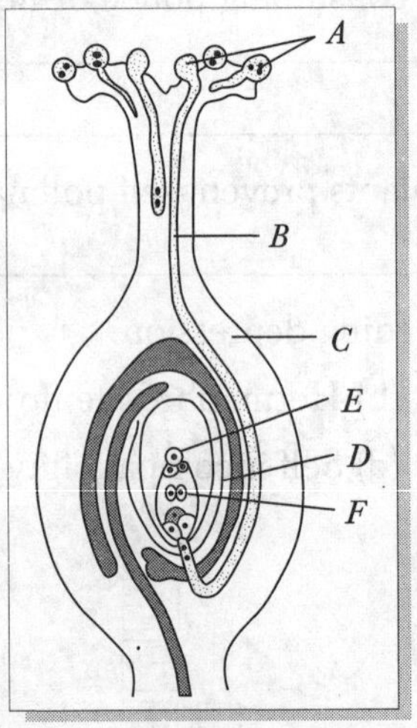

A ______________________

B ______________________

C ______________________

D ______________________

E ______________________

F ______________________

***110.** Diagram given belows shows the entry of pollen tube to the embryo sac, identify the parts labelled as *A* to *G*.

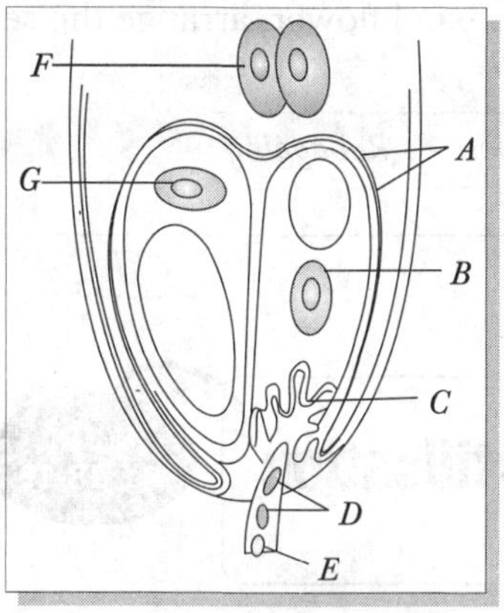

A. ____________________

B. ____________________

C. ____________________

D. ____________________

E. ____________________

F. ____________________

G. ____________________

111. In plants that shed their pollen at 2-celled stage, the way to fertilisation is guided by

(a) Synergids ☐ (b) Filiform apparatus ☐

(c) Stigma ☐ (d) Central cell ☐

112. Diagram given below shows discharge of gametes in the egg apparatus. Identify the parts labelled as *A* and *B*.

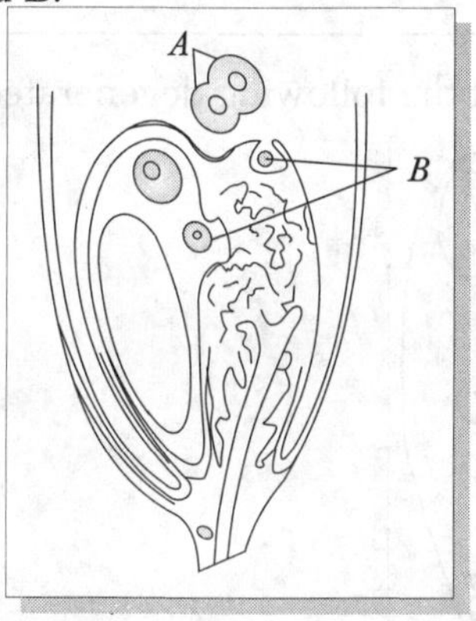

A. ____________________

B. ____________________

113. Name the interaction that occurs from pollen deposition to pollen tube entry into the ovule.

____

114. The pistil alone does not have ability to recognise the compatibility of pollen.

True ☐ False ☐

***115.** Pollen pistil recognition promotes the ____________________ events.

***116.** Pollen-pistil interaction is a __________________________ (dynamic/not worthy) process in the hybridisation technique.

117. __________________________ is the effective pollination between flowers of different species of the same genus or between different genera.

118. Removal of anthers from flower before anther dehiscence is called

____

119. Give reason why 10% sugar solution is used for pollen grain germination on glass slide. _

____

120. ____________ (Promotion/Inhibition) of germ tube from pollen occurs when there is genetic compatibility between pollen and stigma.

121. For artificial hybridisation experiment in bisexual flower, arrange the sequence in correct order

Cross-pollination → Bagging → Emasculation → Rebagging

____

TOPIC 3

Double Fertilisation and Post-Fertilisation Structure and Events

NCERT Pg. 18-19

122. Pollen tube releases ____________ (one/two/three) male gametes into the cytoplasm of synergid.

123. Zygote is a triploid structure .

True ☐ False ☐

***124.** Name the structure formed by the fusion of a male gamete and polar nuclei in the central cell. ____________

***125.** Consider the following structure. Which of the following degenerates post-fertilisation?

R

P

Q

(a) Only P ☐ (b) Q and R ☐

(c) Only Q ☐ (d) P and Q ☐

126. Write the ploidy of the PEN ____________

***127.** Write the number of chromosomes of the following if the haploid number in a flowering plant is 14.

(i) Integuments ____________

(ii) Embryo ____________

(iii) Endosperm ____________

***128.** If the endosperm mother cell of an angiosperm has 24 chromosomes, the same in megaspore mother cell would be ____________

***129.** PEN formation involves fusion of three ____________ (haploid/diploid) nuclei and therefore it is called ____________ fusion.

130. The fertilisation in flowering plants is termed as ________________ fertilisation as it involves two types of fusion, namely ______________ and ______________.

***131.** How can you justify the name triple fusion?

(a) Fusion of three haploid nuclei ☐

(b) Three fertilisation events ☐

(c) Fusion sperm, egg and polar nuclei ☐

(d) Endosperm is triploid ☐

132. The fusion of one male gamete with egg cell is called ________ (xenogamy/syngamy).

133. Identify the parts labelled as *A*, *B* and *C*.

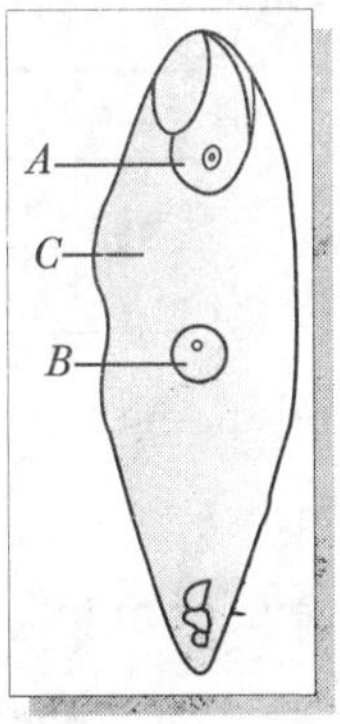

A. ____________________

B. ____________________

C. ____________________

134. If endosperm has 36 number of chromosomes then find out the chromosome number of male and female gamete. ____________________

***135.** Consider the following statements.

Statement I Events of endosperm and embryo development, maturation of ovules into seeds and ovary into fruit are a part of post-fertilisation events.

Statement II Cells of endosperm are filled with reserve food material for nourishing the developing embryo.

Choose the correct option from the following.

(a) Statement I is true, but statement II is false ☐

(b) Statement I is false, but statement II is true ☐

(c) Both statements I and II are true ☐

(d) Both statements I and II are false ☐

***136.** Coconut water from a tender coconut is ____________________

137. Post-fertilisation events do not include seed and fruit formation.

True ☐ False ☐

138. ______________ (Embryo/Endosperm) development precedes ______________ (endosperm/embryo) development.

139. Write the stage of endosperm development where PEN undergoes successive nuclear division to give rise to free nuclei. ____________________

***140.** The white coconut kernel is made up of ____________________

***141.** Write any two seeds in which endosperm is completely consumed by the developing embryo. ____________________

TOPIC 4

Embryo, Seed and Fruit Formation

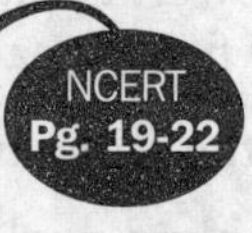

142. The study of embryo development is known as ____________

***143.** Identify the different stages of embryogenesis (*A* to *G*) in the given diagram.

A. ____________
B. ____________
C. ____________
D. ____________
E. ____________
F. ____________
G. ____________

144. Embryogeny are different in both monocots and dicots.

True ☐ False ☐

145. Write the following words in the sequence of development.

Heart-shaped embryo, Mature embryo, Globular embryo, Endosperm development, Proembryo.

____

146. Identify the parts labelled as *A* to *E* in the following diagram of a typical dicot embryo.

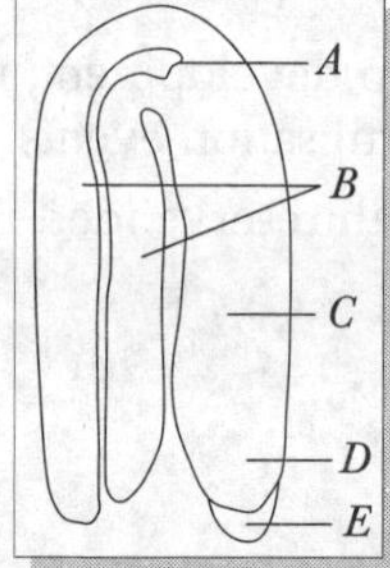

A. ____________
B. ____________
C. ____________
D. ____________
E. ____________

147. In the figure given below, find out the type of seed and identify which labelled parts represent coleoptile, coleorhiza and epiblast.

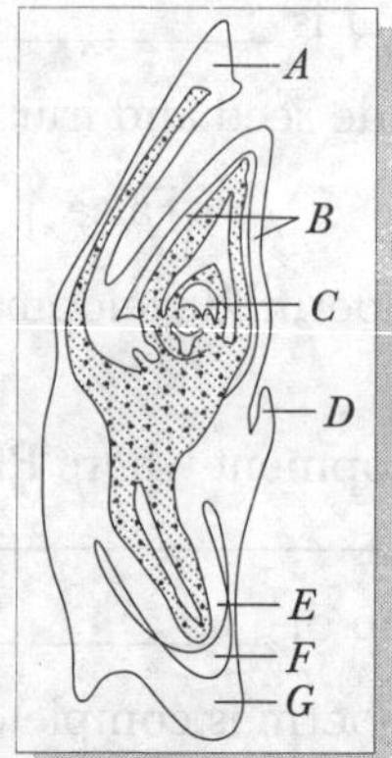

____

***148.** A typical dicotyledonous embryo consists of an ____________ axis and ____________ cotyledons. The portion of embryonal axis above the level of cotyledons is ____________ which terminates with the ____________ or stem tip.

149. The cylindrical portion below the cotyledons is ____________ .

150. Complete the following analogy.

Epicotyl : ____________ : : Plumule : Radicle

151. Name the structure covering the radicle. ____________

152. Write other name for cotyledons in grass family. ____________

153. The sheath covering the radicle and root cap in monocots is known as ____________

154. Name the foliar hollow structure enclosing leaf primordia and a shoot apex. ____________

155. Seed is a fertilised ovary.

True ☐ False ☐

156. Find the odd one out.

Seed coat, Cotyledons, Pericarp, Embryonal axis

____

***157.** Endosperm is not completely consumed during embryo development in non-albuminous seeds.

True ☐ False ☐

158. Write two examples of the albuminous seeds. ____________

159. Find the odd one out.

Castor, Pea, Wheat, Rice

____

***160.** Identify the incorrect set of statements.

I. Seed is the final product of sexual reproduction.

II. Epicotyl consists of shoot apex and a few leaf primordia enclosed in coleoptile.

III. The cylindrical portion below the level of cotyledons is epicotyl.

IV. Scutellum in the grass family is present towards the dorsal side of embryonal axis.

V. Cotyledons are generally thick and swollen structures.

Codes

(a) I, IV and V ☐ (b) II, III and V ☐

(c) I and III ☐ (d) III and IV ☐

***161.** The persistent residual nucellus is known as ____________

162. The diagram given below shows structural details of a dicot seed. Study the diagram and answer the questions that follow.

(i) Identify the structures labelled as *A* to *E*.

A. ________
B. ________
C. ________
D. ________
E. ________

(ii) Name the plant from which this seed is obtained. ________

(iii) Write the function of seed parts labelled as *A* and *B*.

____

***163.** Identify the parts labelled as *A* to *D* in structure of seed given below.

A. ________
B. ________
C. ________
D. ________

164. The seed shows dormancy when seed is ________ and its seed coat is ________ .

165. The wall of <u>ovule</u> develops into wall of the fruit.
(*Rewrite the statement after correcting the underlined word.*)

____

***166.** Match the following columns.

Column I (Seeds / Fruits)	Column II (Examples)
A. Parthenocarpic fruit	1. Banana
B. True fruit	2. Mango
C. False fruit	3. Cashew

A.________ B.________ C.________

***167.** Give a common term for the following.

(i) Fruits developing from ovary only. ________

(ii) Fruits developing from both ovary and thalamus. ________

168. Write two examples of false fruits. ________

169. Write the scientific name for the fruits developed without fertilisation. ________

170. Parthenocarpic fruits are seedless.

True ☐ False ☐

171. Parthenocarpy can be induced by ______________________________.

172. Seeds generate new genetic combinations.

True ☐ False ☐

173. ______________ and ______________ of mature seeds are important for storage of seeds and hence find importance in the agricultural field.

174. *Phoenix dactylifera* (date palm) is an example showing ______________ years old seed to be viable.

175. What is the common seed characteristics of the plants given in the box.

Orobanche, Striga, Ficus, Orchids

____

176. Write the scientific name of the plant having oldest viable seed excavated from Arctic Tundra.

____

TOPIC 5

Apomixis and Polyembryony

NCERT Pg. 22-23

***177.** Name the mechanism by which seeds are produced without fertilisation. __________

178. Asteraceae and grasses usually adapt apomixis.

True ☐ False ☐

179. ______________ is an asexual reproduction that mimics sexual reproduction.

***180.** Give the name for the occurrence of more than one embryo in a seed.

____

181. Write two examples of fruits exhibiting polyembryony. ______________

182. Name the cell which protrudes into the embryo sac and develops into the embryo during polyembryony.

____

183. Find odd one out with respect to fruit development.

Orange, Papaya, Apple, Pomegranate

____

184. Cultivation of hybrid has tremendously ______________ (increased/decreased) productivity.

185. Seeds collected from hybrids do not maintain ______________ characters.

186. There is segregation of characters in the hybrid progeny when the hybrids are made into apomicts.

True ☐ False ☐

187. A farmer who wishes to grow hybrid seeds all throughout the year, without the need to purchase the costly seeds, would preferably use the technique of

(a) Apomixis ☐ (b) Polyembryony ☐
(c) Parthenocarpy ☐ (d) Emasculation ☐

Assertion-Reason Questions

The following questions consist of two statements- Assertion (A) and Reason (R). Answer these questions by selecting the appropriate option given below.
(a) Both A and R are true and R is the correct explanation of A
(b) Both A and R are true, but R is not the correct explanation of A
(c) A is true, but R is false
(d) A is false, but R is true

1. **Assertion** (A) The sporogenous tissue lying at the centre of microsporangium is called a pollen mother cell.

Reason (R) Microspores arise by meiotic division of sporogenous tissue to form microspore tetrads.

(a) ☐ (b) ☐ (c) ☐ (d) ☐

2. **Assertion** (A) Pollen grain exine has prominent apertures called germ pores where sporopollenin is absent.

Reason (R) Sporopollenin is one of the most resistant organic material that cannot be degraded by acid or alkali.

(a) ☐ (b) ☐ (c) ☐ (d) ☐

3. **Assertion** (A) Pollen tube enters the embryosac through micropylar end.

Reason (R) Filiform apparatus secretes chemotactic substances in order to attract and guide the entry of pollen tube.

(a) ☐ (b) ☐ (c) ☐ (d) ☐

4. **Assertion** (A) After the 4-nucleate stage, cell wall is laid down to form a functional embryo sac.

Reason (R) The mitotic divisions of the functional megaspore lead to multinucleate condition of the embryo sac.

(a) ☐ (b) ☐ (c) ☐ (d) ☐

***5.** **Assertion** (A) The chance of genetic variability is poor in cleistogamous flowers.

Reason (R) Cleistogamous flowers produce assured seed-set even in the absence of pollinators.

(a) ☐ (b) ☐ (c) ☐ (d) ☐

6. **Assertion** (A) Water hyacinth despite being an aquatic plant, is not pollinated by water currents.

Reason (R) In most aquatic plants flowers emerge above the water level and are pollinated by insects.

(a) ☐ (b) ☐ (c) ☐ (d) ☐

***7.** **Assertion** (A) Castor plants are dioecious and can prevent both autogamy and geitonogamy.

Reason (R) Self-incompatibility can prevent inbreeding depression that results from continued autogamy.

(a) ☐ (b) ☐ (c) ☐ (d) ☐

8. **Assertion** (A) Not all types of pollen that lands on the stigma, germinates to form the pollen tube.

Reason (R) Chemical interactions between the pollen and the anther leads to pollen acceptance.

(a) ☐ (b) ☐ (c) ☐ (d) ☐

9. **Assertion** (A) For artificial hybridisation, it is important to emasculate a flower before the anther dehisces.

Reason (R) Emasculation ensures that the flower is protected against unwanted pollen contamination.

(a) ☐ (b) ☐ (c) ☐ (d) ☐

10. **Assertion** (A) Fertilisation event in angiosperms is called double fertilisation.

Reason (R) Two types of fusion, syngamy and triple fusion take place in embryo sac.

(a) ☐ (b) ☐ (c) ☐ (d) ☐

***11.** **Assertion** (A) Post fertilisation, micropyle persists as a small pore in the seed coat.

Reason (R) Seeds coats are formed from protective integuments of the ovule post fertilisation.

(a) ☐ (b) ☐ (c) ☐ (d) ☐

12. **Assertion** (A) Apomixis results in the formation of seedless varities of fruits.

Reason (R) In apomixis, the egg cell does not undergo meiotic cell division.

(a) ☐ (b) ☐ (c) ☐ (d) ☐

Case Based Questions

1. Amit when tried cutting a transverse section of an anther, observed the following under a microscope. Identify the slide and answer the questions by choosing the right answer from options below.

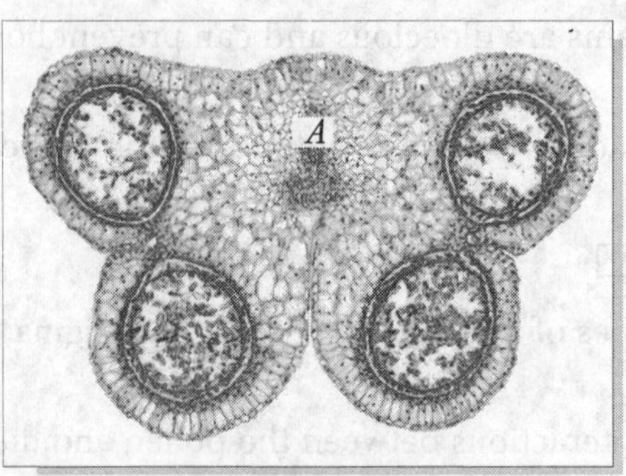

(i) What conclusion can be drawn from the above slide?

(a) The connective is non-functional ☐
(b) Anther is mature and ready to dehisce ☐
(c) Anther is bisporous and dithecous ☐
(d) Label A represents microsporangia ☐

(ii) The cells of innermost wall layer called ____________ possess __________ and are ________

(a) Sporogenous tissue, scarce cytoplasm, uninucleate ☐
(b) Tapetum, dense cytoplasm, enucleate ☐
(c) Tapetum, dense cytoplasm, multinucleate ☐
(d) Sporogenous tissue, dense cytoplasm, enucleate ☐

(iii) Label A represents

(a) Pollen sac ☐ (b) Microcporangium ☐
(c) Dead microspores ☐ (d) Connective ☐

(iv) Which term will be used to describe an anther that matures early in comparison to the time taken by stigma to become receptive?

(a) Protandry ☐ (b) Protogyny ☐
(c) Heterostyly ☐ (d) Dehiscence ☐

2. A farmer wants to grow a superior variety of tomatoes. He chose one variety (Plant A)that show pest resistance and another variety (Plant B) that is temperature tolerant. The new variety would have the combined properties of both and would thus be a hybrid superior variety. For this he emasculated plant A and left it open in the fields. This was followed by dusting pollen grains from plant B. However, the progeny plants formed by this method were not hybrids, which confirmed something was wrong with the process. With reference to the given information answer the following.

(i) Which of the structures is absent from plant after emasculation?

(a) Stigma ☐ (b) Anther ☐
(c) Filament ☐ (d) Ovary ☐

(ii) Why did the process fail to yield desired result?

(a) Emasculated flowers did not dehisce ☐

(b) Emasculated flowers were not mature ☐

(c) Stigma did not attain receptivity ☐

(d) Emasculated flowers were not bagged ☐

(iii) What is the disadvantage of prolonged self pollination?

(a) Increased genetic variability ☐ (b) Increased mutation ☐

(c) Inbreeding depression ☐ (d) Decreased fertilisation capacity ☐

COMPETITION EDGE UP

1. *Identify the set of correct statements.* **[NCERT Pg. 13, NEET 2024]**

A. *The flowers of Vallisneria are colourful and produce nectar.*

B. *The flowers of water lily are not pollinated by water.*

C. *In most of water-pollinated species, the pollen grains are protected from wetting.*

D. *Pollen grains of some hydrophytes are long and ribbon like.*

E. *In some hydrophytes, the pollen grains are carried passively inside water.*

Choose the correct answer from the options given below.

(a) *C, D and E only* ☐

(b) *A, B, C and D only* ☐

(c) *A, C, D and E only* ☐

(d) *B, C, D and E only* ☐

2. *Identify the correct description about the given figure.* **[NCERT Pg. 13, NEET 2024]**

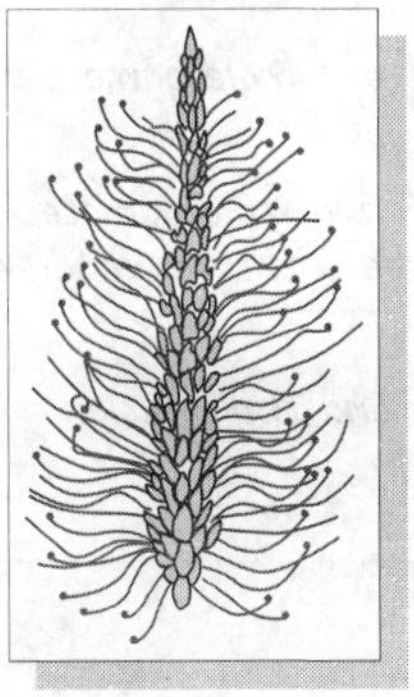

(a) *Wind pollinated plant inflorescence showing flowers with well exposed stamens.* ☐

(b) *Water pollinated flowers showing stamens with mucilaginous covering.* ☐

(c) *Cleistogamous flowers showing autogamy.* ☐

(d) *Compact inflorescence showing complete autogamy* ☐

3. *What is the function of tassels in the corn cob?* **[NEET 2023]**

(a) *To trap pollen grains* ☐

(b) *To disperse pollen grains* ☐

(c) *To protect seeds* ☐

(d) *To attract insects* ☐

4. *In angiosperm, the haploid, diploid and triploid structures of a fertilised embryo sac sequentially are* **[NCERT Pg. 18, NEET 2023]**

(a) *Antipodals, synergids and primary endosperm nucleus* ☐

(b) *Synergids, zygote and primary endosperm nucleus* ☐

(c) *Synergids, antipodals and polar nuclei* ☐

(d) *Synergids, primary endosperm nucleus and zygote* ☐

5. *Given below are two statements.*

Statement I *Cleistogamous flowers are invariably autogamous.*

Statement II *Cleistogamy is disadvantageous as there is no chance for cross-pollination.*

In the light of the above statements, choose the correct answer from the options given below. **[NCERT Pg. 12, NEET 2022]**

(a) Both statement I and statement II are incorrect

(b) Statement I is correct, but statement II is incorrect

(c) Statement I is incorrect, but statement II is correct

(d) Both statement I and statement II are correct

6. Which part of the fruit, labelled in the given figure makes it a false fruit? **[NCERT Pg. 20, NEET 2022]**

(a) B → Endocarp
(b) C → Thalamus
(c) D → Seed
(d) A → Mesocarp

7. The plant part which consists of two generations, one within the other **[NEET (Sep.) 2020]**

I. Pollen grains inside the anther.
II. Germinated pollen grain with two male gametes.
III. Seed inside the fruit.
IV. Embryo sac inside the ovule.

(a) I, II and III (b) III and IV
(c) I and IV (d) Only I

8. Which of the following is incorrect for wind pollinated plants? **[NCERT Pg. 13, NEET (Oct.) 2020]**

(a) Well exposed stamens and stigma
(b) Many ovules in each ovary
(c) Flowers are small and not brightly coloured
(d) Pollen grains are light and non-sticky

9. What is the fate of the male gametes discharged in the synergid? **[NCERT Pg. 18, NEET 2019]**

(a) One fuses with the egg and other fuses with central cell nuclei
(b) One fuses with the egg, other(s) degenerates in the synergid.
(c) All fuse with the egg
(d) One fuses with the egg, other(s) fuses with synergid nucleus

10. What type of pollination takes place in Vallisneria? **[NCERT Pg. 13, NEET (Odisha) 2019]**

(a) Pollination occurs in submerged condition by water
(b) Flowers emerge above surface of water and pollination occurs by insects
(c) Flowers emerge above water surface and pollen is carried by wind
(d) Male flowers are carried by water currents to female flowers at the surface of water

11. Which is the most common type of embryo sac in angiosperms? **[NCERT Pg. 10, Odisha NEET 2019]**

(a) Tetrasporic with one mitotic stage of divisions
(b) Monosporic with three sequential mitotic divisions
(c) Monosporic with two sequential mitotic divisions
(d) Bisporic with two sequential mitotic divisions

12. Double fertilisation is **[NCERT Pg. 18, NEET 2018]**

(a) fusion of two male gametes with one egg
(b) fusion of one male gamete with two polar nuclei
(c) fusion of two male gametes of pollen tube with two different eggs
(d) syngamy and triple fusion

Chapter 02

Human Reproduction

Scan and take Chapter Test

TOPIC 1

The Male Reproductive System

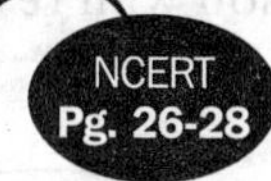

NCERT Pg. 26-28

1. The male reproductive system located in the ______ region includes all of the given except __________

(a) thoracic; ovum ☐ (b) pelvis ; ovum ☐

(c) pelvis ; external genitalia ☐ (d) thoracic ; accessory ducts ☐

2. Name the pouch in which testes are suspended outside the abdominal cavity. ____________________

3. The ____________________ (scrotum/hypothalamus) helps in the maintenance of low temperature (34-35°C) necessary for spermatogenesis.

4. Answer the following questions in numbers only.

(i) The length of each testis. ____________________

(ii) The width of each testis. ____________________

(iii) The number of testicular lobules in each testis. ____________________

(iv) The number of seminiferous tubules in each lobule. ____________________

5. The seminiferous tubules of the testis are lined on its inside by <u>spermatids</u> and Sertoli cells. (*Rewrite the statement after correcting the underlined word.*)

____

6. ____________ provides nutrition to the developing male germ cells.

***7.** The region outside the seminiferous tubules called interstitial spaces contain small blood vessels and masses of cells called ____________________

8. Name the testicular hormones synthesised and secreted by the Leydig cells.

____

9. Which of the following cells present in the mammalian testes form the sperms?

Leydig cells, Spermatogonia, Interstitial cells, Sertoli cells

____

*Concepts of all questions bearing * are important for NEET & CUET*

***10.** The seminiferous tubules of the testis open into the vasa efferentia by rete testis.

True ☐ False ☐

11. The vasa efferentia leave the testis and open into epididymis along the anterior surface of each testis.

True ☐ False ☐

12. Choose the incorrect pair.

(a) Leydig cells – Secrete LH and FSH ☐

(b) Vasa efferentia and epididymis – Accessory ducts ☐

(c) Vas deferens – Loops over the urinary bladder ☐

(d) Ejaculatory duct – Store and transport sperms from testis to the outside ☐

***13.** Choose the correct option with respect to the given diagram.

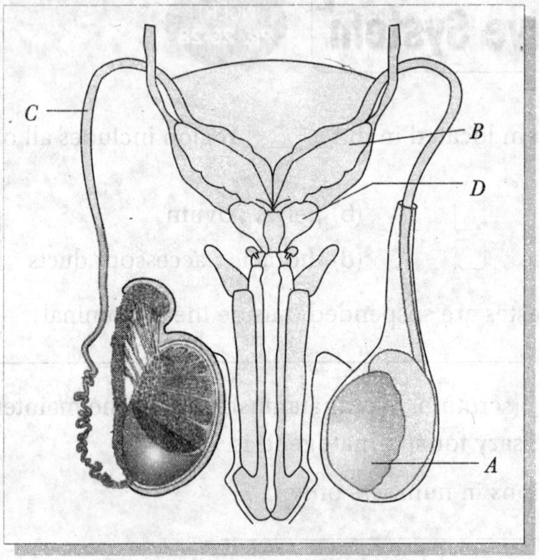

(a) *A*– Testis–possesses 3-4 testicular lobules ☐

(b) *B*– Seminal vesicle–storage of sperm ☐

(c) *C*– Vas deferens–helps in sperm transfer ☐

(d) *D*– Prostate gland–secretes seminal fluid ☐

***14.** Complete the sequence for transport of sperm cells in male reproductive system.

Seminiferous tubules → ________ → Vasa efferentia → Epididymis → ________ → Ejaculatory duct → Urethra → ________.

15. The shared terminal duct of the reproductive and urinary system in the human male is ________________

16. Identify the accessory reproductive gland found in males.

Seminal vesicles, Testis, Hypothalamus

____

17. The given diagram refers to TS of testis showing sectional view of a few seminiferous tubules. Identify the parts labelled as *A-D*.

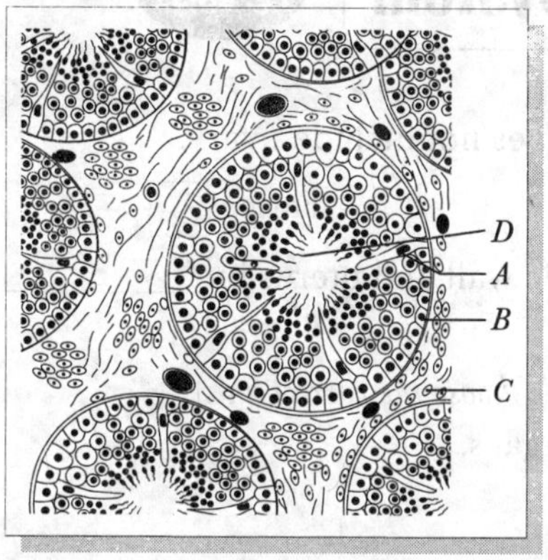

A. ____________________

B. ____________________

C. ____________________

D. ____________________

18. Study the given image and mark the answer that correctly represents the function of *X*.

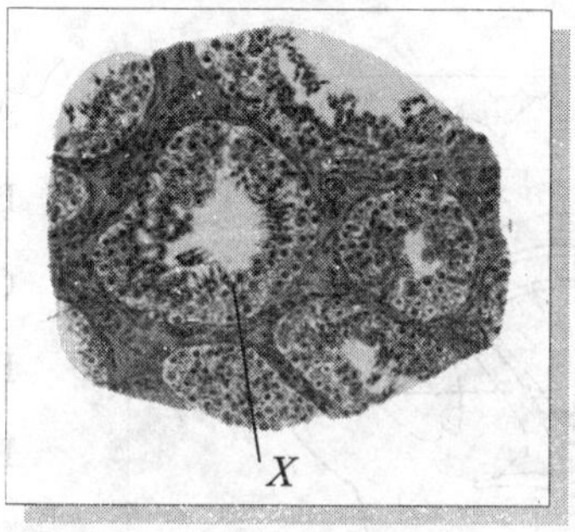

(a) Secretes male androgens ☐
(b) Gives rise to spermatozoa ☐
(c) Provides nutrition to germ cells ☐
(d) Secretes seminal fluid ☐

19. Glans penis is covered by a loose fold of skin called ____________________

20. Seminal vesicle is paired, while prostate is an unpaired gland.

True ☐ False ☐

21. Find odd one out.

Rete testis, Vasa efferentia, Epididymis, Vas deferens, Seminiferous tubule

____

22. Consider the following statements.

Statement I The seminal plasma of males is rich in fructose, calcium and enzymes.

Statement II Secretions of the prostate gland helps in lubrication of the penis.

Choose the correct option from the following.

(a) Statement I is true, but statement II is false ☐
(b) Statement I is false, but statement II is true ☐
(c) Both statements I and II are true ☐
(d) Both statements I and II are false ☐

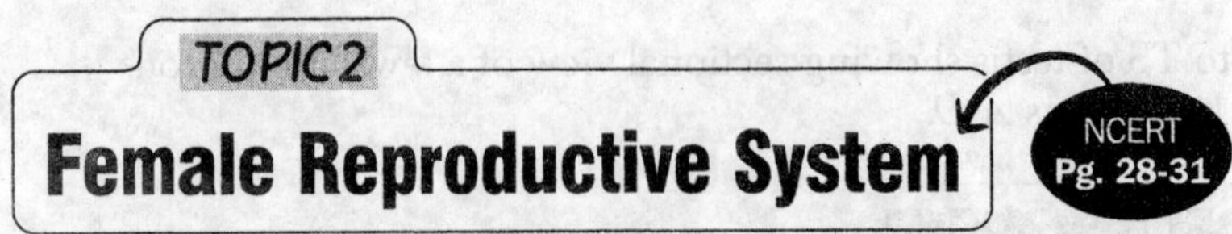

TOPIC 2
Female Reproductive System
NCERT Pg. 28-31

23. The female external genitalia does not include ovary.

True ☐ False ☐

24. Ovary is connected to the pelvic wall and uterus by ______________ (ligaments/ovarian stroma).

25. The ovaries of human females (*Choose the correct one.*)

(i) are the primary female sex organs.

(ii) produce FSH and LH.

____

26. The following diagram refers to female reproductive system of human. Identify the labelled parts as *A* to *E*.

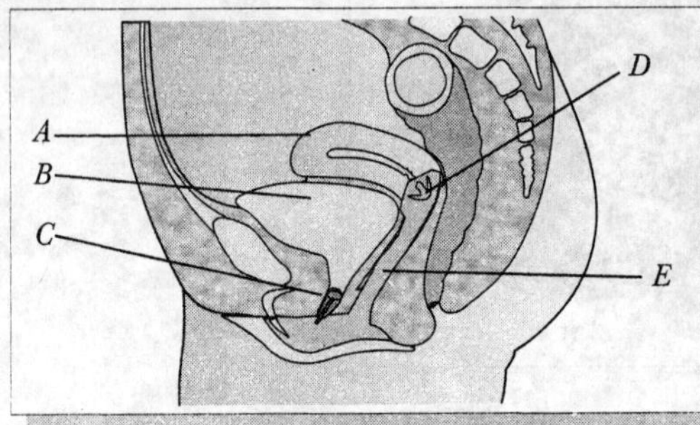

A. ______________

B. ______________

C. ______________

D. ______________

E. ______________

27. Give a collective term for oviducts, uterus and vagina. ______________

***28.** Consider the figure given below and identify the parts which are incorrectly labelled.

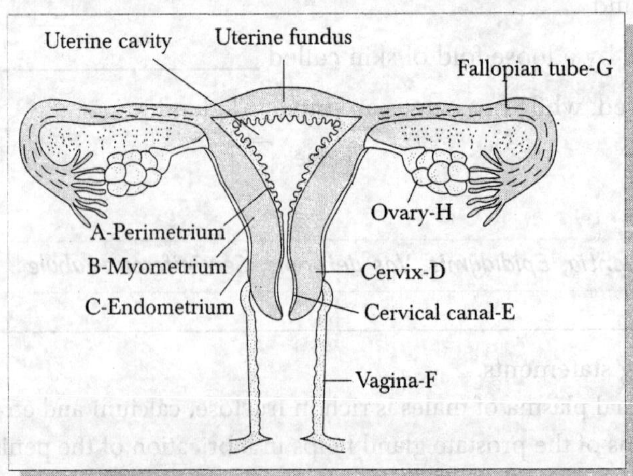

____

***29.** Consider the following statements.

Statement I The infundibulum collects the ovum after its release from the ovary.

Statement II Fusion of the male and female gametes take place in the infundibulum.

Choose the correct option from the following.

(a) Statement I is true, but statement II is false

(b) Statement I is false, but statement II is true

(c) Both statements I and II are true

(d) Both statements I and II are false

30. Write the scientific name for the following.

(i) Finger-like projections on the edges of infundibulum. ____________

(ii) Last part of oviduct with a narrow lumen joining the uterus. ____________

(iii) The part through which uterus opens into the vagina. ____________

***31.** Consider the following image and choose the correct combination of structure and function.

(a) X – Uterine contraction ; Y – Site of fertilisation

(b) P – Uterine contraction ; Q – Site of fertilisation

(c) M – Uterine contraction ; N – Site of fertilisation

(d) A – Uterine contraction ; B – Site of fertilisation

32. Find the odd one out.

Mons pubis, Pubic Symphysis, Labia majora, Labia minora

____

***33.** Consider the following statements.

Statement I Labia minora surrounding the vagina extends from the mons pubis.

Statement II Clitoris lies at the upper junction of the two labia minora above the urethral opening.

Choose the correct option from the following.

(a) Statement I is true, but statement II is false

(b) Statement I is false, but statement II is true

(c) Both statements I and II are true

(d) Both statements I and II are false

34. The membrane which partially covers the opening of vagina is known as <u>clitoris</u>.
(*Rewrite the statement after correcting the underlined word.*)

___

35. Choose the incorrect pair.
(a) Cushion of fatty tissue covered by pubic hair –Mons pubis ☐
(b) Single, inverted pear–shape structure-Uterus ☐
(c) Finger-like structure above the urethral opening –Clitoris ☐
(d) Uterine layer exhibiting strong contraction during delivery–Endometrium ☐

***36.** The presence or absence of hymen is a reliable indicator of virginity or sexual experience.
True ☐ False ☐

37. Pick the odd one out from each series given below.
I. Ampulla, isthmus, Fallopian tube, vas deferens. ___
II. Ovary, uterus, vagina, ejaculatory duct. ___
III. Bulbourethral gland, Graafian follicle, corpus luteum, cervix. ___
IV. Cervical canal, myometrium, endometrium, perimetrium.

38. The main tissue present in breast is ___ tissue.

39. The diagrammatic sectional view of mammary gland is given below. Identify the parts labelled as *A, B, C* and *D*.

A. ___ B. ___ C. ___ D. ___

40. Which of the following best identifies the course of breast milk pathway after its formation?
(a) Alveoli-mammary tubules-mammary duct-mammary ampulla-lactiferous duct ☐
(b) Alveoli-mammary ampulla-mammary tubules-mammary lactiferous ducts ☐
(c) Mammary ampulla-alveoli-mammary duct-mammary tubules-lactiferous ducts ☐
(d) Mammary ampulla-mammary tubules-mammary duct-alveoli-lactiferous ducts ☐

41. Match the following columns.

Column I (Parts of mammary gland)	Column II (Characteristics)
A. Mammary duct	1. Join to form mammary ampulla
B. Lactiferous duct	2. Secrete milk
C. Mammary tubules	3. Duct through which milk is sucked out
D. Cells of alveoli	4. Alveoli open into it

A. ______________ B. ______________ C. ______________ D. ______________

TOPIC 3

Gametogenesis

NCERT Pg. 31-33

42. The primary sex organs ____________ in males and ____________ in females, produce gametes *via* ____________

(a) scrotum, ovaries, gametogenesis

(b) penis, infundibulum, gametogenolysis

(c) testis, ovaries, gametogenesis

(d) testis, cervical canal, gametogenolysis

***43.** Spermatogenesis is initiated in the male testis with the beginning of ____________ (puberty/foetal stage).

44. Number of chromosomes present in spermatogonium is ____________

45. Which cell comes earliest in the sequence of sperm production?

Spermatozoa, Spermatocyte, Spermatid, Spermatogonia

____

***46.** ____________ (Mitosis/Meiosis) is involved in the formation of secondary spermatocytes from primary spermatocytes.

47. Number of chromosomes present in secondary spermatocyte is ____________

48. During spermatogenesis, which cells are the first to contain haploid number of chromosomes? ____________

***49.** Sperms are released from the <u>Sertoli cells</u> by a process called spermiation. (*Rewrite the statement after correcting the underlined words.*)

____

***50.** Consider the given image and identify the structure *P* and the process.

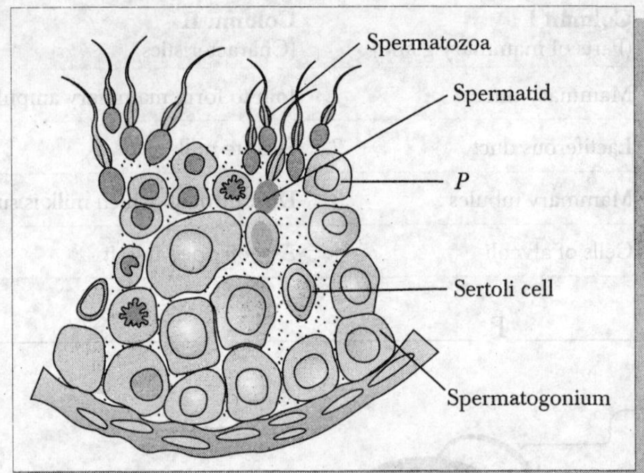

(a) *P* – Primary spermatocyte, Spermatogenesis

(b) *P* – Primary spermatocyte, Spermiogenesis

(c) *P* – Secondary spermatocyte, Spermiogenesis

(d) *P* – Secondary spermatocyte, Spermiation

***51.** Complete the following flowchart of sperm formation.

Spermatogonia ⟶ *A* ⟶ Spermatid ⟶ *B*

A. ______________ B. ______________

52. Increase in the GnRH hormone secretion leads to spermatogenesis.

True ☐ False ☐

53. Name two hormones stimulated by GnRH during spermatogenesis. ______________

***54.** Identify the processes *A, B, C* and *D* in the schematic representation of spermatogenesis given below.

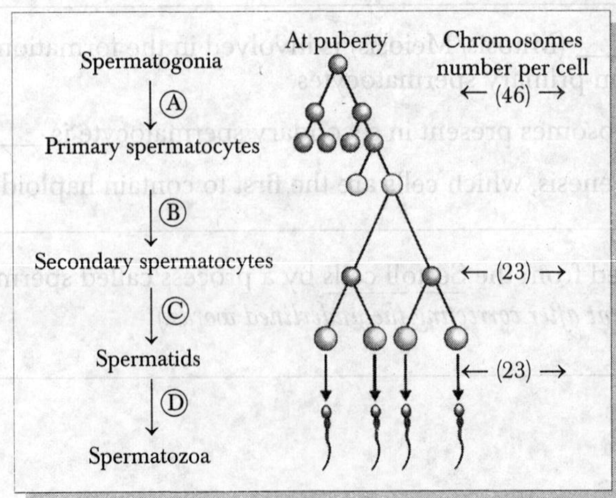

A. ______________ B. ______________ C. ______________ D. ______________

55. Consider the following statements.

Statement I The spermatids in human males formed from secondary spermatocytes contain 23 chromosomes .

Statement II Sertoli cells stimulate the process of spermiogenesis under the influence of FSH hormone.

Choose the correct option from the following.

(a) Statement I is true, but statement II is false ☐

(b) Statement I is false, but statement II is true ☐

(c) Both statements I and II are true ☐

(d) Both statements I and II are false ☐

56. Complete the following analogy given below.

Luteinizing hormone : Leydig cells : : ______________ : Sertoli cells.

***57.** Give the name of two hormones *A* and *B* in the figure given below.

[*A*] $\xrightarrow{\text{Acts on}}$ Leydig cells $\xrightarrow{\text{Secrete}}$ [*B*] $\longrightarrow$ Stimulate spermatogenesis

A. ______________ B. ______________

***58.** Consider the following statements.

Statement I The secretions of the interstitial cells under the action of LH, stimulates spermatogenesis.

Statement II The hypothalamus plays no role in the development of spermatozoa from spermatocytes.

Choose the correct option from the following.

(a) Statement I is true, but statement II is false ☐

(b) Statement I is false, but statement II is true ☐

(c) Both statements I and II are true ☐

(d) Both statements I and II are false ☐

59. ________ is filled with enzymes that help in fertilisation of the ovum.

60. Mitochondria are spirally arranged in sperm at the region of middle piece.

True ☐ False ☐

61. Match Column I with Column II.

Column I	Column II
A. Acrosome	1. Haploid nucleus
B. Tail	2. Movement
C. Middle piece	3. Penetration into ovum
D. Head	4. Energy production

	A	B	C	D	
(a)	3	2	4	1	☐
(b)	3	2	1		☐
(c).	1	2	4		☐
(d)	1	2	3	4	☐

62. For normal fertility, ______________ % of sperm ejaculate must exhibit vigorous motility and ______________ sperms must have normal shape and size.

***63.** In the given figure of structure of sperm, identify the incorrect labellings.

Plasma membrane-*A*
Head-*B*
Middle piece-*C*
Tail-*D*
Mitochondria-*E*

64. Secretions of epididymis, vas deferens, seminal vesicle and prostate are essential for ______________ (acrosome reaction/maturation and motility of sperms).

***65.** Choose the incorrect pair.

(a) Acrosome – Enzymes filled cap-like structure on sperm head ☐
(b) Middle piece – Possesses numerous mitochondria ☐
(c) Sperm tail – Facilitates sperm motility essential for fertilisation ☐
(d) Semen – Contains only sperms ☐

66. The function of male sex accessory ducts and glands is maintained by androgens.

True ☐ False ☐

67. Gamete mother cells (oogonia) start division and get arrested at ______________ stage of meiotic division as ______________ oocytes.

***68.** At puberty, only 60,000-80,000 primary follicles are left in each ovary.

True ☐ False ☐

***69.** Consider the following statements.

Statement I During the foetal stage, the primary oocyte gets arrested in prophase-II of meiosis.

Statement II Primary oocyte develops into secondary oocyte by completing meiosis-II.

Choose the correct option from the following.

(a) Statement I is true, but statement II is false ☐
(b) Statement I is false, but statement II is true ☐
(c) Both statements I and II are true ☐
(d) Both statements I and II are false ☐

***70.** In the given figure, label the structures *A, B, C* and *D.*

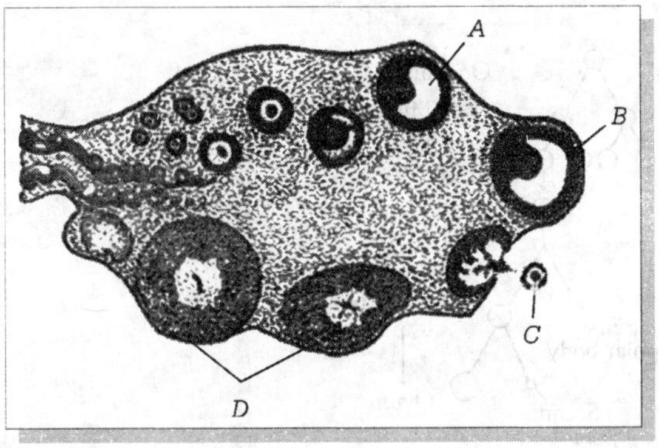

A. ______________

B. ______________

C. ______________

D. ______________

71. The primary follicles get surrounded by more layers of ________ and a new theca and are called

____

72. Formation of antrum is a characteristic of which stage of female gamete development?

(a) Primary follicle ☐ (b) Graafian follicle ☐

(c) Secondary follicle ☐ (d) Tertiary follicle ☐

73. Write the ploidy of the following cells.

(i) Secondary oocyte ________

(ii) Polar body ________

(iii) Primary oocyte ________

74. During oogenesis, one functional ________ and two tiny ________ are produced.

75. Large size of the ovum is due to the large amount of reserve food.

True ☐ False ☐

76. Find the odd one out.

Cowper's gland, Primary oocyte, Antrum, Polar bodies

____

77. Structure consisting of ova with their surrounding tissues is called ________

78. Name the membrane surrounding the secondary oocyte.

____

***79.** Rupture of zona pellucida releases the secondary oocyte from the ovary.

(*Rewrite the statement after correcting the underlined words.*)

____

80. Ovulation in mammals refers to the release of primary oocyte from ovary.

(*Rewrite the statement after correcting the underlined words.*)

____

***81.** Consider the given representation of oogenesis and identify the process X and chromosome number Z.

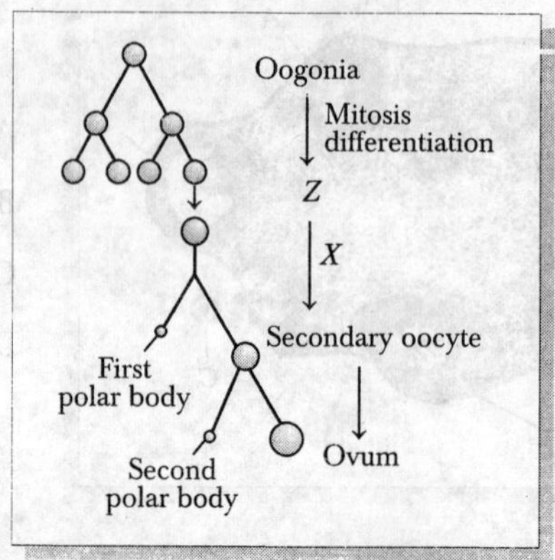

(a) X – Mitosis; Z – 46 ☐ (b) X – Meiosis; Z – 46 ☐

(c) X – Mitosis; Z – 23 ☐ (d) X – Meiosis; Z – 23 ☐

82. Find the odd one out.

Endometrium, Corpus luteum, Acrosome, Graafian follicle

____

83. Mitotic differentiation of oogonia occurs during fetal life.

True ☐ False ☐

***84.** Identify the correct pair among the following.

(a) Secondary oocyte – Diploid ☐ (b) Primary oocyte – Haploid ☐

(c) Ovum – Diploid ☐ (d) Secondary oocyte – Haploid ☐

____

***85.** Consider the given sentences.

I. Tertiary follicle changes into Graafian follicle.

II. The process of addition of oogonia and release of egg continues till the age of 45.

III. Primary follicles get surrounded by more layers of granulosa layer.

IV. At puberty only 60,000 to 80,000 primary follicles remain in the ovary.

How many of the given sentence(s) stand true for oogenesis?

(a) 1 ☐ (b) 3 ☐

(c) 2 ☐ (d) 4 ☐

***86.** Choose the incorrect pair.

(a) Antrum – fluid-filled cavity in primary follicle ☐

(b) Tertiary follicle – primary oocyte completes its I meiotic division inside it ☐

(c) Secondary oocyte – haploid cell formed after I meiotic division ☐

(d) Graafian follicle – mature tertiary follicle which ruptures during ovulation ☐

87. The number of chromosomes in a mature gamete is reduced to half during the formation of first polar body.

True ☐ False ☐

88. Complete the following flowchart of oogenesis.

Primary oocyte → Primary follicle → *A* → Tertiary follicle → *B* → Ovulation

A. ____________ B. ____________

89. Match the following columns.

Column I	Column II
A. Ovum	1. Uterus
B. Endometrium	2. Oogenesis
C. Polar body	3. Secondary oocyte
D. Clitoris	4. Rudimentary erectile tissue

A. ____________ B. ____________ C. ____________ D. ____________

TOPIC 4
Menstrual Cycle
NCERT Pg. 33-35

90. Write the scientific name for the first menstruation at puberty.

____

91. The reproductive cycle repeated at an interval of about__________ days, in human female is called menstrual cycle.

92. When does ovulation occur in a healthy menstruating female?

____

***93.** Endometrium, epithelial glands and connective tissue of uterus are broken due to the lack of progesterone, thus resulting in menstrual flow.

True ☐ False ☐

***94.** What happens in uterus during the follicular phase of menstrual cycle?

____

***95.** During follicular phase, oestrogen is secreted by ____________ (pituitary/growing follicles).

***96.** Rapid secretion of LH in ovulatory phase causes all of the given, except

(a) Rupturing of Graafian follicle ☐

(b) Release of ova ☐

(c) Ovulation ☐

(d) Maintenance of endometrial lining ☐

***97.** Consider the following statements.

Statement I A spike in the levels of LH trigger the rupture of the Graafian follicle to release the secondary oocyte.

Statement II Ovulatory phase is followed by luteal phase where corpus luteum degrades in the absence of fertilisation.

Choose the correct option from the following.

(a) Statement I is true, but statement II is false ☐

(b) Statement I is false, but statement II is true ☐

(c) Both statements I and II are true ☐

(d) Both statements I and II are false ☐

***98.** The corpus luteum secretes large amount of <u>FSH</u> during luteal phase.

(*Rewrite the statement after correcting the underlined word.*)

____

99. No new follicles develop in the luteal phase of the menstrual cycle because

____

100. If the mammalian ovum fails to get fertilised, which of the following is likely to happen?

Corpus luteum will degenerate, Oestrogen secretion further decreases, Primary follicle starts developing, Progesterone secretion rapidly increases

____

***101.** Which of the following is not a correct match?

(a) Proliferative phase–Rupture of Graafian follicle in ovary ☐

(b) Secretory phase–Development of corpus luteum and increased secretion of progesterone ☐

(c) Menstruation–Breakdown of endometrium ☐

(d) Ovulation–LH and FSH attain peak level and cause rupture of Graafian follicle ☐

102. Write the correct sequence of secretions of hormones given in box from the beginning of menstrual cycle to the end.

Progesterone, FSH, Oestrogen

____

***103.** The following graph shows relative concentrations of the four hormones present in the blood plasma of a woman during her menstrual cycle. Identify the hormones *A*, *B*, *C* and *D*.

Increasing concentration of hormone ↑

A *B* *C* *D*

1 2 3 4 5 6 7 8 9 10 11 12 13 14 15 16 17 18 19 20 21 22 23 24 25 26 27 28

Days

A. ____________

B. ____________

C. ____________

D. ____________

***104.** Some important events in the human female reproductive cycle are given below. Arrange the events in proper sequence.

I. Secretion of FSH.

II. Growth of corpus luteum.

III. Growth of the follicle and oogenesis.

IV. Ovulation.

V. Sudden increase in the levels of LH.

____

***105.** Match the following columns.

Column I		Column II
A. Lack of the menstruation	1.	LH surge
B. Secretory phase	2.	Corpus luteum development and increased progesterone
C. Ovulation	3.	Cessation of menstrual cycle
D. Menopause	4.	Indication of pregnancy

A. ________ B. ________ C. ________ D. ________

***106.** The diagram shows the changes that take place in the endometrium during a normal menstruation. Identify *A* and *B*.

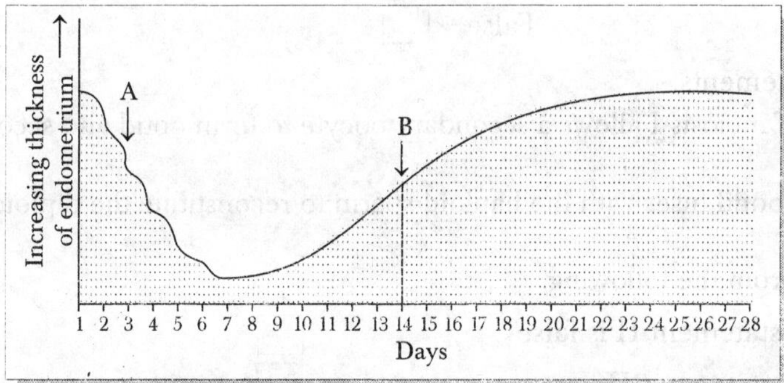

A. ____________

B. ____________

107. After successful fertilisation, a woman shows the presence of elevated levels of progesterone due to

(a) Rupturing of the Graafian follicle ☐

(b) Persistence of the corpus luteum ☐

(c) Release of the secondary oocyte ☐

(d) Shedding of the endometrium ☐

TOPIC 5

Fertilisation and Implantation

NCERT Pg. 35-37

***108.** Fill in the blanks with words provided in the box given below.

Fertilisation, Insemination, Ampullary- Isthmic junction

During copulation, semen is released by the penis into the vagina and this process is called ________________. The ovum released by the ovary is transported to the where ____________ takes place.

109. Fertilisation can only occur if ovum and sperms are transported simultaneously to the ampullary region.

True ☐ False ☐

***110.** Corona radiata ensures that only one sperm can fertilise the ovum.
(*Rewrite the statement after correcting the underlined words.*)

____

111. The secretions of __________________________ help the sperm enter into the cytoplasm of ovum through the zona pellucida and plasma membrane.

112. In females, meiosis-II does not get completed until fertilisation.

True ☐ False ☐

113. Consider the following statements.
Statement I Completion of meiosis-I allows a secondary oocyte to form ootid and second polar body.
Statement II The haploid ootid fuses with the haploid sperm to reconstitute the diploid nature of humans.
Choose the correct option from the following.

(a) Statement I is true, but statement II is false ☐

(b) Statement I is false, but statement II is true ☐

(c) Both statements I and II are true ☐

(d) Both statements I and II are false ☐

114. Secondary maturation of oocyte occurs in the ovary.
(*Rewrite the statement after correcting the underlined word.*)

____

115. Sex of the foetus is decided during fertilisation by male gamete.

True ☐ False ☐

116. Cleavage forms 2-4 to 8-16 cells. These cells are called ____________________

117. Name the structure formed from zygote, with 8-16 cells after successive mitotic division. ____

***118.** Study the given image and mark the option that best represents the process that converts *A* to *B*.

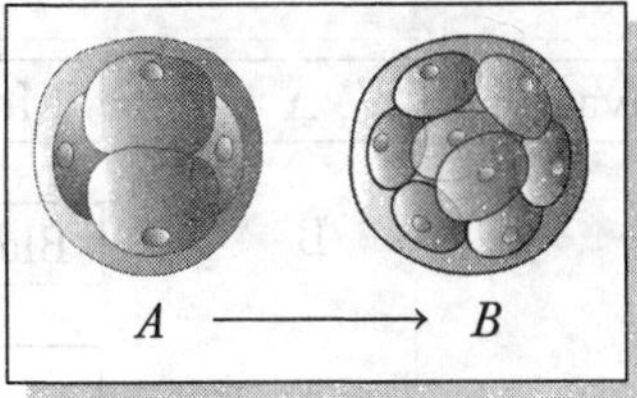

(a) Meiosis-I ☐ (b) Meiosis-II ☐

(c) Mitosis ☐ (d) Differentiation ☐

119. After blastocyst formation, the ______________ gets attached to the endometrium and the ______________ gets differentiated as the embryo.

***120.** Trophoblast of blastocyst attaches to the myometrium.
(*Rewrite the statement after correcting the underlined word.*)

____

121. The given diagram refers to ovum surrounded by few sperms.

(i) Identify the labelled parts as *A*, *B* and *C* in the diagram.

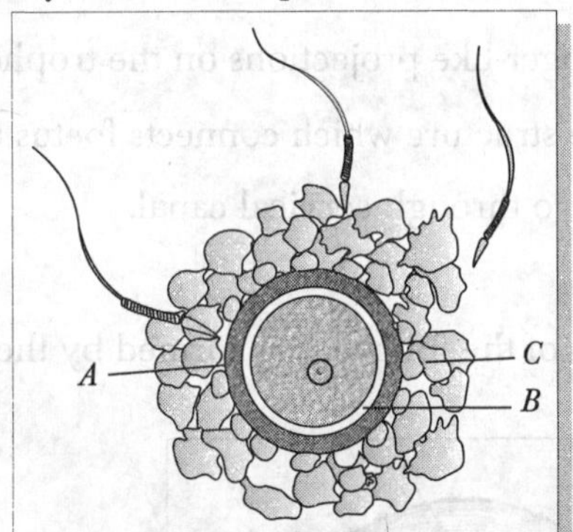

A. ______________

B. ______________

C. ______________

(ii) After a successful fusion the gradual formation of the inner cell mass takes place. This inner cell mass gets differentiated as ___________.

***122.** Refer to the given diagram and identify the structures *A* and *B*.

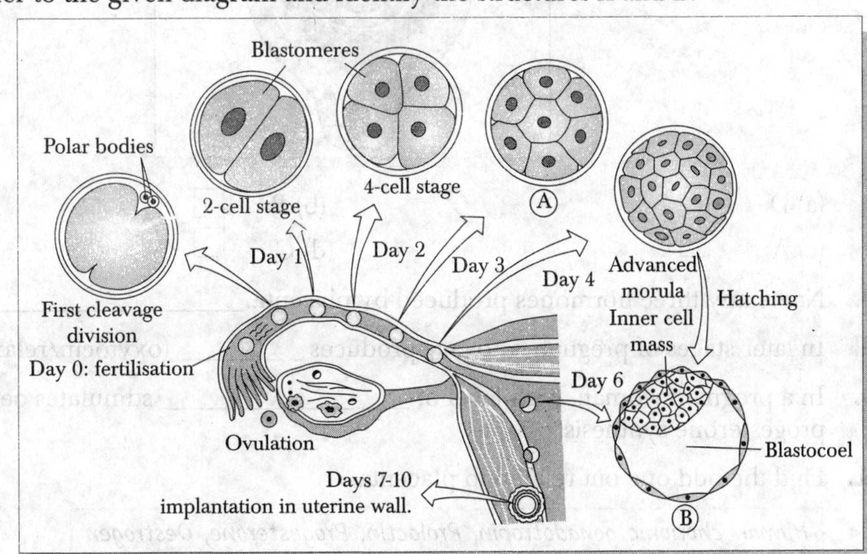

A. ______________________ B. ______________________

***123.** Complete the flowchart according to the sequence of events taking place in fertilisation.

Cleavage → A → Morula → Blastula → C → Embryo → D
Blastula → B

A. ____________
B. ____________
C. ____________
D. ____________

TOPIC 6

Pregnancy and Embryonic Development

NCERT Pg. 37-38

124. Give the scientific name for the finger-like projections on the trophoblast. ____________

125. ____________ is the structure which connects foetus to the maternal body.

126. Placenta is connected to the embryo through cervical canal.

True ☐ False ☐

127. Study the following image. Which of the following is formed by the outer layer of the blastocyst?

A, B, C, D

(a) D ☐ (b) B ☐
(c) A ☐ (d) C ☐

128. Name any three hormones produced by placenta. ____________

129. In later stages of pregnancy, ovary produces ________ (oxytocin/relaxin).

130. In a pregnant woman, high level of ____________ stimulates oestrogen and progesterone synthesis.

***131.** Find the odd one out related to placenta.

Human chorionic gonadotropin, Prolactin, Progesterone, Oestrogen

____

132. Urine test during pregnancy determines the presence of progesterone.

True ☐ False ☐

***133.** Soon after implantation, the inner cell mass differentiates into outer ________, middle ______ and an inner ________.

134. Inner cell mass contains certain cells called ________________ cells which have the potency to give rise to all the tissues and organs.

135. By the end of ____________ trimester, most of the major organ systems are developed.

***136.** The first movement of foetus and appearance of hair on the head are observed during the fourth month.

(Rewrite the statement after correcting the underlined word.)

____

***137.** Which of the following shows an incorrect match pai?

Organ	Time of development in foetus
(a) Heart	– After one month of pregnancy
(b) Body covered with fine hair	– By the end of 24 weeks
(c) External genital organs	– By the end of 26 weeks (second trimester)
(d) First movement of foetus	– During the fifth month

(a) ☐ (b) ☐ (c) ☐ (d) ☐

138. Consider the given situation. The figure below shows a developmental pregnancy with a foetus. If by any chance, the levels of hormones that aid a successful pregnancy e.g. progesterone fluctuate during first trimester which of the following is most expected?

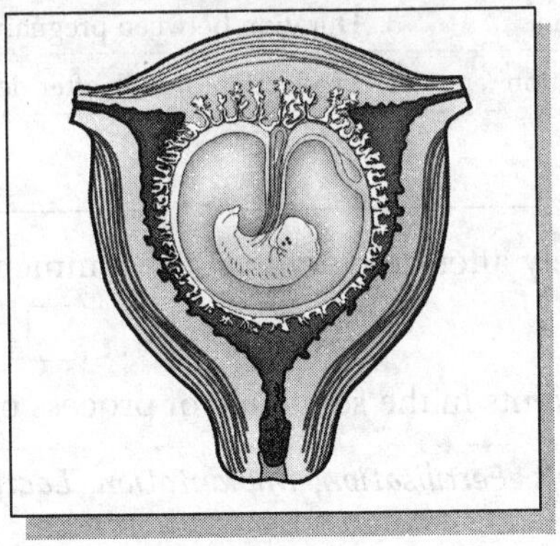

(a) Sustained pregnancy due to counter current FSH mechanism ☐
(b) Successful implantation but pregnancy does not cover complete term ☐
(c) Foetus showing no further growth but implanted ☐
(d) Thickening of uterine lining due to the presence of oestrogen ☐

TOPIC 7

Parturition and Lactation

NCERT Pg. 38

139. Write the scientific name for delivery of developed foetus. ____________

140. The process of parturition is induced by a complex muscular mechanism.
(*Rewrite the statement after correcting the underlined word.*)

____

***141.** Fill in the blanks with words provided in the box given below.

Placenta, Parturition, Oxytocin, Prolactin, Amnion, Foetal ejection reflex

The signals for ____________ originate from the fully developed foetus and ____________, which induces mild uterine contractions called ____________.

***142.** Foetal ejection reflex triggers the release of oxytocin from ____________.

____

***143.** Name the hormone responsible for strong uterine contractions during parturition.

____

144. Colostrum, released from the mammary gland is rich in several antibodies.

True ☐ False ☐

***145.** Match the following columns.

Column I	Column II
A. Gestation	1. Delivery of baby from uterus
B. Lactation	2. Attachment of embryo to endometrium
C. Parturition	3. Duration between pregnancy and birth
D. Implantation	4. Production of milk after delivery

A. ____________ B. ____________ C. ____________ D. ____________

146. Breastfeeding immediately after delivery is not recommended by doctors.

True ☐ False ☐

147. Arrange the following events in the sequence of process of reproduction in humans.

Parturition, Gametogenesis, Fertilisation, Implantation, Lactation

____

***148.** Consider the given statements and identify the correct set.

I. The average duration of mammalian pregnancy is 9 months and is not variable.
II. By the end of first trimester, the external genital organs get developed completely.
III. The mitotic division called cleavage, starts as the zygote moves through isthmus of oviduct, towards the uterus.
IV. GnRH is a hypothalamic hormone that stimulates the secretion of LH and FSH.

Codes

(a) I, II and III ☐ (b) II, III and IV ☐
(c) III and IV ☐ (d) I and III ☐

Assertion-Reason Questions

The following questions consist of two statements Assertion (A) and Reason (R). Answer these questions by selecting the appropriate option given below.
(a) Both A and R are true and R is the correct explanation of A
(b) Both A and R are true, but R is not the correct explanation of A
(c) A is true, but R is false
(d) A is false, but R is true

***1.** **Assertion** (A) The Sertoli cells are present in the interstitial spaces outside the seminiferous tubules.
Reason (R) Sertoli cells are referred to as nurse cells due to their major role in providing nourishment to spermatogonia.

(a) ☐ (b) ☐ (c) ☐ (d) ☐

2. **Assertion** (A) Each breast of a female contains 15-20 mammary lobes that contain milk secreting alveolar cells.
Reason (R) Each alveoli opens into mammary ducts which fuse to form the mammary tubules that open into ampulla.

(a) ☐ (b) ☐ (c) ☐ (d) ☐

3. **Assertion** (A) In males the spermatids formed from second meiotic division contain 23 chromosomes.
Reason (R) In spermiogenesis, spermatids are transformed into spermatozoa by the action of LH.

(a) ☐ (b) ☐ (c) ☐ (d) ☐

***4.** **Assertion** (A) The first meiotic division of the primary oocyte within the tertiary follicle is unequal.
Reason (R) Meiosis I of the primary oocyte forms a large secondary oocyte and a small first polar body.

(a) ☐ (b) ☐ (c) ☐ (d) ☐

***5.** **Assertion** (A) In the absence of fertilisation, the endometrial lining disintegrates thus initiating menstruation.
Reason (R) Corpus luteum degenerates in the absence of fertilisation, thus the progesterone secretion is stopped.

(a) ☐ (b) ☐ (c) ☐ (d) ☐

6. **Assertion** (A) Fertilisation takes place in the isthmus of the Fallopian tube of the female reproductive system.
Reason (R) During fertilisation the acrosomal secretion allows the sperm to penetrate the cytoplasm of ovum.

(a) ☐ (b) ☐ (c) ☐ (d) ☐

7. **Assertion** (A) Blastomeres in a blastocyst are organised into a trophoblast layer and inner cell mass.
Reason (R) The inner cell mass attaches to the endometrium and gets embedded into the uterus.

(a) ☐ (b) ☐ (c) ☐ (d) ☐

***8.** **Assertion** (A) Placenta is formed by interdigitation of chorionic villi and uterine tissue.
Reason (R) Placenta secretes certain hormones like hCG which is secreted only during pregnancy.

(a) ☐ (b) ☐ (c) ☐ (d) ☐

***9.** **Assertions** (A) The innermost layer of the uterus is called endometrium which is glandular in nature.
Reason (R) During delivery of the baby, the endometrium undergoes strong contractions to expel the baby since it is closest to it.

(a) ☐ (b) ☐ (c) ☐ (d) ☐

10. **Assertion** (A) The secretion of maternal oxytocin is essential for development of foetal ejection reflex.
Reason (R) Oxytocin induces uterine contractions which in turn stimulates more oxytocin secretion from pituitary.

(a) ☐ (b) ☐ (c) ☐ (d) ☐

Case Based Questions

1. Sarah, a 19-year old girl, is concerned becasue her menstrual cycle has become irregular from past few months. Previously, her periods arrived every 28-30 days, but now they are either as short as 23 days or as long as 35 days. She wants to know what would be the cause of the irregularity. Based on the situation, answer the questions that follow

(i) In 23 days menstrual cycle, on which day is the ovulation expected?

(a) 13-14 day ☐ (b) 11-12 day ☐
(c) 9-10 day ☐ (d) 14-15 day ☐

(ii) Which of the following conditions is most likely to cause irregular menstrual cycle?

(a) Exessive caffeine consumption ☐ (b) Insufficient calcium intake ☐
(c) Hormonal imbalance ☐ (d) Emotional stress ☐

(iii) Among the following which one is most likely to cause delayed menstruation?

(a) Elevated estrogen levels ☐ (b) Insufficient Progesterone levels ☐
(c) High cortisol levels ☐ (d) Increased FSH secretion ☐

2. A woman was experiencing headache and nausea for a few days. On visiting a doctor, she was taken for some blood and urine analysis. On getting the test result, doctors found the presence of certain compounds in her urine that confirmed her pregnancy. Based on the above situation, answer the following questions:

(i) Which of the following compounds is secreted only by pregnant females?

(a) Estrogen ☐ (b) HCG ☐
(c) Progesterone ☐ (d) LH ☐

(ii) During which month of pregnancy are the first fetal movements typically felt by the mother?

(a) 3rd month ☐ (b) 5th month ☐
(c) 6th month ☐ (d) 7th month ☐

(iii) If the pregnant mother wants to hear her baby's heart beat, she can do so using a stethoscope after

(a) First trimester ☐ (b) Second trimester ☐

(c) Second month of pregnancy ☐ (d) First month of pregnancy ☐

COMPETITION EDGE UP

1. *Identify the correct option (A), (B), (C), (D) with respect to spermatogenesis.*

GnRH → LH → (B) → Androgens →

GnRH → (A) → (C) → Factors → (D)

[NCERT Pg. 31, 32 NEET 2024]

(a) FSH, Leydig cells, Sertoli cells, Spermiogenesis ☐

(b) ICSH, Interstitial cells, Leydig , spermiogenesis ☐

(c) FSH, Sertoli cells, Leydig ce Spermatogenesis ☐

(d) ICSH, Leydig cells, Sertoli cells, Spermatogenesis ☐

2. ***Statement I*** *Vas deferens receives a duct from seminal vesicle and opens into urethra as the ejaculatory duct.*

Statement II *The cavity of the cervix is called cervical canal, which along with vagina forms birth canal.*

In the light of the above statements, choose the correct answer from the options given below. *[NEET 2023]*

(a) Both statement I and statement II are false ☐

(b) Statement I is true, but statement II is false ☐

(c) Statement I is false, but statement II is true ☐

(d) Both statement I and statement II are true ☐

3. *Which of the following statements are correct regarding female reproductive cycle?*

A. In non-primate mammals cyclical changes during reproduction are called oestrus cycle.

B. First menstrual cycle begins at puberty and is called menopause.

C. Lack of menstruation may be indicative of pregnancy.

D. Cyclic menstruation extends between menarche and menopause.

Choose the most appropriate answer from the options given below *[NEET 2023]*

(a) A and B only ☐

(b) A, B and C only ☐

(c) A, C and D only ☐

(d) A and D only ☐

4. *Which of the following statements are true for spermatogenesis, but do not hold true for oogenesis?* *[NCERT Pg. 31 to 33, NEET 2022]*

I. It results in the formation of haploid gametes.

II. Differentiation of gamete occurs after the completion of meiosis.

III. Meiosis occurs continuously in a mitotically dividing stem cell population.

IV. It is controlled by the Luteinising hormone (LH) and Follicle Stimulating Hormone (FSH) secreted by the anterior pituitary.

V. It is initiated at puberty.

Choose the most appropriate answer from the options given below.

(a) II,and III ☐ *(b) II, IV and V* ☐

(c) II, III and V ☐ *(d) III and V* ☐

5. *Receptors for sperm binding in mammals are present on* *[NCERT Pg. 35, NEET 2021]*

(a) Corona radiata ☐

(b) Vitelline membrane ☐

(c) Perivitelline space ☐

(d) Zona pellucida ☐

6. Which of these is not an important component of initiation of parturition in humans? **[NCERT Pg. 38, NEET 2021]**

(a) Increase in oestrogen and progesterone ratio ☐
(b) Synthesis of prostaglandins ☐
(c) Release of oxytocin ☐
(d) Release of prolactin ☐

7. Select the correct option of haploid cells from the following groups. **[NCERT Pg. 32, 33, NEET (Oct.) 2020]**

(a) Primary oocyte, secondary oocyte, spermatid ☐
(b) Secondary spermatocyte, first polar body, ovum ☐
(c) Spermatogonia, primary spermatocyte, spermatid ☐
(d) Primary spermatocyte, secondary spermatocyte, second polar body ☐

8. In human beings, at the end of 12 weeks (first trimester) of pregnancy, the following is observed. **[NCERT Pg. 38, NEET (Oct.) 2020]**

(a) Eyelids and eyelashes are formed ☐
(b) Most of the major organ systems are formed ☐
(c) The head is covered with fine hair ☐
(d) Movement of the foetus ☐

9. Match the following columns and select the correct option. **[NEET (Sep.) 2020]**

Column I	Column II
A. Placenta	1. Androgens
B. Zona pellucida	2. human Chorinoic Gonadotropin (hCG)
C. Bulbourethral glands	3. Layer of the ovum
D. Leydig cells	4. Lubrication of the penis

A B C D
(a) 1 4 2 3 ☐
(b) 3 2 4 1 ☐
(c) 2 3 4 1 ☐
(d) 4 3 1 2 ☐

10. Select the correct sequence for transport of sperm cells in male reproductive system. **[NCERT Pg. 27, NEET (National) 2019]**

(a) Seminiferous tubules → Rete testis → Vasa efferentia → Epididymis → Vas deferens → Ejaculatory duct → Urethra → Urethral meatus ☐
(b) Seminiferous tubules → Vasa efferentia → Epididymis → Inguinal canal → Urethra ☐
(c) Testis → Epididymis → Vasa efferentia → Vas deferens → Ejaculatory duct → Inguinal canal → Urethra → Urethral meatus ☐
(d) Testis → Epididymis → Vasa efferentia → Rete testis → Inguinal canal → Urethra ☐

11. No new follicles develop in the luteal phase of the menstrual cycle because **[NCERT Pg. 35, Odisha NEET 2019]**

(a) follicles do not remain in the ovary after ovulation ☐
(b) FSH levels are high in the luteal phase ☐
(c) LH levels are high in the luteal phase ☐
(d) Both FSH and LH levels are low in the luteal ☐

12. Extrusion of second polar body from egg occurs **[NCERT Pg. 35, 36 NEET 2019, 1993]**

(a) simultaneously with first cleavage ☐
(b) after entry of sperm, but before fertilisation ☐
(c) after fertilisation ☐
(d) before entry of sperm into ovum ☐

13. The difference between spermiogenesis and spermiation is **[NCERT Pg. 31, NEET 2018]**

(a) In spermiogenesis, spermatozoa from Sertoli cells are released into the cavity of seminiferous tubules, while in spermiation spermatozoo are formed ☐
(b) In spermiogenesis, spermatozoa are formed, while in spermiation spermatids are formed ☐
(c) In spermiogenesis, spermatids are formed, while in spermiation spermatozoa are formed ☐
(d) In spermiogenesis, spermatozoa are formed, while in spermiation spermatozoa are released from Sertoli cells into the cavity of seminiferous tubules ☐

Chapter 03

Reproductive Health

Scan and take Chapter Test

TOPIC 1

Reproductive Health : Problems and Strategies

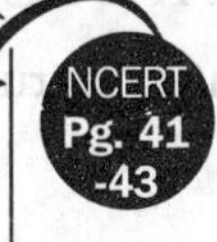

1. According to WHO, reproductive health means a total well-being in all aspects of reproduction, i.e. physical, emotional, behavioural and social.

True ☐ False ☐

2. A reproductively healthy society does not have people with

(i) Physically normal reproductive organs ☐

(ii) Functionally anomalous reproductive organs ☐

(*Tick* ✓ *the most appropriate option*)

3. India was amongst the ________ (first/fifth) country in the world to have launched a National Programme for Family Planning.

4. Family planning programmes were initiated.

True ☐ False ☐

5. Proper information about reproductive organs, adolescence and related changes would help people in ________ age group to lead a reproductively healthy life.

6. Complete the sentence with the words given in the box below.

Reproductive, Physioemotional, Informational, Infrastructural, Economical

Implementation of various action plans to attain ________ health requires strong ________ facilities, professional expertise and material support.

***7.** Give the scientific name for the foetal sex-determination test. ________

***8.** Amniocentesis is based on the chromosomal pattern in the ________ fluid surrounding the developing embryo. It helps us to determine ________ .

*Concepts of all questions bearing * are important for NEET & CUET*

***9.** Which of the following information from amniocentesis can be misused?

(a) Prediction of survivability of foetus ☐

(b) Determination of genetic disorders ☐

(c) Determination of the sex of the child ☐

(d) Cardiac ailments of developing embryo ☐

10. Consider the following statements.

Statement I Statutory ban on amniocentesis has been implemented in India to control the growing cases of female foeticide in rural areas.

Statement II For determining birth defects of the foetus, a part of the placenta is tested in laboratories for dissolved substances in fetal cells.

Choose the correct option from the following.

(a) Statement I is true, but statement II is false ☐

(b) Statement I is false, but statement II is true ☐

(c) Both statements I and II are true ☐

(d) Both statements I and II are false ☐

***11.** Statutory ban on amniocentesis for sex-determination is legalised by the government.

True ☐ False ☐

12. Write the full form of

(i) RCH ____________________

(ii) CDRI ____________________

TOPIC 2

Population Stabilisation and Birth Control

NCERT Pg. 43-46

13. The world population in 2011 was __________ (2.8 billion/7.2 billion).

14. According to the 2011 census report, the population growth rate was ______/ 1000/year.

15. Write the full forms of the following.

(i) MMR ____________________

(ii) IMR ____________________

16. Complete the following diagram.

Decline in death rate → Population Explosion

Decline in (A) → Population Explosion

Decline in (B) → Population Explosion

Increase in number of people in reproducible age → Population Explosion

A. ____________________

B. ____________________

17. Select the main factors affecting the population growth from the box given below.

Industrialisation, Increase in healthcare facilities, Increase in birth rate, Decrease in birth rate, Decrease in death rate

____

18. Decreasing the death rate is the main goal to control population.

True ☐ False ☐

19. The use of prophylactic vaccinations and antibiotics is directly responsible for the current rapid growth in population.

True ☐ False ☐

20. Marriageable age of female is ________ years and males is ________ years in India.

***21.** Give the scientific name of the thoughtful use of artificial methods or techniques to prevent pregnancy. ________________________

22. Write any two requirements for an ideal contraceptive.

(i) ____________________ (ii) ____________________

***23.** Natural methods work on the principle of avoiding chances of ovum and sperm meeting.

True ☐ False ☐

***24.** Give the biological name for the contraceptive method in which couples abstain from coitus.

____

25. Periodic abstinence is also known as rhythm method or calendar method.

True ☐ False ☐

***26.** Fill in the blanks using the words given in the box below.

Abstain, Ovulation, 10-17, Reproductive, Menstrual, Copulation, 8-10

Periodic abstinence is one such method in which the couple avoids or ________ from coitus from ________ days of the ________ cycle when ________ could be expected.

27. Fertilisation is prevented in withdrawal method by avoiding ____________ (insemination/ovulation).

28. The effectiveness of coitus interruption as contraception is least among the other natural methods.

True ☐ False ☐

***29.** Write the scientific name of a natural method of contraception during intense lactation period. ________________________

30. ____________ (Ovulation/Insemination) does not occur during the period of intense lactation following parturition.

31. Chances of conception are almost nil for a breastfeeding mother.

True ☐ False ☐

32. Lactational amenorrhea is effective only upto ________ months following parturition.

***33.** Consider the following statements:

Statement I Withdrawal method has a higher chance of preventing pregnancy as well as STIs like syphilis.

Statement II Natural methods like periodic abstinence and coitus interruptus have zero side effects with a higher failure rate.

Choose the correct option from the following.

(a) Statement I is true, but statement II is false ☐

(b) Statement I is false, but statement II is true ☐

(c) Both statements I and II are true ☐

(d) Both statements I and II are false ☐

34. Barrier method involves preventing physical meeting of ________ and ________ with the help of barriers.

35. Name the barriers made up of thin rubber/latex sheath used for the physical prevention of the meeting of gametes. ________

36. Write the name of the popular brand of condom for the male in India.

________.

37. Use of condoms increased over the years due to its additional benefit of protecting the user from contracting ________ and ________.

38. Find the odd one out regarding condoms.

User friendly, Easily disposable, Self-insertable, Reusable

***39.** Condoms can be used to cover both vagina and cervix in females.

True ☐ False ☐

____

***40.** Consider the given image and choose the option that best defines its mode of action

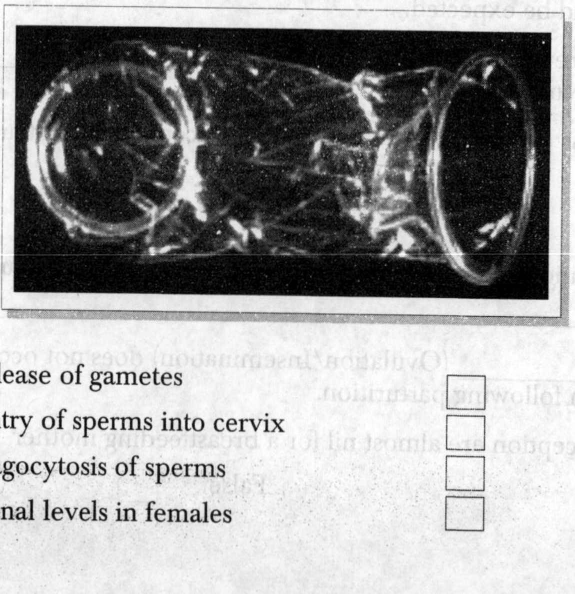

(a) Blocks the release of gametes ☐

(b) Blocks the entry of sperms into cervix ☐

(c) Increases phagocytosis of sperms ☐

(d) Alters hormonal levels in females ☐

***41.** Fill in the blanks with the words given below in the box.

Diaphragms, Cervical caps, Vaults, Condoms, Copper-T

__________ , __________ and __________ are the contraception exclusively for females and are reusable, which block the entry of sperms.

42. Spermicidal creams decrease the contraceptive efficiency.

True ☐ False ☐

43. Write the full form of IUD. __________

44. Condoms should be inserted with help of a doctor or expert nurses.
(*Rewrite the statement after correcting the underlined word.*)

____

***45.** Which of the following pairs are incorrectly matched?
(i) Lippe's loop – Non-medicated IUD.
(ii) Progestasert – Copper releasing IUD.
(iii) LNG-20 – Hormone releasing IUD.

____

***46.** Give a common term for the following.
CU-T, Cu-7, Multiload-375 __________

47. IUDs increase __________ (phagocytosis/pinocytosis) of sperms within the uterus.

48. Cu ions __________ sperm motility and fertilising capacity of sperms.

49. IUDs make the uterus suitable for implantation.

True ☐ False ☐

***50.** Choose the correct combination of the IUDs and their mode of action.
(a) Multiload 375 – cervix hostile to sperms ☐
(b) LNG-20 – suppress sperm motility ☐
(c) Cu7 – decrease fertilising capacity ☐
(d) Lippes loop – promotes implantation ☐

***51.** Match the following columns.

Column I (Contraception methods)	Column II (Features)
A. Condoms	1. Increase sperm phagocytosis in cervix
B. Diaphragms	2. User friendly latex sheath
C. IUDs	3. High chances of failure after a limited period
D. Lactational amenorrhea	4. Self inserted and reusable

A. __________ B. __________ C. __________ D. __________

52. Oral pills used as contraceptives, contain small doses of __________ or combination of __________.

53. Oral administration has to be taken daily for a period of __________ starting within first five days of menstrual cycle.

54. Pills inhibit ______________ and implantation. They also alter the quality of cervical mucus to prevent entry of ____________.

55. Pills are very effective with ______________ (greater/lesser) side effects and are well accepted by ______________ (females/males).

***56.** Consider the following statements.

Statement I Saheli the 'once a week pill' contains a non-steroidal preparation.

Statement II Oral pills inhibit ovulation thus providing a high contraceptive value and no side effects.

Choose the correct option from the following.

(a) Statement I is true, but statement II is false ☐

(b) Statement I is false, but statement II is true ☐

(c) Both statements I and II are true ☐

(d) Both statements I and II are false ☐

57. Progestogen used as implants under skin have longer effective periods.

True ☐ False ☐

58. A woman who underwent a procedure to implant a material under her skin to provide contraceptive effects much longer than oral pills, prevents unwanted pregnancies by which mechanism?

(a) Blocking sperm entry into the cervix ☐

(b) Inhibiting ovulation and implantation ☐

(c) Preventing ovum and sperm to meet ☐

(d) Lowering sperm motility and viability ☐

59. Pills and implants prevent the pituitary from secreting ______________ and ______________ so that ovulation does not occur.

***60.** Emergency pills are taken within ____________ hours after coitus to avoid possible pregnancy.

61. Consider the following statements.

Statement I Emergency contraceptive pills are usually used in cases of rapes or casual unprotected intercourse.

Statement II Progestogen, oestrogen implants work just like oral pills, but their effective periods are much longer.

Choose the correct option from the following.

(a) Statement I is true, but statement II is false ☐

(b) Statement I is false, but statement II is true ☐

(c) Both statements I and II are true ☐

(d) Both statements I and II are false ☐

62. Find the odd one out.

Vasectomy, Tubectomy, Copper-T

63. Complete the following analogy.

Males : Females : : ______________ : Tubectomy

64. Consider the following image and state the part which is removed or altered in terminal contraceptive method?

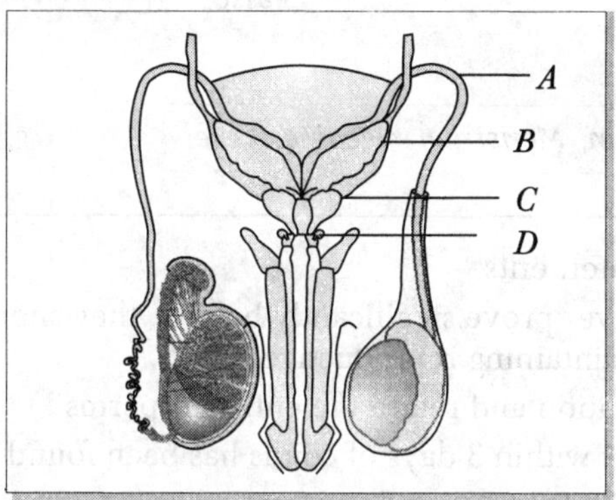

(a) C ☐ (b) D ☐ (c) B ☐ (d) A ☐

65. After vasectomy the semen does not contain sperms.

True ☐ False ☐

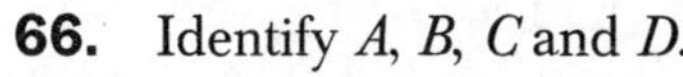

66. Identify *A*, *B*, *C* and *D*.

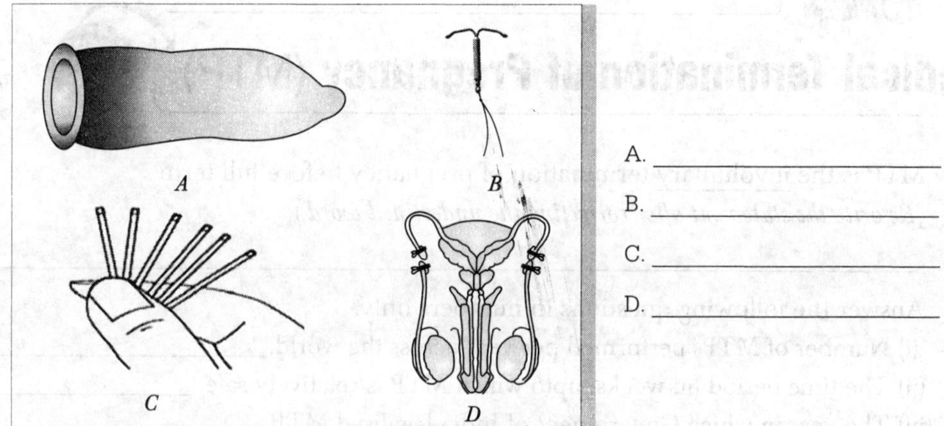

A. ______________________

B. ______________________

C. ______________________

D. ______________________

***67.** Name the process and the reproductive structure involved in the process.

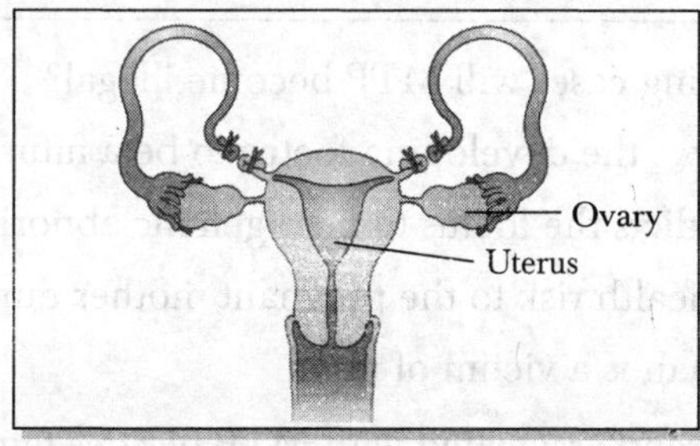

____

68. After tubectomy, ovum would not be found in

(i) Uterus ☐ (ii) Ovaries ☐

(Tick ✓ the most accurate option)

69. Reversibility is high for sterilisation techniques.

True ☐ False ☐

70. Find the odd one out.

Nausea, Abdominal pain, Menstrual bleeding, Fever

____

71. Consider the given statements.

I. Though contraceptives prove significantly helpful, they should not be our regular requirements for maintaining reproductive health.

II. Pills inhibit implantation and retard the entry of sperms.

III. Administering IUDs within 3 days of coitus has been found to be effective in preventing unwanted pregnancies.

IV. IUDs are ideal contraceptives for females who want to space their children.

Identify the set of correct statements.

(a) II and IV ☐ (b) I, II and IV ☐

(c) III and IV ☐ (d) II, III and IV ☐

TOPIC 3

Medical Termination of Pregnancy (MTP)

NCERT Pg. 46-47

72. MTP is the <u>involuntary</u> termination of pregnancy before full term.
(*Rewrite the statement after correcting the underlined word.*)

____

73. Answer the following questions in numbers only.

(i) Number of MTPs performed per year across the world. ______

(ii) The time period (in weeks) upto which MTP is relatively safe. ______

(iii) The year in which Government of India legalised MTP. ______

(iv) The year in which MTP act was enacted by Government of India. ______

(v) Number of opinions required by medical practitioners if MTP has to be performed after 12 weeks. ______

74. In which of the following cases will MTP become illegal?

(a) Amniocentesis shows the developing foetus to be a future girl child. ☐

(b) Amniocentesis predicts the foetus to bear genetic abnormalities. ☐

(c) There is a serious health risk to the pregnant mother during parturition. ☐

(d) The pregnant woman is a victim of rape. ☐

75. Write the dangerous trend associated with MTP besides female foeticide.

____

***76.** The MTP (Amendment) Act 2017, enacted by the Government of India, legalised voluntary abortions considering 16-20 weeks of pregnancy on the opinion of two registered practitioners.

True ☐ False ☐

TOPIC 4

Sexually Transmitted Diseases (STDs)

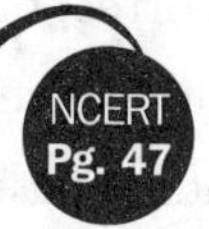

77. Give the scientific term used for diseases or infections that are transmitted through sexual intercourse. ______

78. Write the other names of STDs. ______

***79.** Find the odd one out.

Genital herpes, Syphilis, Trichomoniasis, Amoebiasis

______

80. A man who has never had sexual intercourse with anyone was found to be HIV positive. Which of the following could not be a reason of him contracting the disease?

(a) Blood transfusion ☐
(b) Sharing food with infected person ☐
(c) Sharing needle with infected person ☐
(d) Contaminated surgical instruments ☐

81. Consider the Venn diagram given below and identify the relationship represented by '*P*'

Genital warts | Syphilis | Chlamydia | *P*

______

82. Given below are few symptoms related to STIs

I. Slight pain and swelling in genital region.
II. Fluid discharge.
III. Abdominal pain.
IV. Itching.

How many of these accurately relate to STIs?

(a) 1 ☐ (b) 0 ☐ (c) 3 ☐ (d) 2 ☐

83. Absence of significant symptoms in the early stages of infection and social stigmas attached to the STDs deter the person from getting proper treatment.

True ☐ False ☐

84. Write the age groups most vulnerable to STDs. ______

85. Consider the following statements.

Statement I Hepatitis-B and genital herpes can be completely cured if diagnosed and treated early.

Statement II STIs can never progress to cause pelvic inflammatory diseases or cancer in a person.

Choose the correct option from the following.

(a) Statement I is true, but statement II is false ☐

(b) Statement I is false, but statement II is true ☐

(c) Both statements I and II are true ☐

(d) Both statements I and II are false ☐

86. Identify *A* and *B*.

Avoiding sex with Ⓐ partner → Prevention of STDs ← Using Ⓑ during coitus

A. ____________

B. ____________

87. Early detection and STIs are not given prime importance since they affect less population.

True ☐ False ☐

88. Mention any two complications of STDs in reproductively active women.

____

TOPIC 5

Infertility

NCERT Pg. 47 -48

89. ____________ is the inability of couples in the reproducible age group to produce offspring inspite of unprotected sexual co-habitation.

90. Give the common term for the special assisted techniques to have children.

____

91. IVF stands for *In Vivo* Fertilisation.

True ☐ False ☐

92. Complete the statement by choosing the right words from the box given below.

Fallopian tube, Uterus, ZIFT, IUT

The zygote or embryo, upto eight blastomeres are transferred to the ____________. The process is called ____________.

93. A woman who underwent GIFT was artificially inseminated by semen from a healthy donor. What kind of fertilisation would be observed in this situation?

(a) *In-vitro* fertilisation ☐ (b) Artificial fertilisation ☐

(c) *In-vivo* fertilisation ☐ (d) No fertilisation ☐

***94.** Complete the analogy given below.

8 blastomeres : ____________ :: More than 8 blastomeres : ____________

95. Find the odd one out. *IVF, PID, ZIFT, GIFT*

____

96. Write the full form of GIFT. ______________________________

97. ______________ is a specialised procedure to form an embryo in which a sperm is directly injected into the ovum.

98. Observe the given image carefully and identify the process that represents this technique.

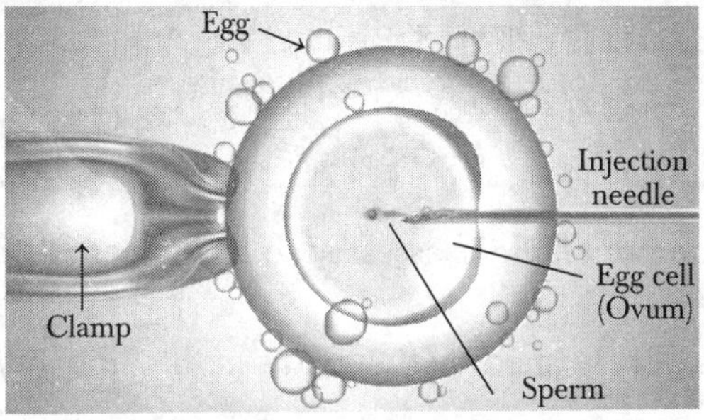

(a) GIFT ☐ (b) IUI ☐ (c) IVF ☐ (d) ICSI ☐

99. IUI is a technique in which semen collected from the husband or a healthy donor is artificially introduced into the cervix.
(*Rewrite the statement after correcting the underlined word.*)

____

100. Consider the following statements.

Statement I If the male partner has a low sperm count, IUI can be used to inseminate the female partner.

Statement II After the completion of ICSI, the embryos can be transferred to the uterus of the female.

Choose the correct option from the following.

(a) Statement I is true, but statement II is false ☐
(b) Statement I is false, but statement II is true ☐
(c) Both statements I and II are true ☐
(d) Both statements I and II are false ☐

***101.** Match the following columns.

Column I		Column II
A. IVF	1.	*In vitro* fertilisation, early embryo transferred into Fallopian tube.
B. ZIFT	2.	*In vitro* fertilisation, followed by embryo implantation into uterus.
C. GIFT	3.	Artificial introduction of semen into vagina of a female.
D. AI	4.	*In vivo* fertilisation, sperm and ova transferred in Fallopian tube.

A. __________ B. __________ C. __________ D. __________

102. Adoption is considered as one of the best methods for couples looking for parenthood.

True ☐ False ☐

Assertion-Reason Questions

The following questions consist of two statements- Assertion (A) and Reason (R). Answer these questions by selecting the appropriate option given below.

(a) Both A and R are true and R is the correct explanation of A

(b) Both A and R are true, but R is not the correct explanation of A

(c) A is true, but R is false

(d) A is false, but R is true

***1. Assertion** (A) The amniotic fluid is assessed to detect genetic disorders like Down's syndrome, haemophilia, etc.

Reason (R) Analysis of cells shed by the foetus in the fluid aids in detecting possible abnormalities.

(a) ☐ (b) ☐ (c) ☐ (d) ☐

2. Assertion (A) The Indian Government is promoting and rewarding smaller families.

Reason (R) There is an alarming growth rate of population in India, which has caused scarcity of basic requirements.

(a) ☐ (b) ☐ (c) ☐ (d) ☐

3. Assertion (A) Use of condoms not only prevent the chances of fertilisation, but also maintains reproductive health.

Reason (R) Condoms prevent the spread of sexually transmitted diseases like AIDS, syphilis, etc. in people.

(a) ☐ (b) ☐ (c) ☐ (d) ☐

4. Assertion (A) Intra-uterine devices (IUDs) are user friendly and can be self inserted by women trying to space children.

Reason (R) IUDs increase phagocytosis of sperms and make the uterus hostile for implantation.

(a) ☐ (b) ☐ (c) ☐ (d) ☐

5. Assertion (A) Oral pills can be used as emergency contraceptives to avoid pregnancy in case of rapes.

Reason (R) Oral contraceptives can inhibit ovulation or alter cervical mucus to retard sperm entry.

(a) ☐ (b) ☐ (c) ☐ (d) ☐

6. Assertion (A) A couple who wants to delay pregnancy can use tubectomy or vasectomy as effective methods.

Reason (R) In sterilisation procedure gamete transport process is blocked which further prevents conception.

(a) ☐ (b) ☐ (c) ☐ (d) ☐

7. Assertion (A) Second trimester pregnancies are often riskier for undergoing MTP.

Reason (R) Foetus becomes intimately associated with maternal tissue.

(a) ☐ (b) ☐ (c) ☐ (d) ☐

8. **Assertion** (A) A female infected with STI like gonorrhoea remains undiagnosed for a long time.

Reason (R) Some STIs can spread through sharing needles or blood transfusion with infected person.

(a) ☐ (b) ☐ (c) ☐ (d) ☐

9. **Assertion** (A) *In-vitro* fertilisation is often followed by transfer of zygote or embryo into the female tract.

Reason (R) Embryos with less than eight blastomeres are transferred into the Fallopian tube of females.

(a) ☐ (b) ☐ (c) ☐ (d) ☐

10. **Assertion** (A) A female having male partner who has a very low sperm count can opt for Artificial Insemination.

Reason (R) Sperms from a healthy donor are artificially introduced into the vagina of the female.

(a) ☐ (b) ☐ (c) ☐ (d) ☐

Case Based Questions

1. The graph given below represents the trend of STDs during COVID times available in a minor section of the country 'B'. Consider the given graph and answer the following questions by choosing the right answer from options below.

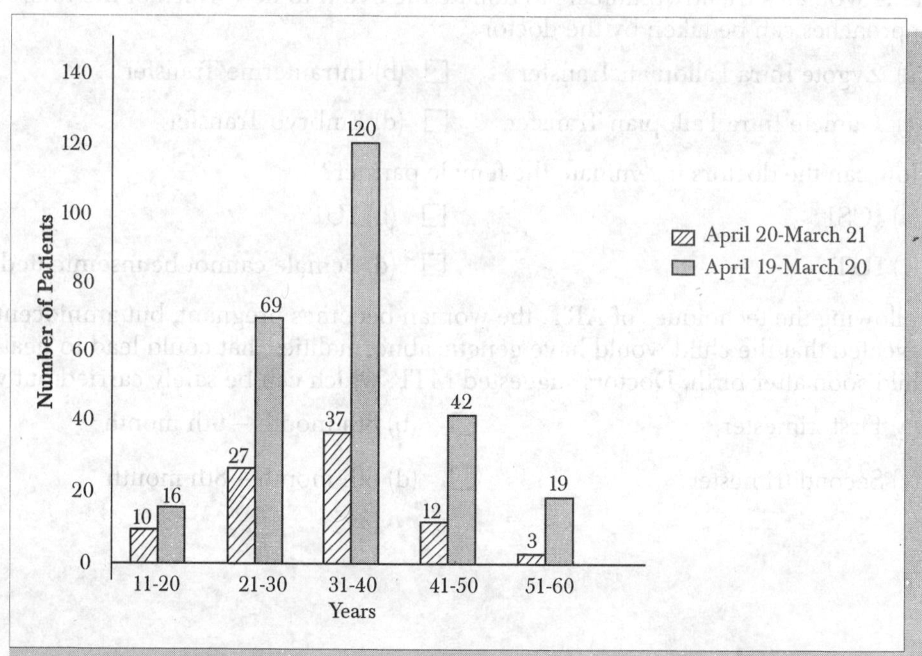

(i) The most possible/accurate reason for the highest peak obtained in graph is

(a) People of the age group are sexually more active and have multiple partners ☐

(b) Members of the age group are immunologically weak due to stressful work conditions ☐

(c) Diet involved results in transmission of these STDs in people of this age group ☐

(d) People of this age group become prone to unhealthy drinking and smoking habits ☐

(ii) A possible drop in case of patients for getting free from STDs/STIs cannot be seen in which of the following?

(a) Use of barriers during coitus ☐

(b) Avoiding sex with multiple/affected partners ☐

(c) Consulting doctor for early treatment if diagnosed ☐

(d) Having multiple male/female partners ☐

(iii) All of the following are examples of sexually transmitted diseases/infections except

(a) Chlamydia ☐ (b) Gonorrhea ☐

(c) Rheumatoid arthritis ☐ (d) Human pappillomavirus ☐

2. A childless couple in USA visited a fertility clinic. After several tests it was found that, the female partner had a healthy uterine environment, but was unable to produce healthy ovum due to cysts in her ovary. The male partner, was unable to inseminate, though the seminal fluid had healthy sperms. The doctor suggested an approach which could help them bear a child. Based on the information provided answer the following questions:

(i) If the woman's friend volunteers to donate the ovum to her, which of the following approaches can be taken by the doctor?

(a) Zygote Intra Fallopian Transfer ☐ (b) Intrauterine Transfer ☐

(c) Gamete Intra Fallopian Transfer ☐ (d) Embryo Transfer ☐

(ii) How can the doctors inseminate the female partner?

(a) ICSI ☐ (b) IUI ☐

(c) IUT ☐ (d) Female cannot be inseminated ☐

(iii) Following the techniques of ART, the woman becomes pregnant, but amniocentesis revealed that the child would have genetic abnormalities that could lead to death of the child soon after birth. Doctors suggested MTP, which can be safely carried out within

(a) First trimester ☐ (b) 8th month – 9th month ☐

(c) Second trimester ☐ (d) 6th month – 8th month ☐

COMPETITION EDGE UP

1. Which of the following is not a natural/traditional contraceptive method? **[NCERT Pg. 44, NEET 2024]**

(a) Coitus interruptus ☐
(b) Periodic abstinence ☐
(c) Lactational amenorrhea ☐
(d) Vaults ☐

2. Match List I with List II.

List I	List II
A. Non-medicated IUD	I. Multiload 375
B. Copper releasing IUD	II. Progestogens
C. Hormone releasing IUD	III. Lippes loop
D. Implants	IV. LNG-20

Choose the correct answer from the option given below: **[NCERT Pg. 44, NEET 2024]**

(a) A-III, B-I, C-II, D-IV ☐
(b) A-I, B-III, C-IV, D-II ☐
(c) A-IV, B-I, C-II, D-III ☐
(d) A-III, B-I, C-IV, D-II ☐

3. Given below are two statements: One is labelled as **Assertion** (A) and the other is labelled as **Reason** (R).

Assertion (A) Amniocentesis for sex-determination is one of the strategies of reproductive and child healthcare programme.

Reason (R) Ban on amniocentesis checks increasing menace of female foeticide.

In the light of the above statements, choose the correct answer from the options given below. **[NEET 2023]**

(a) Both A and R are true, but R is not the correct explanation of A ☐
(b) A is true, but R is false ☐
(c) A is false, but R is true ☐
(d) Both A and R are true and R is the correct explanation of A ☐

4. Match List I with List II.

List I	List II
A. Vasectomy	I. Oral method
B. Coitus interruptus	II. Barrier method
C. Cervical caps	III. Surgical method
D. Saheli	IV. Natural method

Choose the correct answer from the options given below. **[NCERT Pg. 44, 45, 46, NEET 2023]**

(a) A-III, B-IV, C-II, D-I ☐
(b) A-II, B-III, C-I, D-IV ☐
(c) A-IV, B-II, C-I, D-III ☐
(d) A-III, B-I, C-IV, D-II ☐

5. Which one of the following common sexually transmitted diseases is completely curable when detected early and treated properly? **[NCERT Pg. 47, NEET 2023]**

(a) Gonorrhoea ☐
(b) Hepatitis-B ☐
(c) HIV infection ☐
(d) Genital herpes ☐

6. Match the List I with List II.

List I	List II
A. Vaults	1. Entry of sperm through cervix is blocked
B. IUDs	2. Removal of vas deferens
C. Vasectomy	3. Phagocytosis of sperms within the uterus
D. Tubectomy	4. Removal of Fallopian tube

Choose the correct answer from the options given below. **[NCERT Pg. 44, 46, NEET 2021]**

	A	B	C	D	
(a)	4	2	1	3	☐
(b)	1	3	2	4	☐
(c)	2	4	3	1	☐
(d)	3	1	4	2	☐

7. Which of the following STDs are not curable? **[NCERT Pg. 47, NEET (Oct.) 2020]**

(a) Genital herpes, Hepatitis-B, HIV infection ☐
(b) Chlamydiasis, Syphilis, Genital warts ☐
(c) HIV, Gonorrhoea, Trichomoniasis ☐
(d) Gonorrhoea, Trichomoniasis, Hepatitis-B ☐

Chapter 04

Principles of Inheritance and Variation

Scan and take Chapter Test

TOPIC 1

Mendel's Laws of Inheritance

NCERT Pg. 54

1. Select the correct term from the two options provided in the brackets regarding the statements.

(i) Gregor Mendel conducted ____________ (linkage/hybridisation) experiments on garden peas for seven years (1856-1863).

(ii) The characters investigated by Mendel in garden pea were manifested as ____________ (two/four) opposing traits.

2. A true breeding line exhibits stable trait inheritance for several generations.

True ☐ False ☐

***3.** Mendel selected four true breeding characters of pea plant for his experiments.

True ☐ False ☐

***4.** How many characters given below are dominant in pea plants?

Rounded seed, Terminal flower position, Yellow pod colour, White flowers, Yellow coloured seed

____

***5.** Choose the most appropriate answer.

(i) Among the following traits of pea plant, which one was not studied by Mendel?

(a) Seed shape ☐ (b) Seed size ☐

(ii) Inflated pod shape of pea is

(a) Dominant trait ☐ (b) Recessive trait ☐

6. Which is correct about traits chosen by Mendel for his experiment on pea plant?

Terminal pod was dominant, Constricted pod was dominant, Green coloured pod was dominant, Tall plant was recessive

____

*Concepts of all questions bearing * are important for NEET & CUET*

TOPIC 2

Inheritance of One Gene

NCERT Pg. 55-62

7. Mendel crossed true breeding tall and dwarf plant varieties in his experiment. Tallness was the dominant character and dwarfness was recessive. The recessive character appeared in

____

8. *Rewrite the statements after correcting the underlined words.*

(i) While studying inheritance of one gene in pea plant, Mendel found both parental traits appeared in F_2-generation in the proportion 1 : 1.

____

(ii) The recessive trait always appear in F_1-generation in a monohybrid cross.

____

9. How did Mendel obtain recessive (dwarf) character in F_2-generation?

____

10. In the given diagram, what do the steps I and II represent?

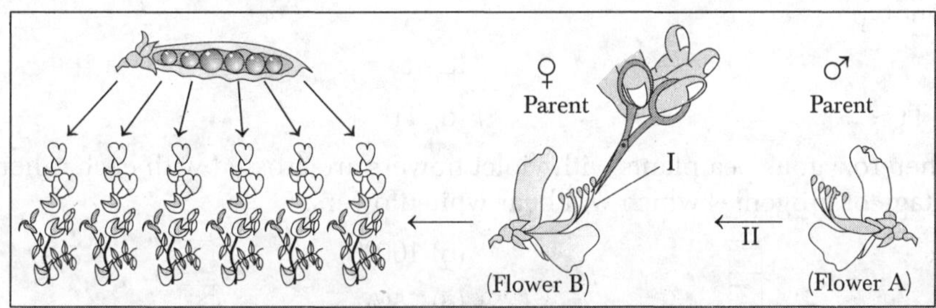

I. ______________________ II. ______________________

11. During his experiments, Mendel used the term factor for ______________________

12. Fill in the blanks.

(i) The alternate forms of a gene at same locus on homologous chromosomes are

____

(ii) Cross between genetically different parents yield generation of hybrids called

____

(iii) ______________________ are the hybrids which contain contrasting alleles.

13. Choose between the two options to answer the questions specified in the brackets.

Genotype or Linkage (Which of the following is predicted using test cross?)

____

14. Choose the incorrect match.

(a) Phenotype – Physical appearance of an organism ☐
(b) Genotype – Expressed genes ☐
(c) Homozygous – Unidentical alleles of a gene present at the same locus ☐
(d) Heterozygous – Genes of an allelic pair are not same ☐

***15.** Consider the following statements.

Statement I A Punnett square a graphical representation of all possible genotypes in a cross, was developed by RC Punnett.

Statement II For monohybrid crosses F_1 progenies show a genotypic ratio of 1:2:1.

Choose the correct option from the following.

(a) Statement I is true, but statement II is false

(b) Statement I is false, but statement II is true

(c) Both statements I and II are true

(d) Both statements I and II are false

16. The F_1-generation of plant of genotype Tt when self-pollinated, produces gametes of two different types T and t in an equal proportion.

True ☐ False ☐

17. Give scientific term for the following statements.

(i) A graphical representation to calculate the probability of all possible offsprings in a genetic cross. ____________

(ii) Cross between the F_1 hybrid and recessive parent. ____________

18. A tall pea plant whose genotype has to be determined, should be crossed with the parent with genotype

(a) TT (b) tt

(c) TT/Tt (d) Tt

19. If two heterozygous pea plants with violet flowers are crossed with each other, find the percentage of progenies which will bear white flowers.

(a) 50% (b) 100%

(c) 25% (d) 75%

20. Consider the given cross.

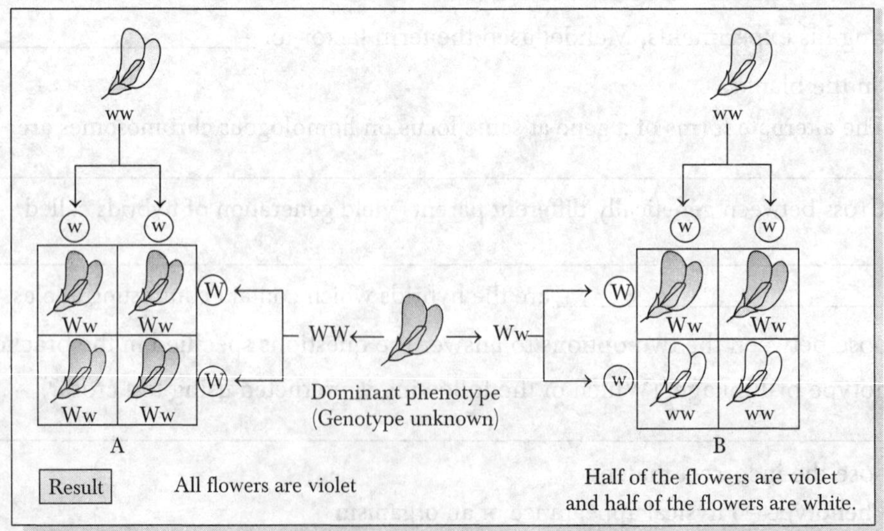

(i) What does the given cross depict?

(ii) What can be interpreted by case B?

____

21. Identify the incorrect statement with respect to inheritance of gene

(a) Genes are units of inheritance

(b) In a true breeding variety, the allelic pair of genes are always heterozygous

(c) Progenies of the test cross can be analysed to predict the genotype

(d) Members of the F_1-generation, as observed, always resemble either of the parents

22. Consider the following statements.

Statement I In order to test the genotype of an organism 'X' the organism is crossed with a recessive parent.

Statement II The organism whose genotype is to be determined is called a test organism.

Choose the correct option from the following.

(a) Statement I is true, but statement II is false

(b) Statement I is false, but statement II is true

(c) Both statements I and II are true

(d) Both statements I and II are false

23. A scientist wanted to test a black mice for its genotype. As per recent reports, black coat colour in mice, dominates brown coat colour. To which of the given below genotypes should the black mice be crossed with?

(a) Bb

(b) bb

(c) BB

(d) Bb followed by selfing with homozygous recessive

***24.** Law of dominance and law of segregation are based on the inheritance pattern in monohybrid cross.

True ☐ False ☐

25. When alleles of two contrasting characters are present together and one of the character expresses itself during the cross, while the other remains hidden gives the

____

26. The law of dominance is applicable in inheritance of starch grain size in pea.
(*Rewrite the statement after correcting the underlined words.*)

____

27. Which of the following cannot be concluded from the Law of dominance?

(a) Characters are controlled by discrete units called factors

(b) Alleles of a pair segregate from each other during gametogenesis

(c) In a dissimilar pair of factors one member of the pair dominates

(d) The dominant allele masks the expression of recessive one

28. Which Mendelian law explains the presence of only one allele in a gamete?

____

29. Mendel's law of segregation is best illustrated by ________ (Bb × Bb / TT × tt).

30. The law based on the fact that the characters do not show any blending and both the characters are recovered as such in F_2-generation although one character was absent in F_1-progeny, is ________________

***31.** Mendel crossed tall and dwarf plants. In F_2-generation, the observed ratio was 3:1 (tall : dwarf). From this result, he deduced

Law of dominance, Law of independent assortment, Law of segregation, Incomplete dominance

***32.** Write the genotype and phenotype of F_1-generation (R–dominant and red, r–recessive and white) in the given cross of snapdragon plant showing incomplete dominance.

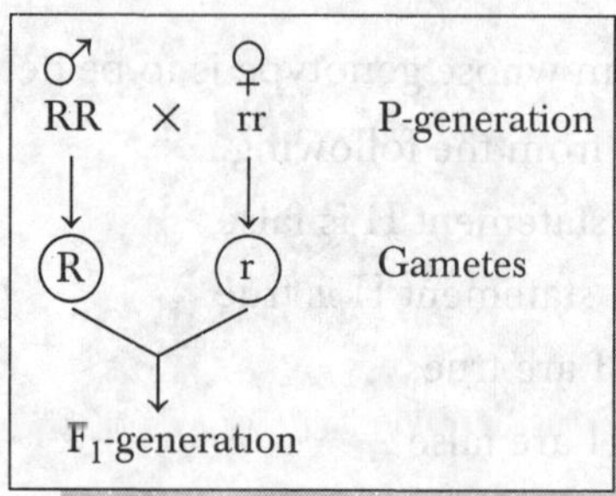

***33.** In ______________, one allele function as normal, while another allele may function as normal, non-functional or less efficient.

***34.** Complete the following flowchart, depicting the inheritance of flower colour in snapdragon.

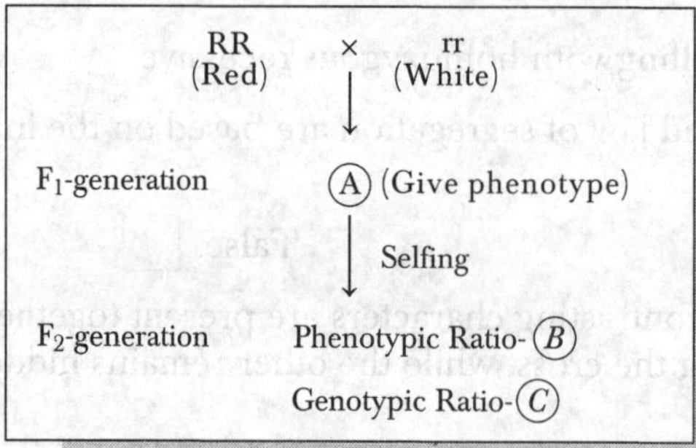

A.__________ B.__________ C.__________

35. Phenotypic and genotypic ratio is similar in case of

(a) Over dominance ☐ (b) Complete dominance ☐
(c) Incomplete dominance ☐ (d) Rest cross ☐

***36.** The __________ trait in case of incomplete dominance is seen due to the non-functional enzyme produced by modified gene or absence of an enzyme.

***37.** The probability of yielding red snapdragon, if a pink snapdragon is crossed to a white snapdragon is ______________ (1/4 / zero).

38. Consider the following statements.

Statement I Snapdragon produces pink flowers on crossing red and white flowers due to incomplete dominance.

Statement II Incomplete dominance occurs when there is a non-functional enzyme or no enzyme at all.

Choose the correct option from the following.

(a) Statement I is true, but statement II is false ☐

(b) Statement I is false, but statement II is true ☐

(c) Both statements I and II are true ☐

(d) Both statements I and II are false ☐

39. TtRr represents a heterozygous tall and pink plant. If this plant is self-crossed then

T-dominant, t-recessive, R-dominant, r-recessive

Choose the correct option.

(i) 25% plants have red flowers.

(ii) 1% plants have white flowers.

(iii) 25% plants have pink flowers.

(iv) 50% plants are tall.

____

***40.** What will be the ratio of offspring in a cross between the red coloured and pink coloured flowers of *Mirabilis jalapa*? ____________________

***41.** Which Mendelian idea is depicted by a cross in which the F_1-generation resembles both the parents? ____________________

42. Incomplete dominance is similar to codominance in having identical ____________________ ratio in F_2-generation.

***43.** Match the following columns.

Column I		Column II
A. Law of dominance	1.	F_1 resembles both the parents
B. Incomplete dominance	2.	F_1 resembles dominant parent
C. Codominance	3.	F_1 exhibits blending inheritance

A.____________ B.____________ C. ____________

***44.** The ABO blood groups are controlled by <u>c-gene</u>.
(*Rewrite the statement after correcting the underlined word.*)

____

45. Out of the three alleles of gene I, the sugar polymers on the plasma membrane of RBCs is controlled by how many alleles? ____________________

46. In human blood group, inheritance of __________ is codominant and __________ is recessive allele.

47. A man with blood group AB marries a woman with blood group O. What will be the probability of their child having blood type A?

(a) 1/2 ☐ (b) 1/4 ☐

(c) 3/4 ☐ (d) 1 ☐

***48.** *Rewrite the statements after correcting the underlined words.*

(i) ABO blood grouping in humans is an example of incomplete dominance.

____

(ii) The genotype of AB blood group is ii. ______________________________

***49.** Complete the table showing genetic basis of blood groups in human population.

Alleles of Parent 1	Alleles of Parent 2	Blood types of offspring
I^A	________	A
I^B	I^A	________
i	i	________

50. Consider the following statements.

Statement I The human blood group is an example of multiple allelism controlled by four alleles.

Statement II Parents with O blood group can produce children having only O blood group.

Choose the correct option from the following.

(a) Statement I is true, but statement II is false ☐

(b) Statement I is false, but statement II is true ☐

(c) Both statements I and II are true ☐

(d) Both statements I and II are false ☐

51. Multiple alleles can be found only when population studies are made.

True ☐ False ☐

52. Give an example of the production of multiple effects by a single gene in pea plant.

____

53. Heterozygous starch synthesising gene in pea plant produce intermediate sized starch grain due to incomplete dominance.

True ☐ False ☐

TOPIC 3

Inheritance of Two Genes

NCERT Pg. 62-68

54. How many round green and wrinkled yellow seeds are produced when round yellow seeds are crossed with wrinkled green seeds?

____

55. In a dihybrid cross, Mendel found that dominant and recessive traits of pea plant were segregated in 3 : 1 ratio in F_2 -generation.

Yes ☐ No ☐

56. If a tall pea plant (TT) with round seeds (RR) is crossed with a dwarf plant (tt) with green seeds (rr), which of the following will not be a gamete produced out of this cross?

(a) RT ☐ (b) Rt ☐

(c) rT ☐ (d) rr ☐

57. Which Mendelian law is based on the study of dihybrid cross?

____

58. The types of gametes formed by the genotype RrYy are ________________ .

***59.** In law of independent assortment, how many factors are involved for a dihybrid cross?

____

60. In Mendel's experiments with garden pea, round seed shape (RR) was dominant over wrinkled shape (rr) and yellow colour (YY) was dominant over green colour (yy). What are the expected phenotypes in the F_1-generation of the cross RRYY × rryy?

____

61. In a cross, between pure breeding pea plants having yellow round (YYRR) and green wrinkled (yyrr) seeds, find out the total seeds (plants) having yellow colour in F_2-generation.

________________ .

62. Consider the following statements.

Statement I In a dihybrid cross alleles of the two genes are always inherited together in a gamete.

Statement II The F_2-generation of a dihybrid cross shows four different genotypes and sixteen phenotypes.

Choose the correct option from the following.

(a) Statement I is true, but statement II is false ☐

(b) Statement I is false, but statement II is true ☐

(c) Both statements I and II are true ☐

(d) Both statements I and II are false ☐

63. In a cross, between plants having yellow round (YYRR) and green wrinkled (yyrr) seeds, what will be the ratio between seeds having yellow and green seed colour?

____

64. Match the following columns.

Column I (Genetic crosses)		Column II (Phenotypic ratios)
A. Test cross	1.	9 : 3 : 3 : 1
B. Monohybrid cross	2.	1 : 1
C. Dihybrid cross	3.	3 : 1

A.____________ B.____________ C. ____________

65. When two pairs of traits are combined in a hybrid, segregation of one pair is independent of the other pair. Does this statement has universal applicability?

Yes ☐ No ☐

66. Mendel published his work on inheritance of characters in __________ but it remained unrecognised till __________.

67. Choose the odd one out with respect to the rediscovery of Mendel's work.

de Vries, Correns, von Tschermak, Reginald C Punnett

____

68. Which two scientists used chromosome movement to explain Mendel's laws in 1902?

____

69. The two alleles of a gene pair are located on the non-homologous sites on homologous chromosomes.
(*Rewrite the statement after correcting the underlined words.)*

____

***70.** Consider the given image and mention which of the following laws derived by Mendel is in accordance with the image ?

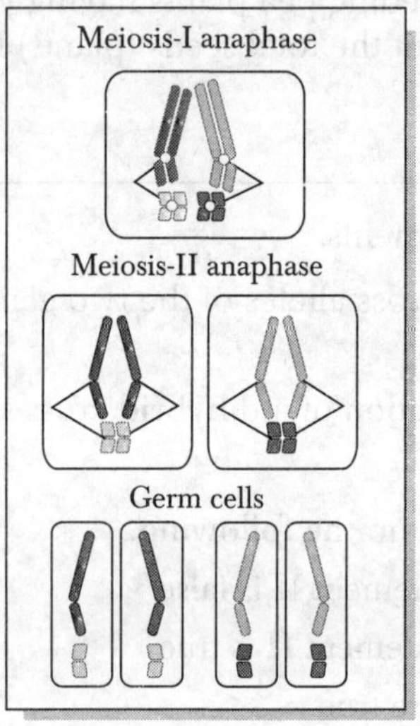

Meiosis-I anaphase

Meiosis-II anaphase

Germ cells

(a) Law of independent assortment ☐ (b) Law of purity of gametes ☐
(c) Law of dominance ☐ (d) Law of segregation ☐

71. Read the following statements.

(i) Both chromosomes and genes occur in pairs.

(ii) Pairing and segregation of a pair of chromosomes lead to the segregation of allelic pair they carry.

Which theory in genetics justify these postulates?

____

***72.** Experimental verification of Sutton and Boveri's theory was given by Thomas Hunt Morgan.

True ☐ False ☐

***73.** The experimental material used by Morgan for his studies was __________ (*Drosophila melanogaster / Pisum sativum*).

74. Out of the listed characteristics, how many are found in *Drosophila melanogaster*?

Hermaphrodite, Several hereditary variations, Two weeks life cycle, Easily grown in laboratory

____

75. Linked genes that were observed by Morgan were present on

____

***76.** Identify the incorrect set of statements from the following.

I. Mendel's approach of using mathematics to explain biological phenomenon was appreciated and acceptable to many biologists of that time.

II. Mendel's concept of genes as stable units that controlled the expression of traits, was not accepted by his contemporaries.

III. Chromosomes are called coloured bodies since they are visualised by staining.

IV. Sutton and Boveri used chromosome movement to explain Mendel's laws.

Codes

(a) II and III ☐ (b) Only I ☐

(c) Only IV ☐ (d) I and IV ☐

***77.** Match the following columns.

Column I	Column II
A. Recombination	1. Non-parental gene combinations
B. Linkage	2. Coloured bodies
C. Chromosomes	3. Physical association of genes

A.__________ B.__________ C. __________

78. Read the following characteristics.

(i) Violation of the law of segregation.

(ii) High proportion of parental gene combinations.

(iii) Deviation of F_2 ratio from 9 : 3 : 3 : 1 ratio.

Which genetic term uphold all the listed characteristics?

____

79. Linked genes are situated on ______________________________ (single chromosome/homologous chromosome).

80. Given below is the percentage of recombinantion between two gene combinations in *Drosophila*.

Gene combination	% Recombination
A. White eyed and yellow bodied	1.3
B. White eyed and miniature winged	37.2

Which gene combination exhibits high linkage? ______________________________

81. Genetic maps were first developed by ____________________

82. The distance between two genes on same chromosome is directly proportional to the strength of linkage between them.

True ☐ False ☐

83. The map distance between various genes is given below.

- *P* and *Q* = 4 nm
- *P* and *R* = 11 nm
- *Q* and *R* = 7 nm

Determine the order of genes on the linkage map.____________________

84. Choose the odd one out with respect to linkage experiment.

AaBb × AaBb,	AAbb × AaBB,
AABB × aabb,	aaBB × aaBB

____

***85.** Observe the image carefully. In which of the following will the recombination frequency be the least?

Chromosorne
Gene 1
Gene 2
A
Gene 1
Gene 2
B
Gene 1
Gene 2
C

(a) Only B ☐ (b) Both B and C ☐
(c) Both A and B ☐ (d) Only A ☐

***86.** Match the following columns.

Column I (Scientists)	Column II (Discoveries)
A. Gregor Mendel	1. Chromosomal theory of inheritance
B. Sutton and Boveri	2. Law of inheritance
C. Alfred Sturtevant	3. Linkage
D. Morgan	4. Genetic maps

A.__________ B.__________ C.__________ D.__________

TOPIC 4

Polygenic Inheritance and Pleiotropy

NCERT Pg. 69

87. The polygenic traits are controlled by

One gene, Two genes, Three or more genes, Mutant genes

____

88. In polygenic inheritance, (*Choose the correct one*).

(i) Traits are influenced by environment. ☐

(ii) Effect of each allele is not expressed. ☐

89. Human skin colour is a polygenic trait in which all dominant and all recessive alleles, respectively show ______________________ phenotype.

90. In human skin colour inheritance, the genotype with three dominant and three recessive alleles will produce intermediate skin colour.

True ☐ False ☐

91. "The effect of each allele is additive". The statement refers to ....

92. Read the following characteristics and identify the gene.

(i) It is a single gene which exhibits multiple phenotypic expressions.

(ii) It shows effect on metabolic pathways, so as to produce various phenotypes.

____

***93.** Phenylketonuria is caused due to

Pleiotropy, Multiple alleles, Codominance, Incomplete dominance

____

94. Phenylketonuria in humans (*Choose the correct one*).

(i) Do not manifest through phenotypic expressions. ☐

(ii) Is characterised by mental retardation, hair reduction and skin pigmentation. ☐

***95.** Which one of the following pairs is wrongly matched?

(a) Phenylalanine hydroxylase – Pleiotropy ☐

(b) ABO blood grouping – Codominance ☐

(c) Starch synthesis in pea – Polygenic trait ☐

(d) TH Morgan – Linkage ☐

***96.** Match the following columns.

Column I (Terms)	Column II (Descriptions)
A. Dominance	1. Many genes govern a single character
B. Codominance	2. In a heterozygous organism, only one allele expresses itself
C. Pleiotropy	3. In a heterozygous organism, both alleles express themselves fully
D. Polygenic inheritance	4. Mutation in gene coding phenylalanine hydroxylase

A. __________ B. __________ C. __________ D. __________

TOPIC 5

Sex-Determination

NCERT Pg. 69-71

97. Henking found X-body in insects while studying ________________ (spermatogenesis/oogenesis).

98. Sex-determination is controlled by ________ and the remaining chromosomes which are not involved in sex-determination are called ________________.

99. If in a given organism males have only X-chromosome and female have a pair of X-chromosome then organism would most likely be

(a) Grasshopper ☐ (b) Owl ☐
(c) Human male ☐ (d) *Drosophila* ☐

***100.** Choose the incorrect pair amongst the following.

(i) Male bird – Homogametic (ii) Female bird – Heterogametic
(iii) Male *Drosophila* – Homogametic

____

101. The number of chromosomes in male and female grasshopper is same.

True ☐ False ☐

102. In human males, counterpart of the X-chromosome is distinctly smaller.

True ☐ False ☐

103. Among the given male organisms, which one is homogametic?

A B C

____

***104.** Female *Drosophila* contains the same sex chromosomes as in female grasshopper and human.

True ☐ False ☐

105. Refer to the genetic cross given below.

Parents (A) ZZ × (B) ZW

Gametes (Z) (Z) (Z) (W)

F_1-generation ZZ ZW ZZ ZW

What is the gender of parents, marked as A and B?

A.________________ B.________________

***106.** Match the following columns.

Column I (Organisms)	Column II (Sex-determination mechanisms)
A. Honeybee	1. ZZ-ZW
B. Pigeon	2. Haplodiploidy
C. *Drosophila*	3. XO-XX
D. True bugs	4. XX - XY

A.________________ B.________________ C.________________ D.________________

107. Choose the odd one out.

XY, XO, ZW

____

108. A human male contains the karyotype ________________ and a human female has ________________ chromosomes.

109. How many pairs of chromosomes are exactly same in human males and females?

____

110. Heterogametes in humans are formed during ________________ (spermatogenesis/oogenesis).

111. The probability of having a girl child, if a couple already has two sons is ________

112. The genetic makeup of the sperm determines the sex of child because ________________ (Y-chromosome is smaller than X-chromosome/males are heterogametic).

113. The given flow chart represents sex determination in honey bees. Choose the correct combination from the following

	Female	Male
Parents	32 ↓ X	16 ↓ Mitosis
Gametes;	16, 16	16
F_1	Male Y	Female 32

(a) X – mitosis; Y – 32 ☐ (b) X – meiosis; Y – 16 ☐

(c) X – meiosis; Y – 32 ☐ (d) X – mitosis; Y – 16 ☐

114. The number of chromosomes in female and male honeybees are ________________

115. The unfertilised eggs in honeybees develop into queen.
(Rewrite the statement after correcting the underlined word.)

____

116. In honeybees, male and female gametes are produced through meiosis and mitosis, respectively.
(*Rewrite the statement after correcting the underlined words.*)

____

117. Males in honeybees have half the number of chromosomes than that of female.

True ☐ False ☐

TOPIC 6

Mutation and Genetic Disorders

NCERT Pg. 72-76

118. Alteration of DNA sequences leading to change in genotype and phenotype of an organism is called ______________________________

119. Mutation arising due to the change in a single base pair of DNA is called frame shift mutation. (*Rewrite the statement after correcing the underlined word*).

____

120. Sickle-cell anaemia is a classical example of ______________________________

121. Give the collective term for these types of mutations.

Insertion, Duplication, Deletion

____

122. Give the scientific term for the analysis of traits in several generations of a family to study the inheritance pattern of a particular trait. ______________________________

123. Pedigree analysis employs the use of ______________________________ (Punnett square/Standard symbols).

124. How many symbols represent affected individuals among those listed below?

■, ◇5, ○, ◆, □—○

____

***125.** Which symbol is used to represent the consanguineous mating in pedigree analysis?

□—○ or □=○
A B

____

126. In pedigree analysis, males are represented by a circle and females by square.

True ☐ False ☐

***127.** Match the following columns.

Column I (Pedigree symbols)	Column II (Refers to)
A. [square–circle connected]	1. Five unaffected offsprings
B. [square–circle with shaded square child]	2. Sex unspecified
C. [diamond]	3. Child affected with disease
D. [diamond with 5]	4. Mating

A.__________ B.__________ C. __________ D. __________

128. Pedigree analysis is employed to study both Mendelian and chromosomal disorders.

True ☐ False ☐

129. Name the common class of genetic disorders to which all of these belong.

Cystic fibrosis, Phenylketonuria, Thalassemia, Colour blindness

____

130. Mendelian disorders are determined by alteration in __________ (single/several) gene(s) and these are transmitted on same lines to offspring.

***131.** Complete the following analogy.

Autosomal dominant trait : Myotonic dystrophy : : Autosomal recessive trait : ______

132. How many mutated copies of genes are involved in autosomal dominant and autosomal recessive disorders? __________

133. Given below is the pedigree analysis of fused ear lobes, which is an autosomal recessive trait.

A

B

C

Identify the genotypes of *A*, *B* and *C*.

A.__________ B.__________ C.__________

134. Mendelian disorders are exclusively recessive.

True ☐ False ☐

135. Choose the odd one out.

Sickle-cell anaemia, Myotonic dystrophy, Colour blindness, Thalassemia

____

***136.** Refer to the given pedigree analysis and identify the type of inheritance pattern shown in it.

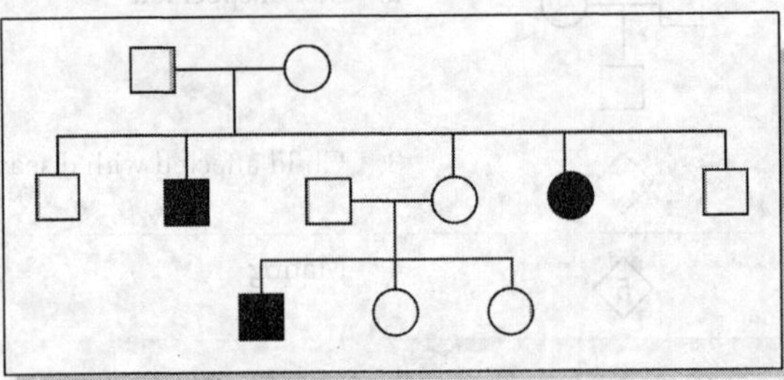

____

***137.** Colour blindness and haemophilia are sex-linked ________________ (dominant/recessive) disorders.

138. X-linked recessive traits like colour blindness occur more frequently in males than females because

(i) Males receive X-chromosomes from mother.

(ii) Females require two-altered copies of genes to get affected.

Most appropriate answer is ________ (Only (i) / Both (i) and (ii))

139. Fathers cannot pass X-linked traits to their sons.

True ☐ False ☐

140. Read the following statements.

(i) Failure to discriminate between red and green colour.

(ii) Mutation in X-linked recessive gene.

(iii) Mostly affect males than females.

These characteristics are indicative of which genetic disorder?

____

141. A marriage between a colourblind man and a normal woman produces ________________ (all carrier daughters and normal sons/all carrier offsprings).

142. Father of a child is colourblind and mother is a carrier. What is the probability that the child would be colourblind? ________________

143. A female is affected by haemophilia when the mother is at least ____________ and father is ________________ .

144. Identify the genotype of the following persons.

(i) Carrier of sickle-cell anaemia. ________________

(ii) Affected by sickle-cell anaemia. ________________

145. Refer to the diagram showing the normal β-chain of haemoglobin.

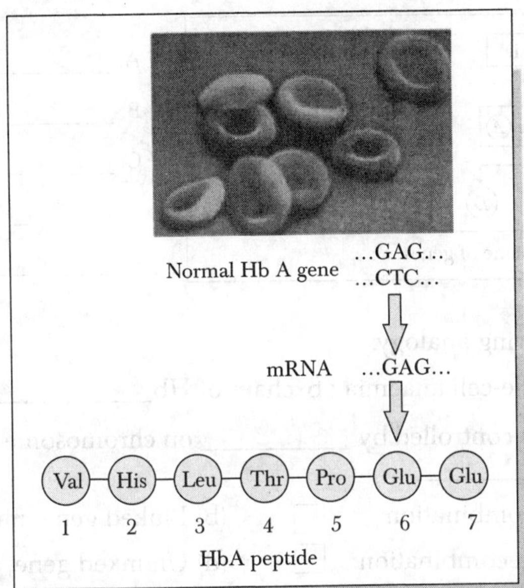

Name the amino acid which gets substituted at position 6 during sickle-cell anaemia.

____

146. Sickle cell anemia occurs due to a change

(a) From Glutamate to Valine ; GAG to GUG ☐

(b) From Valine to Glutamate ; GAG to GUG ☐

(c) From Glutamate to Valine ; GUG to GAG ☐

(d) From Valine to Glutamate ; GUG to GAG ☐

147. During sickle-cell anaemia, under oxygen tension, the shape of RBCs become <u>spherical</u>. (*Rewrite the statement after correcting the underlined word.*)

____

148. An individual affected by phenylketonuria lacks an enzyme that converts the amino acid _______________ into _______________.

149. Name the acid which gets accumulated in the body of an individual affected by phenylketonuria. _______________

150. Mention any two symptoms of phenylketonuria.

(i) _______________ (ii) _______________

151. Accumulation of phenylalanine in brain results in

(a) Kidney disease ☐ (b) Heart disease ☐

(c) Mental retardation ☐ (d) Change in shape of RBCs ☐

152. The transmission of thalassemia from parents to offspring requires _______________ (both carrier parents/only one carrier parent).

***153.** Complete the flowchart given below (*A-E*).

α-thalassemia → Chromosome (A) → (C), (D)

β-thalassemia → Chromosome (B) → (E)

Name of genes

A. ______________

B. ______________

C. ______________

D. ______________

E. ______________

154. Complete the following analogy.

Thalassemia : : Sickle-cell anaemia : β chain of Hb______________

155. Alpha thalassemia is controlled by __________ on chromosome number 16 and may be observed due to __________.

(a) Linked gene, recombination ☐ (b) Linked gene, mutation ☐

(c) Unlinked gene, recombination ☐ (d) Unlinked gene, mutation ☐

156. Name the genetic disorders which are caused due to the absence or excess or abnormal arrangement of one or more chromosomes. ______________

157. Complete the following analogy.

Failure of segregation of chromatids : Aneuploidy : : Failure of cytokinesis : ______

***158.** Both Down's syndrome and Turner's syndrome are the examples of __________ (aneuploidy/polyploidy).

***159.** Choose the odd one out.

Down's syndrome, Turner's syndrome, Klinefelter's syndrome

____

***160.** Refer to the figure given below and identify the genetic disorder.

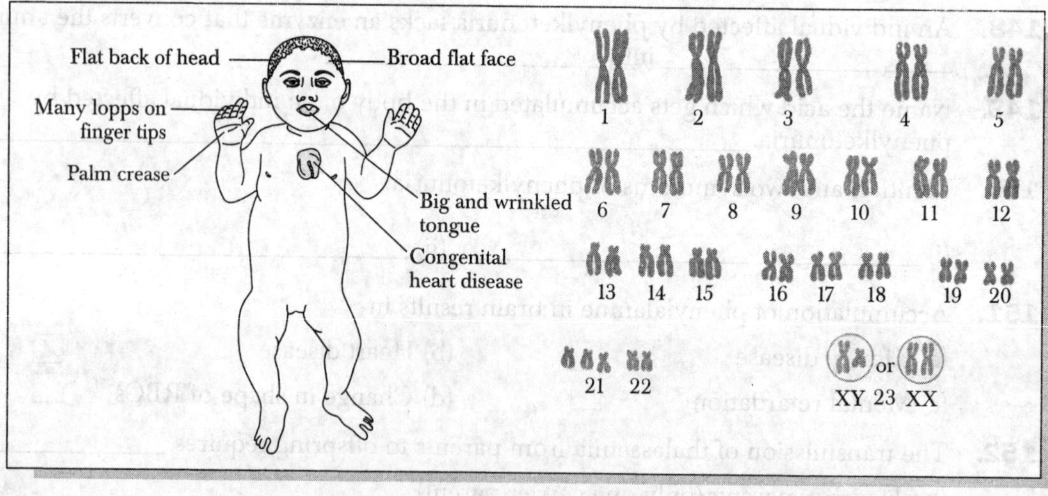

____

***161.** A man suffered from chromosomal aberration that caused a gain of an additional copy of chromosome 4 and chromosome 8. Which of the following shows correct representation of the chromosome?

(a) 46A + XY ☐ (b) 44A + XY ☐
(c) 45A + XY ☐ (d) 48A + XY ☐

162. Give the alternative name of Down's syndrome. ____________

163. How many chromosomes are found in the genetic disorder described by Langdon Down in 1866? ____________

164. Complete the following analogy.
Extra chromosome 21 : Down's syndrome : : Extra X-chromosome : ____________

165. Mention any two symptoms in an individual with karyotype 44 + XXY.
____

166. An individual is suffering from Turner's syndrome. The chromosome complement would be ____________ (44 + XO / 45 + XX).

***167.** Match the following columns.

Column I (Genetical traits)	Column II (Name of disorders)
A. 45 with XO Chromosome	1. Down's syndrome
B. Sex-linked recessive disease	2. Phenylketonuria
C. Inborn metabolic error linked to autosomal recessive trait	3. Haemophilia
D. Additional 21st chromosome	4. Turner's syndrome

A.________ B.________ C. ________ D. ________

168. What do the diagrams *A* and *B* represent?

(*A*) Tall stature with feminine character

(*B*) Short stature and underdeveloped feminine character

A.____________ B. ____________

Assertion-Reason Questions

The following questions consist of two statements- Assertion (A) and Reason (R). Answer these questions by selecting the appropriate option given below.

(a) Both A and R are true and R is the correct explanation of A

(b) Both A and R are true, but R is not the correct explanation of A

(c) A is true, but R is false

(d) A is false, but R is true

***1.** **Assertion** (A) The F_1 progenies in all monohybrid crosses were found to express the phenotype of one of the parent.
Reason (R) In a pair of alleles with contrasting traits of a character, one is completely dominant over the other.

(a) ☐ (b) ☐ (c) ☐ (d) ☐

***2.** **Assertion** (A) In a monohybrid cross the F_1 progenies are heterozygous for genes controlling a single character.
Reason (R) The phenotypic ratio for F_2-generation in a monohybrid cross is 3:1, while the genotypic ratio is 1:2:1.

(a) ☐ (b) ☐ (c) ☐ (d) ☐

3. **Assertion** (A) A test cross can be used to find the genotype of an organism expressing dominant phenotype.
Reason (R) In a test cross, the organism showing dominant phenotype is crossed with either of the parent.

(a) ☐ (b) ☐ (c) ☐ (d) ☐

***4.** **Assertion** (A) The F_2 phenotypic ratio for a monohybrid cross in snapdragon is exactly similar to the Mendelian monohybrid crosses.
Reason (R) The red flowers of the snapdragon are not completely dominant over the white flowers.

(a) ☐ (b) ☐ (c) ☐ (d) ☐

***5.** **Assertion** (A) A couple with blood group A and B can never have a child with blood group O.
Reason (R) ABO blood group is controlled by three genes, out of which two are co-dominant.

(a) ☐ (b) ☐ (c) ☐ (d) ☐

***6.** **Assertion** (A) Chromosomal segregation was independent of the genes that controlled specific characters.
Reason (R) Homologous chromosomes contain same genes at the same loci.

(a) ☐ (b) ☐ (c) ☐ (d) ☐

***7.** **Assertion** (A) The recombination frequency can be used to calculate the distance between genes.
Reason (R) Non-parental combination is quite low for tightly linked genes on the same chromosome.

(a) ☐ (b) ☐ (c) ☐ (d) ☐

8. **Assertion** (A) A person with all dominant alleles for skin colour will have the darkest skin colour.
Reason (R) Certain phenotypes which are controlled by multiple genes are called polygenic traits.
(a) ☐ (b) ☐ (c) ☐ (d) ☐

***9.** **Assertion** (A) A female heterozygous for haemophilia is a carrier of the the disease, but not be affected herself.
Reason (R) A female has two X chromosomes and haemophilia is X-linked recessive genetic disease.
(a) ☐ (b) ☐ (c) ☐ (d) ☐

***10.** **Assertion** (A) Both thalassemia and sickle-cell anaemia are autosomal linked recessive diseases.
Reason (R) Thalassemia is controlled by a single gene HBB on chromosome 12 of each parent whereas sickle cell-anaemia is controlled by a single pair of allele.
(a) ☐ (b) ☐ (c) ☐ (d) ☐

Case Based Questions

1. A cross was made between two pea plants, one had round and yellow seeds while the other had wrinkled and green seeds. The F_1 progenies of such a cross were self crossed to get F_2. The F_2 seeds were grown to obtain 960 progeny plants. It was found that the progenies showed a variation of characters with parental as well as non parental combination. Based on this given information, answer the following questions.

(i) Which type of cross is being performed?
(a) Monohybrid cross with two pairs of contrasting characters ☐
(b) Monohybrid cross with one pair of contrasting character ☐
(c) Dihybrid cross with one pair of contrasting character ☐
(d) Dihybrid cross with two pairs of contrasting characters ☐

(ii) How many F_2 progenies would be round and green?
(a) 270 ☐ (b) 180 ☐
(c) 60 ☐ (d) 540 ☐

(iii) What is the total number of F_2 progenies with wrinkled yellow seeds and wrinkled green seeds?
(a) 240 ☐ (b) 720 ☐
(c) 600 ☐ (d) 960 ☐

2. A young man named Ritik met with a severe accident and lost a significant amount of blood. He arrived at the hospital emergency and needed a blood transfusion immediately. However, the hospital is running low on blood supplies and they only have limited blood type available.
Ritik's mother who is with him, told the doctor about Ritik's blood type, i.e. A^+ positive (A^+).
Based on the following situation, answer the questions that follows

(i) Which type of allelic pattern would be observed in Ritik's blood?
(a) Only i ☐ (b) I^A or i ☐
(c) I^A and I^B ☐ (d) I^A or $I^A i$ ☐

(ii) According to Ritik's blood type (A^+) which blood types can he safely receive without risk of a transfusion reaction?

(a) O^+ only ☐ (b) A^+ and AB^- only ☐

(c) A^-, A^+, O^- and O^+ ☐ (d) A^- only ☐

(iii) Which of the following best describes the immune response when a person receives the wrong blood group during a transfusion?

(a) Production of antibodies against donor red blood cells ☐

(b) Activation of clotting facrters in the bloods tream ☐

(c) Decrease in white blood cell count ☐

(d) Decreased production of platelets ☐

COMPETITION EDGE UP

1. *Which one of the following can be explained on the basis of Mendel's law of dominance?*

A. *Out of one pair of factors one is dominant and the other is recessive.*

B. *Alleles do not show any expression and both the characters appear as such in -generation.*

C. *Factors occur in pairs in normal diploid plants.*

D. *The discrete unit controlling a particular character is called factor.*

E. *The expression of only one of the parental characters is found in a monohybrid cross.*

Choose the correct answer from the options given below. **[NCERT Pg. 58, NEET 2024]**

(a) A, B and C only ☐

(b) A, C, D and E only ☐

(c) B, C and D only ☐

(d) A, B, C, D and E ☐

2. *In a plant, black seed colour (BB/Bb) is dominant over white seed colour (bb). In order to find out the genotype of the black seed plant, with which of the following genotype will you cross it?* **[NCERT Pg. 58, NEET 2024]**

(a) BB ☐ (b) bb ☐

(c) Bb ☐ (d) BB/Bb ☐

3. *As per ABO blood grouping system, the blood group of father is B^+, mother is A^+ and child is O^+. Their respective genotype can be*

A. I^Bi / I^Ai/ii B. I^BI^B/I^AI^A/ii

C. iI^B/iI^A/I^AI^B D. I^Ai/I^Bi/I^Ai

E. iI^B/iI^A/I^AI^B

Choose the most appropriate answer from the options given below. **[NCERT Pg. 61, NEET 2024]**

(a) A only ☐ (b) B only ☐

(c) C and B only ☐ (d) D and E only ☐

4. *Match List I with List II.* **[NCERT Pg. 56, 58, 75, NEET 2024]**

List I	List II
A. Two or more alternative forms of a gene	1. Back cross
B. Cross of F_1 progeny with homozygous recessive parent	2. Ploidy
C. Cross of F_1 progeny with any of the parents	3. Allele
D. Number of chromosome sets in plant	4. Test cross

Codes

	A	B	C	D			A	B	C	D	
(a)	1	2	3	4	☐	(b)	2	1	3	4	☐
(c)	3	4	1	2	☐	(d)	4	3	2	1	☐

5. *Match List I with List II.* **[NCERT Pg. 75, 76, NEET 2024]**

List I	List II
A. Down's syndrome	1. 11th chromosome
B. α-Thalassemia	2. X-chromosome
C. β-Thalassemia	3. 21st chromosome
D. Klinefelter's syndrome	4. 16th chromosome

Codes

	A	B	C	D			A	B	C	D	
(a)	1	2	3	4	☐	(b)	2	3	4	1	☐
(c)	3	4	1	2	☐	(d)	4	1	2	3	☐

6. Frequency of recombination between gene pairs on same chromosome as a measure of the distance between genes to map their position on chromosome, was used for the first time by **[NCERT Pg. 67, NEET 2023]**

(a) Sutton and Boveri ☐
(b) Alfred Sturtevant ☐
(c) Henking ☐
(d) Thomas Hunt Morgan ☐

7. Which of the following statements are correct about Klinefelter's syndrome? **[NCERT Pg. 76, NEET 2023]**

A. This disorder was first described by Langdon Down (1866).
B. Such an individual has overall masculine development. However, the feminine development is also expressed.
C. The affected individual is short statured.
D. Physical, psychomotor and mental development is retarded.
E. Such individuals are sterile.

Choose the correct answer from the options given below

(a) C and D only ☐
(b) B and E only ☐
(c) A and E only ☐
(d) A and B only ☐

8. The recombination frequency between the genes a & c is 5%, b & c is 15%, b & d is 9%, a & b is 20%, c and d is 24% and a and d is 29%. What will be the sequence of these genes on a linear chromosome? **[NCERT Pg. 65, NEET 2022]**

(a) a, d, b, c ☐ (b) d, b, a, c ☐
(c) a, b, c, d ☐ (d) a, c, b, d ☐

9. Given below are two statements, one is labelled as Assertion (A) and the other is labelled as Reason (R).

Assertion (A) Mendel's law of independent assortment does not hold good for the genes that are located closely on the same chromosome.

Reason (R) Closely located genes assort independently.

In the light of the above statements, choose the correct answer from the options given below. **[NCERT Pg. 64, NEET 2022]**

(a) Both (A) and (R) are correct, but (R) is not the correct explanation of (A) ☐
(b) (A) is correct, but (R) is not correct ☐
(c) (A) is not correct, but (R) is correct ☐
(d) Both (A) and (R) are correct and (R) is the correct explanation of (A) ☐

10. The production of gametes by the parents, formation of zygote, the F_1 and F_2-plants, can be understood from a diagram called **[NCERT Pg. 57, NEET 2021]**

(a) Bullet square ☐
(b) Punch square ☐
(c) Punnett square ☐
(d) Net square ☐

11. In a cross between a male and female, both heterozygous for sickle-cell anaemia gene, what percentage of the progeny will be diseased? **[NCERT Pg. 74, NEET 2021]**

(a) 50% ☐
(b) 75% ☐
(c) 25% ☐
(d) 100% ☐

12. Identify the wrong statement with reference to the gene 'I' that controls ABO blood groups. **[NCERT Pg. 61, NEET (Sep.) 2020]**

(a) A person will have only two of the three alleles ☐
(b) When I^A and I^B are present together, they express same type of sugar ☐
(c) Allele 'i' does not produce any sugar ☐
(d) The gene (I) has three alleles ☐

13. Select the correct match. **[NCERT Pg. 74, NEET (Sep.) 2020]**

(a)	Phenylketonuria	-	Autosomal dominant trait
(b)	Sickle-cell anaemia	-	Autosomal recessive trait, chromosome-II
(c)	Thalassemia	-	X-linked
(d)	Haemophilia	-	Y-linked

(a) ☐ (b) ☐
(c) ☐ (d) ☐

Chapter 05

Molecular Basis of Inheritance

Scan and take Chapter Test

TOPIC 1

The DNA : Structure of Polynucleotide Chain

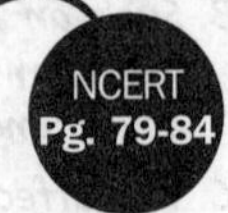

1. Give a scientific term for the following sentence.

The substance that controls the inheritance of traits and also expresses its effects through the formation and functioning of traits. ____________

2. The nature of the putative genetic material was investigated culminating in the realisation that ____________ (deoxyribonucleic acids/proteins) are the genetic material, at least in majority of organisms.

3. Name the genetic material in living organisms mentioned below.

(i) Animals and human beings ____________.

(ii) Viruses ____________

4. DNA mostly functions as a messenger in most living organisms.

True ☐ False ☐

5. Match the following columns.

	Column I (Organisms)		Column II (DNA contents)
A.	$\phi \times 174$	1.	4.6×10^6 bp
B.	Lambda phage	2.	3.3×10^9 bp
C.	Human DNA	3.	48502 bp
D.	*Escherichia coli*	4.	5386 nucleotides

A. ____________ B. ____________ C. ____________ D. ____________

6. DNA is a long polymer of <u>ribonucleotides</u>.

(*Rewrite the statement after correcting the underlined word.*)

____

*Concepts of all questions bearing * are important for NEET & CUET*

***7.** In terms of DNA and RNA structure, what is a nucleotide?

____

***8.** How many of the following are structural components of a polynucleotide chain?

Pentose sugar, Glycerol, Nitrogenous bases, Hexose sugar, A phosphate group

____

***9.** Identify purines from the following bases.

Adenine, Thymine, Guanine, Cytosine, Uracil, Dihydrouridine

____

***10.** Thymine is common for both DNA and RNA and cytosine is present only in DNA.

True ☐ False ☐

***11.** Uracil is present in RNA at the place of ________________.

12. Two types of pentose sugars are shown below, which of the following is found in RNA and DNA, respectively?

(a) 5' $HOCH_2$ O [OH] 1' 4' H H H H 3' 2' OH [OH]

(b) 5' $HOCH_2$ O [OH] 1' 4' H H H H 3' 2' OH [H]

____

***13.** With respect to nucleosides which of the following is paired correctly?

Purine–Adenosine, Thymidine; Pyrimidine – Uridine, Cytidine

____

14. Which of the following correctly describes a nucleoside?

(a) A nitrogenous base attached to a phosphate group ☐
(b) A nitrogenous base attached to pentose sugar and phosphate ☐
(c) A pentose sugar and a phosphate group ☐
(d) Nitrogenous base attached to pentose sugar ☐

15. A nucleotide is formed when phosphate group is linked to ________________ group of deoxythymidine through ________________ linkage.

16. Which of the following is correct with respect to N-glycosidic linkage in nucleoside?

(a) Nitrogenous base is linked to OH at 1'C sugar ☐
(b) Nitrogenous base is linked to OH at 2'C sugar ☐
(c) Nitrogenous base is linked to OH at 3'C sugar ☐
(d) Nitrogenous base is linked to OH at 5'C sugar ☐

17. Consider the given image.

5' phosphate, H, X, P, C, H, H, P, C, H, H, 3' hydroxyl, P, C, OH, H, A, Y, T, G, C

Choose the correct combination of *X* and *Y*

(a) X - N-glycosidic bond, Y - Phosphoester bond ☐

(b) X - N-glycosidic bond, Y - Phosphodiester bond ☐

(c) X - Phosphoester bond, Y - Phosphodiester bond ☐

(d) X - Phosphodiester bond, Y - N-glycosidic bond ☐

18. State whether the following statements are true or false.

(i) In the polynucleotide chain formed using ribose sugar, a free phosphate moiety is present at 5' end and a free —OH at 3'end.

True ☐ False ☐

(ii) In a dinucleotide, two nucleotides are linked through 3′— 5′ phosphodiester linkage.

True ☐ False ☐

19. The backbone in a polynucleotide chain is formed by ______________ .

20. An additional phosphate group at 2' position in the ribose is found in RNA.

(*Rewrite the statement after correcting the underlined words.*)

____

***21.** In a DNA double helix, the bases are held together by ______________ (covalent bonds/hydrogen bonds).

***22.** Match the following columns.

	Column I (Names of scientist)		Column II (Contributions)
A.	Wilkins and Franklin	1.	First identified DNA and named it nuclein
B.	F Meischer	2.	X-ray diffraction of DNA
C.	E Chargaff	3.	Double helix model of DNA
D.	Waston and Crick	4.	Base pairing rules

A. ______________ B. ______________ C. ______________ D. ______________

***23.** Complete the sentence.

Chargaff's rules of base pairing states that the ratio of A + T and G + C ______________ in all tested organisms and______________.

***24.** If a *ds* DNA has 15% of guanine, what will be the percentage of thymine in it?

____

***25.** The base pairing confers a very unique property to the polynucleotide chains as it is complementary.

True ☐ False ☐

26. If each strand from a *ds* DNA acts as a template for synthesis of a new strand, the two double-stranded DNA produced from them would be ______________ (identical/different) to the parental DNA.

27. Which term is used if one chain of *ds* DNA has the polarity $5' \rightarrow 3'$, the other has $3' \rightarrow 5'$ polarity? ______________

***28.** In a *ds* DNA, if the sequence of bases in one strand is 5'- T A C C G A C C A -3', then the sequence of other strand would be ______________

***29.** In the figure given below, identify the correct labelling of *A-E*.

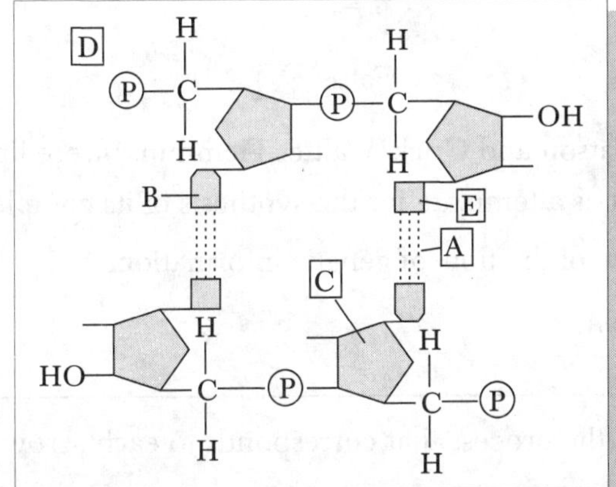

A. ______________

B. ______________

C. ______________

D. ______________

E. ______________

30. How is it so that a purine comes opposite to a pyrimidine in *ds* DNA chain?

____

***31.** Observe the figure given below.

Identify *A* and *B*.

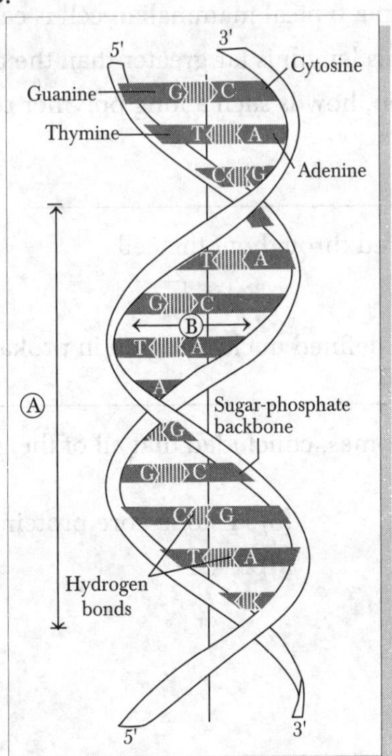

A. ______________

B. ______________

32. The two chains of the DNA strand are coiled in a ______________ (right/left) handed fashion.

***33.** The double helix DNA turns after every 10 base pairs at a distance of 3.4 nm. This distance is known as ______________.

34. If there are 1500 bp in a stretch of DNA, its length will be

(a) 340nm ☐ (b) 3.4 m ☐

(c) 510 nm ☐ (d) 51m ☐

35. The plane of one base pair stacks over the other in double helix, which confers stability of the helical structure.

True ☐ False ☐

36. ______________ (Watson and Crick/Waltter Flemming) were first to suggest that one strand of DNA might act as a template for the synthesis of its complementary strand.

***37.** Arrange them in the sequence of the flow of genetic information.

(i) Protein (ii) DNA (iii) RNA

____

***38.** In the spaces below, indicate the process that corresponds to each arrow.

Ⓐ (circular arrow on DNA) DNA —Ⓑ→ *m*RNA —Ⓒ→ Protein

A. ______________

B. ______________

C. ______________

39. The length of DNA double helix in a typical mammalian cell is calculated and it comes out to be approximately 2.2 m. This length is far greater than the dimension of a typical nucleus (approximately 10^{-6} m). So, how is such a long polymer packaged in a cell? (*Answer in one line.*)

____

40. In prokaryotes, the DNA is scattered throughout the cell.

True ☐ False ☐

41. Give scientific term for the poorly defined nuclear region in prokaryotes.

____

42. Anil while studying about nucleosomes, concluded that all of the given form the components of nucleosome except

(a) DNA ☐ (b) Histone core protein ☐

(c) H_1 linker ☐ (d) RNA ☐

***43.** Observe the figure given below and answer the following questions.

(i) Label the parts *A*-*C*.

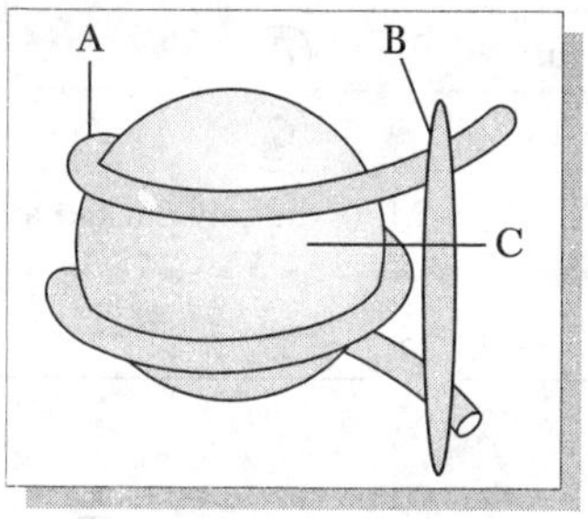

A. ____________

B. ____________

C. ____________

(ii) The figure represents a ____________ .

***44.** The nucleosomes in chromatin appear as ____________ (beads on a string/L, V, X shapes) under electron microscope.

***45.** Basic amino acids help the histones to acquire a ____________ charge on themselves.

***46.** Lysine and arginine - what is common to both these amino acids? ____________

***47.** Give a biological term for the following statements.

(i) A unit of eight molecules formed by histones. ____________

(ii) Thread-like stained (coloured) bodies seen in nucleus. ____________

***48.** Complete the following analogy.

Nucleosome : ____________ :: Histones : Octamer

***49.** The nucleosomes in chromatin are seen as ____________ structures when viewed under ____________.

50. Consider the given image. Which of the following is responsible for stability of the given structure?

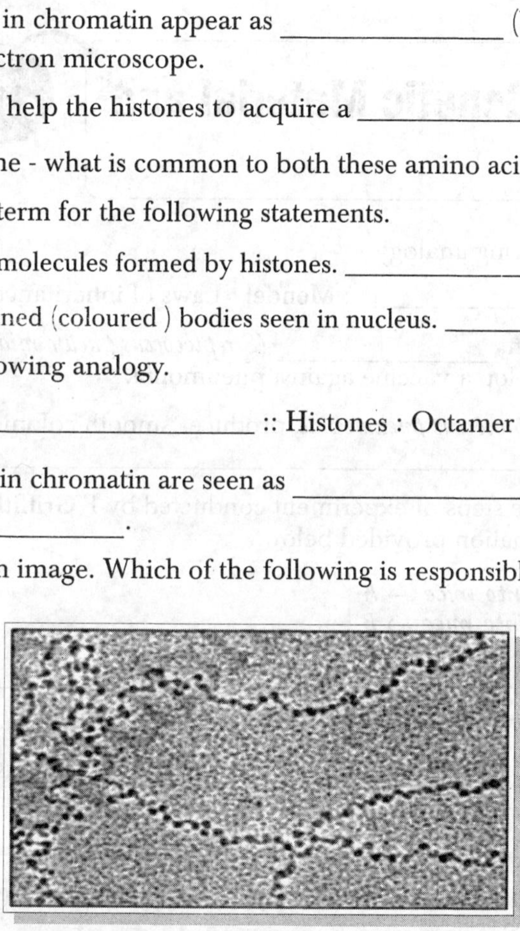

(a) Negative phosphate of DNA and positive arginine of protein ☐

(b) Positive phosphate of DNA and negative glutamate of protein ☐

(c) Negative phosphate of DNA and positive glutamate of protein ☐

(d) Positive phosphate of DNA and negative lysine of protein ☐

***51.** Given below are structures associated with the packaging of DNA helix, paired with their related features. Complete the pairing by filling in the missing terms.

(A)	Nucleosomes
Non-Histone Chromosomal (NHC) proteins	(B)
Euchromatin	(C)
(D)	More densely packed and stains dark

A. __________ B. __________ C. __________ D. __________

***52.** Complete the following analogy.

Euchromatin : Transcriptionally active :: __________ : Transcriptionally inactive

TOPIC 2

The Search for Genetic Material and The RNA World

NCERT Pg. 84-88

***53.** Complete the following analogy.

Frederick Griffith : __________ :: Mendel : Laws of inheritance

54. F Griffith worked on __________ *(Streptococcus pneumoniae/Haemophilus influenzae)* while trying to develop a vaccine against pneumonia.

55. The S-strain of *Streptococcus pneumoniae*, produces smooth colonies. What does this mean?

____

***56.** Given below are the steps of experiment conducted by F Griffith. Answer the questions based on the information provided below.

S-strain → inject into mice → A
R-strain → inject into mice → B

(i) What happens at *A* and *B* ? __________

(ii) Based on the above results, which strain is virulent? __________

57. S-strain (heat-killed) → Injected into mice → Mice lives. In this case, the mice injected with S-strain lives unlike in the original setup. Why so?

____

58. S-strain (heat-killed) + R-strain (live) → inject into mice → *X*. Here, *X* is __________ (mice die/mice lives).

59. Griffith concluded that R-strain bacteria was transformed by the heat-killed S-strain bacteria.

True ☐ False ☐

***60.** On injecting which of the following will the mice be found alive?

(a) Heat killed S-strain + Heat killed R-strain ☐

(b) Heat killed S-strain + Live R-strain ☐

(c) Live S-strain + Heat killed R-strain ☐

(d) Live S-strain + Live R-strain ☐

61. The transforming factor in Griffith's experiment was identified as ______________ (genetic material/polysaccharide capsule).

***62.** The genetic material was thought to be a protein, this assumption was corrected by James Watson. (*Rewrite the statement after correcting the underlined words.*)

____

63. The biochemical nature of 'transforming principle' in Griffith's experiment was determined as ______________ (nucleic acid/glycolipids).

64. Complete the following analogy.
Proteases : Protein digesting enzyme :: ______________ : RNA digesting enzyme

***65.** Consider the following statements.

Statement I Avery, MacLeod and McCarty provided the biochemical characterisation of transforming principle.

Statement II Protease and RNases digestion affected transformation, which proved that DNA is the genetic material

Choose the correct option from the following.

(a) Statement I is true, but statement II is false ☐
(b) Statement I is false, but statement II is true ☐
(c) Both statements I and II are true ☐
(d) Both statements I and II are false ☐

66. Alfred Hershey and Martha Chase (1952) worked with ______________ (bacteria/bacteriophage) to prove that DNA is the genetic material.

67. In Hershey and Chase's experiment, the radioactive labelled elements used were

____

***68.** The steps of Hershey and Chase's experiment are shown below.

(i) Identify the steps *A*, *B* and *C*.

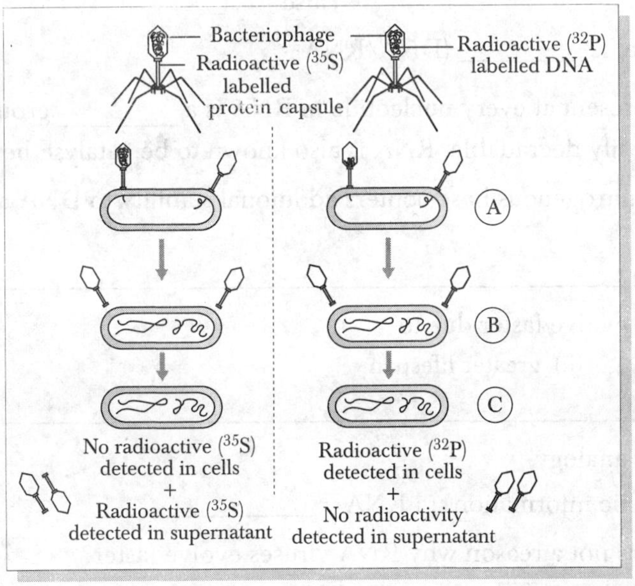

A. ______________
B. ______________
C. ______________

(ii) In which of the above bacterial cells, will the radioactivity be detected?______________

(iii) What conclusion was drawn from this experiment? ______________

69. If phages grown on S^{35} were allowed to infect bacteria, where would radioactivity be detected after centrifugation?

(a) In the bacterial pellet ☐ (b) In the bacterial cell wall ☐
(c) In the supernatant ☐ (d) Both bacteria and supernatant ☐

***70.** Match the following columns.

Column I (Scientists)	Column II (Contributions)
A. Frederick Griffith	1. Confirmed DNA as genetic material
B. Hershey and Chase	2. Central dogma
C. Avery, MacLeod and McCarty	3. Transforming principle
D. Francis Crick	4. Biochemical nature of transforming principle

A. ________ B. ________ C. ________ D. ________

71. Messenger and adapter-these functions are associated with ________

72. For a molecule to act as genetic material, it should be capable of ________ (replication/rapid mutations).

73. Only RNA is capable of directing its duplications.

(*Rewrite the statement after correcting the underlined words.*)

____

74. State whether the following statements are True or False.

(i) RNA is the ideal genetic material due to higher mutation rate that allows evolutionary changes.

True ☐ False ☐

(ii) DNA can express itself in the form of Mendelian characters.

True ☐ False ☐

***75.** The first genetic material is ________ (DNA/RNA).

76. A ________ group present at every nucleotide in RNA is a ________ group and makes RNA ________ and easily degradable. RNA is also known to be catalyst, hence reactive.

77. The presence of which nitrogenous base confers additional stability to DNA as compared to RNA?

____

78. Viruses can mutate and evolve faster due to

(i) RNA genome (ii) greater lifespan

____

79. Complete the following analogy.

DNA : Storage of genetic information : : RNA : ________ .

80. Which of the following is not a reason why RNA viruses evolve faster?

(a) RNA is single stranded ☐ (b) RNA can be translated directly ☐
(c) RNA contains uracil ☐ (d) RNA has catalytic properties ☐

81. Pick the odd one out.

Inheritance, Metabolism, Translation, Splicing

____

82. Consider the following statements about genetic material.

I. Both DNA and RNA have the ability to direct their duplication.

II. Presence of thymine in place of uracil confers additional stability to DNA.

III. DNA proves better as a genetic material due to its storage capacity and the ability to transform genetic material.

IV. DNA being double stranded and having complementary strand resists further changes by evolving a process of repair.

Choose the set of correct statements.

(a) I and II ☐ (b) III, IV and V ☐

(c) I, II and IV ☐ (d) II and III ☐

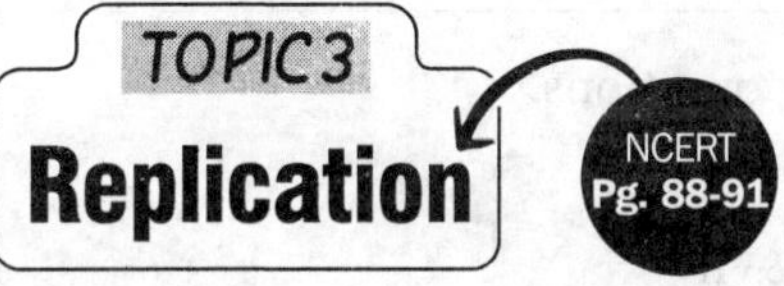

83. Give a biological term for the following statement.
The type of replication where each DNA molecule would have one parental and one newly synthesised strand. ______________________________

84. Answer the questions associated with the figure given below.

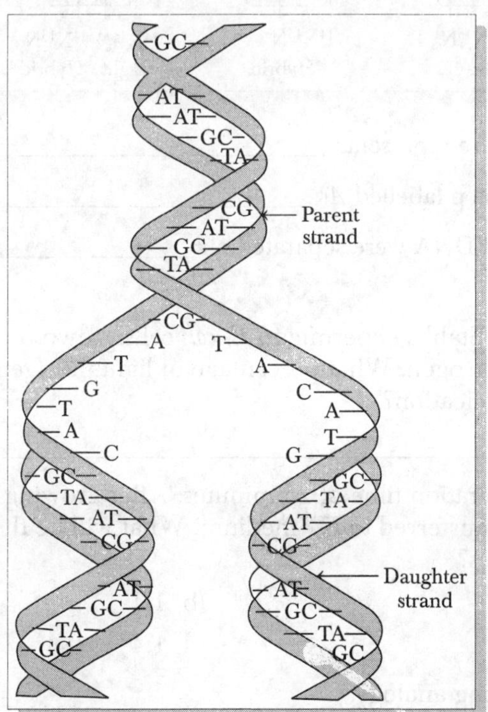

(i) This figure is identified as the semiconservative model of DNA replication.

True ☐ False ☐

(ii) This model of DNA replication was given by Thomas Morgan in 1953.
(*Rewrite the statement after correcting the underlined words.*)

____

(iii) In the figure, parent DNA strands undergo _______________ followed by synthesis of a strand. The parent strand acts as a _______________ in this process.

***85.** "DNA replicates semiconservatively" was first shown in _______________ *(Streptococcus pneumoniae/ Escherichia coli).*

***86.** Waston and Crick, experimentally proved semiconservative mode of replication in DNA in 1958.

(*Rewrite the statement after correcting the underlined words.*)

____

***87.** Observe the figure given below and answer the following questions.

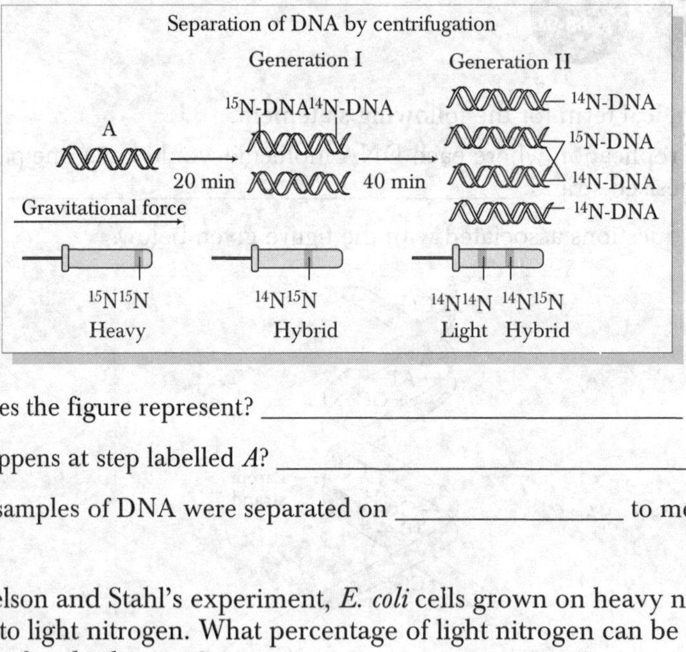

Separation of DNA by centrifugation

Generation I, Generation II

A; ^{15}N-DNA^{14}N-DNA; 20 min; 40 min; ^{14}N-DNA; ^{15}N-DNA; ^{14}N-DNA; ^{14}N-DNA

Gravitational force

^{15}N^{15}N Heavy; ^{14}N^{15}N Hybrid; ^{14}N^{14}N Light; ^{14}N^{15}N Hybrid

(i) What does the figure represent? _______________

(ii) What happens at step labelled *A*? _______________

(iii) Various samples of DNA were separated on _______________ to measure the densities of DNA.

***88.** In the Meselson and Stahl's experiment, *E. coli* cells grown on heavy nitrogen were transferred to light nitrogen. What percentage of light nitrogen can be expected after three generations of multiplication?

____

89. A bacteria has a generation time of 25 minutes. After growing it in N^{14} medium for many generations, it was transferred to N^{15} medium. What will be the ratio of hybrid : heavy DNA after 50 minutes?

(a) 1:2 ☐ (b) 1:1 ☐
(c) 2:1 ☐ (d) 1:4 ☐

90. Complete the following analogy.

E. coli : $^{15}NH_4Cl$: : *Vicia faba* : _______________

91. ______________ are used as substrates in DNA replication, and they also provide energy for polymerisation reaction.

92. What does the efficiency of DNA polymerase activity indicate?

____

***93.** *E. coli* with ____________ completes the process of replication in ______________.

94. DNA polymerisation rate of DNA polymerase is ____________________ (2000 bp per second/5000 bp per second).

95. 'Polymerases have to catalyse the reaction with high degree of accuracy'. What would happen if there is a mistake in polymerisation? ______________

96. In *d*NTPs, the source of energy are the two ______________ (terminal phosphates/ hydroxyl groups).

97. Give one word answer for statement given below.

A small opening of DNA helix in which replication occurs. ______________

98. DNA replication can begin just anywhere on a DNA strand.

True ☐ False ☐

***99.** During replication, ________ strand is formed because the DNA-dependent DNA polymerases catalyse polymerisation only in one direction, i.e. 5' - 3'.

100. Give the correct heading for the differences given below for templates in DNA replication.

A	*B*
Extends 5' - 3' in the direction of replication fork	Synthesised in 5' - 3' direction but discontinuously
No role of DNA ligase	DNA ligase joins the discontinuous fragments of DNA

A. ______________ B. ______________

***101.** Replication of DNA takes place in ______________ direction in ________ manner.

(a) 5′–3′ , template independent ☐ (b) 5′–3′ , template dependent ☐

(c) 3′–5′ , template independent ☐ (d) 3′–5′ , template dependent ☐

102. To form a *ds*DNA, it is necessary to join the DNA fragments for which single-stranded binding proteins are required. (*Rewrite the statement after correcting the underlined words.*)

____

103. A piece of DNA if needed to be propagated during recombinant DNA procedures, requires a vector because it provides

____

104. In eukaryotes, the replication of DNA takes place at G_0-phase of the cell cycle. (*Rewrite the statement after correcting the underlined word.*)

____

105. A cell has just doubled up its DNA content but due to a defect in regulatory mechanism they has stopped undergoing division. What is this condition known as?

____

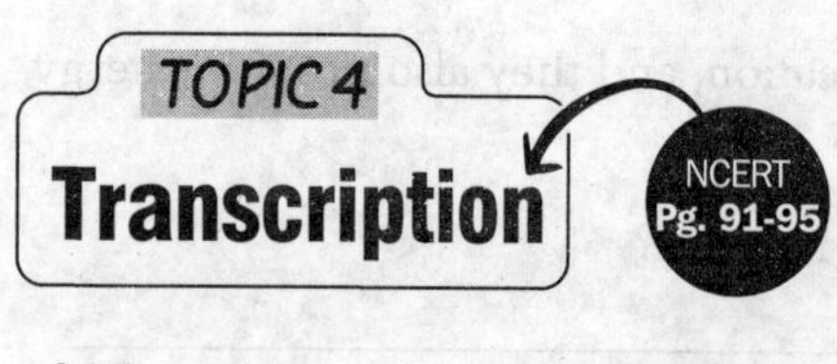

106. Give a scientific term for the following statement.
The process of copying genetic information from one strand of the DNA into RNA.

____

107. Since, RNA is involved, adenine will pair with ____________ while information is being copied from DNA to RNA.

108. In transcription, both segments of DNA are copied into RNA.

True ☐ False ☐

109. If both strands of DNA are transcribed, then two molecules of RNA with <u>similar sequences</u> are produced.
(*Rewrite the statement after correcting the underlined words.*)

110. Another complication arising from transcription of both DNA strands is the formation of *ds*RNA. This renders the exercise of transcription futile, Why?

____

111. Similar to replication, transcription also occurs bidirectionally.

True ☐ False ☐

112. How many of the following are components of a transcription unit?

Promoter, Replication fork, ori, Structural gene, Terminator, RNA coding gene, Ribozymes

____

113. Complete the following analogy with respect to DNA-dependent RNA polymerase.
$3'-5'$ strand : Template:: $5'-3'$ strand : ____________

***114.** Template strand → 3' - ATT-CCC-GGC-GCA-TGC-ATG-CAT-GCA- 5'
Coding strand → 5'- TAA-GGG-CCG-CGT-ACG-TAC-GTA-CGT -3'.
Based on this information, predict the sequence of RNA transcribed from above DNA.

____

115. Identify the structures *A, B, C* and *D* in the representation of a transcription unit.

Transcription start site
Ⓐ Ⓑ Ⓒ Ⓓ
3' 5'
5' 3'

A. ____________ B. ____________ C. ____________ D. ____________

116. With reference to structural genes, indicate the location of
(i) Promoter ____________________
(ii) Terminator ____________________

117. ____________ is a DNA sequence that provides a binding site for RNA polymerase.

118. ________________ usually defines the end of the process of transcription.

119. Give scientific term for the functional unit of inheritance. ____________________

120. Give scientific term for a segment of DNA coding for a polypeptide. ______________

121. Complete the following analogy.
Monocistronic unit : ________________ : : Polycistronic unit : Bacteria

***122.** The genes in eukaryotes are split. What does this mean?

____

***123.** Complete the following analogy.
______________ : Coding sequences : : Introns : Non-coding sequences

***124.** ______________ (Exons/Introns) are said to be those sequences that appear in mature or processed RNA.

125. Considering the following statements, identify the incorrect set of statements from the options below.

I. Introns appear in processed RNA.
II. DNA sequence coding for *t*RNA or *r*RNA molecule defines a gene.
III. Promoter is located towards the 3′-end of the structural gene while terminator is towards 5′-end.
IV. Cistron as a DNA segment codes for a polypeptide.
V. Introns interrupt exons.

Codes
(a) II, III and V ☐ (b) I, II, III and IV ☐
(c) II, IV and V ☐ (d) I and III ☐

126. Which of the following is not true with respect to types of RNA?
(a) *r*RNA – Translates *m*RNA with ribosomal protein ☐
(b) *m*RNA – Primary transcript from DNA ☐
(c) *m*RNA – Encodes amino acid sequence from polypeptide ☐
(d) *t*RNA – Brings amino acid to ribosome during translation ☐

127. Name the RNA that plays a structural and catalytic role during translation.

____

128. DNA dependent <u>DNA polymerase</u> catalyses transcription of all types of RNA in bacteria. (*Rewrite the statement after correcting the underlined words.*)

____

129. To begin the transcription, RNA polymerase recognises nucleotide sequence in ____________________ (promoter region / G -C rich region) of the DNA.

130. In prokaryotes, ________________ (single/three) RNA polymerase (s) is/are present.

131. RNA polymerase requires primer and has the ability to repair mistakes in RNA.

True ☐ False ☐

***132.** The three steps of transcription are depicted below in random order. Rearrange them in their proper sequence.

____

133. After the release of ________________ RNA polymerase core enzyme elongates the chain.

134. RNA polymerase uses ________________________ (deoxyribonucleoside diphosphates/ribonucleotide triphosphates) to elongate the chain.

135. Consider the following statements for initiation factor. Which of the following is correct statement?

(a) Rho is initiation factor ☐

(b) Association with these factor alter specificity for RNA polymerase ☐

(c) Initiation factor bind with DNA polymerase ☐

(d) Initiation factor remain binded throughout the transcription process ☐

***136.** Which of the following is the correct combination with respect to transcription?

(a) Promoter – rho factor ; Terminator – sigma factor ☐

(b) Promoter – sigma factor; Terminator – release factor ☐

(c) Promoter – release factor; Terminator – rho factor ☐

(d) Promoter – sigma factor; Terminator – rho factor ☐

137. Consider the following statements.

Statement I RNA polymerase-II can only catalyse the elongation step of transcription.

Statement II Initiation and termination of transcription requires sigma and rho factors.

Choose the correct option from the following.

(a) Statement I is true, but statement II is false ☐

(b) Statement I is false, but statemet II is true ☐

(c) Both statements I and II are true ☐

(d) Both statements I and II are false ☐

138. Complete the following analogy.

Transcription in bacteria : ________________ : : Transcription in eukaryotes : Nucleus

139. In bacteria, translation begin much before the *m*RNA is fully transcribed because

(i) *m*RNA requires processing to become active.

(ii) Transcription and translation occur in same compartment.

____

140. Name the type of RNA polymerase enzyme associated with functions mentioned below.

(i) Transcribes *r*RNAs ________________

(ii) Transcription of *t*RNA, 5*sr*RNA and *sn*RNAs ________________

(iii) Precursor of *m*RNA and the *hn* RNA ________________

***141.** Apart from having three RNA polymerases, name an additional complexity present in eukaryotic transcription.

____

***142.** Pick the odd one out.

Splicing, Capping, Transformation, Tailing

____

***143.** In post-transcriptional processing, exons are excised and hydrolysed before *m*RNA moves out of the nucleus.

True ☐ False ☐

***144.** Most eukaryotic pre *m*RNAs are matured by undergoing modifications to their ends. Name these modifications.________________________

***145.** Observe the figure given below and answer the following questions.

(i) Name the process depicted by the figure. ________________

(ii) The exons and the introns together make the ________ which is non-functional.

(iii) The introns are removed and exons are joined in a defined order by a process called ________________ .

(iv) *hn*RNA undergoes two additional processes for maturation. In ________, an unusual nucleotide is added to the 5'-end of *hn*RNA. In tailing, ________ residues are added at 3'-end in a template independent manner by the process called ________

***146.** The fully processed *hn*RNA is called exon that is transported out of the nucleus for translation.

True ☐ False ☐

TOPIC 5

Genetic Code

NCERT Pg. 95-98

147. Give the scientific term for the sequence of nitrogenous bases in *m*RNA coding for single amino acid.

____

148. Complete the table given below.

Scientists	Contributions
George Gamow	(A)
(B)	Synthesised RNA molecules with defined combinations of bases
Marshall Nirenberg	(C)
(D)	Enzymatic synthesis of RNA

A. ________ B. ________ C. ________ D. ________

***149.** Mention the characteristic feature of genetic codes associated with the following characteristics.

(i) Three nucleotide bases together make a codon. ________

(ii) A codon specifies same amino acid in all organisms. ________

(iii) A codon is read continuously. ________

(iv) More than one codon codes for one amino acid. ________

***150.** AUG codon performs dual functions.

True ☐ False ☐

***151.** Complete the following analogy.

Initiation codon : AUG :: Termination codon : ________________ .

***152.** Pick the odd one out.

GUG, UAG, UGA, UAA

____

***153.** Degeneracy is due to ________________ (first /last) base in the codon.

***154.** If GUU, GUC, GUA and GUG all code for amino acid valine, it means that the genetic code is

(a) degenerate ☐ (b) universal ☐
(c) triplet ☐ (d) contiguous ☐

155. Stop codons are also called ____________ or ____________ codons.

156. If following is the sequence of nucleotides in *m*RNA, predict the sequence of amino acid coded by it– AUG CUU UUU AAA UGU GGU UUG.

____

***157.** We know that AUG is an initiation codon, while UAA/UAG/UGA are termination codons. A polypeptide cannot be synthesised if it encounters any of the latter codons. On the basis of this information identify the *m*RNA chain that can be translated completely,

(AUG UAU UUC UGC CUC UAG / AUG UUC UCC UGA UGG UUA.)

158. Pick the odd one out.

CUU, CUC, CCA, CUG

____

159. Codon GGU codes for amino acid glycine which is also a function of CGU, UAU and AGG.

(*Rewrite the statement after correcting the underlined phrase.*)

____

160. Give a scientific term for an alternation in the nucleotide sequence of the genome of an organism. ____________________________

161. A change in base sequence alters the phenotype.

True ☐ False ☐

162. A single nucleotide pair is inserted near the 5' end of a protein coding DNA sequence. Its most likely effect will be the production of a protein with

(i) single altered amino acid. ☐
(ii) completely altered sequence. ☐

(*Tick* ☑ *the most accurate option*)

163. Complete the following analogy.

Point mutation : Change in single base : : Frameshift mutation:________________

164. A classical example of __________ mutation is sickle-cell anaemia.

165. A change of single base pair in the gene for ____________ chain results in the change of amino acid residue from glutamate to ____________, resulting in sickle-cell anaemia.

166. Write the correct bases at the 6th position of DNA, RNA and amino acids of the beta chain of haemoglobin which results in sickle-cell anaemia.

____

167. What is a common consequence of insertion and deletion of base pairs in codons?

___

168. Who postulated the presence of an adapter molecule for reading the code and to link it to the amino acids?

___

169. *r*RNA is an adapter molecule.

True ☐ False ☐

170. Complete the sentence and the figure given below

(i) There was a need for an adapter molecule because ________.

(ii) Identify the parts labelled as *A, B* and *C* in the given figure of *t*RNA (an adapter molecule).

A. ________

B. ________

C. ________

171. Consider the following statements.

I. Effects of smaller deletions and rearrangements in a DNA segment are easy to comprehend.

II. Insertion or deletion of one or two bases changes the reading frame from the point of insertion or deletion.

III. There are 3 *t*RNAs for stop codons.

IV. In reality, tRNA appears as a compact molecule which looks like inverted L.

V. *t*RNA has anticodon loop, amino acids and an acceptor molecule.

Choose the set of incorrect statements from the options below.

(a) II and V ☐ (b) I and III ☐

(c) III and IV ☐ (d) IV and V ☐

TOPIC 6

Translation

NCERT Pg. 98-99

172. Give a scientific term for the process of polymerisation of amino acids to form a polypeptide.

___

173. The order and sequence of amino acids are defined by the sequence of bases in the *t*RNA.

True ☐ False ☐

174. During translation, proteins are synthesised by ribosomes using the information on ________________ .

175. Observe the figure given below and answer the questions related to it.

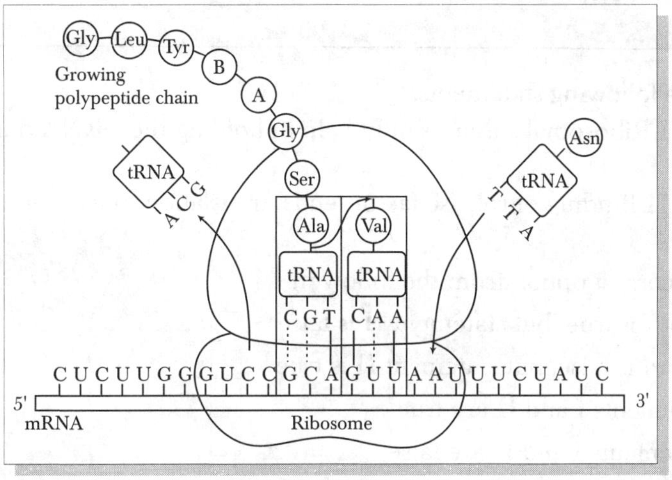

(i) Identify the process shown in the figure. ____________________

(ii) Identify the amino acids *A* and *B* coded by the CUU and UCU codons on *m*RNA chain. ________________________

***176.** Which of the following provides energy for peptide bond formation during translation?

(a) Binding of amino acid to cognate tRNA molecules ☐

(b) Activation of amino acid in the presence of ATP ☐

(c) Base pairing between codon and anticodon arm ☐

(d) Joining of the small and large subunits of ribosome ☐

***177.** Amino acids are linked to their cognate *t*RNA in a process commonly called as *X*. Identify *X*.

____

178. Ribosomes in their inactive state in eukaryotes have two subunits, i.e. a smaller ________________ and a larger ________________ units.

____

179. 23S *r*RNA in bacteria is the enzyme called <u>ribonuclease</u>.

(*Rewrite the statement after correcting the underlined word.*)

____

180. Expand UTR. ____

181. The UTRs on the *m*RNA have additional sequences which are not translated, thus making this region futile.

True ☐ False ☐

***182.** How many of the following are essential requirements for the translation process?

Initiation factors, RNA polymerase, hnRNA, Elongation factors, GTPase, mRNA, tRNA, Aminoacyl tRNA synthetase, Amino acids

____

***183.** Given below are the steps involved in the translation process.

Chain formation, Activation of amino acids, Modifications, Initiation, Termination

Rearrange these steps in the correct sequence of protein synthesis.

____

184. Consider the following statements.

Statement I Ribosomal subunits only help in holding the *m*RNA during translation process.

Statement II Binding of release factor, ends translation, releasing the polypeptide from ribosome.

Choose the correct option from the following

(a) Statement I is true, but statement II is false ☐
(b) Statement I is false, but statement II is true ☐
(c) Both statements I and II are true ☐
(d) Both statements I and II are false ☐

185. Given below is the flowchart depicting the steps of translation.

Initiation begins when the ribosomes bind to *m*RNA at the start codon AUG recognised by (*A*).

↓

(*B*)

↓

Ribosomes move from codon to codon along the *m*RNA

↓

(*C*)

↓

(*D*)

↓

Polypeptide is released from the ribosome.

Identify *A, B, C* and *D*.

A. ____________ B. ____________ C. ____________ D. ____________

TOPIC 7

Regulation of Gene Expression

NCERT Pg. 99-101

186. Gene expression can be regulated at all these levels except

(a) transcriptional level ☐ (b) processing level ☐
(c) translational level ☐ (d) replication level ☐

187. Refer to the reaction given below in *E. coli*,

Lactose $\xrightarrow{(A)}$ Galactose and Glucose. Identify *A*.

____

188. If the bacteria do not have lactose around them to be utilised for energy source

(i) they would require the enzyme needed for lactose metabolism. ☐

(ii) they would not require enzyme. ☐

(*Tick* ✔ *the most accurate option.*)

189. The metabolic, physiological or environmental conditions can regulate the expression of genes.

True ☐ False ☐

190. In a transcription unit, the activity of ________________ polymerase at a given promoter is in turn regulated by interaction with ______________ proteins which affects its ability to recognise start sites.

191. *Lac* operon is a monocistronic structural gene.

(*Rewrite the statement after correcting the underlined word.*)

____

192. Match the following columns.

Column I (Enzymes)	Column II (Functions)
A. Beta galactosidase	1. Attaches a particular chemical group to target molecules
B. Permease	2. Hydrolysis of lactose sugar
C. Transacetylase	3. Increases permeability of the cell to β-galactosidase

A. ______________ B. ______________ C. ______________

***193.** Give a scientific term for a functional unit of transcription and genetic regulation.

____

***194.** Consider the following statements.

Statement I In the presence of glucose, the repressor binds to the operator of *lac* operon.

Statement II Low level of expression of *lac* operon allow lactose to enter into cell by action of permease.

Choose the correct option from the following.

(a) Statement I is true, but statement II is false ☐

(b) Statement I is false, but statement II is true ☐

(c) Both statements I and II are true ☐

(d) Both statements I and II are false ☐

195. Genes that are continually being expressed in mast cells are ______ genes.

(a) repressible ☐ (b) inducer ☐ (c) constitutive ☐ (d) operator ☐

196. Bacterial cells under starvation were provided with allolactose. Which of the following will not take place in such a situation?

(a) RNA polymerase will bind to the promoter of the *lac* operon ☐

(b) Permease would increase the cell's permeability to allolactose ☐

(c) The *i* gene would be switched off and no repressor would be made ☐

(d) β-galactosidase will break lactose to glucose and galactose ☐

***197.** In an inducible operon, a free repressor cannot bind to the operator.

True ☐ False ☐

***198.** Answer the questions related to the diagram.

(i) *Lac* operon as illustrated in the figure is switched ______________ (on/off).

(ii) *X* is the inducer of the given operon. ______________ (True/False).

(iii) To which component of operon, *X* is binding? ______________

(iv) The elucidation of *lac* operon was carried out by ______________ and ______________.

***199.** Observe the figure given below and answer the related questions.

(i) The *lac* operon in figure indicates that lactose is absent in the medium.

True ☐ False ☐

(ii) Name the recognition centre for RNA polymerase in this operon. ______________

(iii) Gene that gives accessibility to RNA polymerase facilitating expression of structural genes is ______________.

(iv) Which gene component produces a repressor protein that binds to the *o*-gene? ______________

***200.** Given below are steps involved in *lac* operon.

A. ______________

B. ______________

***201.** Glucose and galactose cannot act as inducers for *lac* operon because they cannot bind with repressor.

True ☐ False ☐

202. Regulation of *lac* operon by repressor is <u>positive</u> regulation.

(Rewrite the statement after correcting the underlined word.)

____

TOPIC 8

Human Genome Project

NCERT Pg. 102-105

203. The genetic makeup of an organism or an individual lies in his/her DNA sequences.

True ☐ False ☐

204. Name any two techniques of genetic engineering that helped in the launching of human genome sequencing project?

____

205. Expand HGP. ______________________________

206. HGP was launched in year ______________ (1990/1992).

207. Human Genome Project (HGP) was called a mega project. (*Give reason*)

____

208. Human genome contains approximately ________ base pairs.

209. What is total estimated cost of human genome project?

____

210. HGP was closely associated with the rapid development of a new area in biology called biotechnology.

True ☐ False ☐

211. A goal of HGP was to identify all the genes in the human genome which numbered approximately 50,000-55,000 genes.

(*Rewrite the statement after correcting the underlined words.*)

____

212. The information generated from HGP was stored in monographs.

True ☐ False ☐

213. Human genome project was a ________ (13/17) years project.

214. Name the agencies which coordinated the human genome project.

____

215. Which of the following was not a goal of HGP?

Improve manpower for data analysis, Store information in databases

____

216. How many of the following organisms have their genome sequenced?

Bacteria, Yeast, Caenorhabditis elegans, Drosophila, Rice, Arabidopsis, Sparrow

____

***217.** Name the major approaches used in HGP for identifying genes.

____

***218.** Sequencing the entire genome containing all the coding and non-coding sequences and assigning them to different regions in the sequence of functions is associated with ____________ (expressed sequence tags/sequence annotation).

***219.** In order to sequence the human genome, what would have been the first step?

(a) Assign ESTs to the genome ☐ (b) Using automated DNA sequencers ☐

(c) Choose a proper cloning vector ☐ (d) Digest the DNA into fragments ☐

220. Steps of sequencing genome are given below.

Total DNA from a cell is isolated and converted into relatively smaller sized pieces

↓

(A)

↓

Amplification of each piece of DNA fragment using (B)

↓

(C)

↓

(D)

These sequences were subsequently annotated and were assigned to each chromosome. The missing steps are written below, label each of these steps as *A*, *B*, *C* and *D*.

Cloning in a suitable host using specialised vectors, Alignment of these sequences, Fragments were sequenced using automated DNA sequencers, PCR

A. ____________ B. ____________ C. ____________ D. ____________

221. The commonly used hosts for cloning were Drosophila and pea for which YAC and BAC vectors are used.

(*Rewrite the statement after correcting the underlined words.*)

____

222. The last chromosome to be sequenced in HGP was ____________.

223. Genetic and physical maps of genome were generated using the information

(i) derived from all parts of the body.

(ii) on polymorphism of restriction endonuclease recognition sites and satellite DNA.

____

224. Largest known human gene is ____________ that has been sequenced with 2.4 million bases.

225. What per cent of the human genome codes for proteins?

____

***226.** Consider the following statements.

Statement I About 98% of the human genome does not code for any functional protein.

Statement II SNPs are the regions of the human genome with a single base difference.

Choose the correct option from the following.

(a) Statement I is true, but statement II is false ☐
(b) Statement I is false, but statement II is true ☐
(c) Both statements I and II are true ☐
(d) Both statements I and II are false ☐

227. Complete the following analogy.

Chromosome 1 : 2968 genes :: ____________ : 231 genes

228. Expand SNPs.____________

TOPIC 9

DNA Fingerprinting

NCERT Pg. 105-107

229. Almost 99.9 per cent nucleotide bases differ among all people responsible for phenotypic variations.

True ☐ False ☐

***230.** ____________ sequences in our DNA are used for studying chromosomal structure, evolution, etc.

231. Name a quick way to compare the DNA sequences of any two individuals.

____

232. What forms the basis of DNA fingerprinting technique?

____

***233.** Which of the following does not form the basis of classification for satellite DNA?

(a) A:T or G:C rich base composition ☐
(b) Length of segment ☐
(c) Number of repetitive unit ☐
(d) Number of base pair in *m*RNA ☐

***234.** DNA fingerprinting is the basis of paternity testing in case of disputes because

(i) polymorphism in DNA is inheritable. ☐
(ii) Satellite DNA is absent in human genome. ☐

(*Tick* ☑ *the most accurate option.*)

235. Give a scientific term for variations at genetic level.

____

***236.** Polymorphisms arise due to mutations.

True ☐ False ☐

237. A mutation can only spread to offspring when it has occurred in somatic cells of sexually reproducing parents. (*Rewrite the statement after correcting the underlined words.*)

____

238. An inheritable mutation occurring at high frequency is called ____________

***239.** Name the scientist who developed the technique of DNA fingerprinting.

____

240. Expand VNTR. ____________

***241.** VNTRs are ____________ (mini satellites/micro satellites).

242. Steps of DNA fingerprinting technique are indicated in the flowchart given below.

(i) Separation of DNA fragments by electrophoresis.
(ii) Digestion of DNA.
(iii) Transferring of separated DNA fragments to synthetic membranes.
(iv) Isolation of DNA.
(v) Hybridisation using labelled VNTR probe.
(vi) Detection of hybridised DNA fragments by autoradiography.

Arrange these steps in a sequential manner.

____

243. Complete the following analogy with respect to fingerprinting techniques.

Digestion of DNA : ____________ :: Separation of DNA fragments : Electrophoresis

244. The size of VNTRs varies from 10-20 kb.

True ☐ False ☐

245. Blood from crime scene was assessed by a forensic lab and the DNA was matched with the DNA from two possible suspects. The following image gives the gel electrophoresis and autoradiography data. Study the given image and choose the possible criminal.

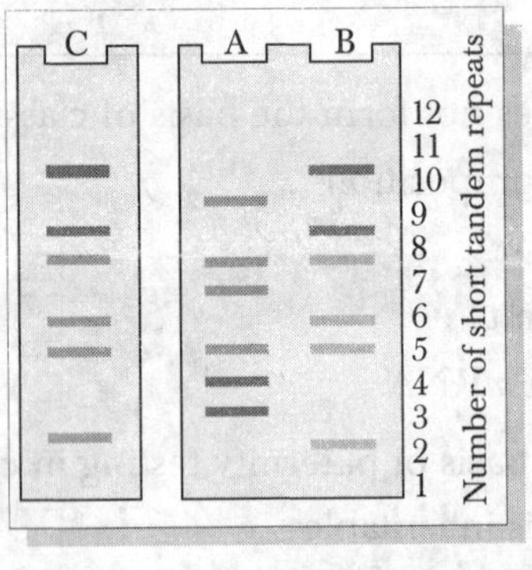

(a) Neither of them is criminal ☐ (b) Both of them are criminals ☐
(c) A is the criminal ☐ (d) B is the criminal ☐

246. Autoradiogram gives many bands of differing sizes. These bands give a characteristic pattern for an individual DNA. It differs from individual to individual in a population except in ____________ .

247. ____________ (PCR/Autoradiography) has increased the sensitivity of fingerprinting technique.

248. Given below is the electrophoretic reading carried out on a DNA sample found at a site of murder.

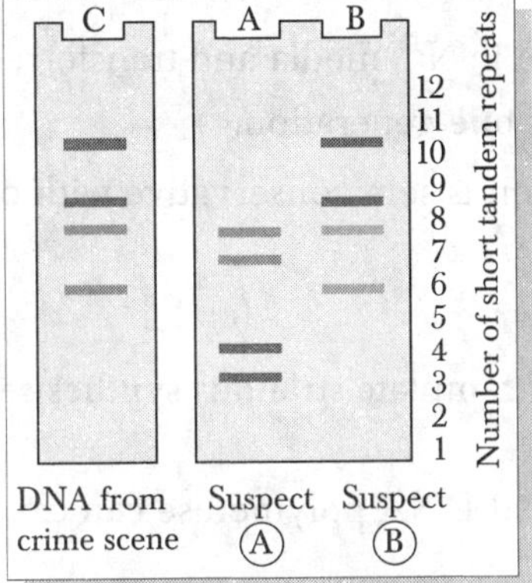

Among the two suspects *A* and *B* which is most likely to have not committed the crime?

Assertion-Reason Questions

The following questions consist of two statements- Assertion (A) and Reason (R). Answer these questions by selecting the appropriate option given below.

(a) Both A and R are true and R is the correct explanation of A

(b) Both A and R are true, but R is not the correct explanation of A

(c) A is true, but R is false

(d) A is false, but R is true

***1.** **Assertion** (A) It is easier to break the bond between adenine and thymine, than between guanine and cytosine.

Reason (R) Adenine pairs with thymine by two hydrogen bonds where as guanine pairs with cytosine by three hydrogen bonds.

(a) ☐ (b) ☐ (c) ☐ (d) ☐

***2.** **Assertion** (A) The assembly of DNA and histone is a stable one, that forms the beads on string structure.

Reason (R) Negatively charged histone proteins are attracted by the positively charged backbone of DNA.

(a) ☐ (b) ☐ (c) ☐ (d) ☐

3. **Assertion** (A) In Griffiths experiment, heat killed S strain could transform the living R strain bacteria.

Reason (R) R strain of bacteria were non virulent as it lacked the smooth polysaccharide coat.

(a) ☐ (b) ☐ (c) ☐ (d) ☐

***4.** **Assertion** (A) DNA and RNA both are able to mutate and can be used for stably storing the genetic information of an organism.

Reason (R) RNA contains a reactive OH group attached to the 2' Carbon atom, which makes it labile.

(a) ☐ (b) ☐ (c) ☐ (d) ☐

***5. Assertion** (A) *E. coli* grown in N^{15} media and transferred to N^{14} media would show intermediate densities after one generation.

Reason (R) DNA replication is semiconservative with one parental and another newly synthesised strand.

(a) ☐ (b) ☐ (c) ☐ (d) ☐

6. Assertion (A) The 3' → 5' template strand is synthesised in a discontinuous manner during replication.

Reason (R) DNA dependent DNA polymerase can catalyse polymerisation only in the direction 5' to 3'.

(a) ☐ (b) ☐ (c) ☐ (d) ☐

7. Assertion (A) For transcription, the 3'→ 5' strand of DNA acts as the template for RNA polymerase.

Reason (R) The DNA strand with polarity 5' → 3' acts as the non-coding strand during transcription.

(a) ☐ (b) ☐ (c) ☐ (d) ☐

8. Assertion (A) Monocistronic genes of eukaryotes undergo splicing post DNA transcription.

Reason (R) Intervening sequences in a monocistronic genes, do not code for functional proteins.

(a) ☐ (b) ☐ (c) ☐ (d) ☐

***9. Assertion** (A) RNA polymerase-II cannot catalyse all three steps of a transcription process.

Reason (R) The sigma factor binds to RNA polymerase and catalyse the initiation of transcription.

(a) ☐ (b) ☐ (c) ☐ (d) ☐

10. Assertion (A) Inserting 2 bases in a reading frame would result in frame shift mutation.

Reason (R) Deleting 3 bases would cause no alteration to the reading frame from the point onwards.

(a) ☐ (b) ☐ (c) ☐ (d) ☐

***11. Assertion** (A) The repressor protein that switches off the *lac* operon is constitutively expressed.

Reason (R) Lactose can bind directly to the operator and stimulate RNA polymerase to transcribe.

(a) ☐ (b) ☐ (c) ☐ (d) ☐

***12. Assertion** (A) VNTRs used during DNA fingerprinting shows high degree of polymorphism.

Reason (R) In forensics, the labelled VNTR probes are hybridised with sample DNA in a membrane.

(a) ☐ (b) ☐ (c) ☐ (d) ☐

Case Based Questions

***1.** The following image shows a famous experiment that was conducted in 1958. Study the image carefully and answer the questions that follow.

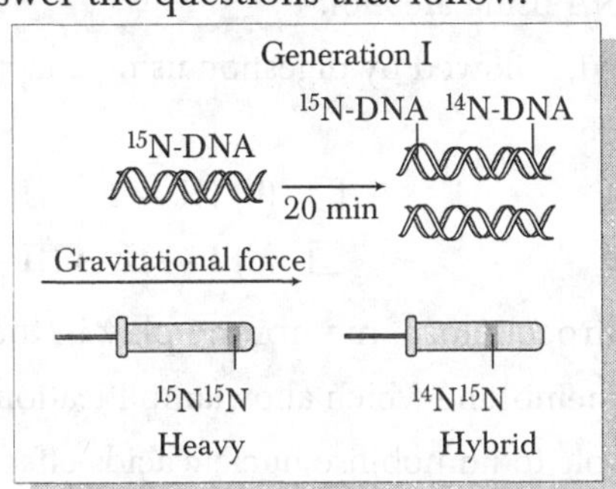

(i) A person can conclude the actual difference between N^{14} and N^{15} DNA by

(a) using autoradiography ☐

(b) using Southern blotting ☐

(c) using density gradient centrifugation ☐

(d) using gel electrophoresis ☐

(ii) What would be the ratio of hybrid to light after 80 minutes in the experiment?

(a) 1:3 ☐ (b) 1:7 ☐ (c) 1:2 ☐ (d) 1:1 ☐

(iii) Which of the following conclusions can be derived from this experiment?

(a) DNA is the genetic material ☐

(b) 99.9 % of DNA is similar in humans ☐

(c) DNA replication is semiconservative ☐

(d) DNA prefers N^{14} over N^{15} ☐

2. The given figure relates to the procedure followed for DNA fingerprinting.

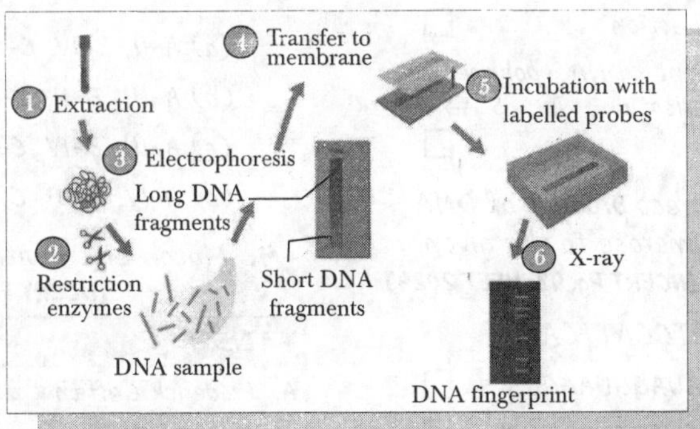

(i) Identify the incorrect statement w.r.t. DNA fingerprinting.

(a) DNA fingerprinting is a chemical test that shows the genetic makeup of an individual ☐

(b) DNA fingerprinting involves identifying differences in some specific regions in DNA sequence called ribosomal DNA ☐

(c) It proves to be a useful technique in case of paternity testing ☐

(d) Polymorphism in DNA sequence is the fundamental basis of DNA fingerprinting ☐

(ii) A scientist working on DNA extraction will follow a specific order of the below given steps.

I. Cell wall lysis and breakdown of nuclear membrane.

II. Using chilled ethanol in order to get DNA in precipitated form.

III. Purification of DNA using alcohol.

IV. Storage, if required, followed by digestion using enzymes.

Identify the correct order.

(a) II → III → I → IV ☐ (b) III → I → II → IV ☐

(c) I → III → II → IV ☐ (d) I → II → III → IV ☐

(iii) What role does the nitrocellulose membrane play in the technique?

(a) These are popular membrane which allow amplification of VNTRs ☐

(b) The membrane is able to immobilise nucleic acids effectively ☐

(c) These catalyse digestion of DNA in efficient manner ☐

(d) Increase the sensitivity of the technique ☐

COMPETITION EDGE UP

1. Which of the following statement is correct regarding the process of replication in E. coli? **[NCERT Pg. 90, NEET 2024]**

(a) The DNA-dependent DNA polymerase catalyses polymerisation in one direction that is 3′ → 5′ ☐

(b) The DNA-dependent RNA polymerase catalyses polymerisation in one direction, that is 5′ → 3′ ☐

(c) The DNA-dependent DNA polymerase catalyses polymerisation in 5′ → 3′ as well as 3′ → 5′ direction ☐

(d) The DNA-dependent DNA polymerase catalyses polymerisation in 5′ → 3′ direction ☐

2. Which one is the correct product of DNA dependent RNA polymerase to the given template? **[NCERT Pg. 92, NEET 2024]**

3‘TACATGGCAAATATCCATTCA5’

(a) 5‘AUGUACCGUUUAUAGGUAAGU3’ ☐

(b) 5‘AUGUAAAGUUUAUAGGUAAGU3’ ☐

(c) 5‘AUGUACCGUUUAAGGGAAGU3’ ☐

(d) 5‘ATGTACCGTTTATAGGTAAGT3’ ☐

3. Match List I with List II.

List I	List II
A. RNA polymerase	I. snRNPs
B. Termination of transcription	II. Promotor
C. Splicing of exons	III. rho factor
D. TATA box	IV. snRNAs, tRNA

Choose the correct answer from the options given below : **[NCERT Pg. 94, 95, NEET 2024]**

(a) A-II, B-IV, C-I, D-III ☐

(b) A-III, B-II, C-IV, D-I ☐

(c) A-III, B-IV, C-I, D-II ☐

(d) A-IV, B-III, C-I, D-II ☐

4. Match List I with List II. **[NCERT Pg. 84, 89, 95, 100, NEET 2024]**

List I	List II
A. Frederick Griffith	I. Genetic code
B. Francois Jacob and Jacque Monod	II. Semi-conservative mode of DNA replication
C. Har Gobind Khorana	III. Transformation
D. Meselson and Stahl	IV. Lac operon

Choose the correct answer from the options given below.

(a) A-III, B-II, C-I, D-IV

(b) A-III, B-IV, C-I, D-II

(c) A-II, B-III, C-IV, D-I

(d) A-IV, B-I, C-II, D-III

5. Given below are two statements.

Statement I In prokaryotes, the positively charged DNA is held with some negatively charged proteins in a region called nucleoid.

Statement II In eukaryotes, the negatively charged DNA is wrapped around the positively charged histone octamer to form nucleosome.

In the light of the above statements, choose the correct answer from the options given below **[NCERT Pg. 83, NEET 2023]**

(a) Both statement I and statement II are false

(b) Statement I is true, but statement II is false

(c) Statement I is false, but statement II is true

(d) Both statement I and statement II are true

6. Given below are two statements.

Statement I RNA mutates at a faster rate.

Statement II Viruses having RNA genome and shorter lifespan mutate and evolve faster. **[NCERT Pg. 87, NEET 2023]**

In the light of the above statements, choose the correct answer from the options given below.

(a) Both statement I and statement II are false

(b) Statement I is true, but statement II is false

(c) Statement I is false, but statement II is true

(d) Both statement I and statement II are true

7. Which one of the following is the sequence on corresponding coding strand, if the sequence on mRNA formed is as follows

5'AUCGAUCGAUCGAUCGAUCGAUCG AUCG 3'? **[NEET 2023]**

(a) 3'UAGCUAGCUAGCUAGCUAGCUAGCUAGC 5'

(b) 5'ATCGATCGATCGATCGATCGATCGATCG 3'

(c) 3'ATCGATCGATCGATCGATCGATCGATCG 5'

(d) 5'UAGCUAGCUAGCUAGCUAGCUAGCUAGC 3'

8. What is the role of RNA polymerase-III in the process of transcription in eukaryotes? **[NCERT Pg. 95, NEET 2023, 21]**

(a) Transcribes rRNAs (28S, 18S and 5.8S)

(b) Transcribes tRNA (5S rRNA and snRNA)

(c) Transcribes precursor of mRNA

(d) Transcribes only snRNAs

9. If a geneticist uses the blind approach for sequencing the whole genome of an organism, followed by assignment of function to different segments, the methodology adopted by him is called as, **[NCERT Pg. 103, NEET 2022]**

(a) gene mapping

(b) expressed sequence tags

(c) bioinformatics

(d) sequence annotation

10. Read the following statements and choose the set of correct statements. **[NCERT Pg. 83, 84, NEET 2022]**

I. Euchromatin is loosely packed chromatin.

II. Heterochromatin is transcriptionally active.

III. Histone octamer is wrapped by negatively charged DNA in nucleosome.

IV. Histones are rich in lysine and arginine.

V. A typical nucleosome contains 400 bp of DNA helix.

Choose the correct answer from the options given below.

(a) I, III and IV (b) II and V

(c) I, III and V (d) II, IV and V

11. If adenine makes 30% of the DNA molecule, what will be the percentage of thymine, guanine and cytosine in it? **[NCERT Pg. 81, NEET 2021]**

(a) T : 20, G : 30, C : 20

(b) T : 20, G : 20, C : 30

(c) T : 30, G : 20, C : 20

(d) T : 20, G : 25, C : 25

Chapter 06

Evolution

Scan and take Chapter Test

TOPIC 1

Origin of Life and Evolution of Life Forms

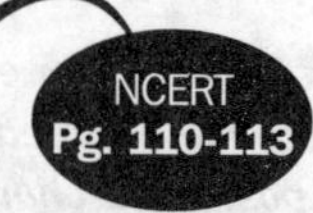

1. Name the branch of science which deals with the study of history of life forms on earth.

____

2. Changes in the flora and fauna on earth in past times can be understood by studying evolution of earth, stars and universe.

True ☐ False ☐

3. Stellar distances are measured in _______________ (kilometers/light years).

4. The stars we see today emitted light _______________ years back.

***5.** Match the following columns.

Column I	Column II
A. Universe	1. 4.5 billion years
B. Earth	2. 4 billion years
C. First life form on earth	3. 20 billion years

A.__________ B.__________ C.__________

6. Name the theory which explains the origin of universe as a singular huge explosion unimaginable in physical terms.

____

7. Arrange the following steps in the sequence of their occurrence during universe formation.

I. Formation of simplest elements, i.e. hydrogen and helium.
II. Cataclysmic eruption of hot, energy rich subatomic particles.
III. Universe expansion and lowered temperature.
IV. Formation of galaxies.
V. Condensation of gases.

____

8. The universe expanded and hence, the temperature came down

True ☐ False ☐

*Concepts of all questions bearing * are important for NEET & CUET*

9. The atmosphere on early earth was rich in oxides and hydrogen.

True ☐ False ☐

***10.** Out of the components listed below,
which of the following did not cover the surface of early earth?

(a) Methane ☐ (b) Carbon dioxide ☐

(c) Ammonia ☐ (d) Oxygen ☐

---

11. Complete the following flowchart by filling the blanks *A, B* and *C* depicting the various reactions that might have occurred on early earth.

Water vapours —Ⓐ→ Escaped hydrogen + Ⓑ

↓

Water + CO_2 + Ammonia + Ⓒ

A.____________ B.____________ C.____________

12. The ________ were formed on earth when ________ layer was cooled and water vapours fell as rain to fill all the depressions.

***13.** Louis Pasteur demonstrated that life comes from pre-existing life and thus, dismissed the <u>theory of biogenesis.</u>

(*Rewrite the statement after correcting the underlined words.*)

***14.** Oparin and Haldane proposed that first form of life could have come from ________________ (Pre-existing, living, inorganic molecules/ Pre-existing, non-living, organic molecules).

***15.** Consider the following statements.

Statement I Chemical evolution states that complex inorganic molecules arose from organic ones.

Statement II High temperature, reducing atmosphere, volcanic storms predominated in early earth.

Choose the correct option from the following.

(a) Statement I is true, but statement II is false ☐

(b) Statement I is false, but statement II is true ☐

(c) Both statements I and II are true ☐

(d) Both statements I and II are false ☐

16. Formation of diverse organic molecules from inorganic constituents occurred during ____________ evolution.

17. According to Oparin and Haldane, chemical evolution occurred after the biological evolution on earth.

True ☐ False ☐

18. How many of the listed conditions were found on the early earth?

Low temperature, Volcanic storms, Reducing atmosphere, CH_4 and NH_3 in atmosphere

____

19. Name the scientist who created early earth conditions in a laboratory scale.

____

***20.** Given below are few statements regarding the famous experiment conducted by Miller. Select the option with the incorrect statement.

I. He created electric discharge in a closed flask containing CH_4, H_2, NH_3 and water vapour at 800°C.

II. He observed the formation of proteins, e.g lysine, isoleucine and valine.

III. He created reducing atmospheric conditions in a laboratory scale.

Codes

(a) Only I ☐ (b) Only II ☐

(c) I and III ☐ (d) II and III ☐

21. Refer to the diagram given below and answer the questions that follow.

(i) Name the three gases in flask labelled as *A*.______________ .

(ii) What was the temperature inside flask *B*, which formed water vapours (H_2O)?

____

(iii) What was formed and observed by Miller in the flask *A*?

____

(iv) In the similar setup, what was formed and observed by other scientists in the flask *A*?

____

22. The compounds formed in Miller's experiment were similar to those in earth's crust. (*Rewrite the statement after correcting the underlined words.*)

____

23. The first non-cellular life forms must have been originated __________ years ago in the form of giant molecules like ____________________.

***24.** The first cellular form of life is believed to have originated about __________ (2000/200) million years ago (mya).

25. Complete the analogy given below.

First non-cellular forms : Giant molecules : : First cellular forms : __________

26. All life forms are believed to have originated on land only.

True ☐ False ☐

27. Give biological term for the formation of first form of life from non-living molecules through slow evolutionary forces.

____

***28.** Match Column I with Column II.

Column I	Column II
A. Theory of Panspermia	1. Life originated from spores
B. Theory of special creation	2. Life arose from non-living molecules through evolutionary force
C. Theory of spontaneous generation	3. Diversity is same since creation
D. Theory of biogenesis	4. Rotting matter created life

	A	B	C	D			A	B	C	D	
(a)	1	3	4	2	☐	(b)	1	4	3	2	☐
(c)	1	2	4	3	☐	(d)	1	3	2	4	☐

29. An incorrect connotations with regard to the theory of special creation is

(i) All existing living organisms were created as such and the diversity was always the same since creation.

(ii) Earth is about 3000 years old.

____

***30.** Charles Darwin observed evolutionary history of earth during a sea voyage in a ship called ____________________.

31. How many of the listed conclusions were drawn by Charles Darwin during his voyage around world?

Similarities of living forms with past forms, Extinction of life forms, Gradual evolution of life forms, Formation of new life forms, No variations in a population.

____

***32.** Consider the following statements.

Statement I An organism who can adapt more, has better chances of survival than others.

Statement II According to Darwin, reproductively fit organisms are selected by nature.

Choose the correct option from the following.

(a) Statement I is true, but statement II is false ☐
(b) Statement I is false, but statement II is true ☐
(c) Both statements I and II are true ☐
(d) Both statements I and II are false ☐

33. According to Darwin, reproductive fitness helps organisms to better fit in an environment and leave more progeny than others.

True ☐ False ☐

34. Give technical term for the phenomenon which acts as mechanism of evolution (according to Darwin).

____

35. Which of the following cannot be concluded from the theory of Natural selection proposed by Darwin?

(a) Variations allow an organism to survive better. ☐
(b) Nature selects organisms with better adaptability ☐
(c) Reproductive fitness allows organisms to have more progenies ☐
(d) Variations occur due to random mutations in a population ☐

36. ____________, a naturalist who worked in Malay Archipelago, concluded that all existing life forms share ____________ ancestors which were present in ____________ periods in the history of earth.

37. The geological history of earth does not coincide with the biological history of earth.

True ☐ False ☐

TOPIC 2

What are the Evidences for Evolution?

NCERT Pg. 113-116

38. Give biological term for the remains of hard parts of life forms found in rocks.

____

39. The rocks in which fossils are found, are called ____________.

40. In the cross-section of earth's crust, the most primitive fossil would be found in ____________ (lower sediments/upper sediments).

41. All new forms of life have arisen at different times in the history of earth called____________.

***42.** Name the method used to determine the age of fossils.

____

43. The study of fossils in different sedimentary layers indicates the Permian period. (*Rewrite the statement after correcting the underlined words.*)

____

44. Which of the following is not true with respect to fossil record?

(a) They are paleontological evidences ☐

(b) They showed life forms varied over time ☐

(c) They indicate geological period of extinct animal ☐

(d) They can tell about genetic composition of extinct animal ☐

45. Refer to the family tree of dinosaurs given below and answer the questions that follow.

(i) Name the organisms labelled as *A*, *B* and *C*.

A. ____________

B. ____________

C. ____________

(ii) The given family tree is showing extinct animals only.

Yes ☐ No ☐

(iii) Name any two modern day counterpart organisms of dinosaurs.

____

46. Which of the following is a flying reptile?

(a) *Pteranodon* ☐ (b) *Brachiosaurus* ☐

(c) *Triceratops* ☐ (d) *Stegosaurus* ☐

47. Who proposed the embryological support for evolution?

____

48. Answer the following question.

The proposal about embryological support for evolution was disapproved by

____

49. Consider the following statements.

Statement I According to Haeckel, certain features during embryonic stage common to all vertebrates are all present in adult.

Statement II Embryological evidences by Haeckel was disapproved and rejected by Karl Ernst von Baer.

Choose the correct option from the following.

(a) Statement I is true, but statement II is false ☐
(b) Statement I is false, but statement II is true ☐
(c) Both statements I and II are true ☐
(d) Both statements I and II are false ☐

50. Comparative anatomy and morphological studies focus on whether common ancestors among organisms were shared or not.

True ☐ False ☐

***51.** Organisms *P* and *Q* are descendents of an organism *A*. Both of them have anatomical similarity of their hindlimbs, but their functions are different. Choose the correct combination of the type of organs and the evolution they follow:

(a) Homologous organs and Convergent evolution ☐
(b) Analogous organs and Convergent evolution ☐
(c) Homologous organs and Divergent evolution ☐
(d) Analogous organs and Divergent evolution ☐

***52.** Refer to the diagram and identify whether these structures are homologous or vestigial.

Thorn
Tendril
Bougainvillea
Cucurbita

____

53. Vertebrate heart or brain show convergent evolution.
(*Rewrite the statement after correcing the underlined words.*)

____

***54.** Complete the following analogy given below.
Homology : Common ancestry :: __________ : Different ancestry.

55. Choose the odd one out with respect to the characteristics of analogous structures.

Anatomically similar, Similar functions, Convergent evolution

____

***56.** How many of the listed examples are of analogous structures?

Wings of birds and butterfly, Flipper of penguin and whale, Eyes of octopus and mammals, Brain of frog and cat

____

***57.** Consider the following statements.

Statement I The wings of butterfly and birds though appear similar, differ anatomically.

Statement II Forelimbs of bats and humans are analogous and show convergent evolution.

Choose the correct option from the following.

(a) Statement I is true, but statement II is false ☐

(b) Statement I is false, but statement II is true ☐

(c) Both statements I and II are true ☐

(d) Both statements I and II are false ☐

58. Give an example of analogous structures in plants.

____

59. Analogous structures are likely to develop in ____________ (similar habitats/different habitats) among different organisms.

60. Similarities in proteins and genes performing a given function indicates __________ ancestry. This biochemical similarity is related to the __________ similarity among diverse organisms.

61. Industrial melanism in moths of England between 1850-1920 support evolution by <u>convergent evolution</u>.

(*Rewrite the statement after correcting the underlined words.*)

____

62. Refer to the given diagram and answer the questions that follow.

A B

(i) Which picture depicts the England situation before the year 1920 ?

____

(ii) What does the light coloured background represent in diagram *A* ?

____

(iii) The condition shown in diagram *A* favoured the survival of ______________ (both moths/light-winged moths).

(iv) The population of ______________ winged moths was more in diagram *B* because they were able to ______________ themselves from predators.

(v) The given diagram depicts industrial melanism where the term melanism is applicable to ______________ (lichens/dark-winged moths).

***63.** Which of the evolutionary ideas is observed in the appearance of melanised moths over white winged ones, post industrialisation?

(a) Theory of spontaneous generation ☐ (b) Natural selection ☐
(c) Mutational theory ☐ (d) Theory of Panspermia ☐

64. Give an example of evolution by anthropogenic actions (other than industrial melanism).

____

65. Evolution by anthropogenic actions occurs in centuries.

True ☐ False ☐

66. Consider the following statements and choose the correct ones.

I. Evolution is a directed process in the sense of determinism.
II. Resistant organisms are appearing in a time scale of centuries and not of month or years.
III. Intensive breeding programme has created breeds that differ from other breeds, but still are of the same group.
IV. Evolution is a stochastic process based on chance events in nature.

(a) I, II and III ☐ (b) III and IV ☐
(c) II and IV ☐ (d) II, III and IV ☐

67. Evolution is a ______________ process based on chance events in nature and chance of ______________ in organisms.

TOPIC 3

What is Adaptive Radiation ?

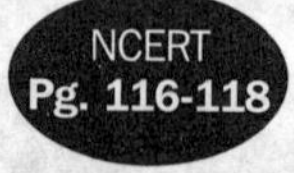

68. Name the islands on which Darwin observed the birds shown in the diagram given below.

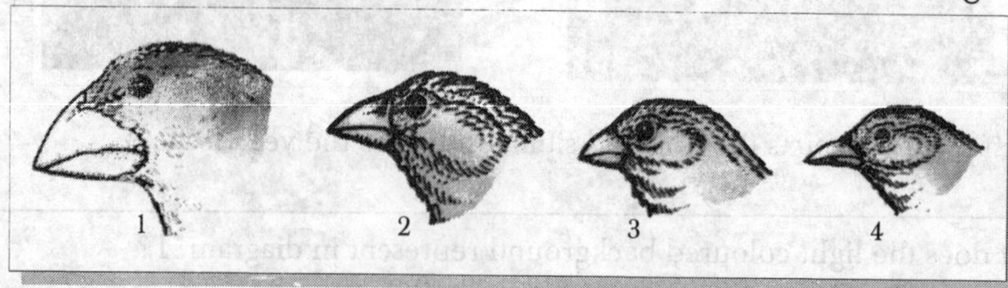

____

69. The varieties of Darwin finches had ________________ (altered beaks/different eye colours).

70. The original (ancestral) Darwin's finches were <u>insectivorous</u>.
(*Rewrite the statement after correcting the underlined word.*)

____

71. The seed eating ancestor finches of Galapagos island gave rise to vegetarian finches only.

True ☐ False ☐

***72.** Give biological term for 'the process of evolution of different species in a given geographical area starting from a point and radiating to other habitats.'

____

***73.** Complete the following analogy given below. ________________

Industrial melanism : Natural selection :: Adaptive radiation : ________________

***74.** Refer to the given diagram and identify the type of evolution shown in it.

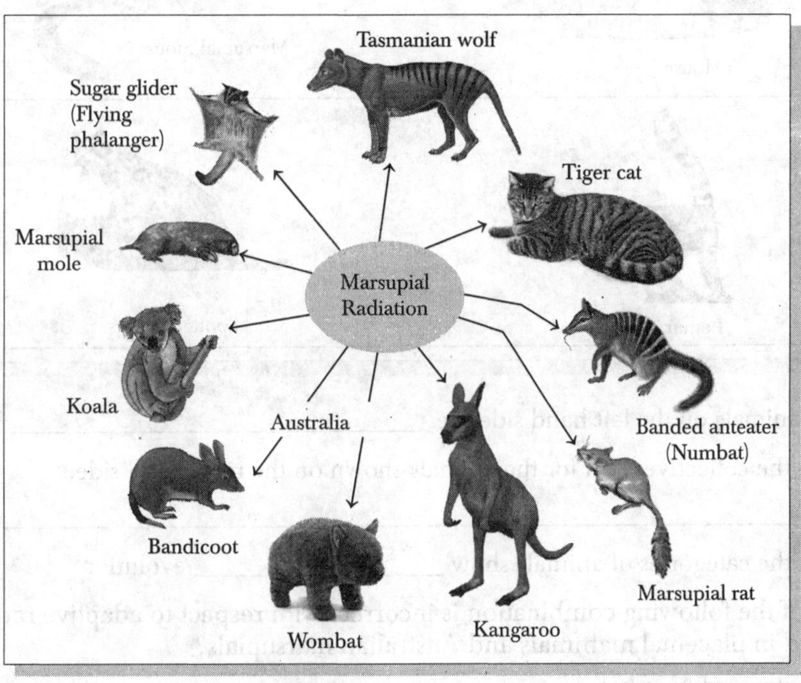

____

75. ________________ evolution occurs when more than one adaptive radiations occur in ________________ geographical area.

76. Refer to the diagram and answer the questions that follow.

Mammals	Marsupials
Mole	Marsupial mole
Anteater	Numbat (anteater)
Mouse	Marsupial mouse
Lemur	Spotted cuscus

(i) The animals on the left hand side are ____________________

(ii) Give the collective term for the animals shown on the right hand side.

____

(iii) Both the categories of animals show ____________ evolution.

***77.** Which of the following combination is incorrect with respect to adaptive radiation observed in placental mammals and Australian marsupials?

(a) Anteater and Numbat ☐

(b) Lemur and Spotted cuscus ☐

(c) Flying squirrel and Flying phalanger ☐

(d) Bobcat and Tasmanian wolf ☐

TOPIC 4

Biological Evolution and its Mechanism

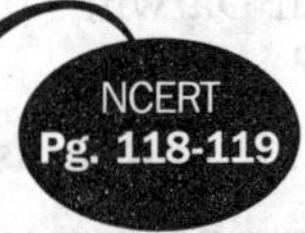

78. The presence of cellular life forms with different metabolic capability on earth represents the evolution by ________________.

79. Refer to the diagrams showing two populations under different conditions.

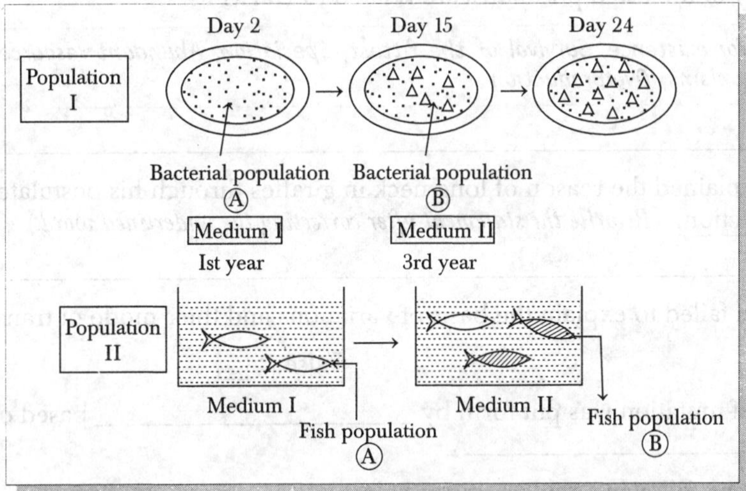

How many of the listed conclusions can be drawn from the above diagrams?

(i) The rate of appearance of new life forms is not related to life cycle of organism.

(ii) Population *B* in both cases (I and II) is better than *A* in terms of fitness.

____

80. Adaptive ability is inherited and ____________ is the end result of the ability to adapt and get selected by nature.

***81.** Name the two key concepts of Darwinian theory of evolution.

____

***82.** Arrange the following steps of Lamarck's theory of use and disuse of organs, in the order of his description.

I. Long neck in giraffes. II. Leaf foraging on tall trees.

III. Acquired character of elongated neck in generations.

____

***83.** Match the following columns.

Column I (Scientists)	Column II (Associated works)
A. Lamarck	1. Nature selects organisms with high reproductive rate
B. Darwin	2. An essay on population
C. Thomas R. Malthus	3. Use and disuse of organs

A.____________ B.____________ C. ____________

84. How can Darwin's principle of natural selection be used to explain the long neck of giraffes?

(a) The use and disuse of an organ creates variations in population ☐
(b) Longer necks provided competitive advantage over other organisms ☐
(c) Sudden random mutations, caused variations in giraffe population ☐
(d) Acquired characteristics were stably passed to offsprings ☐

85. How many of the listed postulates are related to Darwinism?

Struggle for existence, Survival of the fittest, Speciation, Abundant resources, Variations among organisms, Overproduction

____

***86.** Darwin explained the reason of long neck in giraffes through his postulate of overproduction. (*Rewrite the statement after correcting the underlined word.*)

____

***87.** Darwinism failed to explain the basis of variations and their mode of transmission.

True ☐ False ☐

88. The idea of mutation was put forth by _______________ based on his work on _______________.

***89.** Complete the following analogy given below.

Darwin : _______________ : : Hugo de Vries : Mutation causes evolution.

90. In contrast to Darwinian variations, the mutations are _______________ (random and directionless/ small and directional).

***91.** Give the biological term for single step large mutation which causes speciation.

____

***92.** A sudden change in the DNA sequence of a bacterial population, created a new species of bacteria with more virulence and resistance towards antibiotics. Which evolutionary theory best defines this phenomenon?

(a) Natural Selection ☐ (b) Theory of use and disuse ☐
(c) Saltation theory ☐ (d) Survival of the fittest ☐

TOPIC 5

Hardy-Weinberg Principle

NCERT Pg. 120-121

93. Name the principle which helps to find out the frequency of occurrence of alleles of a gene or a locus.

____

***94.** According to Hardy-Weinberg principle, the allele frequency in a population is not stable from generation to generation.

True ☐ False ☐

95. Give biological term for the total genes and their alleles in a population.

___

***96.** The total genes in a population are said to be in genetic equilibrium when sum total of all allelic frequencies is ___(one/zero).

***97.** Hardy-Weinberg principle is calculated by the binominal expansion of $\underline{p^2+q^2}$.
(*Rewrite the statement after correcting the underlined word.*)

___

98. Hardy-Weinberg principle is calculated by the equation $p^2 + 2pq + q^2 = 1$.
Complete the given table based on the representation of each component of equation.

p	Frequency of dominant allele
p^2	(A)
q	(B)
q^2	Percentage of homozygous recessive individuals
$2pq$	(C)

A.___ B.___ C.___

***99.** The genotypes AA, Aa, aa have frequencies 0.5, 0.25 and 0.25, respectively. What will be the frequency of A and a?

___

***100.** The frequency of allele p is 0.6 and q is 0.4 at a particular locus. What would be the frequency of heterozygotes in this population?

___

***101.** In a population of beetles, red color (R) is dominant over green (r). 25% of all beetles are green. What is the percentage of heterozygous beetle population?
(a) 25% ☐ (b) 50% ☐
(c) 100% ☐ (d) 10% ☐

102. The difference between the expected and obtained frequency in Hardy-Weinberg law indicate the extent of ___.

***103.** Out of the factors listed below, which of the following will not affect Hardy – Weinberg equilibrium?
(a) Gentic drift ☐ (b) Gene flow ☐
(c) Genetic recombination ☐ (d) Asexual reproduction ☐

***104.** In a population, Hardy-Weinberg equilibrium can be disrupted due to gene migration.
True ☐ False ☐

105. The migration of a section of population A to a new population B changes the gene frequency in ___ (A only/A and B).

106. Consider the following statements.

I. Change of frequency of alleles in a population will result in mutation.
II. Allele frequencies in a population are stable and constant from generation to generation.

III. According to genetic equilibrium, the gene pool in a population remains constant.
IV. Hardy-Weinberg equilibrium is affected by five factors.

Choose the incorrect statement(s) from the codes given below.

(a) I and III ☐ (b) II and III ☐ (c) Only I ☐ (d) II and IV ☐

***107.** Match the following columns.

	Column I (Factors)		Column II (Explanations)
A.	Mutation	1.	Changes in population's frequencies due to chance alone.
B.	Gene flow	2.	Differences in survival and reproduction among various individuals.
C.	Natural selection	3.	Changes in allele frequency due to immigration and emigration.
D.	Genetic drift	4.	Sources of new alleles.

A.________ B.________ C.________ D.________

108. Name the phenomenon in which change in allele frequencies drift the original population and form new sample of population having different species.

____

***109.** Give biological term for the process of formation of new phenotypes through pre-existing advantageous mutations. ________________

110. ____________ is a process in which heritable variations enable better survival and reproduction rate.

111. How many listed factors result in changed frequency of genes and alleles in future generation?

Mutations, Recombination, Gene flow, Genetic drift

____

***112.** Refer to the givne diagram and answer the questions that follow.

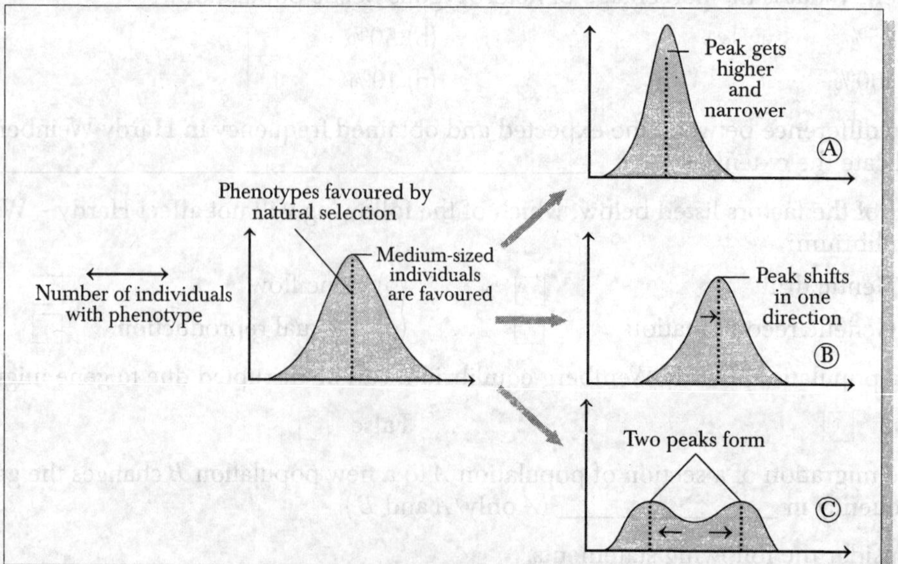

(i) Name the type of natural selection shown in *A*, *B* and *C*.

A.________ B.________ C. ________

(ii) The type of selection shown in A does not promote evolutionary change but maintains phenotypic stability within the population.

True ☐ False ☐

(iii) The B and C types of natural selection occur due to ________________________ ____________________ (stable environment and no selection/selective pressure under changing environment).

***113.** Identify the correct match from the following

(a) Stabalisation – value other than mean character is acquire. ☐

(b) Directional change – individual acquire mean value ☐

(c) Directional change – individual acquire peripheral character ☐

(d) Disruptive change – individual acquire peripheral end value ☐

TOPIC 6

A Brief Account of Evolution

NCERT Pg. 121-124

***114.** When did the first cellular forms of life appeared on earth?

____

115. On early earth, the cells with membranous envelope had the ability to release ______________ . The reaction could have been similar to the ________ reaction in photosynthesis where ________ is splitted with the help of solar energy.

116. Arrange the following organisms with respect to their evolvement on earth.

I. Sea weeds, II. Jawless fish, III. Invertebrates

____

***117.** Name/Give examples for the following.

(i) First organisms that invaded land. ____________________

(ii) Fish organisms that could move on land and in water.

____

(iii) Ancestors of modern day frogs and salamanders. ____________________

(iv) Modern day reptilian descendents of amphibians. ____________________

***118.** Match the following columns.

Column I	Column II
A. Pteridophytes	1. Fish-like reptiles in 200 mya
B. *Ichthyosaurs*	2. Biggest dinosaur with dagger-like teeth
C. *Tyrannosaurus*	3. Formed coal deposits

A.______________ B.______________ C.______________

***119.** Given below is the sketch of evolution of plants forms through geological periods, examine it and answer the questions that follow.

(i) Mention the name of plant types at I and II position.

____

(ii) Bryophytes are likely to be found at position (IV/VII).

____

(iii) Complete the following analogy given below.

VI : Ginkgos : : III : ______________

(iv) Name the type of plants likely to be found at position V.

____

120. Which of the following represents the correct combination of the geological period and the organisms originating?

(a) *Ginkgos*- Triassic ☐ (b) Seed ferns- Permian ☐

(c) *Zosterophyllum*-Silurian ☐ (d) Sphenopsids-Devonian ☐

***121.** About <u>150 mya</u>, the dinosaurs suddenly disappeared from earth. (*Rewrite the statement after correcting the underlined word.*)

____

***122.** The first mammals were like bats.

True ☐ False ☐

123. Mammal's fossils are ______________ sized. They were viviparous, and took over the earth when ______________ came down.

124. The South American mammals resembling horse, bear, rabbit, etc., were over-ridden by North American fauna due to ______________ (recombination/continental drift).

125. Refer to the representative evolutionary history of vertebrates through geological period and answer the questions that follows.

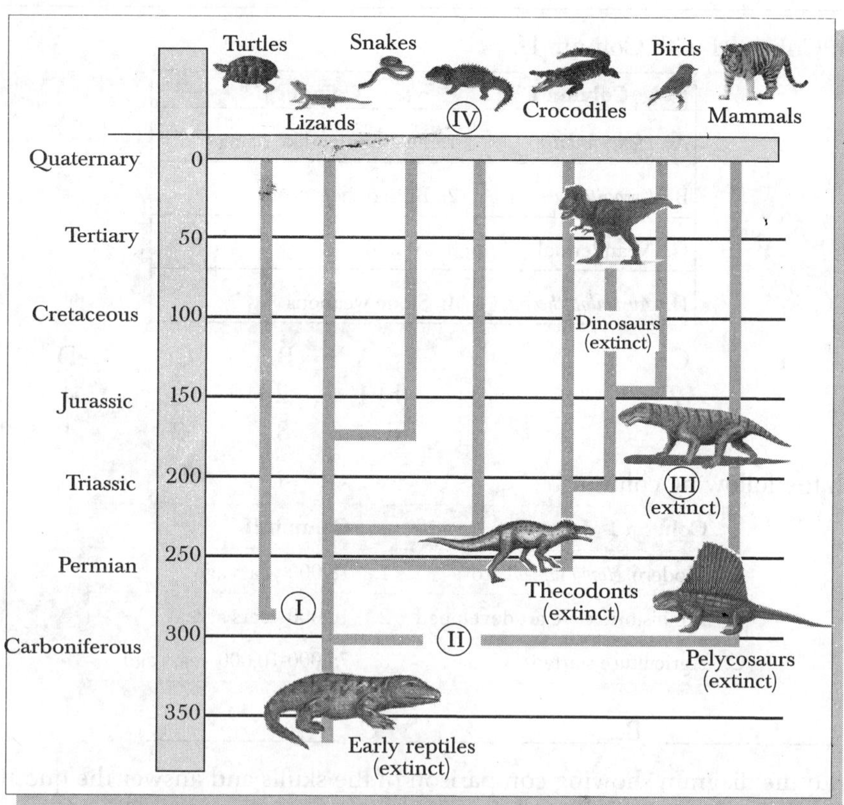

(i) Name the animals labelled as I and II. ______________________

(ii) Tuataras would be found at position (III/IV) ______________________

(iii) ______________________ are not shown in the diagram before early reptiles because there are no specimens of these left with us.

126. Name any two mammals that live wholly in water.

____

***127.** Pouched mammals of Australia survived even after continental drift due to the lack of ______________ from any other mammal.

TOPIC 7

Origin and Evolution of Man

NCERT Pg. 124-125

***128.** Complete the following analogy given below.
Ramapithecus : Man like :: ______________ : Ape-like

129. Few fossils of man like bones have been discovered in Ethiopia and ______________. The hominid features revealed by them reflect that man-like primates walked in ________ about ______________ mya.

***130.** When and where the fossils of *Homo erectus* discovered?

____

131. Where did the *Homo sapiens* arise?

____

***132.** Match Column I with Column II.

Column I	Column II
A. *Homo habilis*	1. First human-like being
B. *Dryopithecus*	2. Buried their dead
C. Neanderthal	3. Ape-like
D. *Australopithecines*	4. Stone weapons

	A	B	C	D			A	B	C	D	
(a)	1	3	2	4	☐	(b)	1	2	3	4	☐
(c)	4	3	1	2	☐	(d	4	3	2	1	☐

***133.** Match the following columns.

Column I	Column II
A. Modern *Homo sapiens* arose	1. 18,000 years ago
B. Pre-historic cave art developed	2. 10,000 years ago
C. Agriculture started	3. 75,000-10,000 years ago

A.______________ B.______________ C.______________

134. Refer to the diagram showing comparison of the skulls and answer the questions that follow.

I

II

III

(i) The skull II and III belong to which animals?

____

(ii) Which one is likely to possess greater cranial capacity? (I/III)

____

135. The Neanderthal man lived in near East and central Asia.

True ☐ False ☐

***136.** Complete the table given below (*A-E*).

Names	Ages of appearance	Cranial capacities	Important features
Ramapithecus	15 mya	–	(*A*)
Australopithecus	5 mya	(*B*)	Hunted with stone weapons and ate fruits
Homo habilis	2 mya	(*C*)	First human-like being the hominid, did not eat meat
Homo erectus	1.5 mya	900 cc	(*D*)
Neanderthal man	100,000-40,000 years	(*E*)	Used hides, burried their dead

A.__________ B.__________ C. __________ D. __________
E.__________

***137.** Complete the flowchart depicting human evolution.

Dryopithecus ⟶ (A) ⟶ *Australopithecus* ⟶ (B)
↓
Homo sapiens ⟵ Cro-Magnon ⟵ (C) ⟵ *Homo erectus*

A.__________ B. __________ C. __________

Assertion-Reason Questions

The following questions consist of two statements–Assertion (A) and Reason (R). Answer these questions by selecting the appropriate option given below.
(a) Both A and R are true and R is the correct explanation of A
(b) Both A and R are true, but R is not the correct explanation of A
(c) A is true, but R is false
(d) A is false, but R is true

***1. Assertion** (A) Chemical evolution is thought to have preceded by biogenesis of life forms.
Reason (R) Organic molecules were synthesised from inorganic ones in the reducing atmosphere.

(a) ☐ (b) ☐ (c) ☐ (d) ☐

2. Assertion (A) Paleontological evidences gives an idea about the geological time scale during which an organism existed.
Reason (R) Fossils are the hard remains of an organism that died during the formation of the particular sediment.

(a) ☐ (b) ☐ (c) ☐ (d) ☐

***3. Assertion** (A) Flippers of dolphins and penguins share similar structural anatomy and share common ancestry.
Reason (R) In convergent evolution, analogous structures have evolved to perform the same function.

(a) ☐ (b) ☐ (c) ☐ (d) ☐

4. **Assertion** (A) Before industrialisation, white winged moths outnumbered the black winged moths in a population.
Reason (R) Due to lesser pollution, lichens covered tree barks against which white winged moths could camouflage.
(a) ☐ (b) ☐ (c) ☐ (d) ☐

*5. **Assertion** (A) The Australian marsupials evolved from a point and then radiated to different habitats.
Reason (R) More than one adaptive radiation in a geography, is indicative of divergent evolution.
(a) ☐ (b) ☐ (c) ☐ (d) ☐

6. **Assertion** (A) Evolution of a new species depends on the reproductive fitness of an organism and their adaptive ability.
Reason (R) Organisms compete with one another for the same resources, and nature selects the better adapted one.
(a) ☐ (b) ☐ (c) ☐ (d) ☐

*7. **Assertion** (A) A shift in the Hardy-Weinberg equilibrium in a given population could indicate evolution.
Reason (R) Huge changes in allele frequency due to genetic drift or gene flow can result in speciation.
(a) ☐ (b) ☐ (c) ☐ (d) ☐

8. **Assertion** (A) Continental drift caused extinction of many mammals while allowing pouched mammals to survive.
Reason (R) Pouched mammals had better reproductive ability than other mammals which allowed them to survive.
(a) ☐ (b) ☐ (c) ☐ (d) ☐

9. **Assertion** (A) *Ramapithecus* was more ape-like and *Dryopithecus* was more man-like.
Reason (R) Few fossils of man-like bones have been discovered in Ethiopia and Tanzania.
(a) ☐ (b) ☐ (c) ☐ (d) ☐

*10. **Assertion** (A) The use of hides for protecting their body was observed in Neanderthal men.
Reason (R) In the evolutionary stages, it was found that *Homo erectus* had highest brain capacity.
(a) ☐ (b) ☐ (c) ☐ (d) ☐

Case Based Questions

*1. During the industrial revolution in England, the peppered moth population dramatically shifted colour. Originally, light-coloured moths were camouflaged against light-coloured tree bark. However, with increased air pollution tree became darker.
Based on the information given above, answer the questions that follow.
(i) How can the change in moth colour could be explained by evolution?
(a) All moths suddenly mutated to a darker colour. ☐
(b) Light-coloured moths preferred darker mates, leading to darker offspring. ☐
(c) Moths with darker variations, better camouflaged on dark bark, survived and reproduced more. ☐
(d) Pollution directly caused moths to turn darker. ☐

(ii) Which of the following best supports the theory of natural selection in the above case?

(a) Darker moths are more visible to birds ☐

(b) Industrial revolution caused mutations directly leading to darker surfaces. ☐

(c) Light-coloured moths prefer to rest on darker surfaces. ☐

(d) Birds preferentially prey on moths that are less camouflaged in their environment. ☐

(iii) During the industrial revolution, what factor most contributed to the increase in the population of dark-coloured peppered moths?

(a) A sudden increase in the mutation rate for dark coloration. ☐

(b) A preference for dark-coloured mates among peppered moths. ☐

(c) Increased air pollution that darkened tree bark, making light-coloured moths more susceptible to predation. ☐

(d) A decrease in the number of birds that preyed on peppered moths. ☐

2. Hardy-Weinberg principle is a fundamental concept in population genetics equilibrium. According to it, allele and genotype frequency in a population remain constant. Based on this answer the questions that follow.

(i) Which of the following conditions must be met for a population to be in Hardy-Weinberg equilibrium?

(a) High mutation ☐ (b) Small population ☐

(c) Non-random mating ☐ (d) No natural selection ☐

(ii) If frequency of homozygous recessive individual is 0.04, then what is the frequency of heterozygous individual

(a) 0.16 ☐ (b) 0.32 ☐

(c) 0.48 ☐ (d) 0.64 ☐

(iii) Which of the following could be a reason for shift of genetic equilibrium if a population moves from region *A* to *B*?

(a) Gene flow ☐ (b) Mutation ☐

(c) Reproduction ☐ (d) Natural selection ☐

COMPETITION EDGE UP

1. *The flippers of the penguins and dolphins are the example of the* **[NCERT Pg. 115, NEET 2024]**

(a) adaptive radiation ☐

(b) natural selection ☐

(c) convergent evolution ☐

(d) divergent evolution ☐

2. *Which one of the following factors will not affect the Hardy-Weinberg equilibrium?* **[NCERT Pg. 121, NEET 2024]**

(a) Genetic recombination ☐

(b) Genetic drift ☐

(c) Gene migration ☐

(d) Constant gene pool ☐

3. *Match List I with List II.*

	List I		List II
A.	Mesozoic Era	I.	Lower invertebrates
B.	Proterozoic Era	II.	Fish and Amphibia
C.	Cenozoic Era	III.	Birds and reptiles
D.	Paleozoic Era	IV.	Mammals

Choose the correct answer from the options given below.
[NCERT Pg. 123, NEET 2024]

(a) A-II, B-I, C-III, D-IV ☐
(b) A-III, B-I, C-II, D-IV ☐
(c) A-I, B-II, C-IV, D-III ☐
(d) A-III, B-I, C-IV, D-II ☐

4. Given below are some stages of human evolution.

Arrange them in correct sequence. (Past to Recent)

A. Homo habilis
B. Homo sapiens
C. Homo neanderthalensis
D. Homo erectus

Choose the correct sequence of human evolution from the options given below.
[NCERT Pg. 124, 125, NEET 2024]

(a) D-A-C-B ☐ (b) B-A-D-C ☐
(c) C-B-D-A ☐ (d) A-D-C-B ☐

5. Select the correct group/set of Australian Marsupials exhibiting adaptive radiation.
[NCERT Pg. 134, NEET 2023]

(a) Numbat, spotted cuscus, flying phalanger ☐
(b) Mole, flying squirrel, Tasmanian tiger cat ☐
(c) Lemur, anteater, wolf ☐
(d) Tasmanian wolf, bobcat, marsupial mole ☐

6. Natural selection where more individuals acquire specific character value other than the mean character value, leads to
[NCERT Pg. 136, NEET 2022]

(a) directional change ☐
(b) disruptive change ☐
(c) random change ☐
(d) stabilising change ☐

7. The factor that leads to Founder effect in a population is [NCERT Pg. 137, NEET 2021]

(a) natural selection ☐
(b) genetic recombination ☐
(c) mutation ☐
(d) genetic drift ☐

8. Match the List I with List II.

List I	List II
A. Adaptive radiation	1. Selection of resistant radiation varieties due to excessive use of herbicides and pesticides
B. Convergent evolution	2. Bones of forelimbs in man and whale
C. Divergent evolution	3. Wings of butterfly and bird
D. Evolution by anthropogenic action	4. Darwin Finches

Choose the correct answer from the options given below.
[NCERT Pg. 131, NEET 2021]

	A	B	C	D	
(a)	4	3	2	1	☐
(b)	3	2	1	4	☐
(c)	2	1	4	3	☐
(d)	1	4	3	2	☐

9. In a species, the weight of newborn ranges from 2 to 5 kg. 97% of the newborn with an average weight between 3 to 3.3 kg survive whereas 99% of the infants born with weights from 2 to 2.5 kg or 4.5 to 5 kg die. Which type of selection process is taking place?
[NCERT Pg. 137 NEET 2021]

(a) Stabilising selection ☐
(b) Disruptive selection ☐
(c) Cyclical selection ☐
(d) Directional selection ☐

10. A hominid fossil discovered in Java in 1891, now extinct having cranial capacity of about 900 cc was
[NCERT Pg. 140, NEET (Oct.) 2020]

(a) Homo erectus ☐
(b) Neanderthal man ☐
(c) Homo sapiens ☐
(d) Australopithecus ☐

Chapter 07

Human Health and Disease

Scan and take Chapter Test

TOPIC 1

Human Health and Common Diseases in Humans

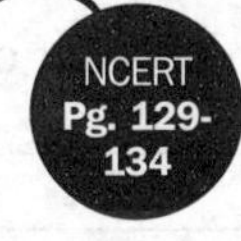

1. The state of complete physical, mental and social well-being is ______________

2. How many factors in the given list are necessary for achieving good health?

Yoga, Drugs, Balanced diet, Vaccination, Alcohols, Hygienic food and Water

____

3. Complete the flowchart given below (*A-D*).

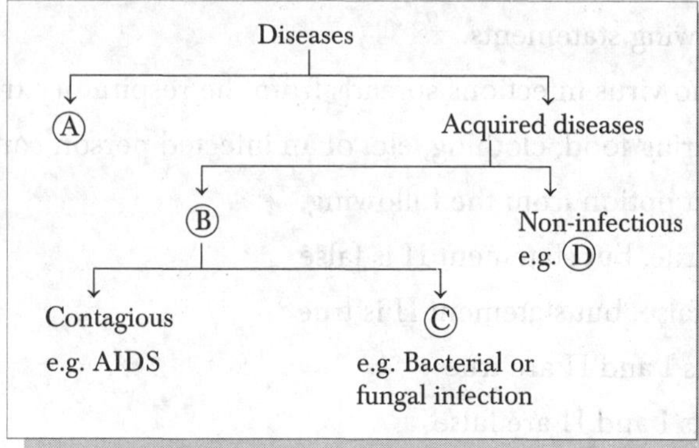

A. ______________ B. ______________ C. ______________ D. ______________

4. The recent pandemic caused due to Covid-19 is an example of ______________ disease.

5. Give the biological term for the disease causing organisms. ______________

6. Pathogenic organisms have the ability to adapt and resist physiological activities within the host body.

True ☐ False ☐

*Concepts of all questions bearing * are important for NEET & CUET*

***7.** Name the causative agent of typhoid fever in human beings.

____

***8.** (i) The pathogenic bacterium which causes typhoid invades in ______________ through contaminated food and water. Its symptoms include sustained high fever, ______________ and ______________. Typhoid fever could be confirmed by ______________ test.

(ii) The lady who continued to spread typhoid for several years through food was

____

***9.** A person who tests positive to the Widal test, can spread the disease through

(a) Food and water ☐ (b Air ☐

(c) Towel ☐ (d) Sexual contact ☐

10. Answer the following questions in context of pneumonia.

(i) Two causative agents ______________

(ii) Infected organ(s) ______________

(iii) Symptoms (Any 4) ______________

(iv) Transmission ______________

***11.** Name the group of viruses which cause the most infectious human ailments, i.e. the common cold. ______________

***12.** Choose the odd one out with respect to the symptoms of disease caused by rhinoviruses.

Nasal congestion, Lung fibrosis, Sore throat, Nasal discharge

____

***13.** Consider the following statements.

Statement I Rhino virus infections spreads from the respiratory tract to the lungs.

Statement II Sharing food, clothing, etc. of an infected person can spread common cold.

Choose the correct option from the following.

(a) Statement I is true, but statement II is false ☐

(b) Statement I is false, but statement II is true ☐

(c) Both statements I and II are true ☐

(d) Both statements I and II are false ☐

____

***14.** Name the common group of viruses to which SARS, MERS and Covid-19 belong.

____

15. *Plasmodium* parasite that causes ______________ (plague/malaria) is neither a virus nor a bacterium.

***16.** Malignant malaria is caused by *Plasmodium malariae.*
(*Rewrite the statement after correcting the underlined words.*)

____

17. Complete the following analogy regarding malarial pathogen.
Intermediate host : Human : : Definitive host : ____________

***18.** (i) Both sexual and asexual life cycle of *Plasmodium* occur in human.
True ☐ False ☐

(ii) *Anopheles* acts as host as well as vector of malarial parasite.
True ☐ False ☐

***19.** Refer to the given diagram and identify *A*, which is being released by female *Anopheles*.

A

***20.** The picture represents the stage of infection of a protozoan that is transmitted by a mosquito vector. Which of the following accurately represents this stage of infection?

(a) Asexual reproduction in the liver cells of humans ☐
(b) Release of haemozoin by bursting of RBCs in humans ☐
(c) Fertilisation of gametocytes in mosquito gut ☐
(d) Maturation of sporozoites in mosquito saliva ☐

***21.** The liver of person infected with malaria contains ____________ stage of parasite. After reproducing ____________, the parasite bursts liver cells and invade RBCs in blood.

***22.** Recurring high fever and chills during malaria is caused due to the release of merozoites from red blood cells.
(*Rewrite the statement after correcting the underlined word.*)

____

***23.** Fertilisation and development of malarial parasite occur in the ____________ (stomach/salivary gland) of mosquito.

***24.** Identify the structure *A* that is found in mosquito and the stage of malarial parasite *B* shown in the diagram given below.

B

A

A. ____________

B. ____________

***25.** Identify the protozoan parasite based on its characteristics given below.

I. Live in large intestine of human and causes amoebiasis.

II. Transmitted through faecal oral route by houseflies.

III. Causes abdominal pain, excess mucus and blood in stools, etc.

____

***26.** Ascariasis is caused due to an ______________ parasite, *Ascaris.*

***27.** Mention any two symptoms of ascariasis.

____

***28.** Consider the following statements.

Statement I *Entamoeba* infects the small intestine of a person and causes abdominal pain.

Statement II Female mosquitoes act as the vectors of diseases like amoebiasis and filariasis.

Choose the correct option from the following.

(a) Statement I is true, but statement II is false

(b) Statement I is false, but statement II is true

(c) Both statements I and II are true

(d) Both statements I and II are false

***29.** The medical condition shown in the given diagram is caused due to a helminthic infection. Consider the diagram and answer the questions that follow.

(i) Name the disease. ______________

(ii) Name the pathogenic organism. ______________

(iii) What is the mode of transmission of this disease?

____

***30.** How many of the given fungal species cause ringworms in human?

Microsporum, Trichophyton, Epidermophyton

____

***31.** A person with dry scaly lesions in the scalp, when shares his towel with another healthy individual, could possibly be transmitting all of the following, except

(a) *Microsporum* (b) *Trichophyton*

(c) *Epidermophyton* (d) *Haemophilus influenzae*

***32.** The pathogen of ringworm grows in the area of human body which is _________________ (hot and moist/cold and dry).

***33.** Find out the incorrect match pair from the options given below.

Column I (Preventive measures)	Column II (Types of disease)
A. Consumption of clean water and food	1. Ringworm
B. Avoid close contact with infected person	2. Pneumonia, common cold
C. Eliminate breeding places of mosquitoes	3. Malaria, filariasis
D. Consumption of clean drinking water	4. Amoebic dysentery

A. _______________ B. _______________ C. _______________ D. _______________

34. Match Column I with Column II.

Column I	Column II
A. *Streptococcus pneumoniae*	1. Dry, scaly lesions on body
B. *Entamoeba histolytica*	2. Lips and finger turn blue
C. *Ascaris lumbricoides*	3. Internal bleeding
D. *Microsporum*	4. Mucous in stool

	A	B	C	D			A	B	C	D
(a)	2	4	3	1		(b)	2	1	3	4
(c)	1	4	3	2		(d)	1	2	3	4

35. (i) Vector – borne disease such as ascariasis can be prevented by spraying of insecticides. (*Rewrite the statement after correcting the underlined word.*)

____

(ii) Tetanus has been eradicated completely through the use of vaccines and immunisation. (*Rewrite the statement after correcting the underlined word.*)

____

36. Consider the following statements.

Statement I *Gambusia* are fishes that feed on mosquito larvae, and control their spread.

Statement II Flowing water is the primary site for breeding of mosquitoes and spread of diseases.

Choose the correct option from the following.

(a) Statement I is true, but statement II is false

(b) Statement I is false, but statement II is true

(c) Both statements I and II are true

(d) Both statements I and II are false

37. The vector of dengue fever is *Aedes aegypti* mosquito.

True ☐ False ☐

38. Which of the following pairs of disease cannot be controlled by use of vaccine?

(a) Polio, tetanus

(b) Diphtheria, smallpox

(c) Amoebiasis, diabetes

(d) Tetanus, smallpox

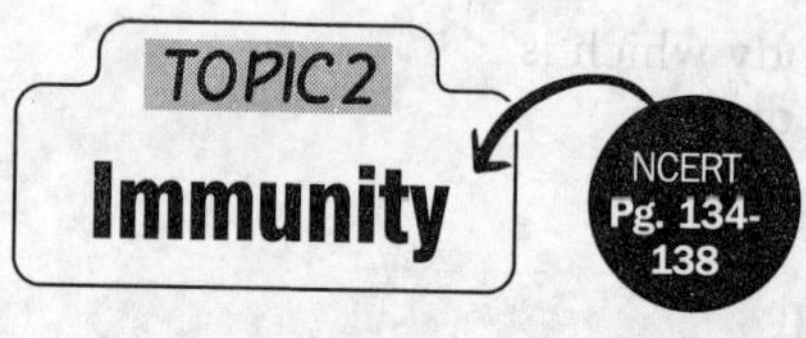

39. The ability of the body to fight the disease causing organisms is called ________________.

40. The non-specific type of defence, that is present at the time of birth is ________________

41. Innate immunity function by acting as a barrier to the entry of foreign agent into body.

True ☐ False ☐

42. Choose the odd one out with respect to the type of innate immunity barrier.

Stomach acid, Mucus coating of respiratory tract, Saliva, Tears

____

43. If a bacterial pathogen in food, manages to reach the stomach of a person, would face which of the following barriers next?

(a) Physical ☐ (b) Cellular ☐

(c) Physiological ☐ (d) Cytokine ☐

44. Complete the following analogy given below.

Skin : Physical barrier : : ________________ : Cellular barrier

45. Monocytes, macrophages and natural killer cells in the blood form ________________ (cellular/physiological) barriers in body.

46. Give the scientific term for the proteins secreted by virus-infected cells.

____

47. Name the type of barrier which protects body against viral infections.

____

48. Match the following columns.

Column I (Types of innate immunity barrier)	Column II (Modes of functioning)
A. Cellular barriers	1. Prevent microbial growth
B. Physiological barriers	2. Fight against viral infections
C. Cytokine barriers	3. Trap microbes
D. Physical barriers	4. Phagocytose and destroy microbes

A. ________ B. ________ C. ________ D. ________

***49.** The pathogen specific immunity, that is characterised by memory is called ________________ immunity.

***50.** An attack by a pathogen for the first time produces high intensity primary response.

True ☐ False ☐

***51.** Anamnestic response is alternatively known as ________________

***52.** Refer to the figure given below and answer the following questions.

(i) Name the parts labelled as *A*, *B* and *C*.

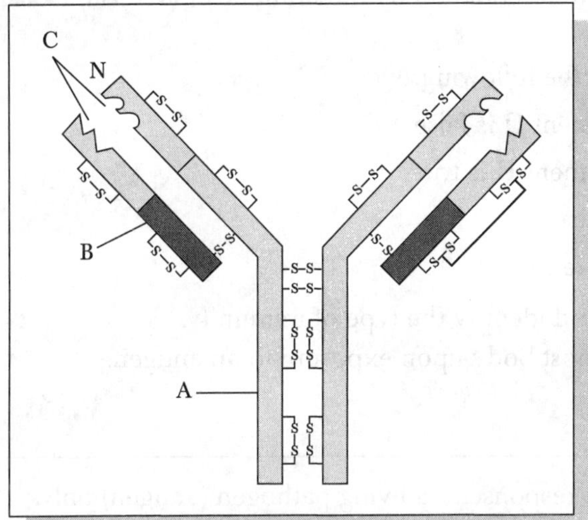

(ii) Name the structure. ________________

(iii) Name the cells which produce this proteinaceous structure. ________________

53. The structure of antibody molecule is represented as ________________ (H_4L_2 / H_2L_2).

____

54. Antibodies or immunoglobulins are synthesised by animals to combat

____

***55.** Complete the flowchart depicting the types of immune response A and B exhibited by different lymphocytes.

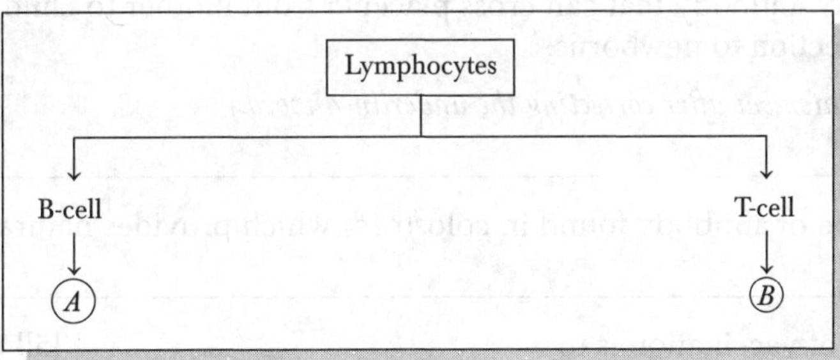

A. ________________ B. ________________

***56.** Humoral immune response is responsible for the graft rejection in humans. (*Rewrite the statement after correcting the underlined word.*)

____

***57.** How many of the listed procedures can be used as the preventive measures of graft rejection?

Tissue matching, Blood-group matching, Immunosuppression,

____

***58.** Consider the following statements.

Statement I T-lymphocytes of humoral immunity is actively involved in antibody production.

Statement II Self and non-self differentiation by the immune system is the basis of graft rejection.

Choose the correct option from the following.

(a) Statement I is true, but statement II is false ☐

(b) Statement I is false, but statement II is true ☐

(c) Both statements I and II are true ☐

(d) Both statements I and II are false ☐

***59.** Read the following statements and identify the type of immunity.

(i) Antibodies are produced in host body upon exposure to an antigen.

(ii) It is slow but long lasting.

____

***60.** Active immunity is generated in response to a living pathogen (antigen) only.

True ☐ False ☐

***61.** Give an example of artificially acquired active immunity.

____

***62.** In passive immunity, ________________ are given to protect the body against foreign agents.

***63.** Choose the odd one out.

Colostrum, Antibody, TAB vaccine

____

64. <u>IgA</u> is the only antibody that can cross placenta from mother to child and provides immune protection to newborns.

(*Rewrite the statement after correcting the underlined word.*)

____

***65.** Name the type of antibody found in colostrum which provides natural passive immunity.

____

***66.** The purpose of vaccination is to ________________ (kill the pathogens /generate memory cells).

***67.** During vaccination, antigens are introduced in the body which later help to elicit anamnestic response on subsequent infection.

True ☐ False ☐

***68.** The treatment given for tetanus and snakebite is based on the principle of <u>active</u> immunity.

(*Rewrite the statement after correcting the underlined word.*)

____

***69.** A person bitten by a venomous cobra, injected with antivenom preparation is comparable to the immunisation

(a) When a person receives a vaccine against tuberculosis ☐

(b) When a person is infected with chicken pox virus ☐

(c) When a person receives oral polio vaccine ☐

(d) When a baby sucks mother's milk during lactation ☐

____

70. The vaccines produced using RDT usually contain ______________

71. Consider the following statements and identify the correct one from the following.

I. The immunity conferred by vaccines is based on the memory of B and T cells.

II. Vaccine production by RDT allow large scale production, but less availability for immunisation.

III. Production of antibodies in the body against antigens would neutralise the pathogenic agents during actual infection.

IV. Hepatitis-B vaccine is being developed from yeast by Recombinant DNA Technology.

Codes

(a) I and II ☐ (b) II, III and IV ☐

(c) III and IV ☐ (d) I, III and IV ☐

72. Give the biological term for the exaggerated response of immune system to certain antigens present in the environment. ______________

73. Name any two allergens which are naturally found in environment.

____

74. Complete the flowchart depicting the process of allergic reaction in human body.

Allergen $\xrightarrow{\text{Bind to}}$ *A* $\xrightarrow{\text{Bind to}}$ Mast cells $\xrightarrow{\text{Release}}$ *B* $\xrightarrow{\text{Causes}}$ Sneezing, Coughing, etc.

A. ______________ B. ______________

75. Adrenaline helps to quickly reduce the symptoms of allergy.

True ☐ False ☐

76. Rheumatoid arthritis is an example of ______________ because the body attacks self-cells.

***77.** Give the collective term used for bone marrow and thymus.

____

***78.** (i) Immature lymphocytes differentiate into antigen sensitive lymphocytes in ______________ (primary/secondary) lymphoid organs.

(ii) ______________ is a lobed lymphoid organ near the heart and beneath breastbone.

79. Which of the following is the incorrect combination?

(a) Peyer's patches – lymphocytes proliferate to form effector cells ☐

(b) Spleen – contains erythrocytes, phagocytes and lymphocytes ☐

(c) MALT – located within the lining of the major tracts of the body ☐

(d) Bone marrow – only site for maturation of B and T lymphocytes ☐

80. Identify the incorrect statement w.r.t lymphoid organs.

(a) Immature lymphocytes differentiate into antigen- sensitive lymphocytes in primary lymphoid organs. ☐

(b) The main lymphoid organ and site for lymphocyte production is spleen. ☐

(c) Thymus, in association with bone marrow provide micro-environments for development of T-lymphocytes. ☐

(d) Lymphocytes post maturation, move to secondary lymphoid organs like tonsils, appendix. ☐

81. Refer to the given figure and answer the following questions.

(i) Name the structure labelled as *A*, *B* and *C*.

A. ____________

B. ____________

C. ____________

(ii) Which structure provides the sites for interaction of lymphocytes with the antigen (*A/B*)? ____________

(iii) ________ (*A/C*) provides micro-environment for the development and maturation of T-lymphocytes.

***82.** Match the following columns.

Column I (Lymphoid organs)	Column II (Characteristics)
A. Bone marrow	1. Trap antigens present in tissue fluid
B. Thymus	2. Site of production of all lymphocytes
C. Spleen	3. Reduces in size with advancing age
D. Lymph nodes	4. Trap blood borne microorganisms

A. ________ B. ________ C. ________ D. ________

83. (i) Lymphoid tissue located within the lining of major tracts like respiratory, digestive, etc., is called ____________. It constitutes ________ per cent of lymphoid tissue in human body.

(ii) ________________ is the large bean-shaped lymphoid organ which contains lymphocytes and ____________.

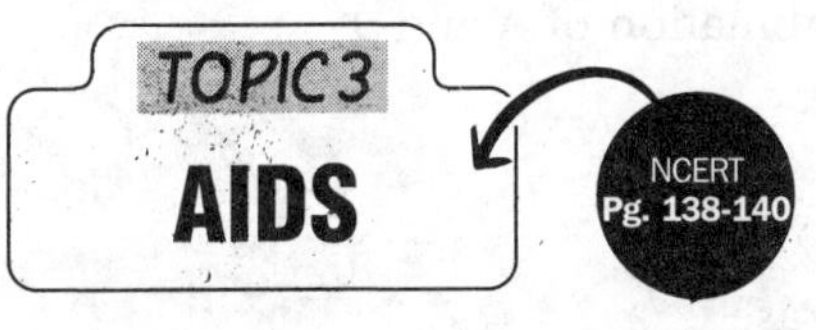

84. AIDS is a congenital disease.

True ☐ False ☐

85. AIDS is associated with the ____________ of immune system. It is known to cause group of symptoms therefore it is a ______________. AIDS was first reported in the year ___________.

86. Name the virus which causes AIDS.

____

87. AIDS causing virus belongs to the group of viruses called adenovirus.
(*Rewrite the statement after correcting the underlined word.*)

____

***88.** The genetic material in HIV is ______________ (naked DNA/enveloped RNA).

89. Choose the odd one out with respect to the transmission of HIV infection.

Sexual contact with multiple partners, Taking drugs intravenously, Repeated blood transfusions, Sharing articles with infected person

____

***90.** Refer to the given diagram showing replication of HIV in human and answer the following questions.

(i) Name the structures labelled as *A* and *B*.

A
Enzyme *X*
B
C
E
D

A. ______________

B. ______________

(ii) Name the enzyme *X* involved in the production of *B*. ______________

(iii) The formations of structure *B* occurs in the ______________ (macrophages/nucleus) of host cells.

(iv) Identify the structures labelled as *C* and *D*.

C. ______________ D. ______________

(v) The infected host cells do not survive after viruses are being replicated and released from them.

True ☐ False ☐

***91.** Consider the given sequence and choose the correct combination of *X* and *Y*

RNA genome $\xrightarrow{Y}$ DNA $\longrightarrow$ *X* $\longrightarrow$ progeny viruses

(a) X – integration into host cell's genome, Y – DNA polymerase ☐

(b) X – release of DNA into host cell, Y – RNA polymerase ☐

(c) X – release of DNA into host cell, Y – DNA polymerase ☐

(d) X – integration of DNA into host cell, Y – Reverse transcriptase ☐

***92.** Helper T-lymphocytes acts as HIV factory in the body of person infected with AIDS. (*Rewrite the statement after correcting the underlined words.*)

***93.** Name the cells which progressively decreases in number in the body of AIDS infected person. ________

94. Various symptoms of AIDS like weight loss, fever, etc. appear when (Viral RNA replicate in macrophages/Helper T-lymphocytes decreases).

95. A widely used diagnostic test for AIDS is ________

96. Expand the following.

(i) NACO ________

(ii) NGO ________

97. How many of the listed measures given below help to prevent AIDS?

Use of disposable syringes, Advocating safe sex, Use of condoms during intercourse, Isolation of AIDS infected person

TOPIC 4 Cancer

NCERT Pg. 140-142

98. Give the biological term for the oncogenic transformation of cells in human body.

99. Cancer cells lack the property of ________ by virtue of which uncontrolled growth is inhibited in normal cells. Continuously dividing cells form masses of cells called ________.

100. Complete the flowchart given below.

Tumors → (A) ; Malignant tumors

A. ________

101. Read the following statements and identify the type of cancer.
(i) Proliferating mass of neoplastic cells.
(ii) Show metastasis.

____

102. How does a malignant cell affect the growth and division process of a normal cell?
(a) By causing mutation in the normal cell ☐
(b) By depriving the normal cell off nutrients ☐
(c) By releasing toxins in their vicinity ☐
(d) By secreting antibodies against normal cell receptors ☐

____

103. Choose the odd one out with respect to the type of carcinogen.

X-rays, Gamma rays, UV-rays

____

104. Tobacco smoke causes lung cancer as it contain __________ carcinogens.

105. Give the biological term for cancer causing viruses. __________

106. Viral oncogenes are the type of __________ (physical/biological) carcinogens.

107. Name the genes in normal cells which, when activated, could lead to oncogenic transformation of the cells. __________

108. Which of the following situations cannot result in oncogenic transformation of proto oncogenes?
(a) α - interferons ☐ (b) X-rays and gamma rays ☐
(c) Nicotine ☐ (d) UV rays ☐

____

109. Complete the following analogy.
Cancer of internal organs : Computed tomography : : __________ : Blood and bone marrow test.

110. Match the following columns.

Column I (Cancer detection techniques)	Column II (Procedures)
A. Biopsy	1. X-rays generate 3D image of organs.
B. CT scan	2. Non-ionising radiations detect pathological changes in living tissue.
C. MRI	3. Piece of suspected tissue is cut into thin sections.
D. Histopathological studies	4. Suspected tissues are observed under microscope.

A. __________ B. __________ C. __________ D. __________

111. Consider the following statements and choose the incorrect one.
I. MRI uses magnetic fields and ionising radiations to accurately detect cancer cells.
II. For cancer treatment, combination of chemotherapy and radiation therapy is used.
III. Early detection of cancer is essential as it helps in the successful treatment of cancer in many cases.

IV. Compound tomography uses gamma rays to generate a three - dimensional image of the internals of an object or an organ.

Codes

(a) II and IV ☐ (b) I and III ☐

(c) I and IV ☐ (d) III and IV ☐

112. Some genes predispose an individual to certain cancers and these can be detected by using the techniques of molecular biology.

True ☐ False ☐

113. In immunotherapy, tumor cells are irradiated lethally without affecting the normal tissues surrounding them.

(*Rewrite the statement after correcting the underlined word.*)

____

114. Side effects like hair loss and anaemia in a cancer patient are most likely to be associated with ______________ (chemotherapy/biopsy).

115. Name the biological response modifiers which activate immune system and destroy tumour.

____

TOPIC 5

Drugs and Alcohol Abuse

NCERT Pg. 142-147

116. The biological substances used to modify or explore physiological or pathological state of body are called ______________

***117.** Name any three commonly abused drugs.

____

118. All the drugs are obtained from fungi.

True ☐ False ☐

***119.** Opioid drugs bind to their specific receptors which are found in CNS and ______________ (respiratory tract/gastrointestinal tract).

***120.** Read the following characteristics and identify the name of opioid drug.

(i) White, odourless, bitter crystalline compound.

(ii) Commonly called smack.

(iii) Obtained by acetylation of morphine.

____

***121.** Consider the following statements.

Statement I Chemical name of heroin, a white, odourless amorphous compound is triacetyl morphine.

Statement II Heroin is an opioid that slows down body functions.

Choose the correct option from the following.

(a) Statement I is true, but statement II is false ☐

(b) Statement I is false, but statement II is true ☐

(c) Both statements I and II are true ☐

(d) Both statements I and II are false ☐

***122.** Identify the correct structure of morphine.

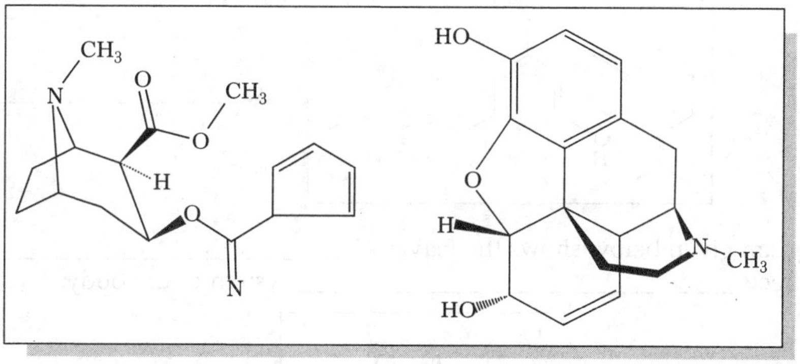

(i) (ii)

____

***123.** Refer to the given figure and answer the following questions.

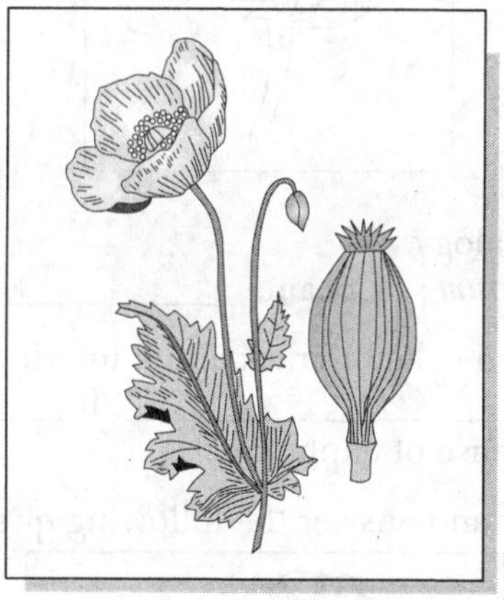

(i) Name the plant (both common and scientific names).

____

(ii) Name the drug obtained from this plant. ______________

(iii) Which part of this plant is used to obtain the drug? ______________

***124.** Choose the odd one out with respect to the mode of taking heroin.

Injection, Snorting, Oraroute

____

***125.** Heroin is a depressant.

True ☐ False ☐

***126.** The cannabinoid receptors are principally found in ______________

***127.** Name the plant and the part from which the cannabinoids are obtained.

____

***128.** Give the common name for the drugs given below.

Marijuana, Hashish, Charas, Ganja

____

***129.** Identify the group labelled as *A* in the structure of cannabinoid molecule given below.

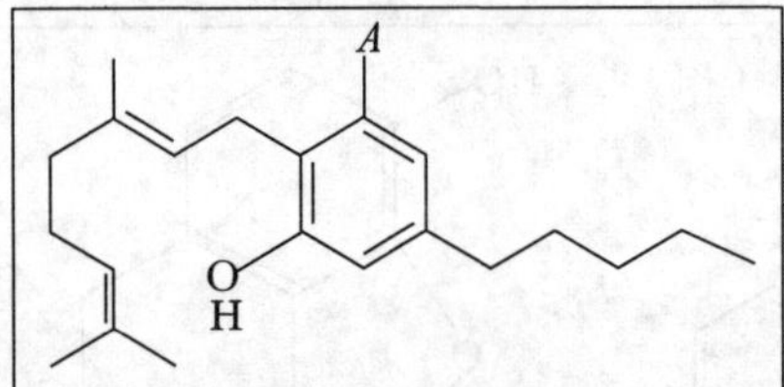

A. ______________________________

***130.** The diagram given below shows the leaves of ______________________________ which affects ______________________________ system of the body.

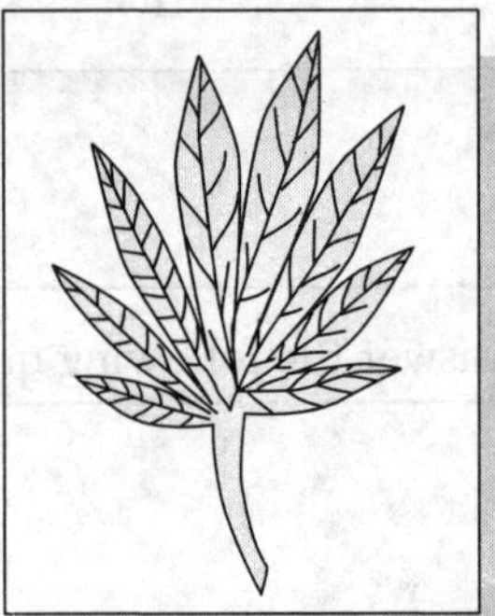

***131.** Complete the following analogy.
Morphine : *Papaver somniferum* : : Cocaine : ______________________________

***132.** Cocaine is commonly called coke or crack and it interferes with the transport of neurotransmitter ______________________________. It ______________________________ the CNS and produces a sense of euphoria.

***133.** Refer to the given diagram and answer the following questions.

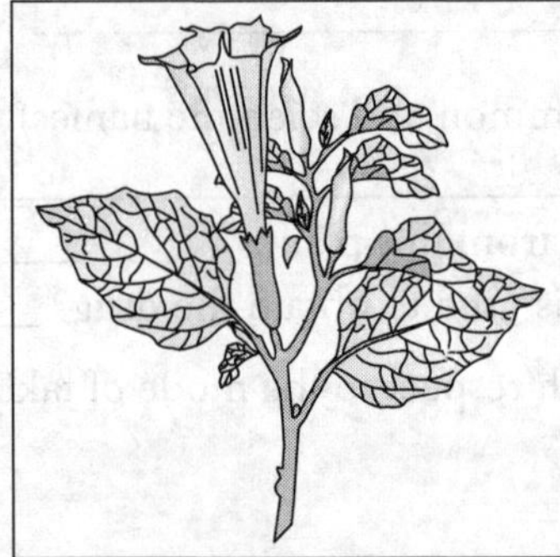

(i) Name the plant. ______________________________

(ii) The given plant has ______________________________ (hallucinogenic/sedative) properties.

(iii) Name the two plants with same properties.

____

134. Choose the incorrect combination from the following.

(a) Opioids – Poppy plant ☐ (b) Hashish - *Cannabis sativa* ☐

(c) Coke - *Atropa belladonna* ☐ (d) Cocaine - *Erythroxylum coca* ☐

***135.** Match the following columns.

Column I	Column II
A. Coke	1. Snorting or by injection
B. Morphine	2. Inhaled or orally ingested
C. Cannabinoid	3. Snorted

A. ________ B. ________ C. ________

***136.** Out of the drugs listed below, which is not used as medicine to help patients cope with mental illness?

(a) Barbiturates ☐ (b) Amphetamines ☐

(c) Hashish ☐ (d) Benzodiazepines ☐

***137.** Sports persons usually abuse <u>cocaine</u>.
(*Rewrite the statement after correcting the underlined word.*)

____

138. Answer the questions with respect to tobacco.

(i) The alkaloid found in tobacco is ________________

(ii) Tobacco smoking can raise blood pressure and heart rate due to the release of hormones ____________ and ____________ from adrenal gland.

(iii) Tobacco smoking increases ________________ content in blood and reduces haembound oxygen.

139. Adolescents are motivated towards drug and alcohol use due to ____________ (excitement/biological demands).

140. All the listed factors might encourage youngsters to consume drugs and alcohol, except

Peer pressure, Social media, Stress, Unsupportive family, Mental illness

____

141. Give technical term for the psychological attachment with drugs and alcohol for certain effects like euphoria.

____

142. Read the following statements and identify the technical term which describes the consequence of alcohol and drug abuse.

(i) Tendency of body to manifest withdrawal symptoms if regular dose of drugs/alcohol is abruptly discontinued.

(ii) Ignoring of all social norms to satiate self needs.

____

143. A person who takes daily doses of diacetylmorphine, is put in a rehabilitation centre. On lowering the doses and sudden discontinuation of the chemical, he shows all of the following symptoms, except

(a) Constant shaking of hands and feet ☐ (b) Anxiety and panic attacks ☐

(c) Increased blood sugar levels ☐ (d) Profuse sweating ☐

144. Choose the odd one out with respect to the symptoms of withdrawal syndrome.

Anxiety, Sweating, Euphoria, Nausea

____

145. Alcohol consumption can cause ______________ (hepatitis-B/cirrhosis).

146. Anabolic steroids help to maintain normal menstrual flow in sports females.

True ☐ False ☐

147. Drug abuse through ______________ route can cause serious infections like AIDS and hepatitis-B.

148. Drug and alcohol abuse may lead to stunted growth due to the premature closure of growth centres of long bones.

True ☐ False ☐

149. Among the listed factors, how many can help to prevent and control drug and alcohol abuse?

Disciplined parenting, Exerting peer pressure, Education, Looking for danger signs

____

150. Can psychologist and psychiatrists help to get rid of drugs and alcohol completely?

Yes ☐ No ☐

Assertion-Reason Questions

The following questions consist of two statements- Assertion (A) and Reason (R). Answer these questions by selecting the appropriate option given below.

(a) Both A and R are true and R is the correct explanation of A

(b) Both A and R are true, but R is not the correct explanation of A

(c) A is true, but R is false

(d) A is false, but R is true

***1.** **Assertion** (A) Common cold, is a highly contagious infectious disease caused by the bacterium *Streptococcus pneumoniae.*

Reason (R) Respiratory problems caused by *Streptococcus pneumoniae* occur due to fluid in the alveoli.

(a) ☐ (b) ☐ (c) ☐ (d) ☐

***2.** **Assertion** (A) Gametocytes of *Plasmodium* develop in the red blood cells of the human host.

Reason (R) Gametocytes develop into infectious sporozoites in the female mosquito's gut.

(a) ☐ (b) ☐ (c) ☐ (d) ☐

***3.** **Assertion** (A) Amoebiasis is caused by protozoan which enters the small intestine of human.

Reason (R) Houseflies are the vector of amoebiasis caused by the pathogen *Entamoeba histolytica.*

(a) ☐ (b) ☐ (c) ☐ (d) ☐

***4.** **Assertion** (A) A person with filariasis shows deformities in the genital organs and lower limbs.

Reason (R) *Wuchereria* lives in the blood vessels of lower limbs causing chronic inflammation.

(a) ☐ (b) ☐ (c) ☐ (d) ☐

5. **Assertion** (A) A cell infected with a virus, is partly responsible for protecting other non-infected cells.

Reason (R) A virus infected cell secretes a group of proteins called interferons to protect the non-infected cells.

(a) ☐ (b) ☐ (c) ☐ (d) ☐

***6.** **Assertion** (A) A person undergoing kidney transplantation is often provided with immune-suppresants.

Reason (R) B-cell of the body distinguish between self and non-self, and are associated with graft rejection.

(a) ☐ (b) ☐ (c) ☐ (d) ☐

***7.** **Assertion** (A) Injecting weakened polio virus in a person to build resistance against the disease is a form of passive immunity.

Reason (R) In passive immunisation, preformed antibodies or antitoxins are provided to the infected person.

(a) ☐ (b) ☐ (c) ☐ (d) ☐

8. **Assertion** (A) Lymphocytes formed in the bone marrow migrate to the thymus for their maturation.

Reason (R) Lymphocytes interact with antigens in the lymph nodes, which causes their activation.

(a) ☐ (b) ☐ (c) ☐ (d) ☐

***9.** **Assertion** (A) HIV infects macrophages and releases their viral DNA genome into the cells.

Reason (R) HIV DNA gets incorporated with the host DNA and replicated to form progeny viruses.

(a) ☐ (b) ☐ (c) ☐ (d) ☐

***10.** **Assertion** (A) A person who snorts coke excessively, often complains of seeing things that are not real.

Reason (R) Cocaine interferes with the transport of dopamine and affects the central nervous system.

(a) ☐ (b) ☐ (c) ☐ (d) ☐

Case Based Questions

1. Natasha was born in U.K and was travelling to India for the first time. As she landed, she took a taxi to her hotel in Delhi. On the way she experienced sneezing and watery eyes. As the symptoms were mild, she did not pay much attention. Later that night, she had to visit the hospital, as she was experiencing repeated sneezing, watery eyes, along with difficulty in breathing. The doctors, after careful examination, rooted the cause to be pollen grains present in air. Based on the information provided, answer the following questions.

(i) Given the situation, under which of the following categories can we place pollen grains?

(a) Antibody ☐ (b) Interferons ☐
(c) Antigen ☐ (d) Cytokines ☐

(ii) Which of the following would be released by mature B-lymphocytes against pollen grains?

(a) Ig-A ☐ (b) Ig-E ☐
(c) Ig-M ☐ (d) Ig-G ☐

(iii) Which of the following will the doctors not employ to relieve Natasha's symptoms quickly?

(a) Antihistamine ☐ (b) Steroid ☐
(c) Adrenaline ☐ (d) α-interferons ☐

***2.** A heavily addicted person started sharing needles with his friends to take smack. Soon he was diagnosed with an infectious disease with no cure. The disease caused him to lose a lot of weight and he became very susceptible to mild infections. Doctors administered certain drugs which could prolong his life , but would not cure him of the disease. Based on the provided information, answer the following questions.

(i) What is the chemical nature of the drug he was abusing?

(a) Diacetylmorphine ☐ (b) Amphetamines ☐
(c) Benzodiazepines ☐ (d) Morphine ☐

(ii) If the infectious disease was viral borne, what would be the genome of the virus?

(a) Single-stranded DNA ☐ (b) Double-stranded DNA ☐
(c) RNA ☐ (d) Protein ☐

(iii) Which immune cells are decreased due to pathogenesis of the virus?

(a) Helper T-cells ☐ (b) B-cells ☐
(c) Monocytes ☐ (d) Polymorphonuclear leukocytes ☐

(iv) How would the doctors confirm the given viral disease in a patient?

(a) Blood test ☐ (b) MRI ☐
(c) ELISA ☐ (d) CT ☐

COMPETITION EDGE UP

1. Given below are two statements; one is labelled as Assertion (A) and the other is labelled as Reason (R).

Assertion (A) Breastfeeding during initial period of infant growth is recommended by doctors for bringing a healthy baby.

Reason (R) Colostrum contains several antibodies absolutely essential to develop resistance for the new born baby.

In the light of the above statements, choose the most appropriate answer from the options given below.

[NCERT Pg. 136, NEET 2024]

(a) Both A and R are correct and R is the correct explanation of A ☐

(b) Both A and R are correct, but R is not the correct explanation of A ☐

(c) A is correct but R is not correct ☐

(d) A is not correct but R is correct ☐

2. Given below are two statements .

Statement I Bone marrow is the main lymphoid organ where all blood cells including lymphocytes are produced.

Statement II Both bone marrow and thymus provide micro environments for the development and maturation of T-lymphocytes.

In the light of above statements, choose the most appropriate answer from the options given below

[NCERT Pg. 137, 138, NEET 2024]

(a) Both statement I and statement II are true ☐

(b) Both statement I and statement II are false ☐

(c) Statement I is true, but statement II is false ☐

(d) Statement I is false, but statement II is true ☐

3. Which of the following are autoimmune disorders?

A. Myasthenia gravis

B. Rheumatoid arthritis

C. Gout

D. Muscular dystrophy

E. Systemic Lupus Erythematosus (SLE)

Choose the most appropriate answer from the options given below.

[NCERT Pg. 137, NEET 2024]

(a) A, B and D only ☐

(b) A, B and E only ☐

(c) B, C and E only ☐

(d) C, D and E only ☐

4. Match List I with List II.

List I	List II
A. Cocaine	I. Effective sedative in surgery
B. Heroin	II. Cannabis sativa
C. Morphine	III. Erythroxylum
D. Marijuana	IV. Papaver somniferum

Choose the correct answer from the options given below

[NCERT Pg. 142, NEET 2024]

(a) A-IV, B-III, C-I, D-II ☐

(b) A-I, B-III, C-II, D-IV ☐

(c) A-II, B-I, C-III, D-IV ☐

(d) A-III, B-IV, C-I, D-II ☐

5. Match List I with List II.

[NCERT Pg. 131, 133 NEET 2023]

List I	List II
A. Ringworm	I. Haemophilus influenzae
B. Filariasis	II. Trichophyton
C. Malaria	III. Wuchereria bancrofti
D. Pneumonia	IV. Plasmodium vivax

Choose the correct answer from the options given below.

(a) A-II, B-III, C-I, D-IV ☐

(b) A-III, B-II, C-I, D-IV ☐

(c) A-III, B-II, C-IV, D-I ☐

(d) A-II, B-III, C-IV, D-I ☐

6. In which blood corpuscles, the HIV undergoes replication and produces progency viruses? **[NCERT Pg. 140, NEET 2023]**

(a) B-lymphocytes ☐

(b) Basophils ☐

(c) Eosinophils ☐

(d) T_H-cells ☐

7. Given below are two statements.

Statement I Autoimmune disorder is a condition where body defence mechanism recognises its own cells as foreign bodies.

Statement II Rheumatoid arthritis is a condition where body does not attack self cells.

In the light of the above statements, choose the most appropriate answer from the options given below.

[NCERT Pg. 137, NEET 2022]

(a) Both statement I and statement II are incorrect ☐

(b) Statement I is correct, but statement II is incorrect ☐

(c) Statement I is incorrect, but statement II is correct ☐

(d) Both statement I and statement II are correct ☐

8. Select the incorrect statement with respect to acquired immunity.

[NCERT Pg. 135, NEET 2022]

(a) Anamnestic response is elicited on subsequent encounters with the same pathogen ☐

(b) Anamnestic response is due to memory of first encounter ☐

(c) Acquired immunity is non-specific type of defence present at the time of birth ☐

(d) Primary response is produced when our body encounters a pathogen for the first time ☐

9. The infectious stage of Plasmodium that enters the human body is

[NCERT Pg. 131, NEET (Sep.) 2020]

(a) Sporozoites ☐

(b) Female gametocytes ☐

(c) Male gametocytes ☐

(d) Trophozoites ☐

10. Identify the wrong statement with reference to immunity.

[NCERT Pg. 136, NEET (Sep.) 2020]

(a) When readymade antibodies are directly given, it is called 'passive immunity' ☐

(b) Active immunity is quick and gives full response ☐

(c) Foetus receives some antibodies from mother, it is an example for passive immunity ☐

(d) When exposed to antigen (living or dead) antibodies are produced in the host's body. It is called 'active immunity' ☐

11. Match the following diseases with the causative organism and select the correct option. **[NCERT Pg. 131, 133 NEET (Sep.) 2020]**

	Column I		Column II
A.	Typhoid	1.	Wuchereria
B.	Pneumonia	2.	Plasmodium
C.	Filariasis	3.	Salmonella
D.	Malaria	4.	Haemophilus

A B C D

(a) 3 4 1 2 ☐

(b) 2 1 3 4 ☐

(c) 4 1 2 3 ☐

(d) 1 3 2 4 ☐

12. The yellowish fluid 'colostrum' secreted by mammary glands of mother during the initial days of lactation has abundant antibodies (IgA) to protect the infant. This type of immunity is called as

[NCERT Pg. 136, NEET (Oct.) 2020]

(a) passive immunity ☐

(b) active immunity ☐

(c) acquired immunity ☐

(d) autoimmunity ☐

13. Identify the correct pair representing the causative agent of typhoid fever and the confirmatory test for typhoid.

[NCERT Pg. 130, NEET (National) 2019]

(a) Streptococcus pneumoniae/Widal test ☐

(b) Salmonella typhi/Anthrone test ☐

(c) Salmonella typhi/Widal test ☐

(d) Plasmodium vivax/UTI test ☐

14. Which of the following immune responses is responsible for rejection of kidney graft?

[NCERT Pg. 136, NEET (National) 2019]

(a) Humoral immune response ☐

(b) Inflammatory immune response ☐

(c) Cell-mediated immune response ☐

(d) Autoimmune response ☐

Chapter 08

Microbes in Human Welfare

Scan and take Chapter Test

TOPIC 1

Basic Concepts and Microbes in Household Products

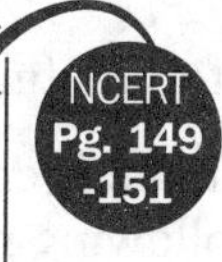

1. The organisms like ________________ are found on places like thermal vents where no other life form is found.

2. The microbes grown on nutritive media to form colonies cannot be seen with naked eyes.

True ☐ False ☐

3. The ____________ (bacteria/virus) and ____________ (fungi/lichen) are the organisms which can be easily grown on culture media.

4. Identify the organisms shown in figures *A* and *B*.

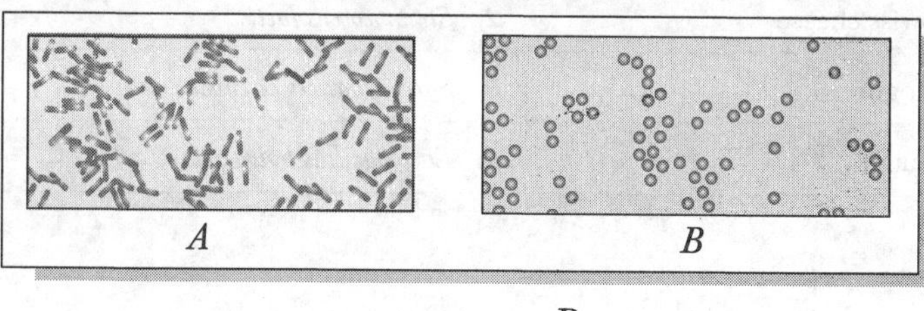

A.________________ B.________________

5. Choose the odd one out with respect to the type of microbes shown in the diagrams given below.

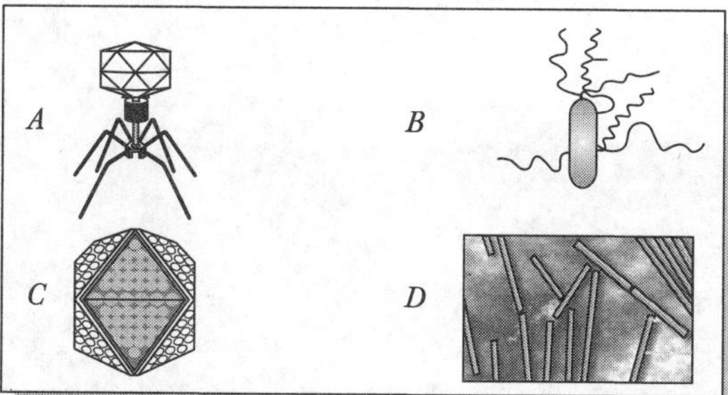

A. ________________

B. ________________

C. ________________

D. ________________

Concepts of all questions bearing * are important for NEET & CUET

6. An example of rod-shaped virus is ____________________ (adenovirus / tobacco mosaic virus).

7. Name one virus that causes respiratory problem.____________________

8. Expand LAB. ____________________

9. Complete the flowchart depicting the formation of curd.

LAB in inoculum ⟶ Produce an acid (from milk sugar) __________ ⟶ Coagulate and partially digest milk protein ⟶ Curd

***10.** LAB improves the nutritional quality of curd by increasing <u>vitamin-A.</u>
(*Rewrite the statement after correcting the underlined word.*)

____

11. The puffing up of idli dough is caused due to the production of __________ during __________ .

12. Name the drink made by fermenting sap from palms in Southern India. __________

13. In the famous cartoon, Tom and Jerry, Jerry is always after a block of cheese with large holes in it. Which of the following microbe is responsible for the production of that cheese?

(a) *Saccharomyces* ☐ (b) *Penicillium* ☐

(c) *Propionibacterium* ☐ (d) *Monascus* ☐

14. Match the following columns.

Column I (Household products)	Column II (Microbes)
A. Bread	1. *Propionibacterium sharmanii*
B. Swiss cheese	2. *Streptococcus lactis*
C. Yogurt	3. *Saccharomyces cerevisiae*
D. Butter	4. *Lactobacillus bulgaricus*

A. __________ B. __________

C. __________ D.__________

15. The particular flavour of Roquefort cheese is imparted by a bacteria.

True ☐ False ☐

TOPIC 2

Microbes in Industrial Products

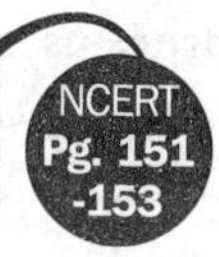

16. Beverages and antibiotics are produced on industrial scale in very large vessels called ____________ .

17. A fermentation plant in shown in the figure given below. Name any two drinks which are formed in these fermentors.

____

***18.** Complete the analogy given below with respect to fermentation
Bread : Baker's yeast : : ____________ : Brewer's yeast

19. Choose the odd one out from the words given below.

Whisky, Brandy, Rum, Wine

____

20. Which of the following combinations is prepared by distillation process?

(a) Wine and beer ☐ (b) Wine and rum ☐
(c) Beer and whisky ☐ (d) Whisky and Rum ☐

21. Give the biological term for the chemical substances, which are produced by some microbes and can kill or retard the growth of other microbes. ____________

22. Given below are certain diseases commonly affecting an average size of population.

I. Plague II. Diphtheria III. Whooping cough
IV. Amoebiasis V. Pneumonia VI. Tuberculosis
VII. Mumps

Which of these can be used for antibiotic treatment?

(a) II, III, V, VII ☐ (b) I, IV, VI, VII ☐
(c) I, II, III, V, VI ☐ (d) IV, V, VI, VII ☐

23. Citric acid is an organic acid which is produced by a bacterium.
(Rewrite the statement after correcting the underlined word.)

____

24. Identify the incorrect statement with respect to antibiotics.

(a) Antibiotics include drugs used to treat diseases caused by bacteria. ☐

(b) These drugs interfere with the formation of bacterial cell wall or its cell contents thereby minimising their growth. ☐

(c) Improper / overuse of antibiotics can render advance protection from the microorganisms. ☐

(d) Antibiotics can cause side effects like nausea, vomiting, diarrhoea. ☐

***25.** Match the following columns.

Column I (Organic acids)	Column II (Microbial sources)
A. Acetic acid	1. *Clostridium butylicum*
B. Lactic aceti	2. *Acetobacter aceti*
C. Butyric acid	3. *Aspergillus niger*
D. Citric acid	4. *Lactobacillus*

A. ________ B. ________ C. ________ D. ________

***26.** Read the following statements and identify the bioactive molecule.

I. Produced by fungus *Trichoderma polysporum*.

II. Used as an immunosuppressive agent in organ transplant patients.

____

***27.** Consider the following statements.

Statement I The oily and greasy stains are removed by lipases present in detergent formulations.

Statement II Streptokinase produced by *Streptococcus* and modified by genetic engineering is used as a clot buster for patients who underwent myocardial infarction.

Choose the correct option from the following.

(a) Statement I is true, but statement II is false ☐

(b) Statement I is false, but statement II is true ☐

(c) Both statements I and II are true ☐

(d) Both statements I and II are false ☐

***28.** Name the microbial source of statins. ________________

***29.** Statins are widely used as cholesterol-synthesising agents.

True ☐ False ☐

***30.** Match column I with column II.

Column I	Column II
A. *Clostridium*	1. Butyric acid
B. Pectinases	2. Statins
C. *Streptococcus*	3. Clarified fruit juices
D. *Monascus purpureus*	4. Clot buster

Choose the correct option.

	A	B	C	D			A	B	C	D	
(a)	1	3	4	2	☐	(b)	1	3	2	4	☐
(c)	1	4	3	2	☐	(d)	1	4	2	3	☐

TOPIC 3

Microbes in Sewage Treatment

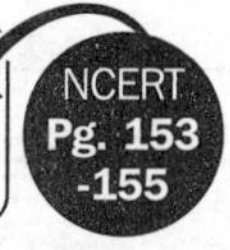

31. Name any two major components in sewage water. ____________

32. Expand STP. ____________

33. Treatment of wastewater is done by ____________ (autotrophic/heterotrophic) microbes which are naturally present in the sewage.

***34.** Complete the following analogy with respect to sewage treatment.
Primary sewage treatment : Physical : : Secondary sewage treatment : ____________

35. During the primary treatment, floating debris is removed by ____________ and then the grit are removed by ____________.

36. Give the biological term for all the solids that settle down during the primary sewage treatment. ____________

37. The secondary sewage treatment is carried out using the supernatant or effluent of primary sewage treatment.

True ☐ False ☐

____

38. Give biological term for the masses of bacteria associated with fungal filaments.

____

39. Flocs are formed in ____________ tanks when effluent is constantly agitated in ____________ environment.

40. How many of the listed components/organisms are found in secondary sewage treatment?

Primary sludge, Flocs, Activated sludge, Grit

____

41. Expand BOD. ____________

42. BOD refers to the amount of the ____________ consumed if all the organic matters in 1L water were ____________ by bacteria. The sewage water is treated till the BOD is ____________.

43. How would you differentiate between two samples, one containing the primary effluent and the other containing the effluent after secondary treatment?

(a) By checking the color ☐
(b) By measuring the BOD ☐
(c) By tasting the water ☐
(d) By checking the pH ☐

44. During secondary sewage treatment, BOD of effluent reduces due to the consumption of <u>CO_2</u> by the flocs.
(*Rewrite the statement after correcting the underlined word.*)

____

45. Greater BOD value indicates ____________(unpolluted/polluted) water.

***46.** The sediment formed by bacterial flocs in secondary settling tank is called ______

47. Arrange the following in the sequence of their requirement during sewage treatment.

I. Large aeration tank　　II. Anaerobic sludge digester

III. Primary settling tank　　IV. Secondary settling tank

______

***48.** Digestion of primary sludge by anaerobic bacteria in anaerobic sludge digester forms biogas.

True ☐　　False ☐

49. The effluent of secondary treatment plant is released into ______ (aeration tank/natural water body).

50. Match Column I with Column II.

Column I	Column II
A. BOD	1. Flocs
B. Secondary treatment	2. Increased in polluted water
C. Dissolved organic matter	3. Large aeration tank
D. Bacterial masses froming mess-like structures	4. Secondary treatment

Codes.

	A	B	C	D			A	B	C	D	
(a)	1	3	4	2	☐	(b)	2	3	4	1	☐
(c)	3	2	1	4	☐	(d)	1	2	4	3	☐

51. Consider the following steps in the treatment of sewage water

I. Growth of aerobic microbes to reduce BOD.

II. Sequential filtration to remove floating debris.

III. Production of gas.

IV. Growth of anaerobic microbes for digestion of bacteria.

(a) II → IV → I → III ☐　　(b) II → I → IV → III ☐

(c) III → I → IV → II ☐　　(d) I → II → IV → III ☐

52. Name the plans initiated by ministry of environment and forests to save major rivers of India from pollution. ______

TOPIC 4

Microbes in Production of Biogas

NCERT Pg. 155-156

53. Biogas is a mixture of gases such as methane, ______ and carbon dioxide.

54. Microbes produce different gases during ______. The type of gas produced depends upon the microbe and ______ they utilise. Fermentation of dough produce ______ gas whereas anaerobic growth of bacteria on cellulosic material produce ______ gas in large amount.

***55.** Read the following statements and identify the group of bacteria.

(i) Methane producing bacteria.

(ii) Helps in the breakdown of cellulose in the rumen of cattle.

____

56. Consider the following statements.

Statement I Human excreta just like that of ruminants contain a hub of methanogens.

Statement II Methanogens are aerobic bacteria that can breakdown cellulosic materials.

Choose the correct option from the following.

(a) Statement I is true, but statement II is false ☐

(b) Statement I is false, but statement II is true ☐

(c) Both statements I and II are true ☐

(d) Both statements I and II are false ☐

57. Choose the odd one out with respect to the methanogens.

Anaerobic sludge, Hydrothermal vents, Human stomach, Cattle's excreta

____

58. Biogas is commonly called ______________.

59. The biogas plant consists of a concrete tank in which ______________ is collected.

60. Refer to the diagram of typical biogas plant and identify the parts labelled as *A, B* and *C*.

Gas

(A) (B) (C)

CH_4+CO_2+

Digester

A. ______________

B. ______________

C. ______________

61. Which of the following pair cannot act as the substrate for methanogens?

(a) Paper, fruit peels ☐ (b) Banana peel, seeds ☐

(c) Vegetable waste, cotton ☐ (d) Fungal colonies, egg shells ☐

62. The spent slurry removed from biogas plant is used as ______________ (fertiliser/cattle feed).

63. Identify the incorrect statement w.r.t. to biogas plant.

(a) Biogas plant consists of a concrete tank 10-15 m deep fed with bio wastes and slurry ☐

(b) The plant has an outlet that supplies gas to nearby houses *via* pipes ☐

(c) Biogas plants are largley found in rural areas due to the easy availability of cattle dung ☐

(d) Biogas plants pose a threat to increasing pollution in the area due to release of CO_2 ☐

64. Expand IARI. ______________________________

65. Expand KVIC. ______________________________

66. IARI and KVIC contributed in the production of ______________________.

TOPIC 5

Microbes as Biocontrol Agents

NCERT Pg. 156 -157

67. Give the scientific term for the use of biological methods for controlling plant diseases and pests. ______________________________

68. Complete the following analogy.
Organic farming : Biocontrol method : : ______________ : Chemical method

69. Organic farmers believe that eradication of pests affect the survival of beneficial predatory and parasitic insects.

True ☐ False ☐

70. If insecticides are used to control insect pests in a given area, which of the following would not be the likely outcome?

(a) Increase in N_2 fixing capacity of plant ☐
(b) Disturbance in the food chains of the area ☐
(c) Loss of biodiversity of the given place ☐
(d) Increased pollution of waterbodies ☐

71. How many of the listed factors are required to be known about pests and predators to develop appropriate means of biocontrol?

Type of pest and predator in field, Life cycles, Feeding habits, Habitat

____

***72.** Match the following columns.

Column I (Biocontrol agents)	Column II (Targets)
A. Ladybird	1. Butterfly caterpillars
B. *Bacillus thuringiensis*	2. Plant pathogens
C. Dragonflies	3. Aphids
D. *Trichoderma*	4. Insects and arthropods
E. Baculoviruses	5. Mosquitoes

A. ____________ B. ____________ C. ____________

D. ____________ E. ____________

73. Consider the following statements.
Statement I Eradicating a pest completely is both possible and desirable.
Statement II *Bt* cotton is resistant to pest larvae due to the engineered gene from *B. thuringiensis.*
Choose the correct option from the following.
(a) Statement I is true, but statement II is false ☐
(b) Statement I is false, but statement II is true ☐
(c) Both statements I and II are true ☐
(d) Both statements I and II are false ☐

74. *Bt* spores are mixed with water and sprayed on to vulnerable plants such as __________. When eaten by insect larvae, *Bt* releases ______________ and the larvae get killed. Plants containing ______________ are insect pests, resistant, e.g. *Bt* cotton.

75. *Trichoderma* species are parasitic fungi in the roots of plants.
True ☐ False ☐

76. *Trichoderma* has proved to be a useful factor in
(a) gene transfer in higher plants ☐
(b) rebuilding of waste lands ☐
(c) biological control of plant pathogens ☐
(d) preventing soil erosion ☐

***77.** Choose the odd one out with respect to baculoviruses.

Species-specific, Broad spectrum insecticides, Pathogenic organisms, Do not affect non-target insects

____

***78.** Expand IPM. ______________________________

***79.** Match Column I with Column II.

	Column I	Column II
A.	*B. thuringiensis*	1. Control mosquitoes
B.	*Nucleopolyhedrovirus*	2. Integrated Pest management
C.	*Trichoderma*	3. Genetically engineered cotton
D.	Dragonflies	4. Free living in root ecosystem

Choose the correct option.

	A	B	C	D			A	B	C	D	
(a)	3	4	2	1	☐	(b)	1	2	4	3	☐
(c)	3	2	4	1	☐	(d)	1	4	2	3	☐

TOPIC 6

Microbes as Biofertilisers

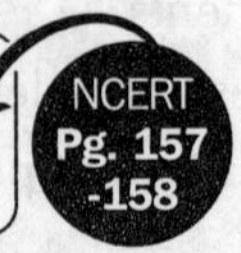

80. Give the scientific term for the organisms that enrich the nutrient quality of the soil.

____

***81.** Choose the odd one out with respect to the source of biofertilisers.

Bacteria, Fungi, Penicillin, Cyanobacteria

____

***82.** Complete the following analogy.
Symbiotic nitrogen-fixing bacteria : *Rhizobium* : : Free-living nitrogen-fixing bacteria :

____

83. Consider the following statements.

Statement I Organic farming employs the use of microbial agents to enrich soil fertility.

Statement II *Azotobacter* is a free living bacteria that can help plants use atmospheric nitrogen.

Choose the correct option from the following.

(a) Statement I is true, but statement II is false ☐

(b) Statement I is false, but statement II is true ☐

(c) Both statements I and II are true ☐

(d) Both statements I and II are false ☐

***84.** Give the biological term for the symbiotic association of fungi with plants.

____

85. Members of genus–*Glomus* do not form mycorrhiza.

True ☐ False ☐

86. In mycorrhizal association, fungal symbiont absorbs _______________ from soil and passes it to associated plant.

87. Do mycorrhizae associated plants show resistance to root borne pathogens and tolerance to salinity and drought?

Yes ☐ No ☐

88. Cyanobacteria are _______________ (autotrophic/heterotrophic) microbes.

***89.** Which of the following bacteria cannot prepare their own food while helping plants absorb organic forms of nitrogen?

(a) *Anabaena* ☐ (b) *Rhizobium* ☐

(c) *Oscillatoria* ☐ (d) *Nostoc* ☐

***90.** Cyanobacteria serve as an important biofertiliser in _______________ (paddy field/wheat plants).

91. Consider the following statements.

I. Ladybird and Dragon flies help us in getting rid of aphids and mosquitoes.

II. Baculoviruses refer to those pathogens which attack insects and other anthropods.

III. Biodiversity promotes sustainability.

IV. *Trichoderma* species are symbiotic fungal species found commonly in the root system.

V. The use of biocontrol measures is appreciable but will not reduce our dependence on chemicals.

Identify the set of incorrect statements.

(a) I, II and III ☐ (b) II, III and V ☐

(c) II and V ☐ (d) IV and V ☐

Assertion-Reason Questions

The following questions consist of two statements– Assertion (A) and Reason (R). Answer these questions by selecting the appropriate options given below.

(a) Both A and R are true and R is the correct explanation of A

(b) Both A and R are true, but R is not the correct explanation of A

(c) A is true, but R is false

(d) A is false, but R is true

***1.** **Assertion** (A) Small amount of curd added as an inoculum, at suitable temperature causes curdling of milk.
Reason (R) Curd contains millions of lactic acid bacteria that curdles and coagulates milk.

(a) ☐ (b) ☐ (c) ☐ (d) ☐

2. **Assertion** (A) Roquefort cheese is known for its specific and unique flavour and is used widely.
Reason (R) The ripening of roquefort cheese is carried out by *Propionibacterium sharmanii.*

(a) ☐ (b) ☐ (c) ☐ (d) ☐

3. **Assertion** (A) Wine and beer are produced by distillation of fermented broth whereas rum does not require distillation.
Reason (R) *Saccharomyces cerevisiae* is used for fermenting malted cereals and fruit juices.

(a) ☐ (b) ☐ (c) ☐ (d) ☐

4. **Assertion** (A) Antibiotics are produced only by fungi and can kill all kinds of bacteria.
Reason (R) Penicillin was the first antibiotic discovered from the mould *Penicillium notatum.*

(a) ☐ (b) ☐ (c) ☐ (d) ☐

***5.** **Assertion** (A) Streptokinase is used to treat people who have undergone myocardial infarction.
Reason (R) Streptokinase, currently used as therapeutic agent is produced by *Streptococcus* and modified by genetic engineering.

(a) ☐ (b) ☐ (c) ☐ (d) ☐

6. **Assertion** (A) Aerobic bacteria in flocs consume huge portion of organic matter present in waste water.

Reason (R) The BOD of the waste water increases upon action of the aerobic bacteria in secondary treatment.

(a) ☐ (b) ☐ (c) ☐ (d) ☐

7. **Assertion** (A) Cow dung is much common in remote areas and contribute maximum towards biogas production.

Reason (R) Dung of cattle contains anaerobic methanogens that produce methane, CO_2 and H_2.

(a) ☐ (b) ☐ (c) ☐ (d) ☐

8. **Assertion** (A) Use of biocontrol agents to control plant disease holds plenty of advantages.

Reason (R) They are easy to use, cost effective and reduce the impact of chemicals and pesticides on human body.

(a) ☐ (b) ☐ (c) ☐ (d) ☐

***9.** **Assertion** (A) In order to control insect pests, organic farmers prefer using baculoviruses rather than insecticides.

Reason (R) Baculoviruses are biocontrol agents that have no negative impacts on non-target insects.

(a) ☐ (b) ☐ (c) ☐ (d) ☐

***10.** **Assertion** (A) Fungal symbionts of mycorrhiza derive phosphorus from the soil and supplies it to the plants.

Reason (R) Plants with mycorrhizal association often are resistant to pathogens and environmental extremities.

(a) ☐ (b) ☐ (c) ☐ (d) ☐

Case Based Questions

1. The graph given below shows the increase in use of a fungal species for obtaining antibiotics named cephalosporins (A) and Penicillin (B) within a time span of 5 years starting from 2015-2020.

Observe the graph and answer the following questions by choosing the correct answer from options below.

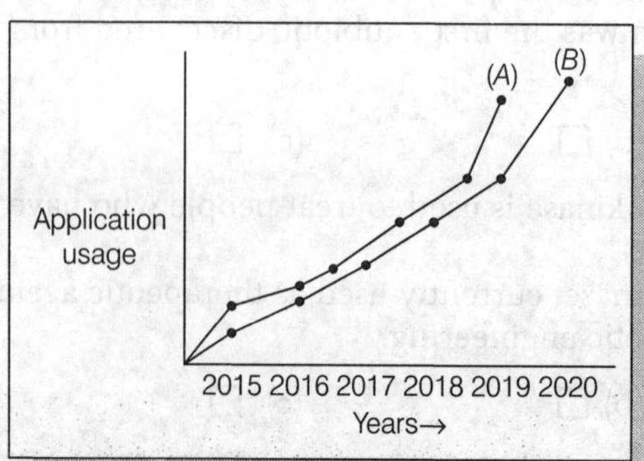

(i) Which of the following represents the correct advantage of using fungi in antibiotic production?

(a) Secretion of antibiotic as a primary metabolite ☐
(b) Easy availability of the species. ☐
(c) Doubling of fungal colonies in minimal time ☐
(d) Colonies can be easily seen ☐

(ii) Identify the correct sources for A and B respectively.

(a) *P. chrysogenum* and *Aspergillus niger* ☐
(b) *Acremonium chrysogenum* and *Penicillium notatum* ☐
(c) *Trichoderma polysporum* and *Aspergillus fumigatus* ☐
(d) *Staphylococci* and *Penicillium notatum* ☐

(iii) The current increase in antibiotic production using fungi will

(a) increase due to the benefits of the fungal species ☐
(b) remain constant after crossing peak value ☐
(c) decrease due to exploitation of the species ☐
(d) undergo no change throughout ☐

2. A small village adjacent to a city, was facing the detrimental impacts of pollution from factories and industries. People living in this village were traditionally farmers. One summer they found that their crops were infested by large flocs of aphids. This resulted in decrease in crop yield. Another challenge was the increasing pollution of water bodies by the run off from fertilisers in the fields. A careful assessment and management of the situation was needed. Based on the given information, answer the following questions:

(i) Which of the following should be used to control the growing number of aphids in the given situation?

(a) Insecticides ☐ (b) Pesticides ☐
(c) Ladybird ☐ (d) *Bt* toxins ☐

(ii) All of the following can be used as an alternative to fertilisers except

(a) *Nostoc* ☐ (b) *Azotobacter* ☐
(c) *Trichoderma* ☐ (d) *Oscillatoria* ☐

(iii) Which of the following is not a nitrogen fixer?

(a) *Anabaena* ☐ (b) *Glomus* ☐
(c) *Azospirillum* ☐ (d) *Rhizobium* ☐

COMPETITION EDGE UP

1. Match List I with List II.

List I	List II
A. Clostridium butylicum	I. Ethanol
B. Saccharomyces cerevisiae	II. Streptokinase
C. Trichoderma polysporum	III. Butyric acid
D. Streptococcus sp.	IV. Cyclosporin-A

Choose the correct answer from the options given below:
[NCERT Pg. 153, NEET 2024]

(a) A-III, B-I, C-II, D-IV ☐
(b) A-II, B-IV, C-III, D-I ☐
(c) A-III, B-I, C-IV, D-II ☐
(d) A-IV, B-I, C-III, D-II ☐

2. Identify the microorganism which is responsible for the production of an immunosuppressive molecule cyclosporin-A. **[NCERT Pg. 152, NEET 2022]**

(a) Clostridium butylicum ☐
(b) Aspergillus niger ☐
(c) Streptococcus cerevisiae ☐
(d) Trichoderma polysporum ☐

3. Match the List I with List II. **[NCERT Pg. 153, NEET 2021]**

List I	List II
A. Aspergillus niger	1. Acetic Acid
B. Acetobacter aceti	2. Lactic Acid
C. Clostridium butylicum	3. Citric Acid
D. Lactobacillus	4. Butyric Acid

Choose the correct answer from the options given below.

	A	B	C	D	
(a)	3	1	4	2	☐
(b)	1	2	3	4	☐
(c)	2	3	1	4	☐
(d)	4	2	1	3	☐

4. Match the following columns and select the correct option. **[NCERT Pg. 153, NEET (Sep.) 2020]**

Column I	Column II
A. Clostridium butylicum	1. Cyclosporin-A
B. Trichoderma polysporum	2. Butyric acid
C. Monascus purpureus	3. Citric acid
D. Aspergillus niger	4. Blood cholesterol lowering agent

	A	B	C	D	
(a)	2	1	4	3	☐
(b)	1	2	4	3	☐
(c)	4	3	2	1	☐
(d)	3	4	2	1	☐

5. Which of the following is put into anaerobic sludge digester for further sewage treatment? **[NCERT Pg. 154, NEET 2020]**

(a) Primary sludge ☐
(b) Floating debris ☐
(c) Effluents of primary treatment ☐
(d) Activated sludge ☐

6. Match the following columns and select the correct option from the codes given below. **[NCERT Pg. 157, NEET (Oct.) 2020]**

Column I	Column II
A. Dragonflies	1. Biocontrol agents of several plant pathogens
B. Bacillus thuringiensis	2. Get rid of aphids and mosquitoes
C. Glomus	3. Narrow spectrum Insecticidal applications
D. Baculoviruses	4. Biocontrol agents of lepidopteran plant pests
	5. Absorb phosphorus from soil

Codes

	A	B	C	D	
(a)	3	5	4	1	☐
(b)	2	1	3	4	☐
(c)	2	3	4	5	☐
(d)	2	4	5	3	☐

7. Match the following organisms with the products they produce **[NCERT Pg. 153, NEET (National) 2019]**

A. Lactobacillus	(i) Cheese
B. Saccharomyces cerevisiae	(ii) Curd
C. Aspergillus niger	(iii) Citric acid
D. Acetobacter aceti	(iv) Bread
	(v) Acetic acid

Select the correct option.

	A	B	C	D	
(a)	(ii)	(iv)	(iii)	(v)	☐
(b)	(iii)	(iv)	(v)	(i)	☐
(c)	(ii)	(i)	(iii)	(v)	☐
(d)	(ii)	(iv)	(v)	(iii)	☐

Chapter 09

Biotechnology : Principles and Processes

Scan and take Chapter Test

TOPIC 1

Principles of Biotechnology and Restriction Enzymes

1. Controlled multiplication of live organisms for deriving products of human welfare is associated with the field of ____________________ (biochemistry/biotechnology).

2. How many processes mentioned below are associated with genetic manipulation?

In Vitro Fertilisation (IVF), Gene therapy, Novel gene synthesis, Translocation, Conjugation

____

3. Expand EFB . ____________________

4. In genetic engineering process, chemistry of genetic material is altered to induce phenotypic change in host.

True ☐ False ☐

5. Fill in the blanks.

(i) ____________________ as a part of biotechnology refers to elimination of all living organisms particularly microbial contamination to enable growth of required organism.

(ii) ____________________ engineering involves maintenance of sterile ambience to enable growth of desired cell.

6. Asexual reproductive mechanism provides opportunities for variations and new genetic combinations.

True ☐ False ☐

*Concepts of all questions bearing * are important for NEET & CUET*

7. In the field of genetic engineering, recombinant DNA (*r*DNA) molecules are formed. The term 'recombinant' here is used in context with

(a) DNA with a piece of foreign DNA ☐

(b) DNA with a piece of RNA ☐

(c) DNA that participates in recombination ☐

(d) DNA not associated with recombination ☐

8. Traditional hybridisation though convenient is not preferred for creating alterations in organisms selected for breeding due to inclusion and multiplication of undesired genes.

True ☐ False ☐

9. Give scientific term for the following statements.

(i) The technique of altering a host's genome by introducing a foreign DNA.

____

(ii) Production of exact copies of a particular gene or DNA sequence.

____

10. A piece of an alien DNA may multiply and be inherited along with the host DNA

(i) When an alien DNA becomes a part of host's genome ☐

(ii) When all palindromic sites are cleaved by restriction enzymes. ☐

(Tick ✓ the most accurate statement)

11. For multiplication in a host cell, an alien piece of DNA should integrate itself with _______________ sequence of the vector.

***12.** *ori* is the _______________ (stop codon/ initiating sequence for replication) in a host cell.

***13.** The sequence that controls copy number of the linked DNA in vector is termed as

(a) gene cloning ☐ (b) plasmid ☐

(c) origin of replication ☐ (d) recombination site ☐

14. Give a biological term for following statement.

An autonomously replicating, circular, extrachromosomal DNA.

____

15. Plasmid used to construct the first *r*DNA was isolated from _______________ (*Escherichia coli* /*Salmonella typhi*).

16. _______________ constructed the first artificial recombinant DNA by linking an _______________ gene with _______________.

17. Complete the following analogy
Restriction enzymes : Molecular scissors :: *ori* : _______________

18. During construction of a recombinant DNA, the linking of antibiotic resistance gene with plasmid is done using *Taq* polymerase.

True ☐ False ☐

19. Plasmids are used as _______________ to deliver an alien piece of DNA into the host organism.

20. The enzyme DNA gyrase acts on cut DNA molecules and joins their ends.
(*Rewrite the statement after correcting the underlined words.*)

____

21. Recombinant DNA when transferred into *Agrobacterium* , a bacterium closely related to *Salmonella,* could replicate using the new hosts's reverse transcriptase enzyme and make multiple copies.

True ☐ False ☐

22. To proceed with the process of genetic modification, first the desired DNA is amplified.
(*Rewrite the statement after correcting the underlined word*.)

____

23. The most common host used in RDT for maintaining the introduced DNA is ______________ (*E. coli / Salmonella*).

24. Consider the following steps of carrying out a genetic modification.

I. Maintenance of introduced gene in the host followed by transfer to progeny.
II. Identification of DNA with desirable gene.
III. Observing the correct functioning and related outputs of the introduced gene.
IV. Introduction of identified DNA into the host.

Choose the correct sequence of the above steps from the options below.

(a) IV → III → II → I ☐ (b) II → III → I → IV ☐
(c) II → I → IV → III ☐ (d) II → IV → III → I ☐

25. Recombinant DNA technology can be accomplished only in the presence of certain key tools. How many of these tools are mentioned in the box given below?

Microscope, Restriction enzymes, Host cells, Polymerase, Vectors, Topoisomerase, Ligases

____

26. Restriction enzymes are lysing enzymes used in RDT.

True ☐ False ☐

27. First restriction enzyme with endonuclease activity was ______________.(*Pst* I/ *Hind* II)

28. More than 150 restriction enzymes have been isolated from over 230 bacterial strains.
(*Rewrite the statement after correcting the underlined word.*)

____

29. Restriction enzymes are a part of defence against bacteriophages in bacteria, which cleave the viral DNA. This system is known as

____

30. While naming restriction enzymes, the first letter of the name comes from the species of host organism.

True ☐ False ☐

31. Identify the incorrect statement with respect to restriction endonuclease.

(a) Restriction enzymes can be thought of as proteins that cleave DNA sequences at certain specific sites ☐

(b) These enzymes are mainly found in bacteria ☐

(c) First letter of the name of enzyme comes from genus and second two letters come from the species of prokaryotic cell from which they are isolated ☐

(d) *Hin*d II always makes a cut in DNA sequence after recognising a specific sequence of 5 bp ☐

32. The source of restriction enzyme *Eco*RI is

(a) *Bacillus thuringiensis* ☐ (b) *Streptomyces albus* ☐

(c) *Escherichia coli* RY 13 ☐ (d) *Escherichia coli* RY 20 ☐

33. Restriction enzymes break ________________ linkages.

***34.** Endonucleases are the class of enzymes that break DNA at specific sites from within.

True ☐ False ☐

35. Enzymes that remove nucleotide one at a time from the ends of DNA molecules are modifying enzymes.

True ☐ False ☐

***36.** Restriction endonuclease cut

(a) *ss* DNA at a specific point after identifying a nuclear localisation signal ☐

(b) *ds* RNA by identifying a nuclear localisation signal ☐

(c) each of the two strands of the double helical DNA, by identifying a specific recognition site ☐

(d) *ss*DNA at a particular point after identifying a signaling molecule ☐

37. Complete the following analogy with respect to *Eco*RI.

R : strain :: *co* : ________________

38. In *Eco*RI, I stand for the <u>number</u> of enzyme isolated from a particular bacterial strain. (*Rewrite the statement after correcting the underlined word.*)

____

39. Some endonucleases are highly specific and operate at specific sites of DNA called ____________.

***40.** Complete the following analogy given below.

Endonuclease : Cuts DNA at palindromic nucleotide sequence : : Exonuclease : ________________.

***41.** Restriction sites are palindromic nucleotide sequences.

True ☐ False ☐

***42.** Each restriction endonuclease functions by

(i) isolating the length of a DNA sequence.

(ii) inspecting the length of DNA sequence.

(Write the correct one in the space below)

____

43. Identify the DNA segment that does not represent a palindromic sequence.

(a) 5′ GCGGCCGC 3′
3′ CGCCGGCG 5′ ☐

(b) 5′ GGATCC 3′
3′ GGTACC 5′ ☐

(c) 5′ GAATTC 3′
3′ CTTAAG 5′ ☐

(d) 5′ CCCGGG 3′
3′ GGGCCC 5′ ☐

44. Restriction enzymes cut each of the two strands of the double helix at specific points in their ____________ backbone.

45. The recognition sequence of restriction enzymes reads the same when read in ____________ direction on either of the strands.

***46.** In the figure given below

(i) Identify the labels *A-C*.

The enzyme cuts both DNA strands at the same site

Restriction enzyme Ⓐ cuts the DNA between bases G and A only when the sequence GAATTC is present in the DNA

Foreign DNA

Ⓑ

G A A T T C
C T T A A G

[I]

A A T T

G
C T T A A

[II]

DNA fragments join at the ends with the help of Ⓒ

Recombinant DNA

A. ____________

B. ____________

C. ____________

(ii) What kinds of ends are formed at I and II? ____________

***47.** Read the sequence of two separate DNA strands

(i) 5′- GTCGAC-3′ (ii) 5′-GAATTC-3′.

What is common to both these sequences?

____

***48.** Consider the given image. Identify which of the following enzymes would recognise the given sequence.

G A A T T C
C T T A A G

(a) *Hind* II ☐

(b) *Eco* RI ☐

(c) *Hind* III ☐

(d) *Bam* HI ☐

***49.** Identify the parts labelled as *A, B* and *C* in the figure given below.

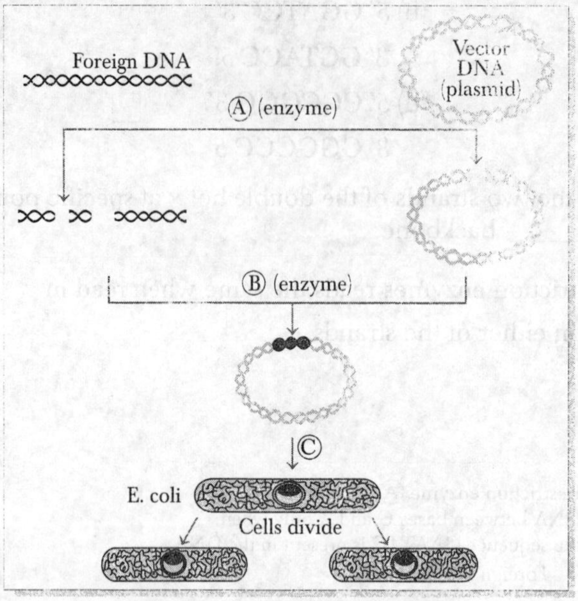

Foreign DNA
Vector DNA (plasmid)
(A) (enzyme)
(B) (enzyme)
(C)
E. coli
Cells divide

A. ______________

B. ______________

C. ______________

50. Why is it necessary to use the same restriction enzyme (*Eco*RI)for cutting the vector and the foreign DNA?

(a) It removes nucleotides from the end and helps in ligation. ☐

(b) It generates different overhangs in the foreign DNA and vector. ☐

(c) It generates the same sticky ends which makes ligation easier. ☐

(d) It is cheaper to use the same restriction enzyme. ☐

51. Ligase enzyme mediates the formation of phosphodiester bonds between adjacent ______________ termini, thereby joining the nicks in double-stranded DNA.

***52.** Fill in the blanks.

*Eco*RI cuts its palindromic sequence which produces overhangs called ________ ends that form __________ bonds with their complementary cut strands.

53. The fragments obtained from vector and host DNA cut by the same restriction enzyme will yield __________, which facilitate the action of __________.

54. Restriction endonucleases are used in genetic engineering processes to

(i) Form recombinant molecules of DNA

(ii) Generate palindromic sites

(*Choose correct one*)

____

55. The resultant DNA fragments have the same kind of sticky ends when cut by the ______________ restriction enzyme.

56. Which enzyme is called as molecular glue?

____

57. Give a scientific term for the following statement.
The process of insertion of *r*DNA in bacterial genome.

___

***58.** Will a vector cut by restriction enzyme 1 and a source DNA cut by restriction enzyme 2 produce a recombinant molecule?

Yes ☐ No ☐

59. When a restriction enzyme recognises its specific sequence in a given DNA segment

(i) It binds to it and generate fragments. ☐

(ii) It first methylate the segment then cleave it. ☐

(*Tick* ✔ *the correct statement.*)

60. Give biological term for following statement.
The technique to separate DNA fragments *in vitro* using natural polymer extracted from sea weeds.

___

***61.** DNA are positively charged molecules.

True ☐ False ☐

***62.** Study the figure given below and answer the following questions.

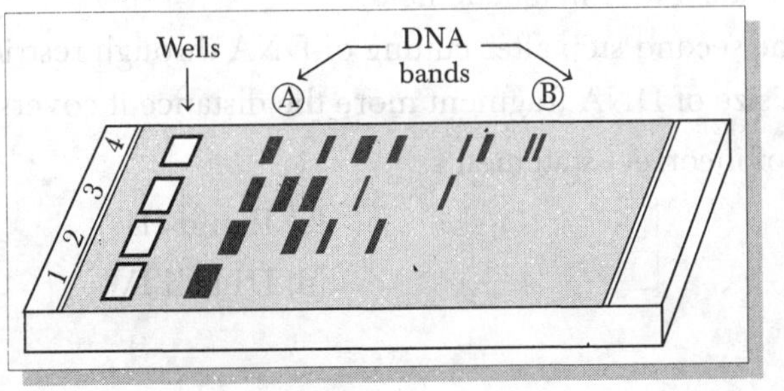

(i) What does the figure respresent? ___

(ii) Identify the type of DNA bands present at *A* and *B*.

A.___ B.___

***63.** The picture represents the process of agarose gel electrophoresis to separate DNA fragments. Study the diagram carefully and answer the question that follows.

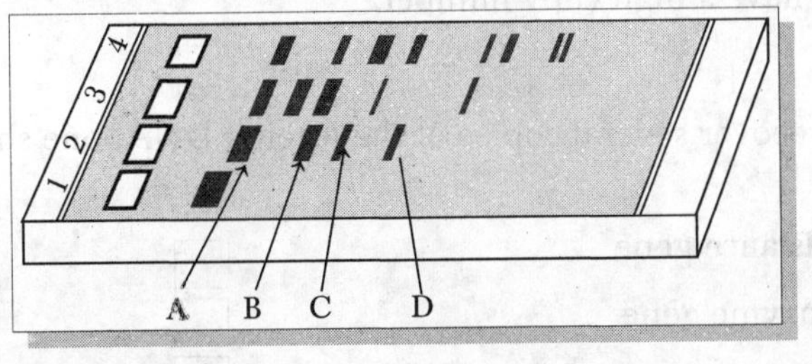

Considering the lane 2, band labelled 'A' shows less distance covered due to

(a) low affinity towards matrix ☐ (b) high affinity towards matrix ☐

(c) high molecular weight ☐ (d) larger size ☐

***64.** Under an electric field, DNA fragments will move towards ____________.

65. The matrix used during electrophoretic segregation of DNA fragments is ____________. (agarose/gelatin)

***66.** The DNA fragments separate based on their size by sieving effect.

True ☐ False ☐

***67.** The dye used to stain separates fragments of DNA is ____________. (aniline blue/ethidium bromide).

***68.** Which of the following steps should be performed by a person in order to visualise bands of DNA, as obtained from gel electrophoresis?

(a) Direct exposure of DNA fragments to UV radiations ☐
(b) Staining the bands with bromophenol blue followed by exposure to UV radiations ☐
(c) Staining the bands with EtBr ☐
(d) Staining the bands with ethidium bromide followed by exposure to UV radiations ☐

***69.** Consider the following statements.

I. The most commonly used matrix is agarose a natural polymer extracted from sea weeds.
II. DNA fragments are negatively charged and can be separated by forcing them to move towards cathode under magnetic field.
III. Elution is the second step after cutting of DNA through restriction enzymes.
IV. Smaller the size of DNA fragment more the distance it covers.

Choose the set of incorrect statements.

(a) I and III ☐ (b) II and III ☐
(c) II and IV ☐ (d) III and IV ☐

TOPIC 2

Cloning Vectors and Competent Host

NCERT Pg. 168-171

70. In recombinant DNA technique, the term vector refers to a ____________.

71. A vector should have a high copy number.

True ☐ False ☐

72. If one wants to recover several copies of the foreign DNA, one should clone the gene in a plasmid with

(a) antibiotic resistance gene ☐
(b) replication enzyme gene ☐
(c) an origin that support high copy number ☐
(d) many restriction sites ☐

73. Apart from helping in linking foreign DNA, vectors can also help in ________________ of recombinant cells.

74. Bacteriophages may have 15-100 copies per cell.
(*Rewrite the statement after correcting the underlined word.*)

____

75. ______________ sequence enables a vector to replicate autonomously and generate multiple copies of itself.

76. An ampicillin resistant gene in a vector is called ________________.

77. Identification and elimination of non-transformed cells is a function of ori.
(*Rewrite the statement after correcting the underlined word.*)

____

***78.** Normal *E. coli* cells carry resistance against ampicillin and kanamycin.

True ☐ False ☐

***79.** Consider the following statements.

Statement I Selectable markers only allow selection of transformants from non-transformants.

Statement II Genes encoding resistance to antibiotics such as kanamycin, etc. are considered useful markers for *Staphylococcus* bacterium.

Choose the correct option from the following.

(a) Statement I is true, but statement II is false ☐
(b) Statement I is false, but statement II is true ☐
(c) Both statements I and II are true ☐
(d) Both statements I and II are false ☐

80. The vector selected for RDT should have ______________ recognition site. The presence of multiple cloning sites generates several DNA fragments which complicate the ______________.

81. The ligation of alien DNA is carried out at restriction site carrying ______________ (*ori* /an antibiotic resistance gene).

82. pBR322 is an artificial cloning vector based on bacteriophages.

True ☐ False ☐

83. Pick the odd one out.

EcoRI, Hind III, pBR322, BamHI, Sal I

____

***84.** Consider the diagram given below and answer the following questions.

Eco RI, Cla I, Hind III, Pvu I, Bam HI, Pst I, (A), (B), Sal I, ori, rop, Pvu II

(i) The figure represents a ______________ (cosmid/plasmid) vector.

(ii) Name this vector. ______________

(iii) This vector has two selectable markers *A* and *B*, whose function is *C*. Identify *A*, *B* and *C*.

A.______________ B.______________ C.______________

(iv) To cut at *Eco*RI restriction site, the recognition sequence at 5′-3′ should be read as ______________

***85.** The recombinant plasmid (pBR322) after losing tetracycline resistance can still be selected from non-recombinants by plating transformants on ________ containing media.

***86.** Transformed bacterial cells grown on tetracycline containing medium, produced 9 distinct colonies. However transferring them on to ampicillin containing media, reduced the number of colonies to 6. Based on this information, which of the following gene was disrupted by insertional inactivation?

(a) Ampicillin resistance gene ☐ (b) Tetracycline resistance gene ☐

(c) Both genes were inactivated ☐ (d) Both genes remain intact ☐

***87.** In blue-white screening, a fluorescent substrate is used to differentiate recombinant cells. (*Rewrite the statement after correcting the underlined word.*)

____

***88.** According to blue-white screening method, recombinants undergo inactivation of enzyme ______________ (β-galactosidase/ transacetylase).

***89.** Give a scientific term for the following statement.
The inactivation of a gene by insertion of DNA sequence within it.

____

90. "Selecting recombinants due to inactivation of antibiotics is a complicated process". Give reason.

____

***91.** Consider the following statements.

Statement I Ligating foreign DNA at the coding region of β-galactosidase allows selection of recombinants.

Statement II The blue colonies formed after addition of chromogenic substrates contain recombinant plasmids.

Choose the correct option from the following.

(a) Statement I is true, but statement II is false ☐

(b) Statement I is false, but statement II is true ☐

(c) Both statements I and II are true ☐

(d) Both statements I and II are false ☐

***92.** For transforming plant cells____________________________ (*Agrobacterium tumefaciens*/adenovirus) is used.

***93.** Plant cells can transform into tumour cells when we insert ________ (B-DNA/ T-DNA) from a known plant pathogen.

***94.** *Agrobacterium* is a plant pathogen of monocot plants like wheat and maize.

True ☐ False ☐

95. Which part of the *Agrobacterium*'s DNA has been modified to be used as a vector for transforming plant cells in genetic engineering?

____

96. The Ti plasmid of *Agrobacterium* is pathogenic as they deliver T-DNA that transforms normal cells to tumour cells. To use the Ti plasmid safely for gene delivery without inducing tumours in host plants, which of the following steps become absolutely necessary?

(a) Restriction digestion of the vector ☐
(b) Ligation of the vector and insert ☐
(c) Insertion of selectable marker genes ☐
(d) Disarming the plasmid DNA ☐

97. ____________ can transform normal cells to cancerous in animals with the help of an enzyme, reverse transcriptase.

98. DNA cannot pass through cell membranes because

(i) it is hydrophobic. ☐ (ii) it is hydrophilic. ☐

(*Tick* ☑ *the most appropriate option*)

99. Give one word answer for following statement.
The bacterial cell which can uptake a foreign DNA from the surrounding medium.

____

100. While working in a laboratory, Aakash tried to incorporate a foreign DNA into a bacterial cell. To speed up the process, which of the following methods should be chosen by him so that host cell incorporates DNA at a faster rate?

(a) PCR ☐
(b) Transduction ☐
(c) Treatment with divalent cation followed by heat shock ☐
(d) Gene gun ☐

101. Heat shock (at 42°C) creates ________________ in the cell membrane of host cells and facilitates uptake of foreign DNA.

102. Competent cells in an experiment were made to undergo transformation by heat shock method. Which of the following steps in the transformation went wrong?

(a) Cells were incubated with recombinant DNA on ice ☐
(b) Reaction mixture was heated to 60° C for few seconds ☐
(c) The experiment was performed under sterile conditions ☐
(d) After heat shock, cells were put back in ice ☐

103. Pick the odd one out.

Plant tumours, Viruses, Gene gun, Retroviruses

____

104. Complete the following analogy.
Animal cells: ______________ : : Plant cells: Biolistics

***105.** High velocity microparticles delivered into plant cells for transformation are made up of ____________ (gold or tungsten/ lead).

106. Disarmed pathogen vectors have been genetically modified to eliminate their ________ .

107. Disarmed pathogen vectors transfer DNA without any risk of infection in host cells.
True ☐ False ☐

108. Consider the following statements.

I. Alternative selectable markers have been developed in order to differentiate recombinants from non-recombinants based on their ability to produce colour in the presence of chromogenic substances.

II. *Agrobacterium*-mediated plant transformation is a highly evolved process that involves genetic determinants of both the bacterium as well as the host plant cell.

III. Retro viruses are able to integrate efficiently into the genome of plant cells and replicate followed by their transfer to all the progeny.

IV. Once a gene or a DNA fragment has been ligated into a suitable enzyme it is transferred into a bacterial, plant or animal host.

Identity the incorrect statements.

(a) I, II, III and IV ☐ (b) II and III ☐

(c) III and IV ☐ (d) II, III and IV ☐

TOPIC 3

Processes of Recombinant DNA Technology

NCERT Pg. 171-173

***109.** Arrange the following process involved in *r*DNA technology as per their correct sequence.

I. Isolation of DNA
II. Ligation of DNA into vector
III. Fragmentation of DNA
IV. Transfer of *r*DNA in host
V. Extraction of desired product
VI. Isolation of desired plasmid DNA fragment
VII. Culturing host cells at large scale

____

110. Biochemically, the genetic material in most organisms is ________ (protein/ nucleic acid).

111. Match the following columns.

Column I (Enzymes)	Column II (Target cells)
A. Lysozyme	1. Plant cells
B. Cellulase	2. Bacterial cells
C. Chitinase	3. Fungal cells

A. ______________ B. ______________ C. ______________

112. When we break open a cell to extract DNA, we also obtain many other constituents. How many of the following can be identified as the same?

RNA, Lipids, Carbon, Proteins, Polysaccharides, Bile, Vitamins

____

113. Complete the following analogy with respect to molecules given.
RNA : _______________ : : Proteins : Protease

***114.** To remove DNA from the extract, we can use <u>$CaCl_2$</u>.
(*Rewrite the statement after correcting the underlined word.*)

____

115. Consider the following figure.

The above figure represents the separation of DNA by a method called _______________.

116. Fragmentation of DNA is facilitated by incubation with lyases.

True ☐ False ☐

117. To check the progression of DNA digestion we use <u>SDS-PAGE</u>.
(*Rewrite the statement after correcting the underlined word.*)

____

118. Complete the following analogy.
Ligation of vector DNA to host: Ligase: : Amplification of desired DNA: _______________

***119.** Answer the following questions based on figure given below.
Identify the processes occurring at *A*, *B* and *C*.

Region to be amplified
5′ 3′ *ds* DNA
3′ 5′
Heat (A)
5′ 3′
3′ 5′ (B)
5′ 3′
3′ 5′
DNA polymerase
(*Taq* polymerase)
+ deoxynucleotides
5′ 3′
5′ 3′ (C)
3′ 5′
3′ 5′
30 cycles
3′
Amplified
(~1 billion times)

A. _______________

B. _______________

C. _______________

120. How many of the following are essential requirements of PCR?

Primers, Ribonuclease, DNA template, Restriction enzymes, Taq polymerase, dNTPs

____

***121.** Consider the following statements.

Statement I The denaturation step of PCR is performed at high temperatures to separate the DNA strands.

Statement II PCR primers are oligonucleotides that are extended in the extension step by *Taq* polymerase.

Choose the correct option from the following.

(a) Statement I is true, but statement II is false ☐

(b) Statement I is false, but statement II is true ☐

(c) Both statements I and II are true ☐

(d) Both statements I and II are false ☐

***122.** The *Taq* polymerase is thermostable as it remains active during ____________ (denaturation/extension).

***123.** *Taq* polymerase is isolated from ____________.

***124.** In PCR, the *Taq* polymerase unwinds the DNA strands.

True ☐ False ☐

125. By using PCR, approximately <u>100</u> copies of desired DNA can be obtained. (*Rewrite the statement after correcting the underlined word.*)

____

126. Typically a PCR is run for 30 cycles.

True ☐ False ☐

127. Molecular diagnosis, DNA fingerprinting, Palaeontology use ____________ to amplify limited amount of DNA.

128. The following represents the steps to clone a foreign gene into a bacterial system.

I. Restriction digestion of the foreign gene and the plasmid.
II. PCR amplification of the isolated foreign gene.
III. Selection by plating in antibiotic containing media.
IV. Incubation of the foreign gene and plasmid with ligase.
V. Calcium treatment and transformation of host bacteria.

Which of the following represents the correct order of the steps?

(a) I → II → IV → V → III ☐ (b) II → I → IV → V → III ☐

(c) IV → II → I → V → III ☐ (d) IV → II → I → III → V ☐

129. The ultimate aim of RDT is to produce a desired protein.

True ☐ False ☐

130. Give a scientific term for the following statement.
Protein encoded by a gene in a heterologous host.

____

TOPIC 4

Bioreactors and Downstream Processing

NCERT Pg. 173-175

131. To produce a recombinant protein at large scale ______________ (bioreactors / small culture vessels) are used.

132. In ______________ culture system used medium is drained and fresh medium is added.

133. Continuous culture techniques produce less biomass leading to higher yield of desired proteins.

True ☐ False ☐

134. In continuous cultures, the cells are maintained in their ______________ (lag/exponential) phase.

135. In the figure given below which apparatus is shown?

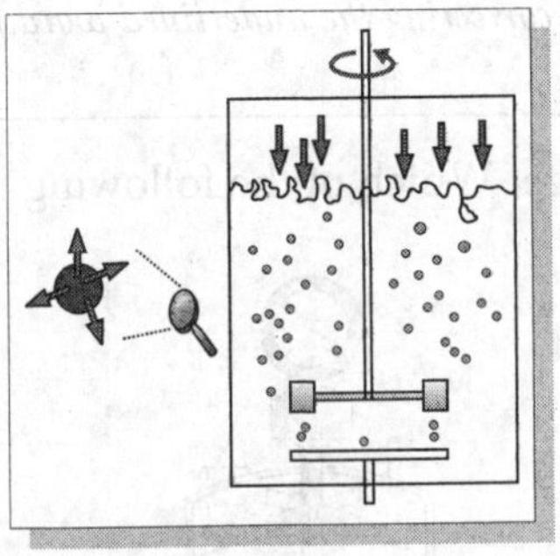

____

136. Consider the following statements.

Statement I In bioreactors, media can be reused as it would allow cells to retain their log phase of growth.

Statement II The only function of the stirrer is to mix the nutrient media evenly in a stirred tank bioreactor.

Choose the correct option from the following.

(a) Statement I is true, but statement II is false ☐

(b) Statement I is false, but statement II is true ☐

(c) Both statements I and II are true ☐

(d) Both statements I and II are false ☐

137. What is the role of bubbles present in the bioreactor?

____

138. Observe the figure given below and answer the following questions.

(i) In the figure given below, label all the essential parts (A to E).

A. ____________

B. ____________

C. ____________

D. ____________

E. ____________

(ii) This type of bioreactor is known as ____________

(iii) In this bioreactor, bubbles facilitate the mixing of contents.
(*Rewrite the statement after correcting the underlined word.*)

____

***139.** Consider the provided image. Which of the following function would be altered if the part labelled as *X* is damaged?

(a) Sterilisation of the media ☐ (b) Breakdown of the foam ☐

(c) Aeration and homogenisation ☐ (d) pH of the growth media ☐

***140.** Complete the following table given below.

Components of bioreactor	Functions
(A)	Mixes the growth media, breaks any clumps
Oxygen delivery system	(B)
(C)	Prevent contamination in fermentation process
Sampling ports	(D)
(E)	To ensure better dispersal of air
Impellers	(F)

A. ____________ B. ____________ C. ____________

D. ____________ E. ____________ F. ____________

141. Give scientific term.

The process of separation and purification of recombinant proteins.

____

142. Before commercially releasing the recombinant product, clinical trials are undertaken to ensure

____

143. Consider the following statements.

Statement I Downstream processing deals with separation and purification of the product along with addition of preservatives and its marketing.

Statement II Dung need to pass through clinical trials before they are made available in markets.

Choose the correct option from the following.

(a) Statement I is true, but statement II is false ☐

(b) Statement I is false, but statement II is true ☐

(c) Both statements I and II are true ☐

(d) Both statements I and II are false ☐

Assertion-Reason Questions

The following questions consist of two statements– Assertion (A) and Reason (R). Answer these questions by selecting the appropriate options given below.

(a) Both A and R are true and R is the correct explanation of A

(b) Both A and R are true, but R is not the correct explanation of A

(c) A is true, but R is false

(d) A is false, but R is true

***1. Assertion** (A) For creating recombinant plasmid it is necessary to cut the plasmid and foreign DNA with the same restriction enzyme.

Reason (R) Restriction enzymes binds to the recognition sequence and cut each of the two strands at a specific point.

(a) ☐ (b) ☐ (c) ☐ (d) ☐

***2. Assertion** (A) Agarose gel electrophoresis allows separating DNA fragments based on their molecular weight.

Reason (R) The seggregated smaller pieces of DNA on an agarose gel cover maximum distance while larger ones travel the least.

(a) ☐ (b) ☐ (c) ☐ (d) ☐

***3. Assertion** (A) A foreign antibiotic resistance gene when introduced simply into *E. coli* would not replicate on its own.

Reason (R) Replication of DNA requires the presence of the origin of replication from where DNA synthesis starts.

(a) ☐ (b) ☐ (c) ☐ (d) ☐

*4. **Assertion** (A) Non-recombinants produce white colonies, while the recombinants produce blue colonies.

Reason (R) Insertional inactivation of specific gene sequences allows the selection of recombinants from non-recombinants.

(a) ☐ (b) ☐ (c) ☐ (d) ☐

5. **Assertion** (A) To allow the host cells take up the recombinant plasmid, the cells are treated with a divalent cation.

Reason (R) Competent host cells are given a heat shock for a few seconds followed by transferring into ice.

(a) ☐ (b) ☐ (c) ☐ (d) ☐

6. **Assertion** (A) For isolating DNA from a plant cell it is necessary to treat the cells with enzymes.

Reason (R) Plant cells can be degraded by chitinase enzymes which makes the isolation easier.

(a) ☐ (b) ☐ (c) ☐ (d) ☐

*7. **Assertion** (A) PCR reactions can only be carried out by *taq* polymerase enzymes.

Reason (R) *Taq* polymerase is stable to high temperature mediated denaturation step of PCR.

(a) ☐ (b) ☐ (c) ☐ (d) ☐

8. **Assertion** (A) Repeated amplification is done preferably using *taq* polymerase.

Reason (R) *Taq* polymerase is capable of functioning at higher temperatures with constantly maintained efficiency.

9. **Assertion** (A) In a sparged stirred type bioreactor sterile air bubbles are sparged.

Reason (R) Stirred tank bioreactor has a curved base to facilitate mixing of reactor contents.

(a) ☐ (b) ☐ (c) ☐ (d) ☐

10. **Assertion** (A) The process of downstream requires separation, purification and formulation of products with suitable preservatives.

Reason (R) Downstream processing and quality control testing are same for all the products manufactured.

(a) ☐ (b) ☐ (c) ☐ (d) ☐

Case Based Questions

*1. pBR322 is a plasmid and one of the first widely used *E. coli* cloning vectors. It was found to be the most versatile and thus was considered suitable. Now, study the image of the plasmid carefully and try to understand the following situation. You as a researcher have to insert a foreign gene at the *Bam*H I restriction site in order to carry our further steps in the process. Analyse the given plasmid and answer the questions that follow

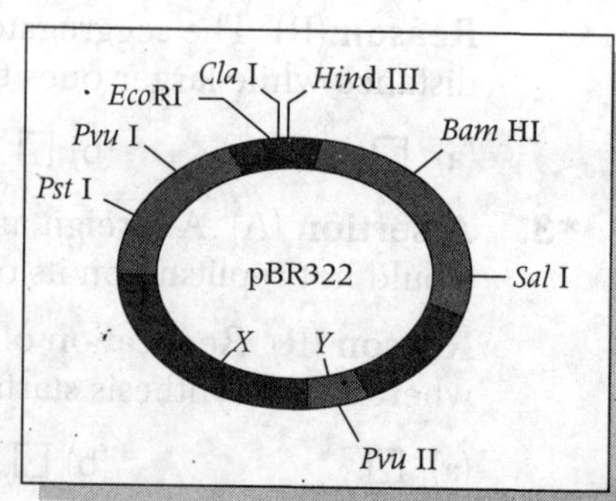

(i) In the given plasmid a gene is inserted using *Pvu*I restriction site. This in turn makes the amp^R gene non-functional, but the recombinant is tetracycline resistant. This concludes that

(a) insertion of gene has given tetracycline resistant properties to pBR322 ☐

(b) pBR322 has both amp^R and tet^R genes ☐

(c) tetracycline resistant property of pBR322 functions only in absence of ampicillin resistant gene ☐

(d) the plasmid must have undergone high temperature treatment ☐

(ii) Transformed recombinant plasmid would grow on media containing

(a) Both ampicillin and tetracycline ☐ (b) Only tetracycline ☐

(c) Only ampicillin ☐ (d) None of the antibiotics ☐

(iii) If foreign gene is ligated in the *Pvu* I restriction site, which of the following genes would show insertional inactivation?

(a) *Pvu* I restriction endonuclease ☐ (b) *Pst* I restriction endonuclease ☐

(c) Ampicillin resistance ☐ (d) Tetracycline resistance ☐

2. A scientist has to isolate a foreign DNA from *Salmonella typhi* bacterium. He next plans on amplifying the foreign DNA before ligating it with a suitable plasmid to create a recombinant plasmid. Based on this information, answer the following questions.

(i) Which of the following enzymes would not be used for isolation of foreign DNA from the bacterium?

(a) Lysozyme ☐ (b) RNases ☐

(c) Proteases ☐ (d) Ligase ☐

(ii) Which organism is the source of the enzyme needed for amplification of the foreign DNA?

(a) *E. coli* ☐ (b) *Salmonella typhi* ☐

(c) *Thermus aquaticus* ☐ (d) *Bacillus* ☐

(iii) Once the recombinant plasmid is created it becomes necessary to make the host cell accept the *r*DNA. Which of the following ions can be used to make the host cells accept the recombinant DNA?

(a) Calcium ☐ (b) Chloride ☐

(c) Sulphate ☐ (d) Phosphate ☐

COMPETITION EDGE UP

1. *What is the fate of a piece of DNA carrying only gene of interest which is transferred into an alien organism?* **[NCERT Pg. 164, NEET 2024]**

A. The piece of DNA would be able to multiply itself independently in the progeny cells of the organism.

B. It may get integrated into the genome of the recipient.

C. It may multiply and be inherited along with the host DNA.

D. The alien piece of DNA is not an integral part of chromosome.

E. It shows ability to replicate.

Choose the correct answer from the options given below.

(a) A and B only ☐

(b) D and E only ☐

(c) B and C only ☐

(d) A and E only ☐

2. *Hind II always cuts DNA molecules at a particular point called recognition sequence and it consists of* **[NCERT Pg. 165, NEET 2024]**

(a) 8 bp ☐

(b) 6 bp ☐

(c) 4 bp ☐

(d) 10 bp ☐

3. *The following diagram shows restriction sites in E. coli cloning vector pBR322. Find the role of 'X' and 'Y' genes.* **[NCERT Pg. 169, NEET 2024]**

Cla I
Hind III
*Eco*RI
Pvu I
Bam HI
Pst I
pBR322
Sal I
X
Y
Pvu II

(a) The gene 'X' is responsible for resistance to antibiotics and 'Y' for protein involved in the replication of plasmid. ☐

(b) The gene 'X' is responsible for controlling the copy number of the linked DNA and 'Y' for protein involved in the replication of plasmid. ☐

(c) The gene 'X' is for protein involved in replication of plasmid and 'Y' for resistance to antibiotics. ☐

(d) Gene 'X' is responsible for recognitions sites and 'Y' is responsible for antibiotic resistance. ☐

4. *During the purification process for recombinant DNA technology, addition of chilled ethanol precipitates out* **[NCERT Pg. 171, NEET 2023, 21]**

(a) DNA ☐

(b) histones ☐

(c) polysaccharides ☐

(d) RNA ☐

5. *In the following palindromic base sequences of DNA, which one can be cut easily by particular restriction enzyme?* **[NCERT Pg. 167, NEET 2022]**

(a) 5' G A A T T C 3'; 3' C T T A A G 5' ☐

(b) 5' C T C A G T 3'; 3' G A G T C A 5' ☐

(c) 5' G T A T T C 3'; 3' C A T A A G 5' ☐

(d) 5' G A T A C T 3'; 3' C T A T G A 5' ☐

6. *Which one of the following statement is not true regarding gel electrophoresis technique?* **[NCERT Pg. 168, 170 NEET 2022]**

(a) The separated DNA fragments are stained by using ethidium bromide ☐

(b) The presence of chromogenic substrate gives blue coloured DNA bands on the gel ☐

(c) Bright orange coloured bands of DNA can be observed in the gel when exposed to UV light ☐

(d) The process of extraction of separated DNA strands from gel is called elution ☐

7. *Which of the following is not a desirable feature of a cloning vector?* **[NCERT Pg. 169, NEET 2022]**

(a) Presence of a marker gene ☐

(b) Presence of single restriction enzyme site ☐

(c) Presence of two or more recognition sites ☐

(d) Presence of origin of recognition sites ☐

8. *Given below are two statements, one is labelled as Assertion (A) and the other is labelled as Reason (R).*

Assertion (A) Polymerase chain reaction is used in DNA amplification.

Reason (R) The ampicillin resistant gene is used as a selectable marker to check transformation.

In the light of the above statements, choose the correct answer from the options given below. **[NCERT Pg. 165, 172 NEET 2022]**

(a) Both (A) and (R) are correct, but (R) is not the correct explanation of (A). ☐

(b) (A) is correct, but (R) is not correct. ☐

(c) (A) is not correct, but (R) is correct. ☐

(d) Both (A) and (R) are correct and (R) is the correct explanation of (A). ☐

9. Plasmid pBR322 has Pst I restriction enzyme site within gene amp^R that confers ampicillin resistance. If this enzyme is used for inserting a gene for β-galactoside production and the recombinant plasmid is inserted in an E.coli strain **[NCERT Pg. 169, NEET 2021]**

(a) It will not be able to confer ampicillin resistance to the host cell ☐

(b) The transformed cells will have the ability to resist ampicillin as well as produce β-galactoside ☐

(c) It will lead to lysis of host cell ☐

(d) It will be able to produce a novel protein with dual ability ☐

10. During the process of gene amplification using PCR, if very high temperature is not maintained in the beginning, then which of the following steps of PCR will be affected first? **[NCERT Pg. 172, NEET 2021]**

(a) Annealing ☐

(b) Extension ☐

(c) Denaturation ☐

(d) Ligation ☐

11. In gel electrophoresis, separated DNA fragments can be visualised with the help of **[NCERT Pg. 168, NEET (Sep.) 2020]**

(a) ethidium bromide in UV radiation ☐

(b) acetocarmine in UV radiation ☐

(c) ethidium bromide in infrared radiation ☐

(d) acetocarmine in bright blue light ☐

12. In recombinant DNA technology antibiotics are used **[NCERT Pg. 169, NEET Oct.) 2020]**

(a) to keep medium bacteria-free ☐

(b) to detect alien DNA ☐

(c) to impart disease-resistance to the host plant ☐

(d) as selectable markers ☐

13. Match the following techniques or instruments with their usage. **[NCERT Pg. 168, NEET (Oct.) 2020]**

Column I		Column II
A. Bioreactor	(i)	Separation of DNA fragments
B. Electrophoresis	(ii)	Production of large quantities of products
C. PCR	(iii)	Detection of pathogen, based on antigen-antibody reaction
D. ELISA	(iv)	Amplification of nucleic acids

Select the correct option.

	A	B	C	D	
(a)	(iii)	(ii)	(iv)	(i)	☐
(b)	(ii)	(i)	(iv)	(iii)	☐
(c)	(iv)	(iii)	(ii)	(i)	☐
(d)	(ii)	(i)	(iii)	(iv)	☐

14. First discovered restriction endonuclease that always cuts DNA molecule at a particular point by recognising a specific sequence of six base pairs is **[NCERT Pg. 165, NEET (Oct.) 2020]**

(a) EcoRI ☐

(b) Adenosine deaminase ☐

(c) Thermostable DNA polymerase ☐

(d) Hind II ☐

15. The specific palindromic sequence which is recognised by EcoRI is **[NCERT Pg. 166, NEET 2020]**

(a) 5′-GAATTC-3′ 3′-CTTAAG-5′ ☐

(b) 5′-GGAACC-3′ 3′-CCTTGG-5′ ☐

(c) 5′- CTTAAG-3′ 3′-GAATC-5′ ☐

(d) 5′-GGATCC-3′ 3′-CCTAGG-5′ ☐

Chapter 10

Biotechnology and Its Applications

Scan and take Chapter Test

TOPIC 1

Biotechnological Applications in Agriculture

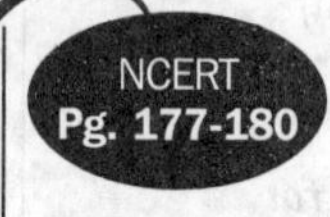

1. How many of the given processes are applications of biotechnology?

Waste treatment, Bioremediation, Genetically modified crops, Conventional hybridisation, Energy generation

____

2. Downstream processing of recombinant products aims to provide the best catalyst, i.e. either an enzyme or a microbe in biotechnological processes.

True ☐ False ☐

3. Read the following statements given below.

I. Tripling of the food supply.

II. Increased use of agrochemicals.

III. Improved crop varieties and yields.

These statements can be correlated with which major phenomenon in India?

____

4. Due to which factor did the food supply increase during the phase of green revolution?

____

5. An alternate way to maximise the agricultural output without involving the agrochemicals is ______________.

6. Using conventional breeding methods, we can increase the yield of crops with the existing varieties.

True ☐ False ☐

*Concepts of all questions bearing * are important for NEET & CUET*

7. Consider the following statements.

Statement I The nutrient media in which the explants are cultured should contain a carbon source.

Statement II Totipotent cells have the capacity to give rise to all different cell types in a plant.

Choose the correct option from the following.

(a) Statement I is true but statement II is false ☐

(b) Statement I is false but statement II is true ☐

(c) Both statements I and II are true ☐

(d) Both statements I and II are false ☐

8. A sugarcane plant infected with a viral pathogen can be used to grow progeny plants which are genetically identical by culturing which part of the plant?

(a) Flower ☐ (b) Meristem ☐ (c) Xylem tissue ☐ (d) Bark ☐

9. Fusing two protoplasts from two different plant varieties will yield hybrids which are called

(a) Somatic hybrids ☐ (b) Somaclones ☐

(c) GMO ☐ (d) Transgenics ☐

10. Consider the following statements.

Statement I Somatic hybrids are genetically similar to the parent plants.

Statement II The naked protoplast of plant cells are free of their cell membranes.

Choose the correct option from the following.

(a) Statement I is true, but statement II is false ☐

(b) Statement I is false, but statement II is true ☐

(c) Both statements I and II are true ☐

(d) Both statements I and II are false ☐

11. Give scientific term for the following statement.

Plants, bacteria, fungi and animals whose genes have been altered by manipulation.

____

12. As a result of genetically modified crops, chemicals use on an agricultural lands have gone up significantly.

True ☐ False ☐

13. Genetically modified plants are more tolerant to abiotic stresses than their conventional forms.

True ☐ False ☐

***14.** An example of a tailor made crop to supply an enhanced level of vitamin- A is ____________.

15. An important objective of biotechnology in agriculture is ____________ (production of insect resistance /to decrease the seed number) in plants.

16. All these plants share a common characteristic very essential to agriculture. Name it.

Bt cotton, Bt corn, Bt rice, Bt tomato and Bt potato.

____

17. *Bt* toxin is obtained from bacterium called ____________ *(Bacillus thermus aquaticus/Bacillus thuringiensis)*.

***18.** An insect belonging to order ____________ (Dermaptera/Lepidoptera) is harmed by the strains of *Bacillus thuringiensis.*

19. *Bt* toxin has been cloned in a virus and expressed in plants to reduce the addition of agricultural chemicals.
(*Rewrite the statement after correcting the underlined word.*)

____

20. Match the following columns.

Column I (Orders of class-Insecta)	Column II (Examples of insects)
A. Dipterans	1. Armyworm
B. Coleopterans	2. Flies
C. Lepidopterans	3. Ladybugs

A. ____________ B. ____________ C. ____________

21. Genetically modified crops containing *cry* gene were intended to
(i) introduce natural insect resistance in plants.
(ii) increase vitamin content in plants.
(*Choose the correct one.*)

____

***22.** Fill in the blanks.
(i) During its particular growth phase, *B. thuringiensis* forms a special ____________ protein crystal which can kill insects of certain orders, but not their host.
(ii) *Bt* toxin exists as ____________ in host bacteria due to which it remains unaffected.

***23.** Which factor is responsible for activation of the inactive protoxin as it reaches the target insect's body?

____

***24.** The *Bt* toxin kills the target insects by inhibiting an essential metabolic pathway.
(*Rewrite the statement after correcting the underlined phrase.*) ____________

***25.** *Bt* toxins are not insect group specific.

True ☐ False ☐

26. *Bt* toxin in *B. thuringiensis* is encoded by a ____________ (*cry*/ *CRY*) gene.

27. Specific *Bt* toxin genes have been isolated from *Bacillus thuringiensis* and incorporated into how many of the plants mentioned in the box?

Cotton, Pea, Corn, Rice, Radish, Potato, Pumpkin and Soyabean

____

***28.** Complete the following analogy.
cry IAc : Cotton bollworms :: __________________ : Corn borer

29. Study the given image carefully and answer the question that follows

Introduction of which of the following genes in (b) will prevent them to develop the condition in (a)?

(a) *cry*IAb ☐ (b) *cry*IAc ☐
(c) *cry*IIAb ☐ (d) Both (b) and (c) ☐

30. ____________________ is a nematode known to infect the roots of tobacco plant and cause great reduction in yield.

31. Which strategy was implemented to prevent parasitic infections in tobacco plants?

____

32. RNAi is a method of cellular defence in all prokaryotic organisms.

True ☐ False ☐

***33.** Consider the following statements.

Statement I Protection against *Meloidegyne incognitia* can be conferred by silencing the pathogen *m*RNA.

Statement II The ssRNA in RNAi is complementary to the pathogen *m*RNA and thus silences them.

Choose the correct option from the following.

(a) Statement I is true, but statement II is false ☐
(b) Statement I is false, but statement II is true ☐
(c) Both statements I and II are true ☐
(d) Both statements I and II are false ☐

***34.** The sequence specific ________________ *via* RNAi promises an effective management of agricultural pests.

***35.** One way in which the *ds*RNA can gain entry into eukaryotic cells and cause RNA interference is an infection caused by ____________________.

36. Silencing with reference to RNAi indicates prevention of <u>transcription of *r*RNA</u> due to its complementary *ds*RNA.
(*Rewrite the statement after correcting the underlined words.*)

____

37. Most genetically modified plants are produced with the help of *Xanthomonas citri.* (*Rewrite the statement after correcting the underlined words.*)

____

38. Using vectors derived from *E. coli*, nematode specific genes are introduced in the host plant.

True ☐ False ☐

***39.** RNA interference is a strategy to produce plants with herbicide tolerance.

True ☐ False ☐

***40.** Complete the following analogy with respect to insect and pest diseases and its host.

Bt cotton : Insect resistance :: ______________ : Pest resistance

***41.** In pest resistant plants, the nematode parasite cannot survive due to ______________________.

TOPIC 2

Biotechnological Applications in Medicine

NCERT Pg. 181-183

42. There are atleast ______________ different proteins being produced using ______________ which serves as therapeutic agents for human beings.

43. How many of the below mentioned substances are recombinant DNA derived therapeutic agents?

Insulin, Growth hormone, α-1-antitrypsin, Ligase, Golden rice

____

***44.** Insulin is used in the treatment of liver damage.

(*Rewrite the statement after correcting the underlined words.*) ______________

45. Insulin extracted from animal sources other than human body is just as effective in the treatment of concerned disease.

True ☐ False ☐

46. Insulin derived from animal sources caused ______________ (kidney damage/allergic reactions) in human body.

47. Which organism has been employed for the large scale production of insulin by RDT?

______________________.

48. In mammals, insulin is synthesised as a prohormone due to the presence of A-peptide (*Rewrite the statement after correcting the underlined word.*)

____

49. Name the biotech company which commercially manufactured the first recombinant human insulin. ______________

50. The given image represents the immature form of human insulin. Which of the following chains would be linked in its mature form?

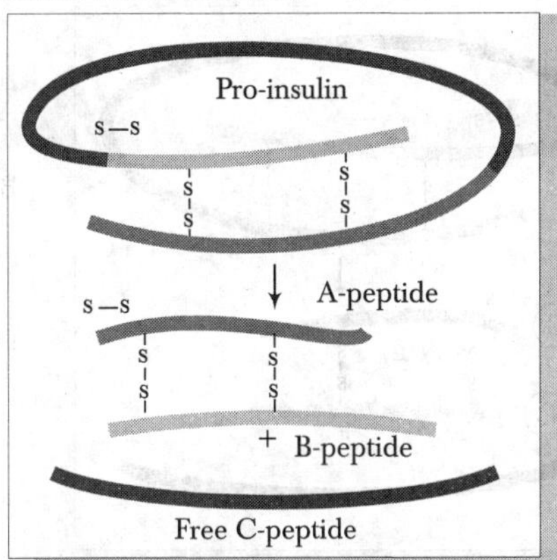

(a) A and B chains ☐ (b) B and C chains ☐
(c) A, B and C are inter linked ☐ (d) A and C chains ☐

51. Mature insulin consists of four polypeptide chains.

True ☐ False ☐

***52.** Consider the following statements.

Statement I Insulin needs to be processed before it becomes a fully mature and functional hormone.

Statement II The C peptide present in inactive proinsulin, is absent in its mature active form.

Choose the correct option from the following.

(a) Statement I is true, but statement II is false ☐
(b) Statement I is false, but statement II is true ☐
(c) Both statements I and II are true ☐
(d) Both statements I and II are false ☐

53. The polypeptide chains of human insulin are linked together by ________ (covalent bonds/disulphide bridges).

54. Which of the following is not involved in preparation of genetically engineered insulin?

(a) Preparation of DNA sequences specific to insulin A and B chains ☐
(b) Introduction of insulin chain genes into suitable *E.coli* vector ☐
(c) Expressing the insulin chain genes in a suitable host ☐
(d) Combining of chains A and B by hydrogen bonding between them ☐

***55.** Arrange the following steps (I–VI) in the order of stages involved in the production of *r*-insulin *via* genetic engineering.

I. Identification of gene required. II. Joining of chains A and B.
III. Extraction of gene and plasmid. IV. Gene inserted into plasmid.
V. Transformation in *E. coli*. VI. Production of insulin.

____

56. Study the diagram and identify the labels marked as *A-D.*

A. ____________________

B. ____________________

C. ____________________

D. ____________________

57. The presence of which 2 chains is essential for the formation of mature insulin? ________

58. The main challenge faced by companies for the artificial production of mature insulin using genetic engineering techniques was ____________________.

59. If a person is born with a hereditary disorder, he/she is can be cured by ____________________.

60. Correction of genetic disorders involves the repair of non-functional gene.

True ☐ False ☐

***61.** In 1990, first clinical gene therapy was provided for

62. What is common to all the diseases mentioned in the box given below?

ADA deficiency, Cystic fibrosis, Emphysema, Haemophilia-B, Sickle-cell anaemia

____

63. Enzyme ADA is crucial for normal functioning of which system in human body?

____

***64.** Consider the following statements and find out the option with correct one.

I. A person with ADA deficiency lacks the gene encoding Adenosine Deaminase.

II. Enzyme replacement therapy can completely cure a person with ADA deficiency.

III. ADA is caused due to deletion of the gene for adenosine deaminase.

IV. First clinical gene therapy was given in 1980 to a 4-year old girl.

(a) I and III ☐ (b) III and IV ☐

(c) II, III and IV ☐ (d) I and IV ☐

____

65. In treatment of Adenosine Deaminase (ADA) deficiency disorder, thrombocytes are extracted by doctors for culturing *in vitro*.
(*Rewrite the statement after correcting the underlined word.*)

____

66. As an alternate to gene therapy, ADA deficiency can also be cured by transplantation of ____________________ (blood / bone marrow).

67. In some patients, functional ADA is directly injected as a part of somatic gene therapy.

True ☐ False ☐

68. How many of the following can be used as vectors in gene therapy?

Retroviruses, Bone marrow cells, Cosmids

____

69. A patient with ADA deficiency needs the assistance of gene therapy. In the corrective therapy, a functional copy of ADA gene is delivered into the lymphocytes of the patient. Which of the following can act as a vector for transferring the ADA gene into the lymphocytes?

(a) pBR322 ☐ (b) *Agrobacterium* ☐
(c) Retrovirus ☐ (d) Bacteriophage ☐

70. Why does the ADA deficiency patient require periodic infusion of genetically engineered lymphocytes?

____

***71.** Gene therapy can be a permanent cure for ADA deficiency disorder if

(i) gene producing ADA is introduced at early embryonic stages.

(ii) bone marrow containing functional lymphocytes is transplanted in adults.

(*Choose correct one.*)

____

***72.** Urine and serum analysis are ______________ methods of diagnosis.

73. Pick the odd one out.

ELISA, ECG, PCR, RDT

____

***74.** Give one word for technique of selective amplification of nucleic acids.

____

***75.** Expand ELISA. ______________________________

76. ______________ is used to detect HIV in patients suspected of AIDS.

77. Consider the following and identify the option with correct statements.

I. Very low concentration of the corona virus can be detected in a person by PCR.

II. HIV tests make use of PCR and ELISA for detecting the viral DNA and protein.

III. Presence of pathogen is suspected only when the pathogen has produced a disease symptom.

IV. High concentration of bacteria or virus cannot be detected by amplification of their nucleic acid by PCR.

(a) I, II and IV ☐ (b) II, III and IV ☐
(c) I, II and III ☐ (d) II and IV ☐

78. Give scientific term for the following sentence.

A single strand of DNA/RNA tagged with radioactive molecule used as diagnostic tool.

____

79. Hybridisation of radioactivity tagged DNA/RNA with its *c*DNA can be confirmed using _______________.

80. A radioactive probe was made complementary to a normal gene X that codes for a growth factor. In a clone of cells expressing the growth factor, the probe was allowed to hybridize with the complementary DNA sequences. Autoradiography presented an anomalous result, where none of the clones appeared on the photographic film. What could have been the possible reason behind the same?

(a) The probe did not hybridize properly ☐

(b) The clone of cells were dead ☐

(c) Cloned cells had mutated version of the gene ☐

(d) Cloned cells appeared more in number ☐

***81.** ELISA technique is based on which principle?

____

TOPIC 3

Transgenic Animals

NCERT Pg. 183-184

82. Give scientific term for following statement.

Animals whose genome is manipulated to allow expression of a foreign gene.

____

83. How many animals have been transgenically created?

Rabbits, Pigs, Sheep, Fish, Crocodile, Frogs

____

84. 95% of all existing transgenic animals are _______________ (mice/sheep).

85. Novel transgenics are created to study the affect of genes on normal body functions.

True ☐ False ☐

86. Pick the odd one out.

Dolly, Bt tobacco, Rosie, Transgenic fish

____

87. Transgenic models exists for how many of the following diseases?

Cancer, Diabetes, Cystic fibrosis, Rheumatoid arthritis, AIDS, Hepatitis-A, Alzheimer's disease

____

***88.** A human protein α-1 antitrypsin is used for treatment of _______________. (emphysema/cystic fibrosis).

89. The first transgenic cow is Dolly that produced human protein enriched milk.

True ☐ False ☐

90. The milk produced by first transgenic cow was enriched in antithrombin III. (*Rewrite the statement after correcting the underlined word.*)

____

91 For what purpose transgenic mice and transgenic monkeys are used during vaccine production?

____

92. Match Column I with Column II.

Column I	Column II
A. Transgenic models	1. Emphysema
B. Polio vaccines	2. Transgenic mice
C. Rosie	3. Cancer
D. α-1-antitrypsin	4. Human alpha-lactalbumin

	A	B	C	D			A	B	C	D	
(a)	3	2	4	1	☐	(b)	3	1	4	2	☐
(c)	2	3	4	1	☐	(d)	2	4	3	1	☐

93. Transgenic animals are more sensitive to toxic substances than their non-transgenic forms due to the presence of transgenes.

True ☐ False ☐

TOPIC 4 Ethical Issues

NCERT Pg. 184-185

94. GEAC stands for _______________

95. CSIR is the organisation responsible for validating the GM research in India. (*Rewrite the statement after correcting the underlined word.*)

____

96. Introduction of food/medicines developed through genetic engineering are not much desirable due to

(i) danger of the entry of virus or toxins with transgenic crops.

(ii) low productivity of these products. (*Choose correct one.*)

____

97. Genetically modified organisms can have unpredictable effects on ecosystem.

True ☐ False ☐

***98.** Give scientific term for following statement.

Intellectual property right granted by government to an individual for novel scientific inventions.

____

99. Patents are granted for all research works.

True ☐ False ☐

100. India has faced patent related issues for how many of the following products?

Ghee, Turmeric, Rice, Sugar, Neem, Cotton

____

101. Which of the following Indian items have not been targeted to obtain a patent by multinational companies in an unethical manner?

(a) Basmati ☐ (b) Tulsi ☐ (c) Turmeric ☐ (d) Neem ☐

102. In 1997, an American company got patent rights on Basmati rice, which was produced by crossing ______________________________

103. Approximately ______________ (200,000/27) varieties of rice exist in India alone.

104. Give the scientific term for the following statement.

Illegal use of resources and traditional knowledge without proper authorisation from concerned person.

____

105. ______________ (Indian patents bill/Cartagena protocol) protects the patent rights research and development initiative, etc., of people and protect against biopiracy.

Assertion-Reason Questions

The following questions consist of two statements- Assertion (A) and Reason (R). Answer these questions by selecting the appropriate option given below.

(a) Both A and R are true and R is the correct explanation of A
(b) Both A and R are true, but R is not the correct explanation of A
(c) A is true, but R is false
(d) A is false, but R is true

1. **Assertion** (A) Micropropagation techniques can be used to develop genetically dissimilar plants.
Reason (R) Tissue culture relies on the ability of totipotent cells to regenerate a whole plant from an explant.

(a) ☐ (b) ☐ (c) ☐ (d) ☐

***2.** **Assertion** (A) Somatic hybridization is a valuable tool for plant breeding.
Reason (R) It allows the creating of hybrids that cannot be produced through sexual reproduction.

(a) ☐ (b) ☐ (c) ☐ (d) ☐

***3.** **Assertion** (A) The *Bt* toxins kill lepidopterans however the *Bacillus* producing them are protected against their effects.
Reason (R) The *Bt* toxins are produced as inactive protoxins and become activated by the acidic pH of the insect gut.

(a) ☐ (b) ☐ (c) ☐ (d) ☐

***4. Assertion** (A) Plants can be protected from nematode pathogen by using RNA interference and *Agrobacterium* vectors.
Reason (R) RNA interference for gene silencing has evolved as a defence strategy in all eukaryotic organisms.
(a) ☐ (b) ☐ (c) ☐ (d) ☐

***5. Assertion** (A) Insulin as a pro-hormone lacks the C-peptide which is present in the mature form.
Reason (R) Using *r*DNA, chain A and B of insulins were separately produced and linked by disulfide bonds.
(a) ☐ (b) ☐ (c) ☐ (d) ☐

6. Assertion (A) ADA deficiency patients require periodic infusion of genetically engineered lymphocytes.
Reason (R) By genetic engineering ADA cDNA is introduced into the lymphocytes, but the cells are not immortal .
(a) ☐ (b) ☐ (c) ☐ (d) ☐

7. Assertion (A) One application of biotechnology is to create transgenic animals for drug testing and vaccine safety.
Reason (R) Transgenic animals are developed by introducing DNA that codes for α-1 trypsin to treat emphysema .
(a) ☐ (b) ☐ (c) ☐ (d) ☐

8. Assertion (A) Biopiracy discourages the conservation of biodiversity in developing countries.
Reason (R) Local communities have less incentive to protect resources that can be exploited without their benefit.
(a) ☐ (b) ☐ (c) ☐ (d) ☐

Case Based Questions

1. A farmer in India has been cultivating Bt cotton for the past three years. He has observed an increase in his crop yield and a decrease in the usage of chemical pesticide.
Based on the above case answer the following questions

(i) What is the primary advantages of *Bt* cotton for farmers?
(a) Reduced water consumption ☐ (b) Resistance to bollworm pests ☐
(c) Enhanced cotton fiber quality ☐ (d) Faster growth rate ☐

(ii) Which gene is introduced into cotton plants to make them Bt cotton?
(a) *cry IAc* gene from *Bacillus thuringiensis* ☐
(b) *cry IAb* gene from *Bacillus thuringiensis* ☐
(c) *cry IIAc* gene from *E. coli* ☐
(d) *cry IAc* gene from *E. coli* ☐

(iii) The *Bt* toxin does not kill the *Bacillus* because the *Bt* toxin protein exist as inactive
(a) lipid ☐ (b) protoxin ☐
(c) protein ☐ (d) toxoid ☐

2. Maria, a 62 year-old woman, has been diagnosed with type-I diabetes. Her doctor prescribes a genetically engineered human insulin medication to regulate her blood sugar levels

Based on the above situation, answer the questions that follow.

(i) Maria, diagnosed with type-I diabetes is prescribed humulin which is a type of

(a) medication that can completely cure type-I diabetes ☐

(b) medication that helps manage blood sugar levels in type-I diabetes ☐

(c) dietary supplement that can reverse the effects of type-I diabetes ☐

(d) preventive medication to stop someone from developing type-I diabetes ☐

(ii) What advantage does genetically engineered insulin have over animal-derived insulin?

(a) It is less expensive to produce ☐

(b) It is less likely to cause allergic reactions ☐

(c) It is more potent ☐

(d) It has a longer shelf life ☐

(iii) What is the role of recombinant DNA technology in the production of human insulin?

(a) To clone the human insulin gene and insert it into a bacterial plasmid ☐

(b) To extract insulin free bacterial cultures ☐

(c) To synthesize insulin chemically ☐

(d) To identify mutations in the insulin gene ☐

COMPETITION EDGE UP

1. *Given below are two statements.*

Statement I *Bt toxins are insect group specific and coded by a gene cry IAc.*

Statement II *Bt toxin exists as inactive protoxin in B. thuringiensis. However, after ingestion by the insect. The inactive protoxin gets converted into active form due to acidic pH of the insect gut.*

In the light of the above statements, choose the correct answer from the options given below. ***[NCERT Pg. 179, 180, NEET 2024]***

(a) Both Statement I and Statement II are true ☐

(b) Both Statement I and Statement II are false ☐

(c) Statement I is true but Statement II is false ☐

(d) Statement I is false but Statement II is true ☐

2. *Match List I with List II.*

List I	List II
A. $\alpha-1$ antitrypsin	I. Cotton bollworm
B. cry IAb	II. ADA deficiency
C. cry IAc	III. Emphysema
D. Enzyme replacement therapy	IV. Corn borer

Choose the correct answer form the options given below. ***[NCERT Pg. 180, 182, 184, NEET 2024]***

(a) A-II, B-I, C-IV, D-III ☐

(b) A-III, B-I, C-II, D-IV ☐

(c) A-III, B-IV, C-I, D-II ☐

(d) A-II, B-IV, C-I, D-III ☐

3. *Which one of the following techniques does not serve the purpose of early diagnosis of a disease for its early treatment?* ***[NCERT Pg. 182-183, NEET 2023]***

(a) Serum and urine analysis ☐
(b) Polymerase Chain Reaction (PCR) technique ☐
(c) Enzyme Linked Immuno-Sorbent Assay (ELISA) technique ☐
(d) Recombinant DNA technology ☐

4. Transposons can be used during, which one of the following? **[NCERT Pg. 180, NEET 2022]**

(a) Polymerase chain reaction ☐
(b) Gene silencing ☐
(c) Autoradiography ☐
(d) Gene sequencing ☐

5. Statements related to human insulin are given below. Which statement(s) is/are correct about genetically engineered insulin? **[NCERT Pg. 181-182, NEET 2022]**

I. Pro-hormone insulin contains extra stretch of C-peptide.
II. A-peptide and B-peptide chains of insulin were produced separately in E.coli, extracted and combined by creating disulphide bond between them.
III. Insulin used for treating diabetes was extracted from cattles and pigs.
IV. Pro-hormone insulin needs to be processed for converting into a mature and functional hormone.
V. Some patients develop allergic reactions to the foreign insulin.

Choose the most appropriate answer from the options given below.

(a) Only II ☐
(b) III and IV ☐
(c) III, IV and V ☐
(d) I, II and IV ☐

6. In gene therapy of Adenosine Deaminase (ADA) deficiency, the patient requires periodic infusion of genetically engineered lymphocytes because **[NCERT Pg. 182, NEET 2022]**

(a) retroviral vector is introduced into these lymphocytes ☐
(b) gene isolated from marrow cells producing ADA is introduced into cells at embryonic stages ☐
(c) lymphocytes from patient's blood are grown in culture, outside the body ☐
(d) genetically engineered lymphocytes are not immortal cells ☐

7. Now-a-days it is possible to detect the mutated gene causing cancer by allowing radioactive probe to hybridise its complimentary DNA in a clone of cells, followed by its detection using autoradiography because **[NCERT Pg. 183, NEET 2021]**

(a) mutated gene does not appear on photographic film as the probe has complementarity with it ☐
(b) mutated gene partially appears on a photographic film ☐
(c) mutated gene completely and clearly appears on a photographic film ☐
(d) mutated gene does not appear on a photographic film as the probe has no complementarity with it ☐

8. When gene targeting involving gene amplification is attempted in an individual's tissue to treat disease, it is known as **[NCERT Pg. 182, NEET 2021]**

(a) biopiracy ☐
(b) gene therapy ☐
(c) moleuclar diagnosis ☐
(d) safety testing ☐

9. With regard to insulin choose the correct options.

I. C-peptide is not present in mature insulin.
II. The insulin produced by rDNA technology has C-peptide.
III. The pro-insulin has C-peptide.
IV. A-peptide and B-peptide of insulin are interconnected by disulphide bridges.

Choose the correct answer from the options given below. **[NCERT Pg. 181-182, NEET 2021]**

(a) II and IV ☐ (b) II and III ☐
(c) I, III and IV ☐ (d) I and IV ☐

10. RNA interference is used for which of the following purposes in the field of biotechnology? **[NCERT Pg. 180, NEET (Oct.) 2020]**

(a) To develop a plant tolerant to abiotic stresses ☐
(b) To develop a pest-resistant plant against infestation by nematode ☐
(c) To enhance the mineral usage by the plant ☐
(d) To reduce post harvest losses ☐

Chapter 11

Organisms and Populations

Scan and take Chapter Test

TOPIC 1

Population Attributes and Population Growth

NCERT Pg. 191-196

1. Name the area of ecology that links ecology to population genetics and evolution.

______

2. If in a pond, there are 20 lotus plants of last year and through reproduction 8 new plants are added then the birth rate would be ______.

3. Write the technical name for the ratio of male to female individuals in a population.

______

4. Write the technical term for the following sentence.
Graphical representation of age distribution (per cent individuals of a given age group).

______

***5.** Write the growth status of the following populatio`ns.

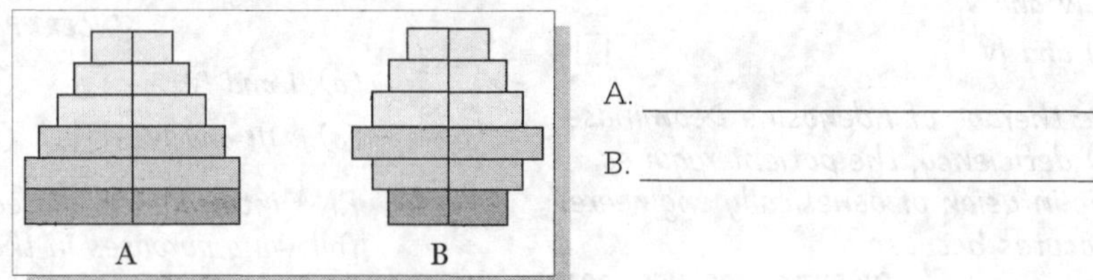

A. ______
B. ______

***6.** Identify the parts labelled as *A, B* and *C* as per their reproductive phase.

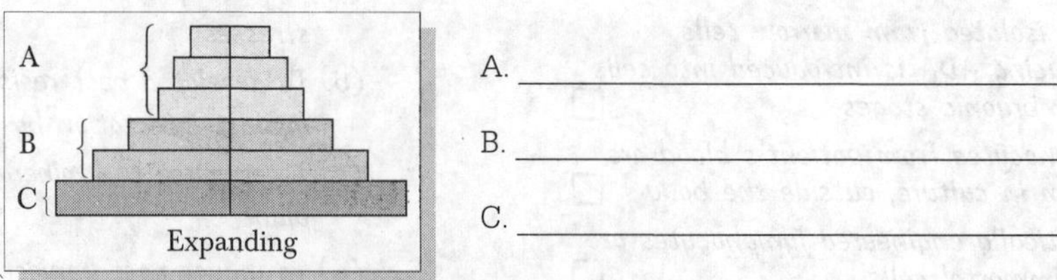

A. ______
B. ______
C. ______

*Concepts of all questions bearing * are important for NEET & CUET*

7. Consider the given images of the age pyramids and identify the incorrect statement from the following options.

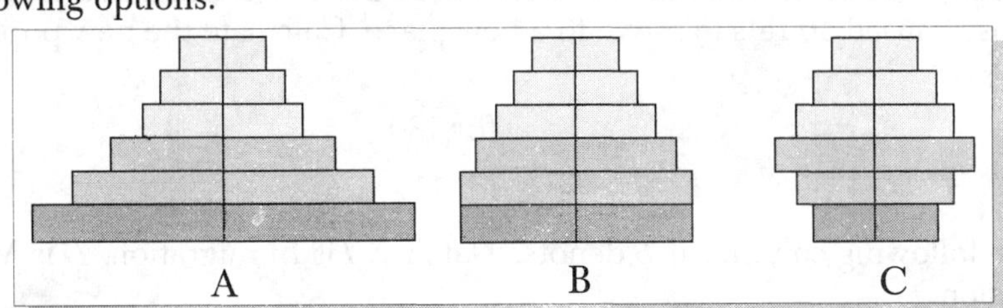

(a) Pyramid A shows expanding population pyramid since it has a larger percentage of younger age groups ☐

(b) Pyramid C is declining population age pyramid with a narrow base and is usually urn shaped ☐

(c) Pyramid A has equal number of young or pre-reproductive and reproductive individuals ☐

(d) Pyramid B is stable showing somewhat equal proportion of population in each age group. ☐

8. Name the process by which tiger census is done in our national parks and tiger reserves.

____

9. In population ecology, 'N' refers to ______________________________

10. Write the technical name for population size.

____

11. The size of a population for any species is a static parameter.

True ☐ False ☐

12. Consider the following statements.

Statement I Ecology as a study is concerned with four levels of biological organisation-organisms, populations, communities and biomes.

Statement II Emigration and immigration as processes are irreversible and affect the population density.

Choose the correct option from the following.

(a) Statement I is true, but statement II is false ☐

(b) Statement I is false, but statement II is true ☐

(c) Both statements I and II are true ☐

(d) Both statements I and II are false ☐

13. The number of deaths in a population during a given period is called ______________.

***14.** Complete the following flowchart.

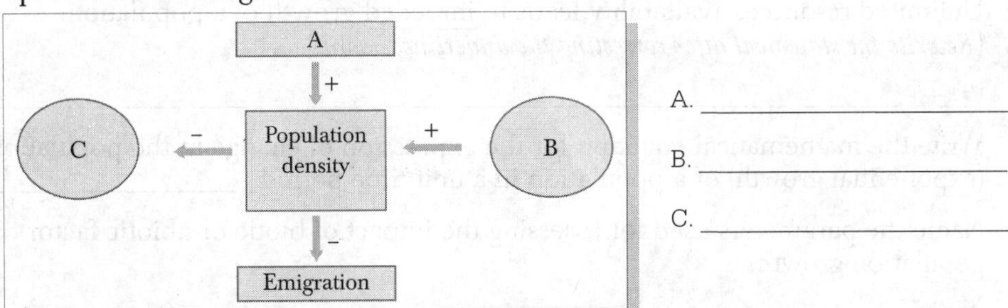

15. The population of rats in an area in during 2019 was 900. Within a span of one year, about 230 new rats were born while 50 rats were killed due to a sudden natural disaster. The disaster also caused 40 rats to move to a new place. Calculate the new population density after one year.

(a) 1040 ☐ (b) 580 ☐
(c) 1220 ☐ (d) 1140 ☐

***16.** Match the following columns if *B* denotes Natality, *I* is Immigration, *D* is Mortality and *E* is Emigration.

Column I (Characteristics of population)	Column II (Equation related to characteristics of population)
A. Stable population	1. $B + I > D + E$
B. Population is increasing	2. $B + I = D + E$
C. Decreasing population	3. $B + I < D + E$

A.________ B.________ C.________

17. Write an equation which correlates population density at time t+1, Emigration, Immigration, Natality and Mortality.

____

18. Increase in the number of births and immigration would leads to ________ (increase/decrease) of population density.

19. For a new colony, birth rate would contribute more to population growth than the immigration.
(*Rewrite the statement after correcting the underlined words.*)

____

20. Match the following columns.

Column I (Population attributes)	Column II (Characteristic features)
A. Emigration	1. Number of births during a given period
B. Mortality + Emigration	2. Number of individuals leaving habitat
C. Natality	3. Increase in population
D. Natality + Immigration	4. Decrease in population

A.________ B.________ C.________ D.________

21. Write the two models of population growth.

____

22. Unlimited resources availability leads to impeded growth of a population.
(*Rewrite the statement after correcting the underlined word.*)

____

23. Write the mathematical equation for the expression of change in the population size (exponential growth) of a population in a unit time period________

24. Name the parameters used for assessing the impact of biotic or abiotic factor on population growth.

____

25. In 1981, the '*r*' value for human population in India was 0.0205.

True ☐ False ☐

26. Write the shape of the curve obtained in a plot between population density and time for exponential growth.

____

27. Write the integral form of exponential growth equation.

____

***28.** Any species growing ______________ (exponentially/logistically) under unlimited condition can reach enormous population density.

29. A limited resource would lead to ______________ in many individuals.

30. Write biological term for the following sentence.

The limit of a possible number of a population in a given habitat beyond which no further growth is possible. ______________

31. Complete the following paragraph by using the words given below in the box.

Deceleration, Growth, Log, Carrying capacity, Lag, Population density

A population in a habitat with limited resources show initially a ______________ phase, followed by phases of acceleration and ______________ and finally an asymptote, when the population density reaches the ______________.

***32.** '*K*' stands for *K*-selected species in the Verhulst-Pearl logistic growth equation.

True ☐ False ☐

33. Carrying capacity of a population is determined by limiting resources.

True ☐ False ☐

34. A plot of *N* in relation to time '*t*' when resources are limited is ______________ curve.

***35.** Write the Verhulst-Pearl logistic growth equation.

____

***36.** Identify the growth models given below.

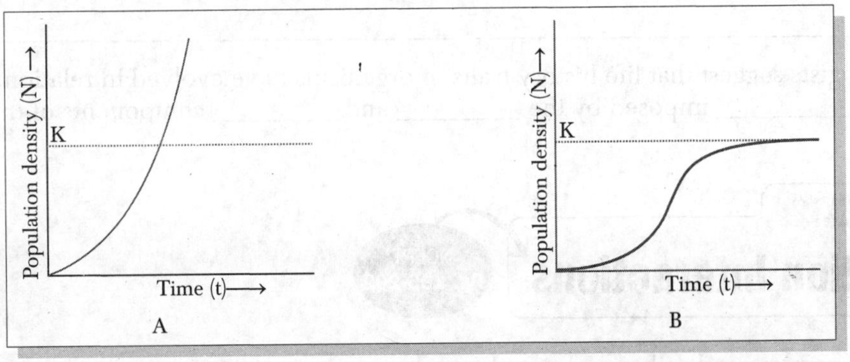

A. ______________ B. ______________

37. Name the growth model which is considered as a realistic one.

____

***38.** Consider the given image of population growth curve. Which of the following regions represent saturation of population due to carrying capacity?

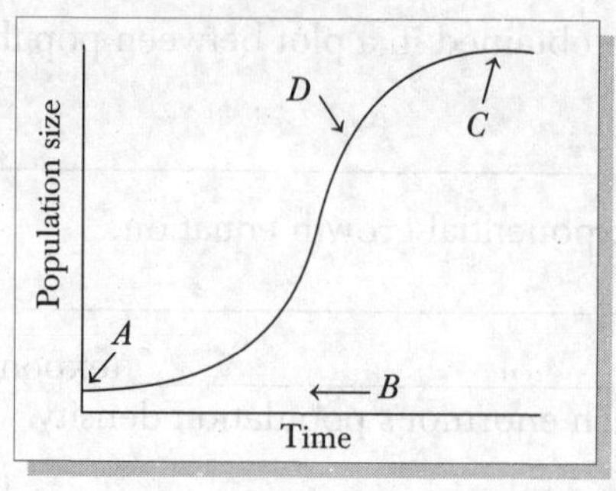

(a) D ☐ (b) C ☐ (c) A ☐ (d) B ☐

39. Consider the following statements

I. Any species growing exponentially under unlimited resources conditions often reach enormous population densities in short span of time.

II. Both food and space availability is essential for a restricted growth of a population.

III. The Verhulst Pearl Logistic Growth is represented by the equation $\frac{dN}{dt} = \mu N\left(\frac{k-N}{k}\right)$.

IV. In reality carrying capacity of nature allows a population to grow only upto a definite size.

Identify the set of correct statements.

(a) I, II and IV ☐ (b) II, III and V ☐

(c) I, III and IV ☐ (d) III and V ☐

40. Darwin fitness has ____________ (high/low) r value in the habitat in which they live.

41. Write any two organisms which breed only once in their lifetime.

____

42. Select the incorrect pair.

(i) Small number but large-sized offspring–Birds/mammals

(ii) Breeds many times – Mammals

(iii) Small-sized but many offspring – Prey birds/Raptors

____

43. Ecologists suggest that life history traits of organisms have evolved in relation to the ____________ imposed by the __________ and __________ components of the habitat.

TOPIC 2

Population Interactions

NCERT Pg. 196-202

44. Plant species need soil microbes to breakdown ____________ matter in soil and to return the ________________ nutrients for absorption.

45. Organisms can live in isolation in nature.

True ☐ False ☐

46. Interspecific interactions occur from <u>separation of population of two similar species.</u>
(*Rewrite the statement after correcing the underlined phrase.*)

____

***47.** Write the type of interactions assigned by the following symbols.

(i) + _______________

(ii) 0 _______________

***48.** _______________ is the type of population interaction in which both the species are harmed.

***49.** In amensalism, one species is harmed and the other is unaffected.

True ☐ False ☐

50. The interaction where one species is benefitted and the other is neither benefitted nor harmed is called <u>mutualism.</u>
(*Rewrite the statement after correcting the underlined word.*)

____

***51.** Table given below shows the positive interaction (+) and negative interaction – between the species *A* and species *B*. Study the table and complete the missing words *A* to *D*.

Species A	Species B	Interaction
+	+	Ⓐ
–	Ⓑ	Amensalism
Ⓒ	0	Commensalism
+	–	Ⓓ

A.__________ B.__________ C.__________ D.__________

52. Find odd one out with respect to the population interaction.

Predation, Parasitism, Commensalism, Competition.

____

53. Sparrow eating any seed is an example of predation.

True ☐ False ☐

***54.** Predators act as conduits for _______________ transfer across the trophic levels.

55. A new species becomes invasive due to the unavailability of its natural predators.

True ☐ False ☐

56. Name the cactus that became invasive in Australia.

____

57. _______________ control methods are based on the ability of predator to control its prey population.

58. Extinction of prey population ultimately leads to the extinction of _______________

59. Which of the following is not an effect produced by predation on a particular prey species?

(a) Controls the prey population in an area

(b) Maintains species biodiversity

(c) Hinders the energy transfer process

(d) Reduces inter specific competition

60. Name the butterfly which becomes distasteful to its predator bird.

61. Write the source of the chemical which protects the monarch butterfly from its predator species.

62. Consider the following statements.

Statement I The loss of invertebrates in the absence of starfish in the Pacific coast was due to loss of mutualism between the two species.

Statement II Monarch butterfly caterpillars feed on poisonous weed as a defence mechanism to escape predation.

Choose the correct option from the following.

(a) Statement I is true, but statement II is false

(b) Statement I is false, but statement II is true

(c) Both statements I and II are true

(d) Both statements I and II are false

63. Write the scientific name for the insects feeding on plant sap.

64. Write two plants that have thorns as a morphological means of defence.

65. Name the scientific name of the weed that produces highly poisonous cardiac glycosides.

66. Identify the incorrect statement with respect to predation.

(a) If a predator is too efficient or dominates the prey population, the latter possibly gets extinct

(b) Cattle or goat varieties are not found feeding over *Calotropis* due to the thorns present in latter for its defence

(c) Predators help in maintaining species diversity in a community

(d) Predators prove to be of much importance when prey population control is talked about

67. Find odd one out with respect to chemical defence substances found in plants against grazers.

Nicotine, Caffeine, Opium, Chloroquine

***68.** Competition occurs among closely related species competing for limited resources.

True ☐ False ☐

***69.** In competition, intrinsic rate of increase of one species is lowered due to the presence of another species.

True ☐ False ☐

70. Abingdon tortoise in Galapagos island became extinct due to parasitism.

True ☐ False ☐

***71.** Match the following columns.

Column I (Interacting organisms)	Column II (Interactions)
A. Flamingo and fishes	1. Commensalism
B. Egret and cattle	2. Competition
C. *Nepenthes*	3. Predator
D. Liver fluke	4. Parasite

A.________ B.________ C. ________

***72.** The Abingdon tortoise in Galapagos Islands became extinct within a decade after goats were introduced on the island.

True ☐ False ☐

73. Write the scientific name of the following.

(i) Superior barnacle ____________

(ii) Smaller barnacle ____________

74. Carnivores are more affected than herbivores by competition.

True ☐ False ☐

75. Name the principle which states that two closely related species competing for same resources cannot co-exists.

____

76. Consider the following statements.

Statement I Competition between two species creates a negative impact on both of them.

Statement II If resources are abundant, closely related species share resources to co-exist.

Choose the correct option from the following.

(a) Statement I is true, but statement II is false ☐

(b) Statement I is false, but statement II is true ☐

(c) Both statements I and II are true ☐

(d) Both statements I and II are false ☐

77. Name the mechanism of adapting different times for foraging among two species competing for same resource.

____

78. Which of the following phenomena would happen when a species spreads across a geographical area due to removal of a superior species from that area?

(a) Competitive release ☐ (b) Competitive exclusion ☐
(c) Resource partitioning ☐ (d) Natural selection ☐

***79.** Match the following columns.

Column I (Types of principle)	Column II (Scientist's names)
A. Struggle for existence	1. MacArthur
B. Competitive exclusion principle	2. Darwin
C. Resource partitioning	3. Gause

A.__________ B.__________ C. __________

80. Niche overlap indicates two different parasites on the same host.

True ☐ False ☐

81. Parasites evolved special adaptations such as loss of __________, high reproductive capacity and presence of __________ to cling to host.

82. Human liver fluke has __________ (one/two/three) intermediate hosts.

83. __________ are the parasites that feed on external surface of the host organism.

84. Find odd one out from the following species.

Lice, Ticks, Copepods, Fluke

____

85. Write the scientific name of the parasitic plant that had lost its chlorophyll and leaves.

____

86. Which of the following is an endoparasite?

(a) *Cuscuta* ☐ (b) Lice ☐
(c) Tick ☐ (d) *Plasmodium* ☐

87. Female mosquito is not considered as a parasite. (*Give reason*)

____

88. Endoparasites emphasize more on their reproductive potential.

True ☐ False ☐

89. Select ectoparasites among the following.

Lice, Copepods, Cuscuta, Taenia, Ascaris, Liver fluke, Ticks.

____

***90.** The parasitism in which cuckoo bird lays its eggs on the crow nest during breeding season is called __________.

91. Given below is a Venn diagram with '*P*' showing the type of interaction observed in two cases. Identify '*P*'

Orchid growing on a mango tree	*P*	Barnacles growing on the back of the whale

(a) Parasitism ☐ (b) Commensalism ☐
(c) Predation ☐ (d) Brood Parasitism ☐

92. Match the following columns.

Column I	Column II
A. Cattle egret	1. Clown fish
B. Orchid	2. Pseudoscorpions
C. Sea anemone	3. Livestock
D. Beetles	4. Mango tree

A.________ B.________ C. ________ D.________

***93.** The mutualistic relationship between a fungus and photosynthesising algae or cyanobacteria is called ____________.

***94.** Name the association between fungi and roots of higher plants.

____

95. Write any two rewards plants offers for pollinators.

____

96. Co-evolution of the mutualists can be found between fig species and wasp species.

True ☐ False ☐

97. Female wasp uses the fig inflorescence as an ____________ site.

98. Give the scientific name for the orchid which employs sexual deceit to get pollination done.

____

99. In Mediterranean orchid, the flower petal resembles the female bee.

True ☐ False ☐

100. Consider the following statements.

Statement I The female wasp deceives by using the fig plants for oviposition but does not provide any benefit.

Statement II The Mediterranean orchid resemble bees so that they can get pollinated during the act of pseudocopulation.

Choose the correct option from the following.

(a) Statement I is true, but statement II is false ☐

(b) Statement I is false, but statement II is true ☐

(c) Both statements I and II are true ☐

(d) Both statements I and II are false ☐

101. Match column I with column II

Column I	Column II
A. Mutualism	1. Egret and cattle
B. Commensalism	2. Female wasp and fig
C. Parasitism	3. Prickly pear and moth
D. Predation	4. Liver fluke and humans

	A	B	C	D			A	B	C	D	
(a)	2	1	4	3	☐	(b)	2	3	4	1	☐
(c)	1	3	4	2	☐	(d)	1	2	4	3	☐

COMPETITION CONNECT

Topic 1. Organism and Its Environment [NCERT (Old) Pg. 220-226]

***1.** ____________ is a subject which studies the interactions among organisms and between the organism and its environment.

2. Write the four levels of biological organisation.

____

3. The variations in the intensity and duration of temperature and precipitation account for the formation of biomes.

True ☐ False ☐

4. Match the following columns.

Column I (Name of biomes)	Column II (Temperture ranges)
A. Tropical forest	1. – 12-2°C
B. Arctic and Alpine tundra	2. 20-25°C
C. Coniferous forest	3. – 2-22°C
D. Temperate forest	4. 0-12°C

A.____________ B.____________ C. ____________ D. ____________

***5.** Select the major biomes of India from the box given below .

Coniferous forest, Tropical rainforest, Deciduous forest, Sea coast, Temperate forest, Alpine tundra, Desert

____

6. Find odd one out with respect to abiotic factors of ecosystem.

Temperature, Water, Soil, Plants

____

7. Find odd one out with respect to biotic components of ecosystem.

Pathogens, Predators, Parasites, Light

____

8. Over the years, organisms involved adaptations to optimise its survival and reproduction in its habitat through genetic drift.

(*Rewrite the statement after correcting the underlined words.*)

____

9. The average temperature ______________ (decreases/increases) progressively from the equator towards poles.

10. Average temperature exceeds 50°C in deep sea thermal vents.

True ☐ False ☐

11. Name any two countries where mango trees cannot grow. ______________

12. The ______________ (temperature/moisture) does not affect the basal metabolism of living organisms.

13. The abiotic factor which determines the species geographical distribution is ______________ (wind/temperature).

14. Life on earth originated in water.

True ☐ False ☐

15. The productivity and distribution of plants is dependent on ______________

16. Arrange the following in the increasing order of salinity.

Sea water, Hypersaline lagoons, Inland water

____

17. Identify the water bodies which show the given salinity in parts per thousand.

(i) 30-35 ______________ (ii) < 5 ______________

18. Consider the following statements.

Statement I Most animals can tolerate wide range of temperatures and are stenothermal.

Statement II Photoperiod of a plant depends on intensities and duration of light.

Choose the correct option from the following.

(a) Statement I is true, but statement II is false ☐

(b) Statement I is false, but statement II is true ☐

(c) Both statements I and II are true ☐

(d) Both statements I and II are false ☐

19. Organisms that can tolerate narrow range of temperature and wide range of salinity are called

(a) Stenothermal and euryhaline respectively ☐

(b) Stenohaline and eurythermal respectively ☐

(c) Eurythermal and stenohaline respectively ☐

(d) Eurythermal and Stenohaline respectively ☐

20. Match the following columns.

Column I (Categories of organisms)	Column II (Examples)
A. Stenohaline	1. Salmon
B. Eurythermal	2. Shark
C. Euryhaline	3. *Artemisia*
D. Stenothermal	4. Coconut

A.________ B.________ C. ________ D. ________

21. Herbs and shrubs in forests cannot perform photosynthesis at high light conditions.
(*Rewrite the statement after correcting the underlined words.*)

____

22. Which of the following represents the correct decreasing order of light intensities required for productivity in a forest?

(a) Trees, shrubs, herbs ☐ (b) Shrubs, herbs trees ☐

(c) Herbs, shrubs, trees ☐ (d) Trees, herbs, shrubs ☐

23. Complete the following sentence by using the words in the box given below.

Diurnal, Nocturnal, Photoperiod, Photosynthesis, Migratory, Respiratory, Foraging, Hunting

The diurnal and seasonal variations in light intensity and ____________ are the area of animals for ________, reproductive and ________ activities.

24. Radiation below the visible light, i.e. infrared is useful to some organisms.
(*Rewrite the statement after correcting the underlined words.*)

____

25. The nature and properties of soil depend on the ____________, ____________ process and how soil development occurred.

26. Soil composition, grain size and aggregation determine the ____________ and ____________ of soil.

27. Find odd one out with respect to vegetation cover of an area.

pH, Topography, Mineral composition, Types of animal

____

28. Sediment characteristics often determine the type of benthic animals in the soil environment.
(*Rewrite the statement after correcting the underlined word.*)

____

29. Name the process in which the organism should try to maintain constancy of its internal environment.

____

30. __________ are organisms which maintain their body temperature despite of change in temperature of their environment.

31. Write biological term for the sentence.

Process of maintaining constant osmotic concentration. __________

32. __________ regulate their temperature up to certain extent.

33. Consider the following statements.

Statement I Constant internal body conditions require a constant internal temperature as well as fluid balance.

Statement II Success of mammals is related to their homeostasis irrespective of the habitat they are living in.

Choose the correct option from the following.

(a) Statement I is true, but statement II is false ☐
(b) Statement I is false, but statement II is true ☐
(c) Both statements I and II are true ☐
(d) Both statements I and II are false ☐

34. In summer, sweating gives a cooling effect to an animal.

True ☐ False ☐

35. Complete the following analogy given below.

Summer : Sweating : : __________ : Shivering

36. Plants have a mechanism to maintain internal temperature.

True ☐ False ☐

37. Give two examples of regulators. __________

38. 99% of animals are regulators which are also referred as ectotherms.

True ☐ False ☐

39. Write the biological term used for plants and animals whose internal environment changes with the ambient environmental conditions. __________

40. Which of the following only consists of conformers ?

(a) Snakes, lizards, crocodiles, eagle ☐ (b) Eagle, sparrow, kangaroo, rats ☐

(c) Snake, crocodile, fish, frog ☐ (d) Fish, lizard, sparrow, cockroach ☐

41. Thermoregulation is thermodynamically expensive for many organisms.
(*Rewrite the statement after correcting the underlined word.*)

____

42. Name any two small animals which cannot afford thermoregulations.

____

43. Heat gain or heat loss is a function of ______________________________

44. Small animals have ____________ (smaller/larger) surface area relative to their volume.

45. Small animals have to expend ____________ (less/more) energy to generate body heat through metabolism.

46. Very small animals are rarely found in polar regions. (*Give reason*)

____

47. Write the two other alternatives that organism adopt for a short duration stressful condition.

____

***48.** Identify the parts labelled as *A, B, C* and *D* in this diagrammatic representation of organismic response.

A ↑
C
Regulators
D
B ⟶

A. ____________

B. ____________

C. ____________

D. ____________

49. Consider the following statements.

Statement I Organisms migrate if the stressful external condition persists for longer duration.

Statement II Migratory birds often fly from Siberia to Rajasthan to avoid stressful conditions.

Choose the correct option from the following.

(a) Statement I is true, but statement II is false ☐

(b) Statement I is false, but statement II is true ☐

(c) Both statements I and II are true ☐

(d) Both statements I and II are false ☐

50. Name the very famous National Park in India which hosts the migratory birds from Siberia.

____

51. Thick-walled spore formation during unfavourable condition is seen in bacteria and fungi.

True ☐ False ☐

52. Write a biological term for the sentence.

A state of reduced metabolic activity observed in seeds to tide over the period of stress conditions.

____

53. Write the scientific name of escape in time exhibited by bears during winter.

____

54. ______________ is a escape from summer related heat and desiccation problems.

55. Match the following columns.

Column I (Names of animals)	Column II (Adaptations)
A. Snail	1. Hibernation
B. Zooplankton	2. Aestivation
C. Bear	3. Diapause

A.__________ B.__________ C. __________

56. Name the stage of suspended development in planktons. ______________

57. ______________ is any attribute of an organism which enables the organism to survive and reproduce in its habitat.

58. Write the three major attributes of adaptation found in animals.

____

***59.** Write the attribute (behavioural/physiological/morphological) of adaptation for the following .

(i) Lizard basking in sun in cold climates. ______________

(ii) Increased haemoglobin in high altitude people. ______________

(iii) Increased breathing rate due to less oxygen availability. ______________

(iv) *Opuntia's* leaves are reduced to spines. ______________

60. Survival of Archaebacteria in hot deep sea hydrothermal vents is an example of ______________ (behavioural/ physiological adaptations).

61. Internal fat oxidation is metabolic reaction in kangaroo rat to meet its fat requirement.

(*Rewrite the statement after correcting the underlined words.*)

____

62. All of the following are adaptations in a kangaroo rat except

(a) Internal fat oxidation ☐ (b) Low water output ☐

(c) Long and muscular legs ☐ (d) Concentrated urine ☐

63. Write the two beneficiary adaptations of internal fat oxidation.

(i) ______________________

(ii) ______________________

64. Thick cuticle on leaf and stomatal arrangement in deep pits is to ________________ (maximise/minimise) water loss through ______________ .

***65.** Name the plants which carry special photosynthetic pathway in which the stomata remain closed during daytime.

____

66. Complete the following analogy with respect to adaptation in *Opuntia*.

Stem : __________ : : Leaves : ______________

***67.** Consider the following statements.

Statement I. Certain desert plants close their stomata during the day and open at night.

Statement II. In *Opuntia* photosynthesis is performed by leaves at night when the stomata opens.

Choose the correct option from the following.

(a) Statement I is true, but statement II is false ☐

(b) Statement I is false, but statement II is true ☐

(c) Both statements I and II are true ☐

(d) Both statements I and II are false ☐

***68.** *Opunita* has a special photosynthetic pathway (CAM) that enables its stomata to remain closed during day time.

True ☐ False ☐

69. Name the rule which assumes mammals from colder climates have shorter ears and limbs to minimise heat loss.

____

70. Seals have a thick layer of fat called ________________ below thin skin and acts as an ________________ to reduce body heat.

71. Write a common term for the following.

Nausea, Fatigue, Heart palpitations

____

72. Write the two mechanisms by which body compensates for the low oxygen availability.

(i) ____

(ii) ____

***73.** People living in high altitudes have lower RBCs than the people living in plains.

(*Rewrite the statement after correcting the underlined words.*)

74. Biochemical adaptations are seen in organisms in great depths of the ocean to face ________________________ .

75. Desert lizard lacks the physiological condition to deal with high temperature of their habitat and cannot manage to keep their body temperature fairly constant by behavioural means.

True ☐ False ☐

76. Consider the following statements.

Statement I Organisms can show behavioural changes as a means to adapt to the external conditions.

Statement II Desert lizards often bask in the sun to absorb heat if the body temperatures fall below comfort levels.

Choose the correct option from the following.

(a) Statement I is true, but statement II is false ☐
(b) Statement I is false, but statement II is true ☐
(c) Both statements I and II are true ☐
(d) Both statements I and II are false ☐

Assertion-Reason Questions

The following questions consist of two statements- Assertion (A) and Reason (R). Answer these questions by selecting the appropriate option given below.
(a) Both A and R are true and R is the correct explanation of A
(b) Both A and R are true, but R is not the correct explanation of A
(c) A is true, but R is false
(d) A is false, but R is true

1. **Assertion** (A) The availability of light on land is closely linked with that of temperature.

Reason (R) Sun acts as common source for both light and temperature.

(a) ☐ (b) ☐ (c) ☐ (d) ☐

***2.** **Assertion** (A) Desert plants like *Opuntia* are adapted to live in dry conditions by following CAM pathway and leaves reduced to spines.

Reason (R) The adaptation promotes minimal loss of water.

(a) ☐ (b) ☐ (c) ☐ (d) ☐

3. **Assertion** (A) The population of a bacteria growing in a petri plate is often determined by its density.

Reason (R) It is sometimes difficult and irrelevant to calculate population of a species by its number.

(a) ☐ (b) ☐ (c) ☐ (d) ☐

***4.** **Assertion** (A) Natality and mortality rate are the positive attributes that causes an increase in population density.

Reason (R) Population density of a place is affected by the immigration and emigration of a particular species.

(a) ☐ (b) ☐ (c) ☐ (d) ☐

*5. **Assertion** (A) If food and resources become unlimited, a population shows geometric growth or exponential growth.

Reason (R) In an exponential growth curve, the value of 'r' indicates the impact of any biotic or abiotic factor on population density.

(a) ☐ (b) ☐ (c) ☐ (d) ☐

*6. **Assertion** (A) The logistic growth curve is the realistic curve in nature that shows a sigmoid curve.

Reason (R) Resources in nature are not unlimited and the earth has its own carrying capacity.

(a) ☐ (b) ☐ (c) ☐ (d) ☐

7. **Assertion** (A) Exotic species when introduced in an area can become invasive and spread faster.

Reason (R) Often predators are introduced in an area to control invasive prey species.

(a) ☐ (b) ☐ (c) ☐ (d) ☐

8. **Assertion** (A) Quinine obtained from plants is of commercial importance to humans.

Reason (R) Quinines are produced by plants to promote their growth in developmental stage.

(a) ☐ (b) ☐ (c) ☐ (d) ☐

9. **Assertion** (A) In an association observed between sea anemone and clown fish, both the species benefit one another .

Reason (R) Sea anemones keep the predators of the clown fish away due to the presence of their stinging tentacles.

(a) ☐ (b) ☐ (c) ☐ (d) ☐

10. **Assertion** (A) The Mediterranean orchid does not provide any floral reward to the bees but uses sexual deceit to get pollinated.

Reason (R) One of the petal of *Ophrys* resembles the female bee, which attracts male bees that pseudocopulates with it.

(a) ☐ (b) ☐ (c) ☐ (d) ☐

Case Based Questions

1. In a given geographical area characterised by grassland, a given deer species is prevalent. Few tigers were also introduced to this area in the year 2022. Population density studies conducted over a period of five years showed the following numbers as tabulated below.

Year	Population (Number of deer)
2019	375
2020	470
2021	485
2022	405
2023	382

Based on the given information answer the following questions

(i) Which of the following growth curve would be followed by the deer population, considering that resources are not unlimited?

(a) Exponential growth curve ☐ (b) J-shaped growth curve ☐
(c) Sigmoid growth curve ☐ (d) Geometric growth curve ☐

(ii) Why does the fall in deer population coincide with the introduction of tigers in the area?

(a) Competition ☐ (b) Mutualism ☐
(c) Predation ☐ (d) Ammensalism ☐

(iii) If the deer population falls, despite the absence of any predator species or invasive species, what could be the possible reason behind it?

(a) Interspecific competition ☐ (b) Inability to adapt ☐
(c) Climatic conditions ☐ (d) Parasitism ☐

2. Consider two trees A and B. Tree A has three species living in it, designated as S1, S2 and S3. Tree B also has three different species S6, S7 and S8 living in it. It was found that after a given time period of one year, tree A showed the presence of all three species, however tree B showed only species S7 and S8. S6 was completely eliminated. It is to be noted that there was no predator or parasite of the species in either of the plants. Based on this ecological situation answer the following questions:

(i) The limiting factor-that affected species population in tree B by giving rise to....

(a) Climate; intraspecific competition ☐
(b) Food; interspecific competition ☐
(c) Temperature; intraspecific competition ☐
(d) Rainfall; interspecific competition ☐

(ii) Which of the following ecological principles was observed in tree B?

(a) Competitive exclusion ☐ (b) Survival of the fittest ☐
(c) Competitive release ☐ (d) Resource partitioning ☐

(iii) How did all the three species survive in tree A?

(a) Mutualism ☐ (b) Symbiosis ☐
(c) Resource partitioning ☐ (d) Competition release ☐

COMPETITION EDGE UP

1. The equation of Verhulst-Pearl logistic growth is $\frac{dN}{dt} = rN\left[\frac{K-N}{K}\right]$.

[NCERT Pg. 195, NEET 2024]

From this equation, K indicates

(a) intrinsic rate of natural increase ☐
(b) biotic potential ☐
(c) carrying capacity ☐
(d) population density ☐

2. Given below are two statements.

Statement I Gause's competitive exclusion principle states that two closely related species competing for different resources cannot exist indefinitely.

Statement II According to Gause's principle, during competition, the inferior will be eliminated. This may be true if resources are limiting.

In the light of the above statements, choose the correct answer from the options given below.

[NCERT Pg. 199, NEET 2024]

(a) Both statement I and statement II are true ☐
(b) Both statement I and statement II are false ☐
(c) Statement I is true, but statement II is false ☐
(d) Statement I is false, but statement II is true ☐

3. Match List I with List II.

	List I		List II
A.	Logistic growth	I.	Unlimited resource availability condition
B.	Exponential growth	II.	Limited resource availability condition
C.	Expanding age pyramid	III.	The per cent individuals of pre-reproductive age is largest followed by reproductive and post-reproductive age groups
D.	Stable age pyramid	IV.	The per cent individuals of pre-reproductive and reproductive age group are same

Choose the correct answer from the options given below

[NCERT Pg. 192 to 195, NEET 2023]

(a) A-II, B-III, C-I, D-IV ☐
(b) A-II, B-IV, C-I, D-III ☐
(c) A-II, B-IV, C-III, D-I ☐
(d) A-II, B-I, C-III, D-IV ☐

4. Given below are two statements.

Statement I Gause's 'competitive exclusion principle' states that two closely related species competing for the same resources cannot co-exist indefinitely and competitively inferior one will be eliminated eventually.

Statement II In general, carnivores are more adversely affected by competition than herbivores.

In the light of the above statements, choose the correct answer from the options given below

[NCERT Pg. 199, NEET 2023]

(a) Both statement I and statement II are false ☐
(b) Statement I is true, but statement II is false ☐
(c) Statement I is false, but statement II is true ☐
(d) Both statement I and statement II are true ☐

5. Match List I with List II.

	List I (Interaction)		List II (Species A and B)
A.	Mutualism	I.	+(A), 0(B)
B.	Commensalism	II.	−(A), 0(B)
C.	Ammensalism	III.	+(A), −(B)
D.	Parasitism	IV.	+(A), +(B)

Choose the correct answer from the options given below.

[NCERT Pg. 197, NEET 2023]

(a) A-IV, B-I, C-II, D-III ☐
(b) A-IV, B-III, C-I, D-II ☐
(c) A-III, B-I, C-IV, D-II ☐
(d) A-IV, B-II, C-I, D-III ☐

6. Match List I with List II.

List I (Interacting species)	List II (Name of interaction)
A. A leopard and a lion in a forest/grassland	I. Competition
B. A cuckoo laying egg in a crow's nest	II. Brood parasitism
C. Fungi and root of a higher plant in mycorrhizae	III. Mutualism
D. A cattle egret and a cattle in a field	IV. Commensalism

Choose the correct answer from the options given below. **[NEET 2023]**

(a) A-I, B-II, C-IV, D-III ☐
(b) A-III, B-IV, C-I, D-II ☐
(c) A-II, B-III, C-I, D-IV ☐
(d) A-I, B-II, C-III, D-IV ☐

7. If '8' Drosophila in a laboratory population of '80' died during a week, the death rate in the population is ......individuals per Drosophila per week. **[NCERT Pg. 191, NEET 2022]**

(a) 10 ☐ (b) 1.0 ☐
(c) zero ☐ (d) 0.1 ☐

8. While explaining interspecific interaction of population, (+) sign is assigned for beneficial interaction, (–) sign is assigned for detrimental interaction and (0) for neutral interaction. Which of the following interactions can be assigned (+) for one species and (–) for another species involved in the interaction ? **[NCERT Pg. 197, NEET 2022]**

(a) Amensalism ☐
(b) Commensalism ☐
(c) Competition ☐
(d) Predation ☐

9. Match List I with List II. **[NCERT (Old) Pg. 226, NEET 2021]**

List I	List II
A. Allen's Rule	I. Kangaroo rat
B. Physiological adaptation	II. Desert lizard
C. Behavioural adaptation	III. Marine fish at depth
D. Biochemical adaptation	IV. Polar seal

Choose the correct answer from the options given below.

	A	B	C	D	
(a)	(IV)	(III)	(II)	(I)	☐
(b)	(IV)	(II)	(III)	(I)	☐
(c)	(IV)	(I)	(III)	(II)	☐
(d)	(IV)	(I)	(II)	(III)	☐

10. Match the items in Column I with those in Column II. **[NCERT Pg. 198 to 201, NEET (Oct.) 2020]**

Column I		Column II
A. Herbivores-Plants	(i)	Commensalism
B. Mycorrhiza-Plants	(ii)	Mutualism
C. Sheep-Cattle	(iii)	Predation
D. Orchid-Tree	(iv)	Competition

Select the correct option.

	A	B	C	D	
(a)	(iv),	(ii),	(i),	(iii)	☐
(b)	(iii),	(ii),	(iv),	(i)	☐
(c)	(ii),	(i),	(iii),	(iv)	☐
(d)	(i),	(iii),	(iv),	(ii)	☐

11. Secondary metabolites such as nicotine, strychnine and caffeine are produced by plants for their **[NCERT Pg. 198, NEET (Sep.) 2020]**

(a) growth response ☐
(b) defence action ☐
(c) effect on reproduction ☐
(d) nutritive value ☐

12. Pinus seed cannot germinate and establish without fungal association. This is because **[NEET (National) 2019]**

(a) it has obligate association with mycorrhizae ☐
(b) it has very hard seed coat ☐
(c) its seeds contain inhibitors that prevent germination ☐
(d) its embryo is immature ☐

Chapter 12

Ecosystem

Scan and take Chapter Test

TOPIC 1

Ecosystem : Structure and Function, Productivity and Decomposition

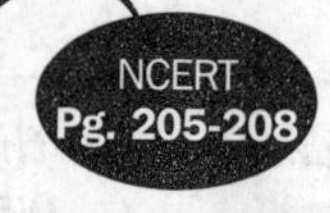

1. An ecosystem is a ______________ unit of nature, where living organisms interact among themselves and also with the surrounding ______________.
2. Name the two basic categories of ecosystem. ______________
3. Choose the odd one out with respect to the type of ecosystem.

   Forest, Estuary, Grassland, Desert

   ____
4. Give two examples of man-made ecosystem. ______________
5. The physical structure of an ecosystem is formed by the interaction of its plants and animals.
   (*Rewrite the statement after correcting the underlined words.*)

   ____
6. ______ and ______ of plant and animal species of an ecosystem gives its species composition.
7. Consider a forest ecosystem where there are trees, shrubs, herbs, bushes, climbers, etc. What would you designate to the distribution of the plants to different layers in the forest?
   (a) Productivity ☐ (b) Stratification ☐
   (c) Succession ☐ (d) Energy Flow ☐
8. In a forest ecosystem, trees occupy ______________ vertical strata, shrubs the second and herbs and ______________ occupy the bottom layers.
9. How many of the listed aspects functions as a unit in an ecosystem?

   Productivity, Decomposition, Energy flow, Stratification, Biome, Nutrient cycling

   ____
10. All the four basic functional components of an ecosystem are found in a pond having shallow water.

    True ☐ False ☐

*Concepts of all questions bearing * are important for NEET & CUET*

11. Complete the flowchart given below.

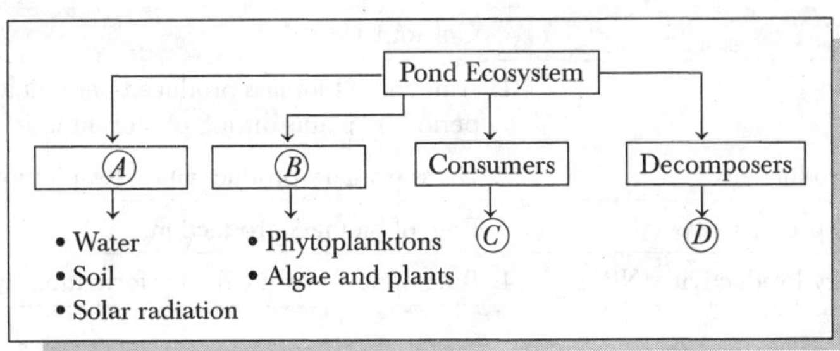

A. __________ B. __________ C. __________ D. __________

12. Identify the components of pond ecosystem based on the given characteristics/functions.
(i) Name the component which contains all dissolved inorganic and organic substances.

____

(ii) Name the component which converts inorganic into organic material.

____

(iii) Name the component which is especially abundant in the bottom of the pond.

____

13. Name the two processes by which matter is released from dead remains and made available to autotrophs in a pond ecosystem.

____

14. In a pond ecosystem, there is __________ movement of energy towards the __________ trophic levels. It is accompanied by energy dissipation and loss as __________ to the environment.

15. The unit of productivity is __________ (gm^{-2} yr^{-1}/gm^2/yr^{-1}).

16. The available biomass for the consumption of heterotrophs is Gross Primary Productivity (GPP). (*Rewrite the statement after correcting the underlined words.*)

____

17. If the gross primary productivity in a desert ecosystem is 1500 (k cal m^{-2}) yr^{-1}, and the available biomass to the heterotrophs is 1100 (k cal m^{-2}) yr-1, then calculate the loss suffered due to respiration.

(a) 100 (k cal m^{-2}) yr^{-1} ☐ (b) 2600 (k cal m^{-2}) yr^{-1} ☐
(c) 400 (k cal m^{-2}) yr^{-1} ☐ (d) 1400 (k cal m^{-2}) yr^{-1} ☐

18. Consider the following statements.
Statement I Primary productivity refers to the biomass production by producers of a food chain.
Statement II Consumers are responsible for the secondary productivity in a food chain.

Choose the correct option from the following.

(a) Statement I is true, but statement II is false ☐
(b) Statement I is false, but statement II is true ☐
(c) Both statements I and II are true ☐
(d) Both statements I and II are false ☐

19. Match the following columns.

Column I	Column II
A. Productivity	1. Amount of biomass produced per unit area over a time period by plants during photosynthesis.
B. Primary productivity	2. Gross primary productivity – Respiration losses.
C. Secondary productivity	3. Rate of biomass production.
D. Net Primary Productivity (NPP)	4. Rate of new organic matter formation by consumers.

A. ________ B. ________ C. ________ D. ________

20. How many listed factors can affect the primary productivity of an ecosystem?

Plant species habitat, Environmental factors, Presence of decomposers, Nutrient availability, Photosynthetic capacity of plants

____

21. Primary productivity of different ecosystem varies, and oceans are highly productive as they occupy 70% of the surface.

True ☐ False ☐

22. Complete the following analogy with respect to productivity.

Annual NPP of biosphere : 170 billion tons : : Annual NPP of oceans : ________

23. Name the biological process in which an organism breaks down complex organic matter into inorganic substances. ________

24. Name the detritivore which is referred to as farmer's friend.

____

25. Choose the odd one out with respect to the composition of detritus.

Dead leaves and flowers, Faecal matter, Inorganic substances, Dead remains of animals

____

26. The raw material for decomposition is called detritivore.
(*Rewrite the statement after correcting the underlined word.*)

____

27. The organisms which carry out the process of decomposition are known as ________.

28. Consider the following statements.

Statement I Inorganic materials by the process of leaching precipitate into available salts.

Statement II Humus acts as the substrate for few microbes that return nutrients back into the soil.

Choose the correct option from the following.

(a) Statement I is true, but statement II is false ☐

(b) Statement I is false, but statement II is true ☐

(c) Both statements I and II are true ☐

(d) Both statements I and II are false ☐

29. Humus is highly susceptible to microbial action and undergoes decomposition at faster rate.

True ☐ False ☐

30. Being colloidal in nature, __________ (humus/detritus) serves as a reservoir of nutrients.

31. Which of the following is not a property of humus?

(a) Resistant to microbial action ☐ (b) High rate of decomposition ☐

(c) Colloidal in nature ☐ (d) Reservoir of nutrients ☐

32. Refer to the given list and answer the questions that follow.

I. Leaching, II. Catabolism, III. Humification, IV. Mineralisation, V. Fragmentation

(i) Arrange the following steps in the order of their occurrence during the process of decomposition. __________

(ii) How many of these steps operate simultaneously on the detritus? __________

(iii) How many of these steps occur during decomposition in the soil? __________

33. Match the following columns.

Column I (Steps of decomposition)	Column II (Characteristics)
A. Fragmentation	1. Inorganic nutrients seep into soil.
B. Humification	2. Humus release inorganic nutrients due to the action of microbes.
C. Leaching	3. Breakdown of detritus into smaller particles.
D. Mineralisation	4. Nutrient rich dark-coloured amorphous substance is formed.
E. Catabolism	5. Detritus is broken down by bacterial and fungal enzymes.

A. __________ B. __________ C. __________ D. __________

E. __________

***34.** What does the diagram given below represent?

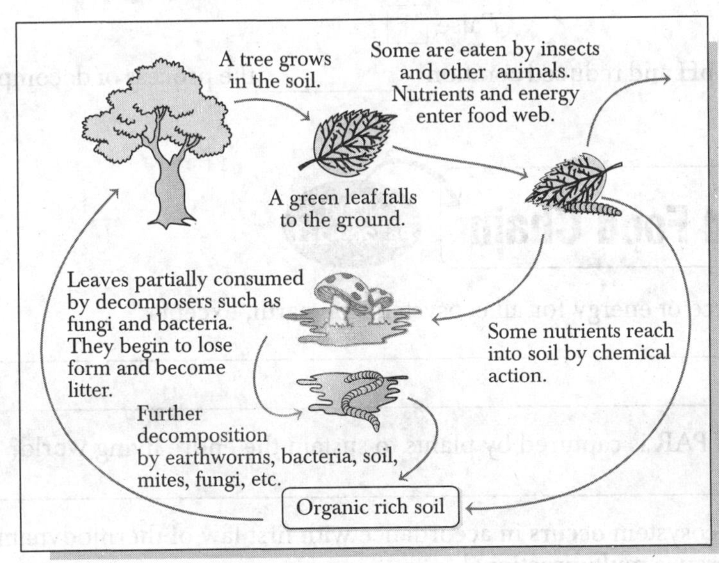

____

***35.** Decomposition is largely an ____________ requiring process. The rate of decomposition is controlled by ____________ of detritus and ____________ factors.

***36.** Which of the following will make the detritus decompose at a slower rate?

(a) High chitin composition ☐ (b) Aerobic conditions ☐
(c) Warm and humid weather ☐ (d) Low lignin composition ☐

***37.** Complete the analogy given below with respect to process of decomposition.
Slower decomposition rate : Lignin and chitin in detritus : : Faster decomposition rate: ____________

***38.** Name any two climatic factors that regulate decomposition through their effects on the activities of soil microbes.

____

39. Choose the odd one out with respect to their effects on the rate of decomposition.

Warm environment, Anaerobiosis, Moist environment

____

40. Consider the following statements.
Statement I Decomposition of the detritus is accelerated under anaerobic conditions.
Statement II Presence of sugar and nitrogen in the detritus lowers decomposition rate.
Choose the correct option from the following.

(a) Statement I is true, but statement II is false ☐
(b) Statement I is false, but statement II is true ☐
(c) Both statements I and II are true ☐
(d) Both statements I and II are false ☐

41. Low temperature inhibits the process of decomposition, resulting in build up of organic material.

True ☐ False ☐

42. The soil with acidic pH and reduced aeration ____________ the process of decomposition.

TOPIC 2
Energy Flow and Food Chain

NCERT Pg. 209-211

43. Sun is the only source of energy for all ecosystems on earth, except

____

44. Expand PAR. ____________

45. What percentage of PAR is captured by plants to sustain the entire living world?

____

46. Energy flow in an ecosystem occurs in accordance with first law of thermodynamics because flow of energy is <u>multidirectional</u>.
(*Rewrite the statement after correcting the underlined word.*)

____

47. Ecosystems are exempted from the second law of thermodynamics, as they do not need a constant supply of energy to synthesise the molecules.

True ☐ False ☐

48. Give the common term for the following words.

Herbaceous and woody plants, Phytoplanktons, Algae

____

49. Give the biological term for the sequence of species through which the food energy pass in a community.______________________________

50. Food chains always start with a ________________ (producer/consumer), an organism that makes food.

51. Consider the following statements.

Statement I During the process of photosynthesis plants can capture only 2-10 % of PAR.

Statement II Once a consumer feeds on a producer, energy gets trapped indefinitely in them.

Choose the correct option from the following.

(a) Statement I is true, but statement II is false ☐

(b) Statement I is false, but statement II is true ☐

(c) Both statements I and II are true ☐

(d) Both statements I and II are false ☐

52. Some common herbivores in terrestrial ecosystem include insects, birds and mammals.

True ☐ False ☐

***53.** Match the following columns.

Column I	Column II
A. Primary consumers	1. Top of food chain
B. Secondary consumers	2. Flesh-eating animals
C. Tertiary consumers	3. Herbivores

A. ____________ B. ____________ C. ____________

***54.** How many of the listed herbivores are found in terrestrial ecosystem?

Insects, Birds, Mammals, Molluscs

____

***55.** Complete the following analogy given below with respect to consumers.

Primary carnivores : Secondary consumers : : Secondary carnivores : ____________ .

56. Consider the following statements and identify the option with correct ones.

I. Molluscs, insects, birds and mammals are some common herbivores in terrestrial ecosystem.

II. Ecosystems are exempted from the second law of thermodynamics.

III. Decomposers secrete digestive enzymes that breakdown dead and waste material into simple, inorganic material.

IV. In an aquatic ecosystem, algae and phytoplankton are the major producers.

Codes

(a) I, II and III ☐ (b) II and III ☐

(c) I and IV ☐ (d) III and IV ☐

57. Expand GFC. ____________

***58.** Identify the correct grazing food chain among (i) and (ii) given below.

(i) Grass → Goat → Man

(ii) Cow → Grass → Goat

____

59. A grazing food chain begins with <u>herbivores</u>.
(*Rewrite the statement after correcting the underlined word.*)

____

60. Expand DFC. ____________

61. Detritus food chain derives energy from ____________ (sun/organic matter).

62. Name two organisms which start detritus food chain.

____

63. Read the following statements and identify the type of organisms.

I. Heterotrophic organisms which degrade dead organic matter.

II. They are ecological cleansers that create balance in ecosystem.

____

64. The major conduit of energy in an aquatic ecosystem is ____________ food chain whereas in a terrestrial ecosystem much larger fraction of energy flow through ____________ food chain.

65. Which of the following is correct for the food chain represented below?

Grass ⟶ Grasshopper ⟶ Frog ⟶ Snake ⟶ Owl

(a) Any organism at a point cannot be a part of more than one food chain.

(b) The frogs are the tertiary consumers in the given food chain

(c) The detritus food chain is not operative in this terrestrial network

(d) The major flow of energy takes place through DFC and not by GFC.

***66.** A person who is eating a bowl of curd, can be classified to which trophic and consumer level in the food chain?

(a) Trophic level III, secondary consumer, primary carnivore

(b) Trophic level II, secondary consumer, primary carnivore

(c) Trophic level III, secondary consumer, secondary carnivore

(d) Trophic level II, primary consumer, primary carnivore

67. Give the biological term for the natural interconnections of food chains. ____________

68. Detritus food chain may be connected with the grazing food chain at some levels.

True ☐ False ☐

***69.** Identify the number of grazing food chains in the food web shown below.

Lion

Cow ← Plants → Goat

Grasshopper Man

Frog

____

70. Give the biological term for the specific place of an organism in the food chain based on their nutrition. ____________

***71.** Refer to the flowchart of a typical food chain and answer the following questions.

Ⓐ Primary producers → Ⓑ Primary consumers → Ⓒ Secondary consumers → Ⓓ Tertiary consumers.

(i) Mention the trophic levels of *A* and *D*.

____

(ii) Give the examples of organisms which are likely to be present at first trophic level. ____________

(iii) The organisms found at position *B* are likely to be ____________ (carnivores/herbivores)

(iv) At which position, birds and fishes would be found?

____

(v) Zooplanktons being primary consumers would occupy ____________ trophic level.

***72.** The amount of energy increases at successive trophic levels.

True ☐ False ☐

***73.** The mass of living material at a trophic level at a particular time is known as

____

74. Refer to the given statements and identify the biological term.

I. It is the mass of living matter in a unit area.
II. It is expressed in terms of fresh or dry weight.

____

75. Consider the following statements.

I. Standing crop measures only the biomass in a unit area at particular time.
II. At each trophic level, 10% of the energy passed down is radiated as heat.
III. Organisms at each trophic level depend on those at the lower trophic level for their energy demands.
IV. Standing crop is the certain mass of living material present in each trophic level.

Identify the option with correct set of statements.

(a) I, II and III ☐ (b) II, III and IV ☐
(c) I, III and IV ☐ (d) I and IV ☐

76. Refer to the diagram of energy flow through different trophic levels and answer the following questions.

(i) Identify the type of food chain shown in the given diagram.

____

(ii) What per cent of energy is being transferred from first to second trophic level?

____

(iii) If the plants received 5000 kJ energy from sun, what amount of energy would be received by the top carnivore?

____

(iv) The number of trophic levels in a grazing food chain is limited due to 10% law of energy transfer.

True ☐ False ☐

77. In a given food chain, the primary consumers have 100 J of energy for their utilisation. If plants can use only 1% of the solar radiation, then calculate the energy available to the producers.

(a) 1000 J ☐ (b) 10,000 J ☐
(c) 100000 J ☐ (d) 10 J ☐

TOPIC 3

Ecological Pyramids

NCERT Pg. 211-214

78. Give the biological term for the graphical representation of producer's and consumer's relationship in the form of a pyramid.

____

79. Choose the odd one out with respect to the applicability of ecological pyramids.

Number, Biomass, Energy, Standing Crop

____

80. The base of an ecological pyramid represents top carnivores.
(*Rewrite the statement after correcting the underlined words.*)

____

81. A pyramid of number shows four trophic levels. In a grassland ecosystem, where would you place grasses in the pyramid?

(a) Proximal to the apex ☐ (b) At the apex ☐
(c) Proximal to the base ☐ (d) At the base ☐

82. While calculating energy, biomass or number, all the organisms at a trophic level of pyramid are considered.

True ☐ False ☐

83. The trophic level in ecological pyramids represent ______ (a species/ functional level).

***84.** In most ecosystems, pyramid of number, biomass and energy is ______.

85. What does the ecological pyramid shown in the given diagram represent?

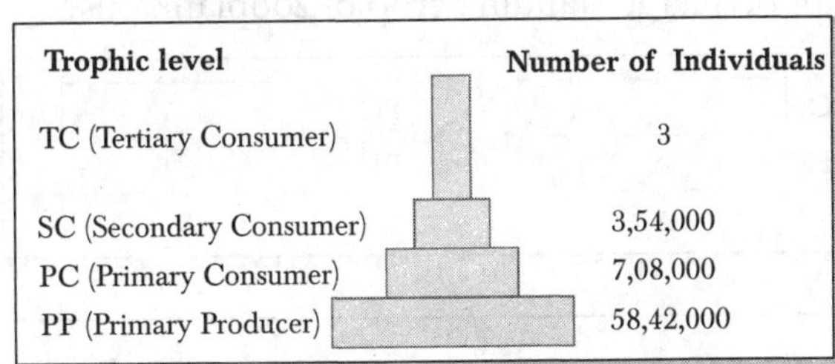

86. What shape of pyramid would you obtain if numerous insects feed on a big tree?

87. If a tree supports number of small birds which inturn are eaten by large birds, then the shape of pyramid of number would be

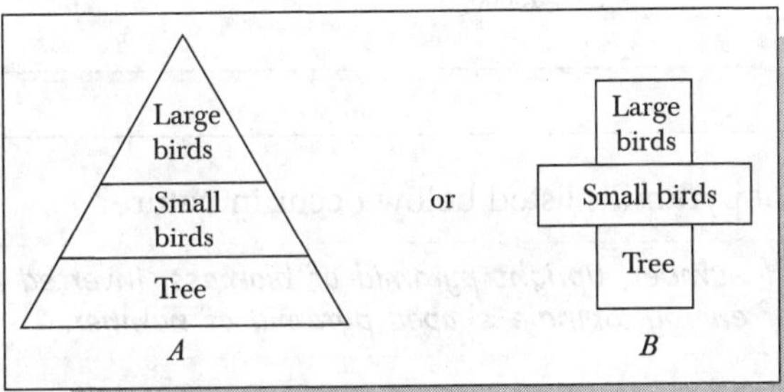

88. Consider the given image and mark the option which does not follow the given pyramid structure.

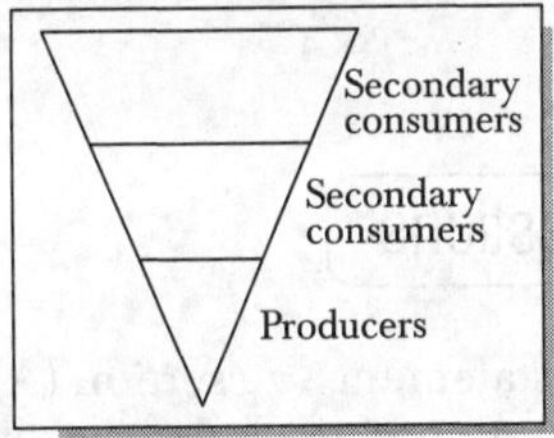

(a) Insects feeding on a tree

(b) Zooplanktons feeding on phytoplanktons

(c) Small fishes feeding on zooplanktons

(d) Snakes feeding on rats in a grassland

89. Refer to the given diagram of pyramid of biomass.

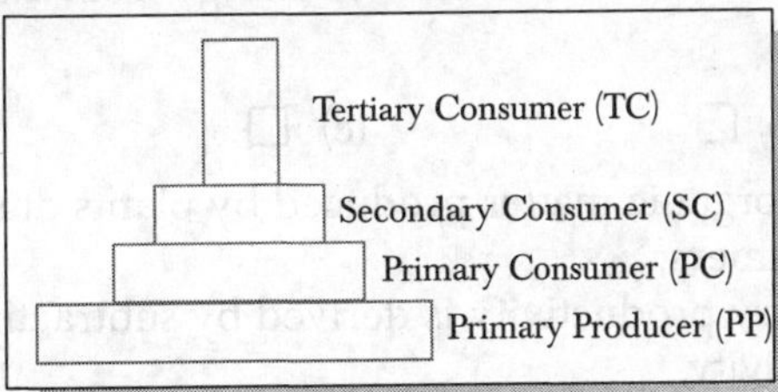

The dry weight (kg m^{-2}) of biomass from PP to TC would ________ (increase/decrease).

90. What shape of pyramid of biomass would you obtain if small standing crop of phytoplanktons supports large standing crop of zooplanktons?

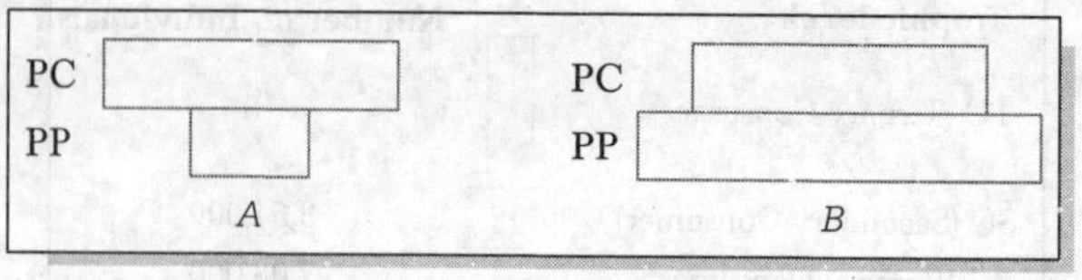

PC PC
PP PP
A B

____

91. In a sea, the pyramid of biomass is ______________ shaped.

92. An ideal pyramid of energy is

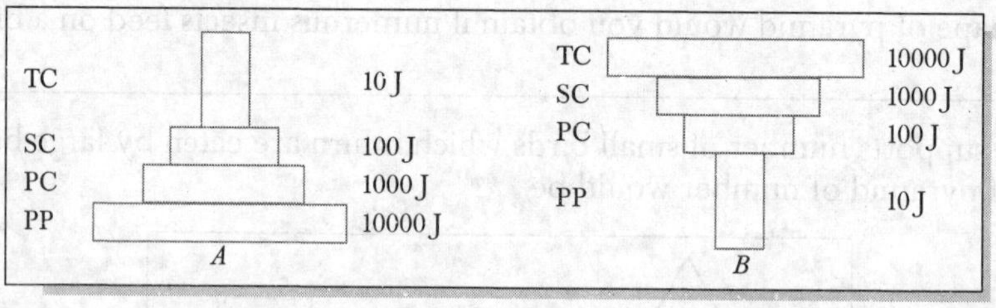

	A		B
TC	10 J	TC	10000 J
SC	100 J	SC	1000 J
PC	1000 J	PC	100 J
PP	10000 J	PP	10 J

____

93. How many types of pyramids listed below occur in nature?

Inverted pyramid of number, Upright pyramid of biomass, Inverted pyramid of biomass, Inverted pyramid of energy, Spindle-shaped pyramid of number.

____

94. Ecological pyramids take into account food ___________ and does not accommodate a food ___________.

95. Ecological pyramids neglect the role of ______________ (saprophytes/herbivores) in the ecosystem.

Assertion-Reason Questions

The following questions consist of two statements- Assertion (A) and Reason (R). Answer these questions by selecting the appropriate option given below.

(a) Both A and R are true and R is the correct explanation of A

(b) Both A and R are true, but R is not the correct explanation of A

(c) A is true, but R is false

(d) A is false, but R is true

1. **Assertion** (A) The consumers are represented by the phytoplanktons that dwell at the bottom of a pond ecosystem.

Reason (R) There is a unidirectional flow of energy from autotrophs to heterotrophs in an ecosystem.

(a) ☐ (b) ☐ (c) ☐ (d) ☐

***2.** **Assertion** (A) All the organic matter produced by plants during photosynthesis is not available for the consumers.

Reason (R) Net primary productivity is derived by subtracting respiration losses from gross primary productivity.

(a) ☐ (b) ☐ (c) ☐ (d) ☐

*3. **Assertion** (A) Detritivores are involved in the catabolism step of decomposition process.
Reason (R) In catabolism, bacteria and fungi degrade the detritus into simple inorganic substances.

(a) ☐ (b) ☐ (c) ☐ (d) ☐

4. **Assertion** (A) Only a small fraction of the solar energy is passed to trophic levels two and three.
Reason (R) There is a unidirectional energy flow in subsequent trophic levels starting with plants.

(a) ☐ (b) ☐ (c) ☐ (d) ☐

5. **Assertion** (A) The number of trophic levels in a grazing food chain is restricted.
Reason (R) 15 % of the total energy receives can be transferred from one trophic level to the other.

(a) ☐ (b) ☐ (c) ☐ (d) ☐

*6. **Assertion** (A) All the ecological pyramids in nature are upright with no exceptions.
Reason (R) The pyramids represent the number of biomass and energy flow in an ecosystem.

(a) ☐ (b) ☐ (c) ☐ (d) ☐

*7. **Assertion** (A) Pyramid of energy operating in an ecosystem is always upright and never inverted.
Reason (R) When energy flows from one trophic level to another, there is loss of some energy as heat.

(a) ☐ (b) ☐ (c) ☐ (d) ☐

Case Based Questions

1. The graphs given below show the relationship between a factor X and primary productivity and that between photosynthesis and primary productivity.

Factor X
Primary Productivity→
(A)

Photo-synthesis
Primary Productivity→
(B)

(i) What conclusion can be drawn from the graph A?

(a) Curve drops down due to respiratory losses ☐
(b) Curve shows a drop due to another influential factor ☐
(c) Factor 'X' is a limiting factor for primary productivity ☐
(d) On further increasing the factor X, the curve of primary productivity will rise further ☐

(ii) Factor 'X' can be any of the following except

(a) essential nutrients ☐ (b) temperature ☐
(c) oxygen levels ☐ (d) water availability ☐

(iii) If in case, there is a sharp decline in one of the factors contributing to photosynthesis the curve of the graph (B) will

(a) Fall sharply ☐ (b) Remain constant ☐

(c) Decline gradually ☐ (d) First rise and then fall ☐

2. In a sea ecosystem, the phytoplanktons are the primary producers. A team of researchers using satellite data discovered that there were about 4 kg/m^2 of phytoplanktons at a depth of 65 m in a sea. In contrast the average biomass of zooplanktons were 11 kg/m^2. The GFC is the major energy conduit in an aquatic ecosystem. Based on the provided information, answer the following questions.

(i) Which of the following represents the pyramid of biomass operating in the sea ecosystem?

(a)

Trophic level	Number of Individuals
TC (Tertiary Consumer)	3
SC (Secondary Consumer)	354000
PC (Primary Consumer)	708000
P (Producer)	5842000

☐

(b)

Trophic level	Dry weight (kg m^{-2})
TC	1.5
SC	11
PC	37
P	809

☐

(c)

PC	21
PP	4

☐

(d)

TC	10 J
SC	100 J
PC	1000 J
P	10.000 J

1,000,000 J of Sunlight

☐

(ii) If 100 J of energy is available to the phytoplanktons, calculate the energy available to the fishes.

(a) 1 J ☐ (b) 10 J ☐

(c) 100 J ☐ (d) 1000 J ☐

(iii) Which of the following is not true about the sea ecosystem?

(a) The energy pyramid in the sea will be upright ☐

(b) The biomass of the phytoplanktons is less than the zooplanktons ☐

(c) Standing crop of phytoplankton is smaller than that of zooplankton ☐

(d) Detritus food chain is not operative in the sea ecosystem ☐

COMPETITION EDGE UP

1. In an ecosystem if the Net Primary Productivity (NPP) of first trophic level is $100 \times (\text{kcal m}^{-2})\text{yr}^{-1}$. What will be the GPP (Gross Primary Productivity) of the third trophic level of the same ecosystem? **[NCERT Pg. 207, NEET 2024]**
   - (a) $\frac{x}{10}(\text{kcal m}^{-2})\text{yr}^{-1}$ ☐
   - (b) $x\,(\text{kcal m}^{-2})\text{yr}^{-1}$ ☐
   - (c) $10x\,(\text{kcal m}^{-2})\text{yr}^{-1}$ ☐
   - (d) $\frac{100x}{3x}(\text{kcal m}^{-2})\text{yr}^{-1}$ ☐

2. Identify the correct statements.
   A. Detritivores perform fragmentation.
   B. The humus is further degraded by some microbes during mineralisation.
   C. Water soluble inorganic nutrients go down into the soil and get precipitated by a process called leaching.
   D. The detritus food chain begins with living organisms.
   E. Earthworms breakdown detritus into smaller particles by a process called catabolism.
   Choose the correct answer from the options given below. **[NCERT Pg. 207, NEET 2023]**
   - (a) B, C and D only ☐
   - (b) C, D and E only ☐
   - (c) D, E and A only ☐
   - (d) A, B and C only ☐

3. Detritivores breakdown detritus into smaller particles. This process is called **[NCERT Pg. 207, NEET 2022]**
   - (a) Fragmentation ☐
   - (b) Humification ☐
   - (c) Decomposition ☐
   - (d) Catabolism ☐

4. Given below are two statements.
   Statement I Decomposition is a process in which the detritus is degraded into simpler substances by microbes.
   Statement II Decomposition is faster if the detritus is rich in lignin and chitin.
   In the light of the above statements, choose the correct answer from the options given below. **[NCERT Pg. 207, NEET 2022]**
   - (a) Both statement I and statement II are incorrect ☐
   - (b) Statement I is correct, but statement II is incorrect ☐
   - (c) Statement I is incorrect, but statement II is correct ☐
   - (d) Both statement I and statement II are correct ☐

5. In the equation GPP – R = NPP GPP is Gross Primary Productivity.
   NPP is Net Primary Productivity. R here is .... **[NCERT Pg. 207, NEET 2023, 2021]**
   - (a) Respiratory quotient ☐
   - (b) Respiratory loss ☐
   - (c) Reproductive allocation ☐
   - (d) Photosynthetically active radiation ☐

6. Which of the following statement is not correct? **[NEET 2021]**
   - (a) Pyramid of biomass in sea is generally inverted ☐
   - (b) Pyramid of biomass in sea is generally upright ☐
   - (c) Pyramid of energy is always upright ☐
   - (d) Pyramid of numbers in a grassland ecosystem is upright ☐

7. In relation to gross primary productivity and net primary productivity of an ecosystem, which one of the following statements is correct? **[NCERT Pg. 207, NEET (Sep.) 2020]**
   - (a) Gross primary productivity is always more than net primary productivity ☐
   - (b) Gross primary productivity and net primary productivity are one and same ☐
   - (c) There is no relationship between gross primary productivity and net primary productivity ☐
   - (d) Gross primary productivity is always less than net primary productivity ☐

8. The rate of decomposition is faster in the ecosystem due to following factors except **[NCERT Pg. 208, NEET (Oct.) 2020]**

(a) detritus rich in sugars ☐
(b) warm and moist environment ☐
(c) presence of aerobic soil microbes ☐
(d) detritus richer in lignin and chitin ☐

9. Match the trophic levels with their correct species examples in grassland ecosystem.

A.	Fourth trophic level	(i)	Crow
B.	Second trophic level	(ii)	Vulture
C.	First trophic level	(iii)	Rabbit
D.	Third trophic level	(iv)	Grass

Select the correct option.
[NCERT Pg. 212, NEET 2020]

	A	B	C	D	
(a)	(ii)	(iii)	(iv)	(i)	☐
(b)	(iii)	(ii)	(i)	(iv)	☐
(c)	(iv)	(iii)	(ii)	(i)	☐
(d)	(i)	(ii)	(iii)	(iv)	☐

10. Which of the following statements is incorrect? **[NEET (Oct.) 2020]**
(a) Biomass decreases from first to fourth trophic level ☐
(b) Energy content gradually increases from first to fourth trophic level ☐
(c) Number of individuals decreases from first trophic level to fourth trophic level ☐
(d) Energy content gradually decreases from first to fourth trophic level ☐

11. Which of the following ecological pyramids is generally inverted?
[NCERT Pg. 212, NEET (National) 2019]
(a) Pyramid of energy ☐
(b) Pyramid of biomass in a forest ☐
(c) Pyramid of biomass in a sea ☐
(d) Pyramid of numbers in grassland ☐

12. What type of ecological pyramid would be obtained with the following data?
Secondary consumer : 120 g
Primary consumer : 60 g
Primary producer : 10 g **[NEET 2018]**
(a) Upright pyramid of numbers ☐
(b) Pyramid of energy ☐
(c) Inverted pyramid of biomass ☐
(d) Upright pyramid of biomass ☐

Chapter 13

Biodiversity and Conservation

Scan and take Chapter Test

TOPIC 1

Biodiversity : Levels and Patterns

NCERT Pg. 216-220

1. On earth, there exists more than 20,000 species of __________ and __________ .
2. The significance of biodiversity existing on earth can be understood by the efforts made by __________ and __________ biologists.
3. Heterogeneity refers to the immense __________ in biosphere, at all the levels of biological organisation.
4. Name the sociobiologist who popularised the term biodiversity. __________
5. Biodiversity refers to the combined diversity at three major levels *viz* __________ (genetic, species, ecological/atomic, molecular)
6. A single species cannot show high diversity at the genetic level over its distributional range.

   True ☐ False ☐
7. The medicinal plant, __________ growing in Himalayan ranges shows genetic diversity in terms of potency and __________ of the active chemical, i.e. __________ produce by it.
8. India has more than 2000 genetically different strains of rice.

   (*Rewrite the statement after correcting the underlined word.*)

   ____
9. More than 2000 genetically different varieties of mango are found in India.

   True ☐ False ☐
10. More amphibian species in Western ghats than the Eastern ghats is an example of

    ____

*Concepts of all questions bearing * are important for NEET & CUET*

11. Consider the following statements.

Statement I There are more than 30,000 species of fishes.

Statement II India is more ecologically diverse than Scandinavian countries like Norway.

Choose the correct option from the following.

(a) Statement I is true, but statement II is false ☐

(b) Statement I is false, but statement II is true ☐

(c) Both statements I and II are true ☐

(d) Both statements I and II are false ☐

12. Ecological diversity increases with the type of ____________ diversity.

13. Scandinavian country like Norway has less coral reefs, estuaries and alpine meadows as compared to India.

True ☐ False ☐

14. Which of the following represents the correct combination?

(a) *Rauwolfia vomitoria* – Ecological diversity ☐

(b) Western ghats – Genetic diversity ☐

(c) Western ghats – Ecological diversity ☐

(d) *Rauwolfia vomitoria* – Genetic diversity ☐

***15.** Expand IUCN.

____

16. According to IUCN, the total number of plant and animal species on earth is about ____________ (1.5 million/15 billion).

17. Species inventories for many taxonomic groups are more complete in <u>tropical</u> countries. (*Rewrite the statement after correcting the underlined word.*)

____

***18.** According to Robert May, the global species diversity on earth is about ____________.

19. Based on current species inventories, more than 70% of all species recorded are plants, while animals comprise about 22% of the total.

True ☐ False ☐

20. Refer to the diagram showing global biodiversity of invertebrates and answer the questions that follow.

(i) Match the following columns with respect to above figure.

Column I (Groups of animal labels)			Column II (Examples of groups)
A.	I	1.	Molluscs
B.	II	2.	Insects
C.	III	3.	Crustaceans

A. __________ B. ____________C. ________________

(ii) According to the given pie chart, most species-rich taxonomic group is I, which make __________________ (70/90) per cent of the total diversity on earth.

21. Which of the following is the incorrect combination from the following?

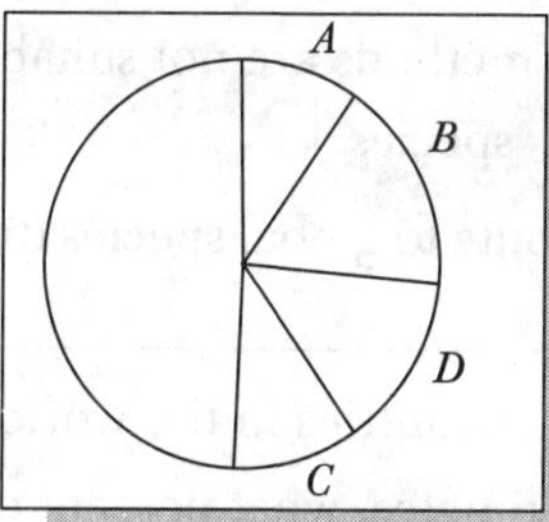

(a) *A* - Mammal, *B* - Bird ☐
(b) *B* - Bird, *D* - Reptile ☐
(c) *C* - Reptile, *D* - Amphibian ☐
(d) *B* - Bird, *C* - Amphibian ☐

22. The number of species of fishes is more than the combined total of the species of birds, amphibians, reptiles and mammals.

True ☐ False ☐

23. Consider the following statements.

Statement I Currently available species inventories show that majority of the recorded species are animals.

Statement II Among the animal kingdom, the most diverse phylum with respect to species is Insecta.

Choose the correct option from the following.

(a) Statement I is true, but statement II is false ☐
(b) Statement I is false, but statement II is true ☐
(c) Both statements I and II are true ☐
(d) Both statements I and II are false ☐

24. Refer to the diagram of global biodiversity of plants on earth and answer the questions that follow.

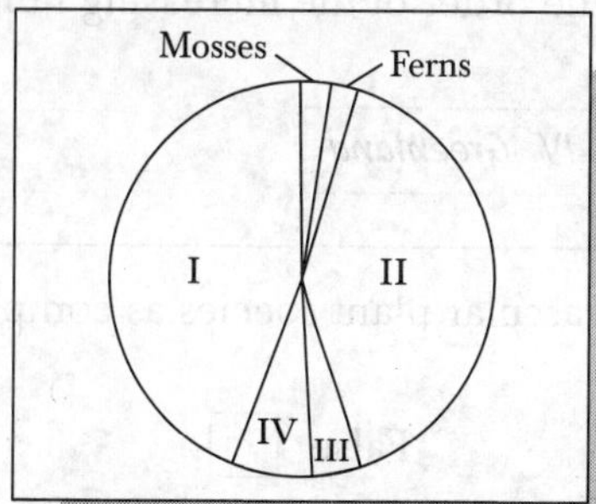

(i) Match the following columns with respect to figure shown above.

Column I (Plant groups labels)	Column II (Examples of plant group)
A. I	1. Lichens
B. II	2. Fungi
C. III	3. Algae
D. IV	4. Angiosperms

A. ______ B. ______ C. ______ D. ______

(ii) The given diagram does not give any figures for ______ (bryophytes/prokaryotes).

25. The conventional taxonomic methods are not suitable to determine the global biodiversity of ______ species.

26. What share does India contribute to global species diversity, if its world's land area is 2.4%?

______

27. The number of megadiversity countries in the world is ______

28. According to May's global estimates, what percent of total species have been recorded so far?

______

***29.** 'The species diversity decreases from the equator towards the poles'. Give the ecological term for this pattern of biodiversity. ______

***30.** The tropics latitudinal range of <u>71°N to 23°S</u> harbour more species than temperate or polar areas.
(*Rewrite the statement after correcting the underlined words.*)

______

***31.** Match the following columns.

Column I (Places)	Column II (Latitudinal gradients)
A. Colombia	1. 41°N
B. New York	2. Tropical latitudes
C. Greenland	3. Near the equator
D. India	4. 71°N

A. ______ B. ______ C. ______ D. ______

32. Arrange the following countries in the order of the increasing number of bird species found in them.

I. India, II. Colombia, III. New York, IV. Greenland

______

33. Equador forest has less number of vascular plant species as compared to the midwest forest of the USA.

True ☐ False ☐

34. Complete the following analogy with respect to regionwise biodiversity.

Forest in tropical region : ____________ :: Forest in temperate region : Midwest of the USA.

***35.** Name the tropical forest in South America which has the greatest biodiversity on earth.

____

36. Match the following columns.

Column I (Species)	Column II (Numbers in Amazonian rainforest)
A. Plants	1. 3000
B. Fishes	2. 378
C. Mammals	3. 40,000
D. Birds	4. 427
E. Reptiles	5. 1300

A.____________ B.____________ C. ____________ D. ____________

E. ____________

37. The number of species of invertebrates in Amazonian rainforest is greater than the combined number of plants and vertebrates.

True ☐ False ☐

38. Which of the following is not a contributory factor for the greater species diversity witnessed in Equador compared to the Midwest of USA?

(a) Relatively low disturbances in the tropical latitudes ☐

(b) More constant and predictable tropical environments ☐

(c) Frequent glaciation in the tropical latitudes ☐

(d) Increased sunlight and higher productivity in tropics ☐

***39.** How many of the listed factors contribute to a greater biological diversity in tropics?

Frequent glaciations, Less seasonal and more constant environment, More solar energy, Niche specialisation, Unpredictable environment, Higher productivity

____

40. Consider the following statements.

I. Constant environments promote niche specialisation and lead to a greater species diversity.

II. The diversity of plants and animals shows an uneven distribution.

III. More than 70% of the species recorded are fungi since they can be found in almost all habitats.

IV. India has more than 5000 genetically different strains of rice and 1000 varieties of mango.

V. With the importance of biodiversity recognised worldwide, the concept of biodiversity and its importance have become issues of international concern.

Identify the set of incorrect statements.

(a) I, III and V ☐ (b) II, III and IV ☐

(c) III and IV ☐ (d) IV and V ☐

***41.** Species-area relationship was proposed by the geographer ______________ during his exploration in the jungles of ______________

***42.** Refer to the graph showing species-area relationship and answer the questions that follow.

(i) Mention the correct labellings of I, II and III.

I. ______________ II. ______________ III. ______________

(ii) As per the given graph, species richness decreases with increasing explored area.

True ☐ False ☐

(iii) For how many of the listed taxa, rectangular hyperbola is obtained?

Angiosperm plants, Bryophytes, Birds, Bats, Freshwater fishes, Porifera

____

***43.** Steeper slopes of the curve plotted with species richness as a function of explored area of the entire continent of Australia indicates a Z value of

(a) 0.1 – 0.2 ☐ (b) 0.6-1.2 ☐ (c) 0.1-0.6 ☐ (d) 1.5-2 ☐

***44.** Study the following equation with respect to species-area relationship graph which becomes linear on log scale and is represented as

$\log S = \log C + Z \log A$

Identify *S*, *C* and *Z* in the equation.

____

***45.** Choose the odd one out with respect to the *Z*-value of species-area relationship.

Plants in Britain, Birds in California, Frugivorous birds in tropical forest, Molluscs in New York

____

***46.** The *Z*-value for the mammals in the tropical forest lies with a steeper line of <u>2</u>. (*Rewrite the statement after correcting the underlined word.*)

____

***47.** Find the value of log '*S*', if log *A* = 4, *Z* = 0.3 and log *C* = 0.8.

____

48. The steeper slope in species-area relationship appear when very large areas are considered.

True ☐ False ☐

TOPIC 2

Importance and Loss of Biodiversity

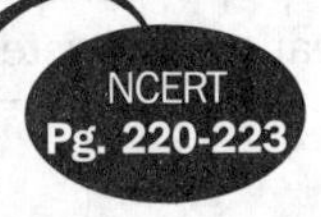

49. Ecologist believed that communities with more species tend to be more _______________ (stable/unstable) than those with less species.

50. Choose the odd one out with respect to the characteristics of a stable community.

Variable productivity, Resistance to natural and man-made disturbances, Resistance to invasion by alien species

____

***51.** According to David Tilman, higher number of species show high year to year variation in total biomass.

True ☐ False ☐

52. In the famous outdoor experiment by David Tilman, which of the following showed resilience to disturbances?

(a) Biomass ☐ (b) Productivity ☐
(c) Energy yield ☐ (d) Diversity ☐

53. 'Increased diversity contributes to higher productivity'. This statement was proposed by _______________ (David Tilman/Haeckel).

54. Name the ecologist who proposed rivet popper hypothesis._______________

55. Complete the following analogy with respect to rivet popper hypothesis.

Ecosystem : Airplane :: _______________ : Rivets.

56. Consider the following statements.

Statement I A stable community is more resilient to periodic disturbances caused by man or nature.

Statement II In the famous analogy by Paul Ehrlich, the rivets of the plane represented ecosystem.

Choose the correct option from the following.

(a) Statement I is true, but statement II is false ☐
(b) Statement I is false, but statement II is true ☐
(c) Both statements I and II are true ☐
(d) Both statements I and II are false ☐

57. According to rivet popper hypothesis, loss of rivets on the wings of airplane is comparable to the loss of _______________ in ecosystem.

58. Rivet popper hypothesis explains that the loss of species affect the proper functioning of ecosystem.

Yes ☐ No ☐

59. As per rivet popper hypothesis, loss of few rivets from which part (I or II) would not pose serious threat to ecosystem, i.e. aeroplane shown below.

II

I

____

60. The colonisation of tropical Pacific Island by humans have led to the extinction of _______ species of native _______.

61. Name the list prepared by IUCN to document the taxa facing risk of extinction.

____

62. How many species of vertebrates, invertebrates and plants have been extinct according to Red list 2004?

____

63. Match the following columns.

Column I (Recent extinctions)	Column II (Countries)
A. Dodo	1. Australia
B. Quagga	2. Mauritius
C. Thylacine	3. Russia
D. Stellar's sea cow	4. Africa

A.______ B.______ C.______ D.______

64. Bali, Javan and Caspian are three extinct subspecies of Rhinoceros.
(*Rewrite the statement after correcting the underlined word.*)

____

65. Name the group of animal which is more vulnerable to extinction.

____

66. Complete the following analogy given below.
Extinct in the wild : Survive in cultivation only : : _______________ : High risk of extinction in the wild in future

67. Arrange the following taxa in the increasing per cent of their threat to extinction.

I. Gymnosperms, II. Mammals, III. Amphibians, IV. Birds

____

68. How many episodes of mass extinction had occurred since the origin and diversification of life on earth? _______________

69. The present extinction episode is considered as the __________ extinction. It is estimated to be 100 to 1000 times __________ than in the pre human times due to __________ activities.

70. Loss of biodiversity leads to __________ in plant production, __________ resistance to environmental perturbations and __________ variability in plant productivity, water use, disease cycle, etc.

71. Give the sorbiquet used to describe the four major causes of biodiversity losses.

____

72. The most important cause of animals and plants being driven to extinction is

____

73. The Amazon rainforest is being cut and cleared for cultivating __________ or for conversion to __________ for raising __________. It leads to the degradation of large habitats into __________.

***74.** How many of the following species have become extinct due to their overexploitation by humans?

Stellar's sea cow, Nile perch, Passenger pigeon, Lantana

____

***75.** Give the common term for the following species.

Parthenium, Lantana, Eichhornia

____

***76.** Complete the analogy given below with respect to alien species invasion.

Nile perch : Cichlid fish : : __________ : Indigenous catfish

***77.** All of the following are probable reasons as to why invasive species cause extinction of native species except

(a) Competition between the invasive and local species ☐
(b) Predatory effect of the invasive species on the local ones ☐
(c) Absence of possible predator of the invasive species ☐
(d) Reduced reproductive ability of the native species ☐

78. Co-extinction results due to the facultative relationship between species.

True ☐ False ☐

79. Match the following columns.

Column I (Causes of biodiversity loss)	Column II (Examples)
A. Habitat loss and fragmentation	1. Overharvesting of marine fishes
B. Over-exploitation	2. Extinction of Cichlid fish due to Nile perch in Lake Victoria
C. Alien species invasion	3. Decreased per cent of land surface covered by tropical forest (14%-6%)
D. Co-extinction	4. Coevolution of plant and pollinator

A.__________ B.__________ C. __________ D. __________

TOPIC 3

Biodiversity Conservation

NCERT Pg. 223-225

80. Narrowly utilitarian, broadly utilitarian and ethical argument are the three categories of biodiversity __________ (pattern/conservation).

81. Choose the odd one out with respect to the type of biodiversity conservation categories.

Drugs, Food, Pollination, Medicinal plants

____

82. Give biological term for exploring molecular, genetic and species level diversity for economically important products.

____

83. Bioprospecting has identified a plant species which produces a therapeutic chemical that has promising effects on cardiovascular diseases. Based on this information alone, which of the following groups should this plant be sorted into?

(a) Narrowly utilitarian ☐ (b) Broadly utilitarian ☐
(c) Ethical ☐ (d) Both (a) and (c) ☐

84. 'The aesthetic pleasure of walking through thick woods is an example of ethical argument'.

(*Rewrite the statement after correcting the underlined words.*)

____

85. Match the following columns.

Column I (Causes of biodiversity conservation)	Column II (Importances)
A. Narrowly utilitarian	1. Ecosystem services provided by nature
B. Broadly utilitarian	2. Every species has an intrinsic value
C. Ethical argument	3. Direct economic benefits from nature

A.__________ B.__________ C.__________

86. Ethical argument of biodiversity conservation apprise to conserve every species even it has no economic value to us.

True ☐ False ☐

***87.** Complete the following analogy

On-site conservation : __________ :: Off-site conservation : *Ex situ*

***88.** Give the biological term for the species confined to particular region and not found elsewhere.

____

***89.** Choose the odd one out with respect to the characteristics of hotspots.

Low species richness, High endemism, Accelerated habitat loss, High biodiversity

____

90. The total number of hotspots in world is ______________________________

91. How many hotspots are found in India? ______________________________

92. All the listed areas are hotspots in India except one, that is

Western Ghats and Sri Lanka, Indo Burma and Himalaya, Madagascar

____

93. All biodiversity hotspots collectively cover less than ____________ per cent of earth's land area. They harbour ____________ number of species. The strict protection of hotspots can reduce ongoing ____________ by almost 30%.

94. Which of the following is not correct about *in situ* conservation?

(a) Key protection to the regions recognized as biodiversity hotspots ☐

(b) Sacred groves and national parks conserve the entire biodiversity of the place ☐

(c) Only selected species in the entire area of the national park are conserved ☐

(d) Hotspots also show a high degree of diversity and endemism ☐

***95.** What type of conservation strategy is employed in biosphere reserves and national parks?

____

***96.** Arrange the following conservation sites in the increasing order of their number in India.

I. National parks, II. Wildlife sanctuaries, III. Biosphere reserves

____

***97.** Give biological term for the protected forest patches having religious and cultural significance. ______________________________

***98.** In Meghalaya, the sacred groves are ____________ for a large number of rare and threatened plants.

***99.** Sacred groves help in *ex situ* conservation of wildlife and threatened plants.

True ☐ False ☐

***100.** Match the following columns.

Column I (Sacred groves)	Column II (Locations)
A. Khasi and Jaintia	1. Rajasthan
B. Aravalli hills	2. Karnataka and Maharashtra
C. Western ghats	3. Madhya Pradesh
D. Sarguja, Chanda and Bastar areas	4. Meghalaya

A. __________ B. __________ C. __________ D. __________

***101.** Which approach of conservation is employed when a species is endangered and need urgent measures to save it from extinction?

____

***102.** In *ex situ* conservation, threatened species are protected in their natural habitats.

True ☐ False ☐

***103.** Give any three examples of *ex situ* conservation.

____

***104.** Animals extinct in the wild are continued to be maintained in national parks.
(*Rewrite the statement after correcting the underlined word*.)

____

***105.** Name the technique used to preserve gametes of threatened species in viable condition for long periods.

____

***106.** Which of the following is not an *ex situ* conservation technique?

(a) Cryopreservation of gametes ☐
(b) *In vivo* conservation of gametes ☐
(c) Tissue culture techniques ☐
(d) Storage in seed banks ☐

***107.** For *ex situ* conservation of gametes, eggs are fertilised __________ and plants are propagated using __________ methods. Seeds of commercially important plants are kept in __________.

***108.** When was 'The Earth Summit' held to take measures for biodiversity conservation?

____

***109.** The Earth Summit was held in __________ which was the historic convention on biological diversity.

***110.** State the measures to be taken by all nations after Earth Summits.

____

***111.** The world summit on sustainable development __________ pledged to reduce the current loss of biodiversity at __________, __________ and __________ levels.

Assertion-Reason Questions

The following questions consist of two statements- Assertion (A) and Reason (R). Answer these questions by selecting the appropriate option given below.

(a) Both A and R are true and R is the correct explanation of A
(b) Both A and R are true, but R is not the correct explanation of A
(c) A is true, but R is false
(d) A is false, but R is true

1. **Assertion** (A) A high degree of species diversity is observed in *Rauwolfia vomitoria* in the Himalaya regions.
Reason (R) The diversity lies in the potency and concentration of reserpine that *Rauwolfia* produces.

(a) ☐ (b) ☐ (c) ☐ (d) ☐

2. **Assertion** (A) The estimates to the number of species as given by taxonomists do not include microbial species.
Reason (R) Most microbial species on this planet are simply not culturable under laboratory conditions.

(a) ☐ (b) ☐ (c) ☐ (d) ☐

3. **Assertion** (A) Tropics have a greater species diversity of the world than the temperate regions.
Reason (R) Tropical Amazonian rain forest in South America has the greatest biodiversity on earth.

(a) ☐ (b) ☐ (c) ☐ (d) ☐

4. **Assertion** (A) Species richness of a place increases with increase in area up to a certain limit.
Reason (R) A plot between species richness of a place and area is a rectangular parabola.

(a) ☐ (b) ☐ (c) ☐ (d) ☐

5. **Assertion** (A) The rivet popper hypothesis explains the reason for greater biodiversity in the tropics.
Reason (R) The species richness of a place contributes towards stability of the ecosystem.

(a) ☐ (b) ☐ (c) ☐ (d) ☐

6. **Assertion** (A) Fragmentation of larger habitats can cause extinction of certain migratory birds.
Reason (R) Breaking of habitats into fragments is caused by natural disasters and not humans.

(a) ☐ (b) ☐ (c) ☐ (d) ☐

7. **Assertion** (A) Extinction of one species can drive the extinction of another in a process called co-extinction.
Reason (R) Some times alien species can become invasive and wipe out the native ones of a place.

(a) ☐ (b) ☐ (c) ☐ (d) ☐

8. **Assertion** (A) The oxygen generation by the Amazon rain forests is the broadly utilitarian reason for its conservation.
Reason (R) Amazon rain forests provide the greatest ecosystem service by providing 20% of the earth's oxygen.

(a) ☐ (b) ☐ (c) ☐ (d) ☐

9. **Assertion** (A) *In situ* conservation is the preferred method for protecting endangered species.
Reason (R) It allows for the preservation of natural behaviour and adaptation within the species ecosystem.

(a) ☐ (b) ☐ (c) ☐ (d) ☐

10. **Assertion** (A) *In situ* conservation is offered to a species that needs urgent measures for protection.
Reason (R) Gametes of threatened species can be cryopreserved and plants can be propagated by tissue culture.

(a) ☐ (b) ☐ (c) ☐ (d) ☐

Case Based Questions

1. Given graph gives a clear illustration on conditions of tiger within a span of 15 years (2007-2022). Analyse the graph and answer the following questions by choosing the right answer from the options below.

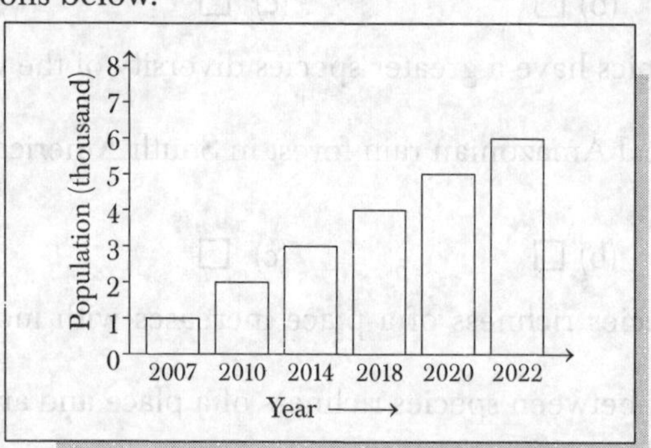

(i) What could be the possible reasons for the smallest bar obtained in 2007?

(a) Intraspecific competition ☐ (b) Hunting and poaching ☐

(c) Competitive release ☐ (d) Ageing and disease ☐

(ii) An increase in number of tigers has been observed, if we head from year 2018 to 2022. Why?

(a) Prey-predation relationship improved ☐

(b) Tigers were provided sufficient food ☐

(c) Efforts made by Government that involve conservation strategies ☐

(d) Tigers are kept in captivity to ensure protection ☐

(iii) One of the *ex situ* conservation for the above scenario is

(a) wildlife sanctuaries ☐ (b) biosphere reserves ☐

(c) cryopreservation ☐ (d) national parks ☐

2. A plant species "X" is threatened due to the human activities in the Amazon forest. This particular species is found exclusively in the tropic Amazonian rainforest and not found any where else. X is a medicinal tree that secretes certain chemicals with antimicrobial properties. The IUCN Red list gives an estimate that only the last 200 plants of this species remain in the world. Following this, they would be added to the pool of extinct species and would be lost from the earth forever. In an attempt to save them, ecologists have identified an approach that uses latest technologies to meet urgent requirements. Based on the provided information, answer the following questions.

(i) Which of the following conservation methods should be adopted by the ecologists?

(a) Sacred groves ☐ (b) National parks ☐

(c) Cryopreservation ☐ (d) Micropropagation ☐

(ii) Which of the following serves as the reason for conservation of 'X'?

(a) Broadly utilitarian ☐ (b) Ethical ☐

(c) Narrowly utilitarian ☐ (d) All of these ☐

(iii) Which of the following best defines the condition of species X?

(a) Endangered and endemic ☐ (b) Vulnerable and extinct ☐

(c) Extinct and endemic ☐ (d) Endangered and vulnerable ☐

COMPETITION EDGE UP

1. List of endangered species was released by **[NCERT, Pg. 217, NEET 2024]**

(a) GEAC ☐
(b) WWF ☐
(c) FOAM ☐
(d) IUCN ☐

2. Tropical regions show greatest level of species richness because

A. tropical latitudes have remained relatively undisturbed for millions of years, hence more time was available for species diversification.

B. topical environments are more seasonal.

C. more solar energy is available in tropics.

D. constant environments promote niche specialisation.

E. tropical environments are constant and predictable.

Choose the correct answer from the options given below. **[NCERT Pg. 219, NEET 2024]**

(a) A, C, D and E only ☐
(b) A and B only ☐
(c) A, B and E only ☐
(d) A, B and D only ☐

3. Match List I with List II.

List I	List II
A. Robert May	I. Species-area relationship
B. Alexander von Humboldt	II. Long term ecosystem experiment using outdoor plots
C. Paul Ehrlich	III. Global species diversity at about 7 million
D. David Tilman	IV. Rivet popper hypothesis

Chooose the correct answer from the options given below. **[NCERT Pg. 217, 220, 221, NEET 2024]**

(a) A-II, B-III, C-I, D-IV ☐
(b) A-III, B-I, C-IV, D-II ☐
(c) A-I, B-III, C-II, D-IV ☐
(d) A-III, B-IV, C-II, D-I ☐

4. These are regarded as major causes of biodiversity loss:

A. Overexploitation
B. Co-extinction
C. Mutation
D. Habitat loss and fragmentation
E. Migration

Choose the correct opton : **[NCERT Pg. 233, NEET 2024]**

(a) A, C, and D only ☐
(b) A, B, C and D only ☐
(c) A, B and E only ☐
(d) A, B and D only ☐

5. The type of conservation in which the threatened species are taken out from their natural habitat and placed in special setting where they can be protected and given special care is called **[NCERT Pg. 224, NEET 2024]**

(a) in situ conservation ☐
(b) biodiversity conservation ☐
(c) semi-conservative method ☐
(d) sustainable development ☐

6. Among The Evil Quartet', which one is considered the most important cause driving extinction of species? **[NCERT Pg. 222, NEET 2023]**

(a) Over exploitation for economic gain ☐
(b) Alien species invasions ☐
(c) Co-extinctions ☐
(d) Habitat loss and fragmentaton ☐

7. Habitat loss and fragmentation, over exploitation, alien-species invasion and co-extinction are causes for **[NCERT Pg. 222, NEET 2022]**

(a) competition ☐
(b) biodiversity loss ☐
(c) natality ☐
(d) population explosion ☐

8. The histotic convention on biological diversity, The Earth Summit was held in Rio de Janeiro in the year **[NCERT Pg. 225, NEET 2022]**

(a) 1992 ☐ (b) 1986 ☐
(c) 2002 ☐ (d) 1985 ☐

9. In situ conservation refers to [NCERT Pg. 225, NEET, NEET 2022]

(a) conserve only high risk species ☐
(b) conserve only endangered species ☐
(c) conserve only extinct species ☐
(d) protect and conserve the whole ecosystem ☐

10. Which of the following is not a method of ex situ conservation? [NCERT Pg. 225, NEET 2022]

(a) National Parks ☐
(b) Micropropagation ☐
(c) Cryopreservation ☐
(d) In vitro fertilisation ☐

11. Which of the following regions of the globe exhibits highest species diversity? [NCERT Pg. 222, NEET (Sep.) 2020]

(a) Madagascar ☐
(b) Himalayas ☐
(c) Amazon forests ☐
(d) Western Ghats of India ☐

12. According to Alexander von Homboldt. [NCERT Pg. 220, NEET (II) 2020]

(a) Species richness goes on increasing with increasing area of exploration ☐
(b) Species richness decreases with increasing area of exploration ☐
(c) Species richness increases with increasing area, but only up to limit ☐
(d) There is no relationship between species richness and area explored ☐

13. According to Robert May, the global species diversity is about [NCERT Pg. 217, NEET 2020]

(a) 20 million ☐
(b) 50 million ☐
(c) 7 million ☐
(d) 1.5 million ☐

14. In the following in each set a conservation approach and an example of method of conservation are given

(i) In situ conservation–Biosphere reserve
(ii) Ex situ conservation–Sacred groves
(iii) In situ conservation–Seed bank
(iv) Ex situ conservation– Cryopreservation

Select the option with correct match of approach and method. [NCERT Pg. 225, NEET (Oct.) 2020]

(a) (i) and (iii) ☐
(b) (i) and (iv) ☐
(c) (ii) and (iv) ☐
(d) (i) and (ii) ☐

15. Decline in the population of Indian native fishes due to introduction of Clarias gariepinus in river Yamuna can be categoriesd as [NCERT Pg. 223, NEET (Odisha) 2019]

(a) co-extinction ☐
(b) habitat fragmentation ☐
(c) over exploitation ☐
(d) alien species invasion ☐

16. Western Ghats have a large number of plant and animals species that are not found anywhere else. Which of the following terms will you use to notify such species? [NCERT Pg. 224, NEET 2019, Odisha]

(a) Keystone ☐ (b) Endemic ☐
(c) Vulnerable ☐ (d) Threatened ☐

NCERT
REVISION WORK BOOK

Answers

Answers

Chapter-1

Sexual Reproduction in Flowering Plants

1. True
2. *A*–Ovary, *B*–Sepal, *C*–Filament, *D*–Petal, *E*–Anther, *F*–Stigma, *G*–Style
3. Female
4. Calyx → Corolla → Androecium → Gynoecium
5. Filament
6. Anther
7. Proximal
8. False. Each lobe in a typical angiospermic anther is dithecous.
9. Four
10. Pollen sacs
11. *A*–Filament (stalk), *B*–Line of dehiscence, *C*–Pollen sacs, *D*–Pollen grain
12. Epidermis → Endothecium → Middle layer → Tapetum.
13. (i) Epidermis, endothecium and middle layer.
    (ii) Tapetum
14. Multinucleate
15. Homogeneous, sporogenous, centre
16. False. The sporogenous tissue undergoes meiotic division to form microspore tetrads.
17. *A*–Connective, *B*–Epidermis, *C*–Endothecium, *D*–Sporogenous tissue, *E*–Tapetum, *F*–Middle layer
18. *A*–Epidermis, *B*–Endothecium, *C*–Middle layers, *D*–Microspore mother cell, *E*–Tapetum
19. Pollen Mother Cell
20. Microsporogenesis
21. Microspore tetrad, pollen grains
22. (d) PMC – 2N, Microspore – N
23. A-3, B-4, C-2, D-1
24. Exine, intine
25. Sporopollenin
26. True
27. (c) Both statements I and II are true
28. (c) Cellulose and pectin
29. Hemicellulose. Rest of the options are the constituents of exine and intine.
30. Vegetative cell, generative cell
31. Vegetative
32. *A*–Pollen tetrad, *B*–Vacuoles, *C*–Nucleus, *D*–Asymmetric spindle, *E*–Vegetative cell, *F*–Generative cell
33. (b) Statement I is false, but statement II is true. Statement I can be corrected as
    The vegetative cell is bigger, has abundant food reserve and a large irregularly shaped nucleus.
34. Generative cell
35. 2-celled stage
36. True
37. *Parthenium*
38. Pollen
39. Poaceae is the odd one out. Rest of the options are the plant families which can maintain pollen viability for months whereas Poaceae members like rice, lose their pollen viability within 30 minutes of their release.
40. (b) Wheat
41. False. Pollen grains can be stored for years in liquid nitrogen at – 196°C.
42. A-2, B-3, C-4, D-1
43. Gynoecium, monocarpellary, multicarpellary
44. *A*-Multicarpellary and syncarpous
    B-Multicarpellary and apocarpous.
45. Stigma
46. (i) Ovary, (ii) style
47. *C*-Ovary
48. Stamen is odd one out as it represents male reproductive part of flower. Rest are female reproductive parts of flower.
49. True
50. Ovule
51. One
52. *A*–Hilum, *B*–Funicle, *C*–Micropyle, *D*–Micropylar pole, *E*–Outer integument, *F*–Inner integument, *G*–Nucellus, *H*–Embryo sac, *I*–Chalazal pole
53. True
54. (a) A-1, B-4, C-3, D-2
55. Embryo sac
56. Embryo sac → Nucellus → Inner integument→ Outer integument
57. (c) Both statements I and II are true
58. Megaspore Mother Cell
59. Meiotic, four, megasporogenesis
60. (a) Diploid and haploid
61. Functional, female, embryo sac, megaspore, monosporic
62. *A*–Nucellus, B–Megaspore Mother Cell (MMC), *C*–Megaspore dyad
63. (i) Meiosis-I
    (ii) Meiosis-II
64. *A*–Meiosis-I, *B*– Meiosis-II, *C*–Mitosis, *D*–Mitosis, *E*–Mitosis, *F*– Cytokinesis
65. (d) Cell wall formation occurs only after 16 nuclear stage.
66. *A*–Synergids, *B*–Egg, *C*–Central cell, *D*–2 polar nuclei, *E*–Antipodal cells
67. Polar
68. (b) I, II and III
69. Synergids, egg cell
70. Filiform apparatus
71. Chalazal
72. 2-1-1-3
73. (d) A typical angiospermic embryo sac is 7-celled and 8-nucleate with a large central cell containing two polar nuclei. The egg apparatus constituted by a group of three cells lies at the micropylar end.
74. *A*-Megaspore dyad,
    B-Megaspore,
    C-7
75. *A*–Filiform apparatus, *B*–Synergids, *C*–Egg, *D*–Central cell, *E*–Polar nuclei, *F*–Antipodal cells
76. Stigma

77. (c) Windstorm and rainpour are natural phenomenon, not considered as external pollinating agents.
78. *A*-Chasmogamous flower *B*-Cleistogamous flower
79. Always closed
80. Open flower
81. True
82. False. Geitonogamy is genetically similar to autogamy.
83. (b) Genetic variability
84. (i) Autogamy, (ii) Xenogamy, (iii) Geitonogamy.
85. Light is odd one out. Rest of the options are agents of pollination.
86. Wind pollinated pollen grains.
87. (i) Large feathery stigma (ii) Compact inflorescence.
88. Corn, wheat
89. Water pollinated
90. True
91. (c) Both statements I and II are true.
92. Mucilaginous
93. Bees
94. (i) Bees, (ii) Flies/Beetles
95. Nectar and pollen grains
96. (i) *Amorphophallus*, (ii) *Yucca*
97. (a) A-3, B-4, C-1, D-2
98. *Yucca*
99. Pollen/nectar robbers
100. Inbreeding depression
101. (i) Non-synchronisation between pollen release and stigma receptivity. (ii) Placement of anther and stigma at different positions.
102. (d) Self-incompatibility
103. (b) Maize-papaya- Dioecious
104. Papaya
105. Autogamy, geitonogamy.
106. True
107. (ii) → (iv) → (i) → (iii)
108. (b) Pollen tube after reaching the ovary, enters the ovule *via* micropyle and then enters one of the synergids through filiform apparatus.
109. *A*–Pollen grains, *B*–Pollen tube, *C*–Ovary, *D*–Ovule, *E*–Antipodal cell, *F*– Polar nuclei
110. *A*–Plasma membrane, *B*–Synergid, *C*–Filiform apparatus, *D*–Male gametes, *E*–Vegetative nucleus, *F*–Central cell, *G*–Egg nucleus
111. (b) Filiform apparatus
112. *A*–Polar nuclei, *B*–Male gametes
113. Pollen-pistil interaction
114. False. The pistil alone have the ability to recognise the compatible and incompatible pollen.
115. Post-pollination.
116. Dynamic
117. Artificial hybridisation
118. Emasculation
119. Sugar solution provides nutrition to germinating pollen.
120. Promotion
121. Emasculation → Bagging → Cross-pollination → Rebagging.
122. Two
123. False. Zygote is a diploid structure.
124. Primary Endosperm Nucleus (PEN)
125. (b) Q (Antipodal) and R (Synergids) degenerate post fetilisation.
126. Triploid
127. (i) 28, i.e. $2n$ (ii) 28, i.e. $2n$ (iii) 42, i.e. $3n$
128. 16
129. Haploid, triple
130. Double, syngamy, triple fusion
131. (a) Since there is fusion of three haploid nuclei.
132. Syngamy
133. *A*-Zygote, *B*- Primary Endosperm Nucleus (PEN), *C*-Primary Endosperm Cell (PEC)
134. Each of them have 12 number of chromosome.
135. (c) Both statements I and II are true
136. Free-nuclear endosperm
137. False. Post-fertilisation events include seed and fruit formation.
138. Endosperm, embryo
139. Free-nuclear endosperm stage
140. Cellular endosperm
141. Pea, groundnut
142. Embryology
143. *A*–2-celled stage, *B*–Globular embryo, *C*–Heart-shaped embryo, *D*–Mature embryo, *E*–Suspensor, *F*–Radicle, *G*–Cotyledon
144. False. The embryogeny is similar in both monocots and dicots.
145. Endosperm development → Proembryo → Globular embryo → Heart-shaped embryo → Mature embryo
146. *A*–Plumule, *B*–Cotyledons, *C*–Hypocotyl, *D*–Radicle, *E*–Root cap
147. Monocot, *B*–Coleoptile, *D*–Epiblast, *G*–Coleorhiza
148. Embryonal, two, epicotyl, plumule
149. Hypocotyl
150. Hypocotyl
151. Root cap
152. Scutellum
153. Coleorhiza
154. Coleoptile
155. False. Seed is a fertilised ovule.
156. Pericarp is odd one out. Rest of the options are parts of a seed. It is a part of a fruit.
157. False. Endosperm is not completely consumed during embryo development in albuminous seeds.
158. Barley, castor
159. Pea is odd one out. Rest of the plants have endospermic seeds.
160. (d) III and IV
161. Perisperm
162. (i) *A*-Seed coat
B-Endosperm
C-Cotyledon
D-Shoot apical meristem
E-Root tip
(ii) Castor (*Ricinus communis*)
(iii) *A*-Seed coat, protects the internal structures of seed.
B-Endosperm provides nutrition to the developing embryo.
163. *A*–Coleoptile, *B*–Plumules *C*–Radicle, *D*–Coleorhiza
164. Dehydrated, hard.
165. Ovary
166. A-1, B-2, C-3
167. (i) True fruits (ii) False fruits
168. Apple and strawberry
169. Parthenocarpic fruit
170. True

171. Growth hormone
172. True
173. Dehydration, dormancy
174. 2000
175. They all produce huge number of seeds.
176. *Lupinus arcticus*
177. Apomixis
178. True
179. Apomixis
180. Polyembryony
181. Orange, mango
182. Nucellar cells.
183. Apple is odd one out. Rest of the options are polyembryonic fruits.
184. Increased
185. Hybrid
186. False. There is no segregation of characters in the hybrid progeny when the hybrids are made into apomicts.
187. (a) Apomixis

Assertion-Reason Questions

1. (a) Both A and R are true and R is the correct explanation of A.
2. (b) Both A and R are true, but R is not the correct explanation of A.
   Pollen grain exine has prominent apertures called germ pores where sporopollenin is absent to facilitate the growth of pollen tube when pollen grain germinates on a receptive stigma.
3. (a) Both A and R are true and R is the correct explanation of A.
4. (d) A is false, but R is true. A can be corrected as
   Cell wall is laid down after the 8-nucleate stage, to form a functional embryo sac.
5. (b) Both A and R are true, but R is not the correct explanation of A.
   The chance of genetic variability is poor in cleistogamous flowers because these flowers do not open at all. The anthers and stigma remain close to one another to support autogamy as there is no chance of cross pollination.
6. (a) Both A and R are true and R is the correct explanation of A
7. (d) A is false, but R is true. A can be corrected as
   Castor plants are monoecious and can prevent autogamy but not geitonogamy.
8. (c) A is true, but R is false. R can be corrected as
   Chemical interactions between the pollen and the pistil leads to pollen acceptance.
9. (c) A is true, but R is false. R can be corrected as
   Bagging ensures that the flower is protected against unwanted pollen contamination.
10. (a) Both A and R are true and R is the correct explanation of A.
11. (b) Both A and R are true, but R is not the correct explanation of A.
    Post-fertilisation, micropyle persists as a small pore in the seed coat to allow the entry of water and gases into the seed.
12. (d) A is false but R is true. A can be corrected as
    Parthenocarpy results in the formation of seedless varieties of fruits.

Case Based Questions

1. (i) (b), (ii) (c), (iii) (d), (iv) (a)
2. (i) (b), (ii) (d), (iii) (c)

Competition Edge Up

1. (d)	2. (a)	3. (a)	4. (b)
5. (d)	6. (b)	7. (c)	8. (b)
9. (a)	10. (d)	11. (b)	12. (d)

Chapter-2

Human Reproduction

1. (b) Pelvis; ovum
2. Scrotum
3. Scrotum
4. (i) 4-5 cm, (ii) 2-3 cm
   (iii) 250, (iv) 1-3
5. Spermatogonia
6. Sertoli cells
7. Interstitial or Leydig cells
8. Androgens
9. Spermatogonia
10. True
11. False. Vasa efferentia open into epididymis along the posterior of each testis.
12. (a) Option (a) represents the incorrect pair as Leydig cells secrete androgens.
13. (c) C-Vas deferens helps in sperm transfer
14. Rete testis, vas deferens, urethral meatus
15. Urethra
16. Seminal vesicle is an accessory gland.
17. *A*–Sertoli cells, *B*–Spermatogonia, *C*–Interstitial cells, *D*–Spermatozoa
18. (c) Provides nutrition to germ cells
19. Foreskin
20. True
21. Seminiferous tubule is odd one out. Rest are parts of male sex accessory ducts.
22. (a) Secretions of the bulbourethral gland help in lubrication of the penis.
23. True
24. Ligaments
25. (i) Are the primary female sex organs.
26. *A*–Uterus, *B*–Urinary bladder, *C*–Urethra, *D*–Cervix, *E*–Vagina
27. Female accessory ducts
28. *A*-Endometrium
    C-Perimetrium
29. (d) The fimbriae collects the ovum after its release from the ovary.
    Fusion of the male and female gametes take place in the ampulla.
30. (i) Fimbriae, (ii) Isthmus, (iii) Cervix
31. (b) P-Uterine contraction; Q-Site of fertilisation.
32. Pubic symphysis is the odd one out. Rest are the structures of female external genitalia.
33. (b) Labia majora surrounding the vagina extends from the mons pubis.
34. Hymen

35. (d) Option (d) is incorrect pair because myometrium exhibits strong contractions during delivery.
36. False. The presence or absence of hymen is not a reliable indicatior of virginity or sexual experience.
37. I-Vas deferens, II-Ejaculatory duct, III-Bulbourethral gland, IV-Cervical canal
38. Glandular
39. *A*–Fat, *B*–Mammary duct, *C*–Lactiferous duct, *D*–Areola
40. (a) Alveoli-mammary tubules-mammary duct-mammary ampulla-lactiferous duct.
41. A-1, B-3, C-4, D-2
42. (c) Testis, ovaries, gametogenesis.
43. Puberty
44. 46
45. Spermatogonia
46. Meiosis
47. 23
48. Secondary spermatocyte
49. Seminiferous tubules
50. (c) P-Secondary spermatocyte, spermiogenesis
51. *A* - Spermatocyte
B - Sperms
52. True
53. Luteinizing Hormone (LH) and Follicle Stimulating Hormone (FSH).
54. *A*-Mitosis and differentiation
B-1st meiotic division
C-2nd meiotic division
D-Differentiation
55. (c) Both statements I and II are true.
56. Follicle Stimulating Hormone (FSH)
57. LH and androgens
58. (a) The hypothalamus plays an important role in the development of spermatozoa from spermatocyte as it releases GnRH which acts at the anterior pituitary gland and stimulates serections of two gonadotrophins, luteinizing hormone and follicle stimulating hormone.
59. Acrosome
60. True
61. (a) A-3, B-2, C-4, D-1
62. 40, 60
63. Incorrect labellings are *B*-Acrosome, *C*-Nucleeus containing chromosomal material, *D*-Middle piece
64. Maturation and motility of sperms.
65. (d) Option (d) is incorrect pair because semen contains sperms, seminal fluid, secretions of prostate glands, etc.
66. True
67. Prophase-I, primary
68. True
69. (d) During foetal stage, primary oocyte gets arrested in prophase-I of meiosis.
Primary oocyte develops into secondary oocyte by completing meiosis-I.
70. *A*-Tertiary follicles showing antrum.
B-Graafian follicle
C-Ovum
D-Corpus luteum
71. Granulosa cells, secondary follicles.
72. (d) Tertiary follicle
73. (i) Haploid,
(ii) Haploid,
(iii) Diploid
74. Ovum, polar bodies
75. True
76. Cowper's gland is odd one out. Rest are structures related to oogenesis.
77. Graafian follicle
78. Zona pellucida
79. Graafian follicle
80. Secondary oocyte.
81. (b) X – meiosis; Z – 46
82. Acrosome is odd one out. Rest are structures related to female reproductive system.
83. True
84. (d) Secondary oocyte-haploid.
85. (b) 3
86. (a) Antrum is fluid filled cavity in primary follicle.
87. True
88. *A* - Secondary follicle
B - Secondary oocyte
89. A-3, B-1, C-2, D-4
90. Menarche
91. 28 / 29
92. Middle of cycle, i.e. 14th -16th day
93. True
94. Endometrium proliferation
95. Growing follicles
96. (d) Maintenance of endometrial lining.
97. (c) Both statements I and II are true.
98. Progesterone
99. Follicles do not remain in the ovary after ovulation.
100. Corpus luteum will degenerate. Oestrogen secretion further decreases.
101. (a) Option (a) is an incorrect match because during proliferative phase, Graafian follicle is formed in ovary.
102. FSH, oestrogen, progesterone
103. *A*-FSH, *B*-Oestrogen, *C*-LH, *D*-Progesterone
104. I→ III→ V→ IV→ II
105. A-4, B-2, C-1, D-3
106. A-Menses, B-Ovulation
107. (b) Peristence of corpus luteum.
108. Insemination, ampullary - isthmic junction, fertilisation
109. True
110. Zona pellucida
111. Acrosome
112. True
113. (b) Completion of meiosis II allows a secondary oocyte to form ootid and second polar body.
114. Fallopian tube
115. True
116. Blastomeres
117. Morula
118. (c) Mitosis
119. Trophoblast, inner cell mass
120. Endometrium
121. (i) *A*–Zona pellucida, *B*–Perivitelline space, *C*–Corona radiata
(ii) Embryo
122. *A*-Morula , *B*-Blastocyst
123. *A*-Blastomere
B-Trophoblast
C-Inner cell mass
D-Implantation
124. Chorionic villi

125. Placenta

126. False. Placenta is connected to the embryo through umbilical cord.

127. (c) A

128. hCG, hPL, Oestrogen

129. Relaxin

130. human Chorionic Gonadotropin (hCG).

131. Prolactin is odd one out. Rest are the hormones produced by placenta.

132. False. Urine test determines the presence of Human Chorionic Gonadotropin (hCG).

133. Ectoderm, mesoderm, endoderm

134. Stem

135. First

136. Fifth

137. (c) External genital organs by the end of 26 weeks

138. (b) Successful implantation but pregnancy does not cover complete term.

139. Parturition

140. Neuroendocrine

141. Parturition, placenta, foetal ejection reflex

142. Maternal pituitary

143. Oxytocin

144. True

145. A-3, B-4, C-1, D-2

146. False

147. Gametogenesis → Fertilisation → Implantation → Parturition → Lactation

148. (b) II, III and IV

Assertion-Reason Questions

1. (d) A is false, but R is true. A can be corrected as
The Leydig cells are present in the interstitial spaces outside the seminiferous tubules.

2. (c) A is true, but R is false. R can be corrected as
Each alveoli open into mammary tubules which fuse to form mammary ducts that open into ampulla.

3. (c) A is true, but R is false. R can be corrected as
In spermiogenesis spermatids are transformed into spermatozoa by the action of FSH.

4. (a) Both A and R are true and R is the correct explanation of A.

5. (a) Both A and R are true and R is the correct explanation of A.

6. (d) A is false, but R is true. A can be corrected as
Fertilisation takes place in the ampulla ary isthmus region of the Fallopian tube of the female reproductive system.

7. (c) A is true, but R is false. R can be corrected as
The trophoblast attaches to the endometrium and gets embedded into the uterus.

8. (b) Both A and R are true, but R is not the correct explanation of A.
Placenta is formed by interdigitation of chorionic villi and uterine tissue as the villi are projections of the trophoblast layer embedded in the uterus.

9. (c) A is true, but R is false. R can be corrected as
During delivery of baby, the myometrium undergoes strong contractions to expel the baby.

10. (a) Both A and R are true and R is the correct explanation of A.

Case Based Questions

1. (i) (c) (ii) (c) (iii) (c)

2. (i) (b) (ii) (b) (iii) (d)

Competition Edge Up

1. (a) **2.** (d) **3.** (c) **4.** (c)
5. (d) **6.** (d) **7.** (b) **8.** (b)
9. (c) **10.** (a) **11.** (d) **12.** (b)
13. (d)

Chapter-3

Reproductive Health

1. True

2. (ii) In a reproductively healthy society, people do not have functionally anomalous reproductive organs.

3. First

4. True

5. Adolescent

6. Reproductive, infrastructural

7. Amniocentesis

8. Amniotic; survivability of foetus.

9. (c) Determination of the sex of the child.

10. (a) In order to determine birth defects of foetus, some of the amniotic fluid of the developing foetus is taken to analyse the fetal cells and dissolved substances.

11. True

12. (i) Reproductive and Child Healthcare
(ii) Central Drug Research Institute

13. 7.2 billion

14. 20

15. (i) Maternal Mortality Rate
(ii) Infant Mortality Rate

16. *A*-Maternal Mortality Rate (MMR)
B-Infant Mortality Rate (IMR)

17. Increase in healthcare facilities, increase in birth rate, decrease in death rate.

18. False. Decreasing the birth rate is the main goal to control population.

19. True

20. 18, 21

21. Contraception

22. (i) Easy availability
(ii) Least or no side effect

23. True

24. Periodic abstinence

25. True

26. Abstains, 10-17, menstrual, ovulation

27. Insemination

28. True

29. Lactational amenorrhea

30. Ovulation

31. True

32. Six

33. (b) Withdrawal or coitus interruptus has a higher rate of preventing pregnancy. However, it does not provide any protection against sexually transmitted infections.

34. Sperm, ova

35. Condom

36. Nirodh

37. STDs, AIDS

38. Reusable is odd one out. Rest of the options are the advantages of using condom as contraceptive.

39. True

40. (b) Blocks the entry of sperms into cervix

41. Diaphragms, cervical caps, vaults
42. False. Spermicidal creams increaser contraceptive efficiency
43. Intra Uterine Device
44. IUDs
45. (ii) is incorrect because progestasert is hormone releasing IUD.
46. Copper-releasing IUDs
47. Phagocytosis
48. Suppress
49. False. IUDs make uterus unsuitable for implantation.
50. (c) Cu-7-decrease fertilising capacity is the correct match.
51. A-2, B-4, C-1, D-3
52. Progestogens, progestogen oestrogen
53. 21 days
54. Ovulation, sperms
55. Lesser, females
56. (c) Both statements I and II are true.
57. True
58. (b) Inhibiting ovulation and implantation.
59. FSH , LH
60. 72
61. (c) Both statements I and II are true.
62. Copper T is odd one out. Rest two are surgical methods of sterilisation.
63. Vasectomy
64. (d) A (Vas deferens)
65. True
66. *A*–Condom, *B*–Copper-T (Cu-T), *C*–Implant, *D*–Vasectomy
67. Process is tubectomy and the structure involved is Fallopian tube.
68. (i) Uterus
69. False. Reversiblity is poor for sterilisation techniques.
70. Fever is odd one out. Rest of the options are mild side effects of using contraceptives.
71. (b) I, II and IV
72. Voluntary
73. (i) 45-50 million, (ii) 12 weeks, (iii) 1971, (iv) 2017, (v) Two
74. (a) Amniocentesis shows the developing foetus to be a future girl child.
75. MTP performed by unqualified quacks, which are unsafe.
76. True
77. Sexually Transmitted Diseases (STDs)
78. Venereal Diseases (VDs) or Reproductive Tract Infection (RTI) or Sexually Transmitted Infection (STI).
79. Amoebiasis is odd one out. Rest of the options are STDs.
80. (b) Sharing food with infected person.
81. Curable STDs.
82. (c) 3
83. True
84. 15-24 years age group
85. (d) Except for Hepatitis-B, genital herpes and HIV infections, other STDs are completely curable if detected early and treated properly.
STIs when not treated on time, can lead to complications like pelvic inflammatory diseases or cancer in a person.
86. *A* - Unknown/Multiple
B - Condoms
87. False. Early detection of STIs are given prime importance.
88. Ecotopic pregnancy and abortion.
89. Infertility
90. Assisted Reproductive Technologies (ARTs)
91. False. IVF stands for *In vitro* fertilisation.
92. Fallopian tube, Zygote Intra Fallopian Transfer (ZIFT)
93. (c) *In-vivo* fertilisation
94. ZIFT, IUT
95. PID or Pelvic Inflammatory Disease is the odd one out. Rest of the options are assisted reproductive technologies.
96. Gamete Intra Fallopian Transfer
97. Intra Cytoplasmic Sperm Injection (ICSI)
98. (d) ICSI
99. Vagina or uterus
100. (c) Both statements I and II are true.
101. A-2, B-1, C-4, D-3
102. True

Assertion-Reason Questions

1. (a) Both A and R are true and R is the correct explanation of A.
2. (a) Both A and R are true and R is the correct explanation of A.
3. (a) Both A and R are true and R is the correct explanation of A.
4. (d) A is false, but R is true. A can be corrected as
Intra-Uterine Devices (IUDs) are inserted by doctors and expert nurses into the uterus through the vagina in women trying to space children.
5. (a) Both A and R are true and R is the correct explanation of A.
6. (d) A is false, but R is true. A can be corrected as
A couple who wants to delay pregnancy can use IUDs but not sterilisation processes as the latter is a permanent method of contraception.
7. (a) Both A and R are true, but R is the correct explanation of A.
8. (b) Both A and R are true and R is not the correct explanation of A.
A female infected with STI like gonorrhoea remains undiagnosed for a long time since most infected females are asymptomatic. Absence or less significant symptoms in the early stages of infection keeps the females undiagnosed at early stages of infection.
9. (b) Both A and R are true, but R is not the correct explanation of A.
In vitro fertilisation is often followed by transfer of zygote or embryo into the female tract, where embryos develop and get embedded into the uterus and develops into a foetus.
10. (b) Both A and R are true, but R is not the correct explanation of A.
Females with their male partners having low sperm count generally opt for artificial insemination as the process delivers sperms directly to cervix or uterus to achieve effective pregnancy.

Case Based Questions

1. (i) (a) (ii) (d) (iii) (c)
2. (i) (c) (ii) (b) (iii) (a)

Competition Edge Up

1. (d) 2. (d) 3. (c) 4. (a)
5. (a) 6. (b) 7. (a)

Chapter-4

Principles of Inheritance and Variation

1. (i) Hybridisation
   (ii) Two
2. True
3. False. Mendel selected 14 true breeding characters
4. 2 (rounded seed and yellow coloured seed).
5. (i) (b) Seed size
   (ii) (a) Dominant trait
6. Green coloured pod was dominant. Terminal and constricted pods were recessive traits and tall plant was dominant trait.
7. F_2-generation
8. (i) 3 : 1
   (ii) Dominant
9. By self-pollinating F_1-generation
10. I–Emasculation, II–Pollination
11. Genes
12. (i) Alleles
    (ii) First filial (F_1) generation
    (iii) Heterozygotes
13. Genotype
14. (c) Option (c) is an incorrect match because in homozygous condition identical alleles of a gene are present at the same locus.
15. (a) Statement I is true, but statement II is false.
    Statement II can be corrected as For monohybrid crosses F_2 progenies show a genotypic ratio of 1 : 2 : 1.
16. True
17. (i) Punnett square
    (ii) Test cross
18. (b) tt
19. (c) 25%
20. (i) Test cross
    (ii) Flower is heterozygous
21. (b) In a true breeding variety allelic pair of genes are always heterozygous.
22. (c) Both statements I and II are true.
23. (b) bb
24. True
25. Law of dominance
26. Seed colour
27. (b) Alleles of a pair seggregate from each other during gametogenesis.
28. Law of segregation (Second law)
29. Bb × Bb.
30. Law of purity of gametes/Law of segregation
31. Law of dominance and segregation
32. Genotype-Rr and Phenotype-pink
33. Incomplete dominance
34. *A* - Pink Rr flowers
    B - 1 : 2 : 1 (Red : Pink : White)
    C - 1 : 2 : 1 (RR : Rr : rr)
35. (c) Incomplete dominance
36. Recessive
37. Zero. Red colour flowers are homozygous dominant (RR) and they cannot appear in the given cross.
38. (c) Both statements I and II are true.
39. (i), Selfing of TtRr would give 25% red flower, 25% white flower and 50% pink flower.
40. Red : Pink = 1 : 1
41. Codominance
42. 1:2:1
43. A -2, B -3, C -1.
44. I-gene
45. Two
46. I^A and I^B, i
47. (a) 1/2
48. (i) Codominance
    (ii) O
49. i or I^A, AB, O
50. (b) The human blood group is an example of multiple allelism controlled by three alleles.
51. True
52. Starch synthesis in pea seeds.
53. True
54. 3 each, as it is an example of typical dihybrid cross which yield 9 round yellow, 3 round green, 3 wrinkled yellow and 1 wrinkled green seeds.
55. Yes
56. (d) rr
57. Law of independent assortment.
58. RY, Ry, rY, ry
59. 2
60. Only round seeds with yellow colour.
61. 12
62. (d) In a dihybrid cross alleles of the two genes segregate independently.
    The F_2-generation of a dihybrid cross shows sixteen different genotypes and four phenotypes.
63. 3 : 1
64. A-2, B-3, C-1
65. No
66. 1865, 1900
67. Reginald C Punnett is odd one out. He was not involved in the rediscovery of Mendel's results on the inheritance of characters.
68. Walter Sutton and Theodore Boveri.
69. Homologous
70. (a) Law of independent assortment
71. Chromosomal theory of inheritance.
72. True
73. *Drosophila melanogaster*
74. 3 (*Drosophila* is not a hermaphrodite).
75. X-chromosome
76. (b) Only
77. A-1, B-3, C-2.
78. Linkage
79. Single chromosome
80. A-White eyed and yellow bodied.
81. Alfred Sturtevant
82. False. Distance between genes is inversely proportional to the strength of linkage between them.

83. The order of the linkage map will be P-Q-R.

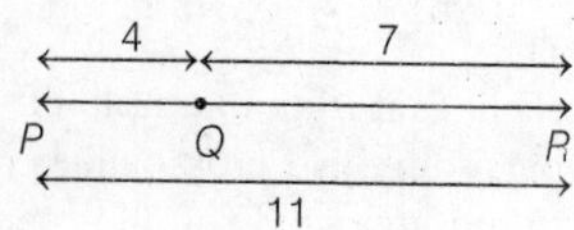

84. AABB × aabb is odd one out as it is the only suitable cross for experiment on linkage as it requires homozygous dominant and homozygous recessive parents. Other crosses are not suitable for this purpose.
85. (d) Only A
86. A-2, B-1, C-4, D-3
87. Three or more genes
88. Option (i) is correct. The polygenic traits are influenced by environment in which effect of each allele is additive.
89. Darkest and lightest
90. True
91. Phenotype reflecting contribution of each allele.
92. Pleiotropic gene
93. Pleiotropy
94. Option (ii) is correct. Phenylketonuria is characterised by mental retardation, hair reduction and skin pigmentation.
95. (c) Option (c) is an incorrect match because starch synthesis in pea shows pleiotropism.
96. A-2, B-3, C-4, D-1
97. Spermatogenesis
98. Allosomes (sex chromosome), autosomes
99. (a) Grasshopper
100. Option (iii) is an incorrect pair because male *Drosophila* is heterogametic.
101. False. Male grasshopper contains 23 and female grasshopper. contains 24 chromosomes.
102. True
103. *C*. In birds, males are homogametic, whereas females are heterogametic.
104. True
105. A–Male, B–Female.
106. A-2, B-1, C-4, D-3.
107. ZW is odd one out as it is the genotype of female bird whereas the rest two are male genotypes in insects *Drosophila* (XY) and grasshopper (XO).
108. 44+XY, 44+XX
109. 22 pairs, i.e. autosomes.
110. Spermatogenesis
111. 50%
112. Males are heterogametic.
113. (b) X-Meiosis; Y-16
114. 32 and 16, respectively.
115. Males
116. Mitosis and meiosis
117. True
118. Mutation
119. Point
120. Point mutation
121. Frameshift mutations
122. Pedigree analysis
123. Standard symbols
124. 2 Affected individuals are represented by shaded-shapes.
125. *B*

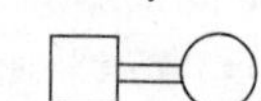

126. False. Male = □, Female = ○.
127. A-4, B-3, C-2, D-1
128. False. Pedigree analysis is employed to study Mendelian disorders.
129. Mendelian disorders
130. Single
131. Sickle-cell anaemia.
132. One and two, respectively
133. *A*-aa, *B*-Aa, *C*-Aa
134. False. Mendelian disorders may be dominant or recessive.
135. Colour blindness is odd one out, as it is a sex-linked trait whereas the other three are autosomal linked trait.
136. Autosomal-recessive trait.
137. Recessive
138. Both (i) and (ii).
139. True
140. Colour blindness.
141. All carrier daughters and normal sons.

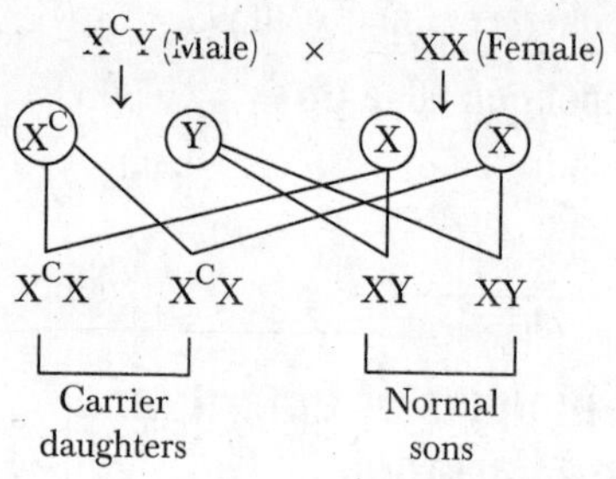

142. 50%. Hint : Workout the cross between X^CY (colourblind father) and X^CX (carrier mother).
143. Carrier, haemophilic
144. (i) $Hb^A\ Hb^S$, (ii) $Hb^S\ Hb^S$
145. Valine
146. (a) From glutamate to valine; GAG to GUG
147. Elongated
148. Phenylalanine, tyrosine
149. Phenylpyruvic acid
150. (i) Mental retardation (ii) Skin pigmentation.
151. (c) Mental retardation
152. Both carrier parents.
153. *A*–16, *B*–11, *C*–HBA1, *D*–HBA2, *E*–HBB
154. Either α or β- chain of Hb.
155. (b) Linked gene, mutation
156. Chromosomal disorder
157. Polyploidy
158. Aneuploidy
159. Turner's syndrome is odd one out as it is an example of monosomy whereas the other two represents trisomy.
160. Down's syndrome
161. (a) 46A + XY
162. Trisomy of 21
163. 47 chromosomes
164. Klinefelter's syndrome
165. Gynaecomastia, sterile individual
166. 44 +XO
167. A-4, B-3, C-2, D-1
168. *A*–Klinefelter's syndrome B–Turner's syndrome

Assertion-Reason Questions

1. (a) Both A and R are true and R is the correct explanation of A.
2. (b) Both A and R are true, but R is not the correct explanation of A. In a monohybrid cross the F_1 progenies are heterozygous for genes controlling a single character as the F_1 progenies inherit one dominant allele from one of the parent and another recessive allele from the other parent.
3. (c) A is true, but R is false. R can be corrected as
In a test cross, the organism showing dominant phenotype is crossed with the recessive parent.
4. (d) A is false, but R is true. A can be corrected as
The F_2 phenotypic ratio for a monohybrid cross in snapdragon is 1:2:1 while that in Mendelian monohybrid cross is 3:1.
5. (d) A is false, but R is true. A can be corrected as
A couple with blood group A and B can have a child with blood group O if the parents are heterozygous for A and B alleles respectively.
6. (d) A is false, but R is true. A can be corrected as
Chromosomal segregation coincided with the segregation of the genes that controlled specific characters.
7. (b) Both A and R are true, but R is not the correct explanation of A.
The recombination frequency can be used to calculate the distance between genes as distant genes have a greater chances of recombination than closely linked genes on the same chromosome.
8. (b) Both A and R are true, but R is not the correct explanation of A.
A person with all dominant alleles for skin colour will have the darkest skin colour as the human skin colour is a polygenic trait where darker skin colour is dominant over lighter skin colour.
9. (a) Both A and R are true and R is the correct explanation of A.
10. (c) A is true, but R is false. R can be corrected as
β-thalassemia is controlled by a single gene HBB on chromosome 11 of each parent whereas sickle cell anaemia is controlled by a single pair of allele.

Case Based Questions

1. (i) (d) (ii) (d) (iii) (a)
2. (i) (d) (ii) (c) (iii) (a)

Competition Edge UP

1. (b)	2. (b)	3. (a)	4. (c)
5. (c)	6. (b)	7. (b)	8. (d)
9. (b)	10. (c)	11. (c)	12. (b)
13. (b)			

Chapter-5

Molecular Basis of Inheritance

1. Genetic material
2. Deoxyribonucleic acids
3. (i) DNA, (ii) RNA
4. False. RNA mostly functions as a messenger in most living organisms.
5. A-4, B-3, C-2, D-1
6. Deoxyribonucleotides
7. A nucleotide is a sugar molecule bounded to phosphate group(s) and a heterocyclic base.
8. 3 (pentose sugar, nitrogenous bases and a phosphate group).
9. Adenine and guanine.
10. False. Cytosine is common for both DNA and RNA and uracil and not thymine is present in RNA.
11. Thymine
12. (a) is ribose, thus it is present in RNA, (b) is deoxyribose sugar present in DNA.
13. The correct pair among these is pyrimidine-uridine, cytidine.
14. (d) Nitrogenous base attached to pentose sugar.
15. 5'– OH, Phosphodiester
16. (a) Nitrogenous base linked to OH at 1'C sugar.
17. (d) X–Phosphodiester bond. Y–N-glycosidic bond
18. (i) True, (ii) True
19. Sugar and phosphates
20. Hydroxyl group (–OH)
21. Hydrogen bonds
22. A-2, B-1, C-4, D-3
23. is constant and equal to 1.
24. According to the Chargaff's rule, A = T and G = C, hence, the d G + C content is 30%.
So, A + T = 70 %
Thus, percentage of thymine is 35 %.
25. True
26. Identical
27. Antiparallel polarity.
28. 3'-A T G G C T G G T 5'
29. *A*–Hydrogen bonds, *B*–Purine base, *C*–Pentose (deoxyribose) sugar, *D*–5' end, *E*–Pyrimidine
30. In a *ds* DNA, adenine always forms two hydrogen bonds with thymine from opposite strand and guanine forms three hydrogen bonds with cytosine and *vice-versa*, which places a purine opposite to pyrimidine base.
31. *A*–3.4 nm, *B*–0.34 nm
32. Right
33. Pitch of the helix.
34. (c) 510 nm
35. True
36. Watson and Crick
37. The genetic information flows from (ii) DNA → (iii) RNA → (i) Protein.
38. *A*–Replication, *B*–Transcription, *C*–Translation
39. This large length of DNA is packaged inside the nucleus by undergoing compaction.
40. False. In prokaryotes, the DNA is not scattered throughout the cell, but held with some proteins around central region.
41. Nucleoid
42. (d) RNA
43. (i) *A*–DNA , *B*–H1 histone, *C*–Histone octamer
(ii) Nucleosome
44. Beads on a string.
45. Net positive
46. These are basic amino acids present in histone proteins.
47. (i) Histone octamer
(ii) Chromatin
48. Chromatin

49. Beads on string, electron microscope

50. (a) Negative phosphate of DNA and positive arginine of protein.

51. *A*–Repeating units of chromatin, *B*–Additional proteins in packaging of chromatin, *C*–Loosely packed and stains light, *D*–Heterochromatin

52. Heterochromatin

53. Transforming principle

54. *Streptococcus pneumoniae*

55. This indicates that the S-strain of this bacterium has a mucous (polysaccharide) coat.

56. (i) *A*–Mice die, *B*–Mice live

(ii) The S-strain is virulent. As a result the mice died from pneumonia, but mice infected with R–strain did not develop pneumonia so the mice lived.

57. In this case, the mice lives because the S-strain has lost its virulence due to heat.

58. *X* – The mice die

59. True

60. (a) Heat killed S-strain + Heat killed R-strain

61. Genetic material

62. Oswald Avery, Colin MacLeod and Maclyn McCarty.

63. Nucleic acid

64. RNases

65. (a) The process of transformation was affected by the enzyme DNase which proved DNA as the genetic material.

66. Bacteriophage

67. Sulphur and phosphorus

68. (i) *A*–Infection by phage, *B*–Blending, *C*–Centrifugation to separate the virus particles.

(ii) Radioactivity will be detected in ^{32}P labelled DNA cells.

(iii) It was concluded that DNA and not protein is the genetic material.

69. (c) In the supernatant.

70. A-3, B -1, C-4, D-2

71. RNA

72. Replication

73. Both DNA and RNA

74. (i) False. Chemically and structurally stable nucleic acid is DNA.

(ii) True

75. RNA

76. 2'-OH, reactive, labile

77. Thymine

78. (i) Viruses having RNA genome and shorter lifespan can mutate and evolve at a faster rate.

79. Transmission of genetic information.

80. (b) RNA can be translated directly.

81. Metabolism is the odd one. The other are specific process related to gene expression or modification.

82. (c) Statements I, II and IV are correct.

83. Semiconservative replication

84. (i) True

(ii) Watson and Crick

(iii) Separation, complementary, template.

85. *Escherichia coli*

86. Matthew Meselson and Franklin Stahl.

87. (i) The figure represents Meselson and Stahl's experiment demonstrating semiconservative replication of DNA.

(ii) At *A*, *E. coli* cells are grown in medium containing heavy isotope of nitrogen.

(iii) CsCl gradient.

88. 75%

89. (b) 1 : 1

90. Radioactive thymidine

91. *d*NTPs (Deoxyribonucleoside triphosphates)

92. Their efficiency indicates the rate of polymerisation of a large number of nucleotides in a very short time.

93. 4.6×10^6 bp, 18 minutes.

94. 2000 bp per sceond.

95. A mistake during replication would result in mutations.

96. Terminal phosphates

97. Replication fork

98. False. DNA replication begins at a specific site called origin of replication (*ori*) in DNA.

99. Discontinuous

100. *A*–Continuous strand, *B*–Discountinuous strand

101. (b) 5'–3', template dependent

102. DNA ligase

103. This is because the vectors provide the origin of replication essential for their propagation within the host genome.

104. S-phase

105. This condition of failure in cell division after DNA replication is called polyploidy.

106. Transcription

107. Uracil

108. False. In transcription, only a segment of DNA and only one of the strands is copied into RNA.

109. Different sequences

110. Formation of double-stranded RNA would prevent RNA from being translated into proteins, thus the exercise of transcription becomes futile.

111. False. Transcription occurs unidirectionally in 5'- 3' direction.

112. 3 (Promoter, structural gene and terminator).

113. Coding strand

114. RNA sequence will be 3' UAA - GGG - CCG - CGU - ACG - UAC - GUA - CGU 5'

115. *A*–Promoter, *B*–Terminator, *C*–Template strand, D–Coding strand.

116. (i) Promoter is located upstream of the structural gene.

(ii) Terminator is located downstream of the structural gene.

117. Promoter

118. Terminator

119. Gene

120. Cistron

121. Eukaryotes

122. Genes in the eukaryotes are sptit means that genes have interrupted coding sequences.

123. Exons

124. Exons

125. (d) I and III

126. (b) *m*RNA – Primary transcript from DNA

127. *r*RNA

128. RNA polymerase

129. Promoter region

130. Single

131. False. RNA polymerase does not require primer and lacks the ability to repair mistakes in RNA.

132. The correct sequence will be (c) chain initiation, (a) chain elongation and (b) chain termination.

133. Sigma factor

134. Ribonucleotide triphosphates

135. (b) Association with these factor alter specificity for RNA polymerase.

136. (d) Promotor–sigma factor; Terminator–rho factor

137. (c) Both statements I and II are true.

138. Cytoplasm

139. (ii) The *m*RNA in bacteria does not require any processing to become active, also transcription and translation take place in the same compartment.

140. (i) RNA polymerase-I
(ii) RNA polymerase-III
(iii) RNA polymerase-II

141. An additional complexity present in eukaryotic transcription is that the primary transcripts contain both the exons and the introns which make it non-functional.

142. Transformation is odd one out. Rest others are post-transcriptional modifications undergone by primary transcripts.

143. False. Introns are excised and hydrolysed during post-transcriptional processing.

144. Capping and Tailing. Addition of a methyl guanosine triphosphate to 5' end, cleavage and polyadenylation to create 3'end.

145. (i) Transcription in eukaryotes
(ii) Primary transcript
(iii) Splicing
(iv) Capping, adenylate, polyadenylation

146. False. The fully processed *hn*RNA is called *m*RNA which is transported out from the nucleus.

147. Genetic code

148. *A*–Proposed that genetic code is a triplet, *B*–Har Gobind Khorana, *C*–Cell free system for protein synthesis, *D*–Severo Ochoa.

149. (i) Triplet
(ii) Universal
(iii) Commaless/Contiguous
(iv) Degenerate

150. True

151. UAA/UAG/UGA

152. GUG is the odd one out because it codes for an amino acid. Rest others are termination codons.

153. Last

154. (a) Degenerate

155. Termination, non-sense

156. Amino acid coded by the given sequence will be Met, Leu, Phe, Lys, Cys, Gly, Leu.

157. The *m*RNA chain that can be translated completely is, AUG UAU UUC UGC CUC UAG.

158. CCA is odd one out as it codes for amino acid proline. Rest others are codes for leucine.

159. GGC, GGA and GGG.

160. Mutation

161. True

162. (ii) An almost completely altered sequence.

163. Change in reading frame of triplet codon

164. Point

165. Beta globin, valine

166. DNA - CAC/GTG, RNA - GUG, Amino acid - valine

167. A common result of insertion and deletion processes is change in the reading frame.

168. Francis Crick

169. False. *t*RNA is an adapter molecule.

170. (i) There was a need of an adapter molecule because amino acids cannot read the code.
(ii) A = 5', B = Anticodon, C = Codon

171. (b) I and III are incorrect.

172. Translation

173. False. The order and sequence of amino acids are defined by the sequence of bases in the *m*RNA.

174. *m*RNA

175. (i) Translation, (ii) *A*–Leucine and *B*–Serine.

176. (b) Activation of amino acid in the presence of ATP.

177. 'X' is charging of *t*RNA or aminoacylation of *t*RNA.

178. 40S and 60S

179. Ribozyme

180. Untranslated region

181. False. The UTRs are required for efficient translation.

182. 7 (Initiation factors, elongation factors, GTPase, *m*RNA, *t*RNA, aminoacyl *t*RNA synthetase, amino acids).

183. The correct sequence is as follows Activation of amino acids, Initiation, Elongation/ Chain formation, Termination and Modifications.

184. (b) Ribosomal subunits by binds to *m*RNAs and holds them in a way that allows formation by joining of amino acids.

185. *A*–Initiator *t*RNA, *B*–Amino acid-*t* RNA, complexes binds sequentially to *m*RNA codons *C*–Sequential translation of amino acids into polypeptide sequence, *D*–Binding of release factors.

186. (d) Replication level.

187. Beta-galactosidase

188. (ii) If bacteria do not have lactose around them to be utilised for energy source, they would no longer require the enzyme beta-galactosidase, since it hydrolyses lactose.

189. True

190. RNA, accessory

191. Polycistronic

192. A-2, B-3, C-1.

193. Operon

194. (c) Both statements I and II are true.

195. (c) Constitutive

196. (c) The i gene would be switched off and no repressor would be made.

197. True

198. (i) Off

(ii) False. X is Repressor

(iii) *X* or repressor binds to operator and prevents RNA polymerase from transcribing the operon.

(iv) Jacob, Monod

199. (i) False. Lactose is present in the medium.

(ii) Promoter gene

(iii) Operator gene

(iv) Regulatory gene

200. *A*-*i* gene, *B* - RNA polymerase gets access to the promoter and transcription proceeds.

201. True

202. Negative

203. True

204. Isolation and cloning of any piece of DNA and determining DNA sequences.

205. Human Genome Project

206. 1990

207. HGP was called a mega project because of its large magnitude and requirements as it involved sequencing storage, retrival and analysis of each and every base pair in the human genome.

208. 3 billion

209. 9 billion US dollars

210. False. HGP was closely associated with bioinformatics.

211. 20,000-25,000 genes

212. False. The information was stored in databases.

213. 13

214. The US Department of Energy and the National Institute of Health.

215. Improving manpower for data analysis was not an objective of HGP.

216. 6 (Bacteria, yeast, *Caenorhabditis elegans, Drosophila,* rice, *Arabidopsis*).

217. Expressed sequence tags and sequence annotation.

218. Sequence annotation.

219. (d) Digest the DNA into fragments.

220. *A*–Cloning in a suitable host using specialised vectors, *B*–PCR, *C*–Fragments were sequenced using automated DNA sequencers, *D*–Alignment of these sequences.

221. Bacteria and yeast

222. Chromosome 1

223. (ii) On polymorphism of restriction endonuclease recognition sites and satellite DNA.

224. Dystrophin

225. Less than 2%

226. (c) Both statements I and II are correct.

227. Y-chromosome

228. Single Nucleotide Polymorphisms

229. False 99.9 per cent of base saquence among humans is the same.

230. Repetitive

231. DNA fingerprinting

232. Satellite DNA that have repeating short stretches of DNA with high degree of polymorphism.

233. (d) Number of base pair in *m*RNA.

234. (i) DNA fingerprinting is the basis of paternity testing in case of disputes because satellite DNA that contributes to polymorphisms are inheritable from parents to children.

235. Polymorphisms

236. True

237. Germ cells

238. DNA polymorphism

239. Alec Jeffreys

240. Variable Number of Tandem Repeat

241. Minisatellites

242. The steps in sequence are (iv) $\rightarrow$ (ii) $\rightarrow$ (i) $\rightarrow$ (iii) $\rightarrow$ (v) $\rightarrow$ (vi)

243. Restriction endonuclease

244. False. The size of VNTR varies in size from 0.1 to 20kb

245. (d) B is the criminal.

246. Monozygotic twins

247. Polymerase Chain Reaction (PCR)

248. Suspect *A* because his DNA does not match the DNA found at the crime scene.

Assertion-Reason Questions

1. (a) Both A and R are true and R is the correct explanation of A.

2. (c) Negatively charged phosphate backbone of DNA is attracted by the positively charged histone proteins.

3. (b) In Griffith's experiment, heat killed S strain could transform the living R strain bacteria, because the genetic material from S strain was responsible for virulence and transformed the living R strain bacteria.

4. (d) DNA can be used for stably storing the genetic information of an organism while RNA is used for information transmission.

5. (a) Both A and R are true and R is the correct explanation of A.

6. (d) The 3' $\rightarrow$ 5' template strand is synthesised in a continuous manner during replication.

7. (c) The DNA strand with polarity 5' $\rightarrow$ 3' acts as the coding strand during transcription.

8. (a) Both A and R are true and R is the correct explanation of A.

9. (b) RNA polymerase-II cannot catalyse all three steps of a transcription process as it requires initiation factor and termination factor for initiation and termination of transcription.

10. (b) Inserting 2 bases in a reading frame would result in frame shift mutation because a codon is made up of three nucleotides and hence adding two bases would shift the reading frame from the point of insertion.

11. (c) Lactose binds with the repressor protein thus preventing it from binding it to the operator. In the absence of operator, RNA polymerase can transcribe the genes.

12. (b) VNTRs used during DNA finger printing shows high degree of polymorphism because these non-coding repetitive DNA sequences can accumulate huge degrees of mutation without affecting the individuals reproductive ability.

Case Based Questions

1. (i) (c) (ii) (b) (iii) (c)
2. (i) (b) (ii) (c) (iii) (b)

Competition Edge Up

1. (d) **2.** (a) **3.** (d) **4.** (b)
5. (c) **6.** (d) **7.** (b) **8.** (b)
9. (d) **10.** (a) **11.** (c)

Chapter-6

Evolution

1. Evolutionary biology.
2. True
3. Light years
4. Million
5. A-3, B-1, C-2
6. Big-Bang theory
7. II → III → I → V → IV
8. True
9. False. There was no atmosphere on the early earth.
10. (d) Oxygen
11. *A*-UV rays, *B*-Oxygen, *C*-Methane.
12. Oceans, ozone
13. Theory of spontaneous generation.
14. Pre-existing, non-living, organic molecules.
15. (b) Chemical evolution states that complex organic molecules arose from inorganic ones.
16. Chemical
17. False. According to Oparin and Haldane, chemical evolution occurred before the biological evolution on earth.
18. 3 (All of them except low temperature). Early earth had high temperature instead of low temperature.
19. SL Miller
20. (b) Only II
21. (i) Methane (CH_4), ammonia (NH_3), hydrogen (H_2).
(ii) 800°C
(iii) Amino acids
(iv) Sugar, nitrogen bases, pigments and fats.
22. Meteorites
23. 3 billion, RNA, protein or polysaccharide
24. 2000
25. Single cells
26. False. All life forms are believed to have originated in water environment only.
27. Abiogenesis
28. (a) A-1, B-3, C-4, D-2
29. Option (ii) is incorrect because according to theory of special creations, earth is about 4000 years old.
30. HMS Beagle
31. 4 (All of them except no variations in a population) Darwin observed built in variations in populations which enable them to survive in natural conditions.
32. (c) Both statements I and II are true.
33. True
34. Natural selection
35. (d) Variations occurs due to random mutation in a population.
36. Alfred Wallace, common, different
37. False. The geological history of earth closely correlates with the biological history of earth.
38. Fossils
39. Sedimentary rocks
40. Lower sediments
41. Paleontological evidences
42. Radioactive dating method.
43. Geological period
44. (d) They can tell about genetic composition of extinct animal.
45. (i) *A-Brachiosaurus*
B-Stegosaurus
C-Pteranodon
(ii) No. The diagram shows both extinct dinosaurs and their living modern day counterparts like crocodiles and birds.
(iii) Birds and crocodiles.
46. (a) *Pterandon*
47. Ernst Haeckel
48. Karl Ernst von Baer
49. (b) According to Haeckel, certain features during embryonic stage common to all vertebrates are absent in adult.
50. True
51. (c) Homologous organs and Divergent evolution.
52. Homologous structures
53. Divergent evolution
54. Analogy
55. Anatomically similar is odd one out, as analogous structures are not similar anatomically.
56. 3 (All of them except brain of frog and cat). Brain of frog and cat is an example of homologous structures.
57. (a) Forelimbs of bats and humans are homologous and show divergent evolution.
58. Potato (stem modification) and sweet potato (root modification)
59. Similar habitats
60. Common, structural
61. Natural selection
62. (i) Diagram *A*, i.e. before industrialisation.
(ii) Light coloured background represents lichens growing on tree trunks.
(iii) Light-winged moths
(iv) Dark, camouflage
(v) Dark-winged (melanised) moths.
63. (b) Natural selection
64. Selection of resistant varieties due to the excessive use of herbicides or pesticides.
65. False. Evolution by anthropogenic actions usually occurs in much lesser time scale of months or years.
66. (b) III and IV
67. Stochastic, mutation
68. Galapagos islands
69. Altered beaks
70. Seed-eater
71. False. The original seed eating ancestor finches of Galapagos island gave rise to insectivorous and vegetarian finches.
72. Adaptive radiation
73. Australian marsupials
74. Divergent evolution
75. Convergent, isolated
76. (i) Placental mammals

(ii) Australian marsupials
(iii) Convergent

77. (d) Bobcat and Tasmanian wolf

78. Natural selection

79. Only one (ii), i.e. population *B* is better than *A*.

80. Fitness

81. Branching descent and natural selection

82. II $\rightarrow$ III $\rightarrow$ I

83. A-3, B-1, C-2

84. (b) Longer necks provided competitive advantage over other organisms.

85. 5 (All of them except abundant resources). Darwin did not considered abundant resources, rather he said that resources remain limited inspite of rapid multiplication of individuals.

86. Survival of the fittest or natural selection

87. True

88. Hugo de Vries, evening primrose

89. Heritable variations causes evolution

90. Random and directionless

91. Saltation

92. (c) Saltation theory

93. Hardy-Weinberg principle

94. False. According to Hardy-Weinberg principle, the allele frequency in a population remains stable and constant from generation to generation.

95. Gene pool

96. One

97. $(p+q)^2$

98. *A* - Percentage of homozygous dominant individuals.
B - Frequency of recessive allele
C - Percentage of heterozygous individuals.

99. $A = AA + \frac{1}{2}Aa$

$= 0.5 + \frac{1}{2}(0.25) = 0.625$

$a = 1 - A = 0.375$

100. Frequency of heterozygotes $= 2pq$
$= 2 \times 0.6 \times 0.4 = 0.48$

101. (b) 50%

102. Evolutionary changes

103. (d) Asexual reproduction

104. True

105. A and B

106. (c) Only I

107. A-4, B-3, C-2, D-1

108. Founder effect

109. Speciation

110. Natural selection

111. 4 (All of them)

112. (i) *A*–Stabilising
B–Directional
C–Disruptive
(ii) True
(iii) Selective pressure under changing environment.

113. (d) Disruptive change – individual acquire peripheral end value.

114. 2000 million years ago (mya)

115. Oxygen, light, water

116. III $\rightarrow$ II $\rightarrow$ I
(500 mya) (350 mya) (320 mya)

117. (i) Plants
(ii) Coelacanth
(iii) Lobefins
(iv) Turtles, tortoises and crocodiles

118. A-3, B-1, C-2

119. (i) I-Tracheophytes ancestors, II-Psilophyton
(ii) Position IV
(iii) Gnetales
(iv) Angiosperms

120. (c) *Zosterophyllum*-Silurian

121. 65 mya

122. False. The first mammals were like shrews.

123. Small, reptiles

124. Continental drift

125. (i) I-Sauropsids, II-Synapsids
(ii) Position IV.
(iii) First amphibians

126. Dolphins, whale, sea cows.

127. Competition

128. *Dryopithecus*

129. Tanzania, Eastern Africa, 3-4

130. In Java, 1891

131. Africa

132. (a) A-1, B-3, C-2, D-4

133. A-3, B-1, C-2

134. (i) II-Baby chimpanzee, III-Adult chimpanzee
(ii) I, i.e. adult human has cranial capacity 1450 cc, whereas it is about 350-450 cc in chimpanzee.

135. True

136. *A*-Hairy and walked like gorilla and chimpanzees, *B*-500 cc, *C*-650-800 cc, *D*-Ate meat, used stone and bone tools, *E*-1400 cc

137. *A-Ramapithecus*, *B-Homo habilis*, *C-Homo sapiens neanderthalensis*

Assertion-Reason Questions

1. (d) A is false, but R is true. A can be corrected as
Biogenesis is thought to have preceded by chemical evolution.

2. (b) Both A and R are true but R is not the correct explanation of A.
Paleontological evidences gives an idea about the geological time scale during which an organism existed as different-aged rock sediment contain fossils of different life-forms who probably died during the formation of the particular sediment

3. (d) A is false, but R is true. A can be corrected as
Flippers of dolphins and penguins have different structural anatomy but serve the same function.

4. (a) Both A and R are true and R is the correct explanation of A.

5. (c) A is true, but R is false. R can be corrected as
More than one adaptive radiation in a geography, is indicative of convergent evolution.

6. (b) Both A and R are true, but R is not the correct explanation of A.
Evolution of a new species depends on the reproductive fitness of organisms and their adaptive ability because only reproductively fit organisms that have greater survival advantage will get selected by nature.

7. (a) Both A and R are true and R is the correct explanation of A.

8. (c) A is true, but R is false. R can be corrected as
Pouched mammals survived better because of lack of competition.

9. (d) A is false, but R is true. A can be corrected as
Ramapithecus was more man-like while *Dryopithecus* was more ape-like.

10. (c) A is true, but R is false. R can be corrected as
In the evolutionary stages, it was found that Neanderthal man had highest brain capacity.

Case Based Questions

1. (i) (c) (ii) (d) (iii) (c)
2. (i) (d) (ii) (b) (iii) (a)

Competition Edge Up

1. (c) 2. (d) 3. (d) 4. (d) 5. (a)
6. (a) 7. (a) 8. (d) 9. (a) 10. (a)

Chapter-7

Human Health and Disease

1. Health
2. 4 (Yoga, balanced diet vaccination, hygienic food and water).
3. *A* – Congenital disease,
B – Infectious disease,
C – Non-contagious,
D – Cancer
4. Infectious
5. Pathogens
6. True
7. *Salmonella typhi*
8. (i) Small intestine, loss of appetite, intestinal perforation, Widal
(ii) Mary Mallon
9. (a) Food and water
10. (i) *Streptococcus pneumoniae* and *Haemophilus influenzae*
(ii) Alveoli of the lungs.
(iii) Bluish lips and nails, fever, cough and headache.
(iv) By inhaling droplets/aerosols released by infected person, sharing utensils and other articles with infected person.
11. Rhinoviruses
12. Lung fibrosis is odd one out, as rhinoviruses infect nose and respiratory passage, but not the lungs.
13. (b) Rhino virus infection spreads from the nose to respiratory passage, but not to the lungs.
14. Corona virus
15. Malaria
16. *Plasmodium falciparum*
17. Female *Anopheles* mosquito
18. (i) False. Only asexual life cycle of *Plasmodium* occurs in human whereas the sexual cycle occurs in *Anopheles* mosquito.
(ii) True
19. Sporozoites
20. (b) Release of haemozoin by bursting of RBC's in human.
21. Sporozoites, asexually
22. Haemozoin (toxin)
23. Stomach
24. *A* - Salivary glands of mosquito,
B - Sporozoites
25. *Entamoeba histolytica*
26. Intestinal
27. Muscular pain, anaemia, blockage of intestinal passage. (any two)
28. (d) *Entamoeba* infects the large intestine of a person and causes abdominal pain.
Female mosquitoes act as the vector of disease like elephantiasis or filariasis.
29. (i) Filariasis or elephantiasis
(ii) *Wuchereria bancrofti and W. malayi*
(iii) Bite by female mosquito vectors
30. 3 (All of them) These fungi are collectively called dermatophytes.
31. (d) *Haemophilus influenzae*
32. Hot and moist.
33. A is incorrect. Diseases like typhoid, amoebiasis, ascariasis can be prevented by consumption of clean water and food.
34. (a) A-2, B-4, C-3, D-1
35. (i) Dengue
(ii) Smallpox
36. (a) Stagnant water is the primary site for breeding of mosquito and spread of diseases.
37. True
38. (c) Amoebiasis and diabetes
39. Immunity
40. Innate immunity
41. True
42. Mucus coating is odd one out, as it is physical barrier. Rest three form physiological barriers.
43. (c) Physiological
44. Polymorpho-nuclear leukocytes
45. Cellular
46. Interferons
47. Cytokine barrier
48. A - 4, B - 1, C - 2, D - 3
49. Acquired
50. False. An attack by a pathogen for the first time produces low intensity primary response.
51. Secondary response
52. (i) *A* - Heavy chain, *B* - Light chain, *C* - Antigen binding site.
(ii) Antibody molecule
(iii) B - lymphocytes
53. H_2L_2
54. Antigens or immunogens.
55. *A*–Humoral immune response
B–Cell-mediated immune response
56. Cell-mediated
57. 3 (All of them).
58. (b) T-lymphocytes of cell-mediated immunity is actively involved in antibody production.
59. Active immunity.
60. False. Active immunity can be generated in response to living or dead pathogen, proteins, etc.
61. Immunisation, vaccination
62. Readymade antibodies
63. TAB vaccine is odd one out, as it provides active immunity whereas the rest two provide passive immunity.
64. IgG
65. IgA
66. Generate memory cells
67. True
68. Passive
69. (d) When a baby sucks mother's milk during lactation.
70. Antigenic polypeptides of pathogen
71. (d) I, III and IV
72. Allergy
73. Pollen and mites.
74. *A*- IgE antibody, *B*- Histamine and serotonin
75. True
76. Auto-immune disease
77. Primary lymphoid organs
78. (i) Primary, (ii) Thymus
79. (d) Bone marrow – only site for maturation of B and T lymphocytes.

80. (b) The bone marrow is the main lymphoid organ where all blood cells, including lymphocytes are produced.

81. (i) *A* - Thymus, *B* - Lymph nodes, *C* - Lymphatic vessels.
(ii) *B*, as it is secondary lymphoid structure.
(iii) *A*, as it is primary lymphoid structure.

82. A - 2, B - 3, C - 4, D - 1.

83. (i) Mucosa-Associated Lymphoid Tissue (MALT), 50
(ii) Spleen, phagocytes.

84. False. AIDS is acquired during the lifetime of an individual.

85. Deficiency, syndrome, 1981.

86. Human Immunodeficiency Virus (HIV)

87. Retrovirus

88. Enveloped RNA

89. Sharing articles with infected person is odd one out, as it does not spread AIDS, while the other listed modes can spread/transmit AIDS through body fluids.

90. (i) *A*–Normal cell infected by retrovirus , *B* –Viral DNA is produced by reverse transcriptase.
(ii) *X*-Reverse transcriptase
(iii) Macrophages
(iv) *C*–Host DNA, *D*–Viral RNA is produced by infected cell.
(v) False. Infected cell can survive even after the replication and release of virus from them.

91. (d) X – integration of DNA into host cell, Y – reverse transcriptase

92. Macrophages

93. Helper T-lymphocytes.

94. Helper T-lymphocytes decreases.

95. Enzyme Linked Immuno-Sorbent Assay (ELISA).

96. (i) National AIDS Control Organisation.
(ii) Non-Governmental Organisation.

97. 3 (All of them except isolation of AIDS infected person, it is not a preventive measure for AIDS).

98. Cancer

99. Contact inhibition, tumors

100. *A*-Benign tumor

101. Malignant tumor

102. (b) By depriving the normal cell off nutrients.

103. UV rays is odd one out, as these are non-ionising carcinogenic radiations, while the other two are ionising carcinogenic radiations.

104. Chemical

105. Oncogenic viruses

106. Biological

107. Proto oncogenes or cellular oncogenes.

108. (a) α-interferons

109. Leukemia

110. A-3, B-1, C-2, D-4

111. (c) I and IV

112. True

113. Radiotherapy

114. Chemotherapy

115. Alpha (α) - interferons

116. Drugs

117. Opioids, cannabinoids, coca alkaloids.

118. False. Majority of drugs are obtained from flowering plants and some from fungi.

119. Gastrointestinal tract

120. Heroin

121. (b) Chemical name of heroin is diactylmorphine.

122. (ii) represents the correct structure of morphine.

123. (i) Opium poppy or *Papaver somniferum.*
(ii) Morphine
(iii) Latex of the plant

124. Oraroute is odd one out, as heroin is not taken in this manner.

125. True

126. Brain

127. Cannabinoids are obtained from inflorescence, flower tops, leaves and resin of the plant *Cannabis sativa.*

128. Cannabinoids

129. *A* - Hydroxyl (OH) group

130. *Cannabis sativa,* cardiovascular

131. *Erythroxylum coca*

132. Dopamine, stimulates

133. (i) *Datura*
(ii) Hallucinogenic
(iii) *Atropa belladonna* and *Erythroxylum* (in excess).

134. (c) Coke – *Atropa belladonna*

135. A-3, B-1, C-2

136. (c) Hashish

137. Cannabinoids

138. (i) Nicotine
(ii) Adrenaline, nor-adrenaline
(iii) Carbon monoxide (CO)

139. Excitement

140. Mental illness

141. Addiction

142. Dependency

143. (c) Increased blood sugar level.

144. Euphoria is odd one out, as it is a sense of happiness and is associated with drug/alcohol consumption.

145. Cirrhosis

146. False. Anabolic steroids are misused by sports persons. In females, these drugs cause abnormal menstrual cycle, facial hair growth, etc.

147. Intravenous

148. True

149. 3 (All of them except exerting peer pressure). One should avoid undue peer pressure to refrain from drug and alcohol abuse.

150. Yes

Assertion Reason Questions

1. (d) A is false, but R is true. A can be corrected as
Common cold, is a highly contagious infectious disease caused by Rhinovirus.

2. (b) Both A and R are true, but R is not the correct explanation of A.
Gametocytes of *Plasmodium* develops in the red blood cells of the human host as the parasite uses two hosts for completing its lifecycle. This will be followed by fertilisation of the gametocytes in the mosquito gut.

3. (d) A is false, but R is true. A can be corrected as
Amoebiasis is caused by protozoan which enters the large intestine of human.

4. (c) A is true but R is false. R can be corrected as
Wuchereria lives in the lymphatic vessels of lower limbs causing chronic inflammation.
5. (a) Both A and R are true and R is the correct explanation of A.
6. (c) A is true, but R is false. R can be corrected as
T-cell of the body distinguish between self and non-self, and are associated with graft rejection.
7. (d) A is false, but R is true. A can be corrected as
Injecting weakened polio virus into a person to develop resistance against the disease is a form of active immunity.
8. (b) Both A and R are true, but R is not the correct explanation of A.
Lymphocytes formed in the bone marrow migrate to the thymus for their maturation as they are the primary lymphoid organs and provide micro-environments for the development of lymphocytes.
9. (a) Both A and R are true and R is the correct explanation of A.
10. (a) Both A and R are true and R is the correct explanation of A.

Case Based Questions

1. (i) (c) (ii) (b) (iii) (d)
2. (i) (a) (ii) (c) (iii) (a) (iv) (c)

Competition Edge Up

1. (a) **2.** (a) **3.** (b) **4.** (d) **5.** (d)
6. (d) **7.** (b) **8.** (c) **9.** (a) **10.** (b)
11. (a) **12.** (a) **13.** (c) **14.** (c)

Chapter-8

Microbes in Human Welfare

1. Bacteria (Microbes)
2. False. The microbes grown on nutritive media to form colonies can be seen with naked eyes.
3. Bacteria, fungi
4. *A*–Rod-shaped bacteria
B–Spherical-shaped bacteria
5. *B* is odd one out, as it is a rod-shaped bacterium showing flagella whereas the rest three are viruses, *A* is Bacteriophage, *C* is Adenovirus and *D* is Tobacco Mosaic Virus.
6. Tobacco mosaic virus
7. Adenovirus
8. Lactic Acid Bacteria
9. Lactic acid
10. Vitamin–B_{12}
11. CO_2 gas, fermentation
12. Toddy
13. (c) *Propionibacterium*
14. A-3, B-1, C-4, D-2
15. False. The particular flavour of Roquefort cheese is imported by a fungi.
16. Fermentors
17. Beer and Whisky
18. Ethanol
19. Wine is odd one out, as it is produced without distillation whereas the other three are produced by the distillation of fermented broth.
20. (d) Whisky and rum.
21. Antibiotics
22. (c) I, II, III, V, VI
23. Fungi
24. (c) Improper/Over use of antibiotics can render advance protection from microorganisms.
25. A-2, B-4, C-1, D-3
26. Cyclosporin-A
27. (c) Both statement I and statement II are true.
28. Yeast, *Monascus purpureus*
29. False. Statins are widely used as cholesterol lowering agents.
30. (a) A-1, B-3, C-4, D-2.
31. Organic matter and microbes.
32. Sewage Treatment Plant
33. Heterotrophic
34. Biological
35. Sequential filtration, sedimentation
36. Primary sludge
37. True
38. Flocs
39. Aeration, aerobic
40. 2 (Flocs and activated sludge). Primary sludge and grit are found in primary sewage treatment.
41. Biochemical Oxygen Demand
42. Oxygen, oxidised, reduced
43. (b) By measuring the BOD
44. Organic matter.
45. Polluted
46. Activated sludge
47. III $\rightarrow$ I $\rightarrow$ IV $\rightarrow$ II
48. False. Digestion of activated sludge by anaerobic bacteria in anaerobic sludge digester forms biogas.
49. Natural water body
50. (b) A-2, B-3, C-4, D-1
51. (b) II $\rightarrow$ I $\rightarrow$ IV $\rightarrow$ III
52. Ganga Action Plan and Yamuna Action Plan
53. Hydrogen sulphide
54. Growth and metabolism, organic substrate, CO_2, methane.
55. Methanogens, e.g. *Methanobacterium.*
56. (d) Methanogens are found in rumen of cattle and in the anaerobic sludge during sewage treatment. These are anaerobic bacteria that can break down cellulosic material.
57. Human stomach is odd one out as methanogens are not found in it while the rest three contain methanogens.
58. Gobar gas
59. Biowaste
60. *A*–Dung + Water
B–Gas holder
C–Sludge
61. (d) Fungal colonies, Egg shells
62. Fertiliser
63. (d) Biogas plants pose a threat to increasing pollution in the area due to the release of CO_2.
64. Indian Agricultural Research Institute
65. Khadi and Village Industries Commission
66. Biogas
67. Biocontrol
68. Conventional farming
69. True
70. (a) Increase in N_2 fixing capacity of plant.
71. 4 (All of them)
72. A-3, B-1, C-5, D-2, E-4
73. (b) Eradicating a pest completely is possible but not desirable as it will adversely affect the predator related to the pest by decreasing its number.
74. *Brassica* and fruit trees, toxins, *Bt* genes.

75. False. *Trichoderma* species are free-living in the roots of plants
76. (c) Biological control of plant pathogens.
77. Broad spectrum insecticide is the odd one out as baculoviruses are narrow spectrum insecticides.
78. Integrated Pest Management
79. (c) A-3, B-2, C-4, D-1
80. Biofertilisers
81. Penicillin is odd one out, as it is an antibiotic while the rest three are the main sources of biofertilisers.
82. *Azotobacter*
83. (c) Both statements I and II are true.
84. Mycorrhiza
85. False. Members of genus–*Glomus* forms mycorrhiza.
86. Phosphorus
87. Yes
88. Autotrophic
89. (b) *Rhizobium*
90. Paddy field
91. (d) IV and V

Assertion-Reason Questions

1. (a) Both A and R are true and R is the correct explanation of A.
2. (c) A is true, but R is false R can be corrected as
The ripening of roquefort cheese is carried out by growing a specific fungi.
3. (d) A is false, but R is true. A can be corrected as
Wine and beer are produced by fermentation of grape juice without distillation whereas whisky, rum and brandy are produced by distilliation.
4. (d) A is false, but R is true.
A can be corrected as
Antibiotics are produced by both bacteria and fungi and can kill or retard the growth of certain bacteria.
5. (b) Both A and R are true, but R is not the correct explanation of A. Streptokinase is used to treat people who have undergone myocardial infarction as it can remove blood clots from blood vessels.
6. (c) A is true, but R is false. R can be corrected as
The BOD of the waste water decreases upon action of the aerobic bacteria in secondary treatment.
7. (a) Both A and R are true and R is correct explanation of A.
8. (a) Both A and R are true and R is the correct explanation of A.
9. (a) Both A and R are true and R is correct explanation of A.
10. (b) Both A and R are true, but R is not the correct explanation of A. Fungal symbionts of mycorrhiza derive phosphorus from the soil and supplies it to the plants as they form symbiotic associations with certain higher plants.

Case Based Questions

1. (i) (c) (ii) (b) (iii) (a)
2. (i) (c) (ii) (c) (iii) (b)

Competition Edge Up

1. (c) 2. (d) 3. (a) 4. (a)
5. (d) 6. (a) 7. (c)

Chapter-9

Biotechnology : Principles and Processes

1. Biotechnology
2. 3(IVF, gene therapy, novel gene synthesis).
3. European Federation of Biotechnology
4. True
5. (i) Sterilisation
(ii) Bioprocess
6. False. Sexual reproductive mechanism provides, opportunities for variations and new genetic combinations.
7. (a) DNA with a piece of foreign DNA.
8. True
9. (i) Genetic engineering
(ii) Gene cloning
10. (i) When an alien DNA becomes a part of the host's genome, it multiples and gets inherited along with the host's DNA.
11. *ori* (origin of replication)
12. Initiating sequence for replication
13. (c) Origin of replication
14. Plasmid
15. *Salmonella typhi*
16. Stanley Cohen and Herbert Boyer, antibiotic resistance, plasmid
17. Initiates replication
18. False. The linking of antibiotic resistance gene with plasmid is done using DNA ligase.
19. Vectors
20. DNA ligase
21. False. The bacterium used is *E.coli* which is similar to *Salmonella.* It uses host's DNA polymerase enzyme.
22. Identified
23. *E. coli*
24. (c) II → I → IV → III
25. 5 (restriction enzymes, host cells, polymerase, vectors and ligases).
26. False. Restriction enzymes are cleavage enzymes.
27. *Hind* II
28. 900
29. Restriction endonuclease enzyme system
30. False. While naming restriction enzymes the first letter of the name comes from genus of host organisms.
31. (d) *Hind* II always makes a cut in DNA sequence after recognising a specific sequence of 6 bp.
32. (c) *Escherichia coli* RY 13
33. Phosphodiester
34. True
35. False. Enzymes that remove nucleotide one at a time from ends of DNA molecules are restriction enzymes.
36. (c) Each of the two strands of double helical DNA, by identifying a specific recognition site.
37. Species
38. Order
39. Restriction sites
40. Remove nucleotide from ends.
41. True
42. (ii) Each restriction endonuclease functions by inspecting the length of a DNA sequence.

43. (b) 5′ GGATCC 3′
3′ GGTACC 5′

44. Sugar-phosphate

45. 5′ → 3′

46. (i) *A*–*Eco* RI, *B*–Vector DNA
C–DNA ligase
(ii) Sticky ends

46. Both (i) and (ii) are palindromic sequences, i.e. they read same when read in 5′ - 3′ direction on both strands.

47. Both are palindromic sequences.

48. (b) *Eco*RI

49. *A*–Restriction endonuclease
B–Ligases join foreign DNA to plasmid
C–Transformation of host cell with *r*DNA

50. (c) It generates the same sticky ends which make ligation easier.

51. 3′ –OH and 5′-phosphate

52. Sticky, hydrogen

53. Sticky ends, DNA ligase.

54. (i) Restriction endonucleases are used in genetic engineering processes to form 'recombinant' molecules of DNA, composed of DNA from different sources.

55. Same

56. DNA ligase

57. Transformation

58. No. A recombinant molecule is formed only when source DNA and the vectors are cut by same restriction enzymes.

59. (i) Restriction enzymes after recognising their specific restriction sites bind to it and make a cut generating fragments of varying lengths.

60. Gel electrophoresis

61. False. DNA is negatively charged molecule.

62. (i) Agarose gel electrophoresis for separation of restriction enzyme digested DNA.
(ii) At *A*- Large size DNA fragments. At *B* - Smallest DNA fragments.

63. (d) larger size

64. Anode (+ve end)

65. Agarose

66. True

67. Ethidium bromide

68. (d) Staining the bands with ethidium bromide followed by exposure to UV radiations.

69. (b) II and III are incorrect

70. Plasmid that transfers DNA into host cell.

71. True. With a high copy number, a foreign DNA can multiply itself equal to the copy number of the vector.

72. (c) an origin that supports high copy number.

73. Selection

74. Plasmids

75. *ori*

76. Selectable marker

77. Selectable marker gene

78. False. Normal *E. coli* cells do not csrry resistamce against ampicillin and kanamycin.

79. (d) Selectable markers help in identifying and eliminating non-transformants and selectively permitting the growth of transformants. Genes encoding resistance to antibiotics such as kanamycin, etc. are considered useful markers for *E. coli*.

80. Single, gene, cloning

81. An antibiotic resistance gene.

82. False. pBR322 is an antificial cloning vector based on plasmids.

83. pBR322 is odd one out as it is a vector, while others are restriction enzymes.

84. (i) The figure represents a plasmid vector.
(ii) pBR322
(iii) *A* - Ampicillin resistance gene, *B*-Tetracycline resistance gene, *C*-Selection of transformed cells.
(iv) To cut at *Eco*RI, the recognition sequence will be 5′ - GAATTC - 3′.

85. Ampicillin

86. (a) Ampicillin resistance gene

87. Chromogenic

88. β-galactosidase

89. Insertional inactivation

90. It requires simultaneous plating on two plates having different antibiotics.

91. (a) Colonies identified as recombinant colonies do not produce any colour.

92. *Agrobacterium tumefaciens*

93. T-DNA

94. False. *Agrobacterium* is a plant pathogen of dicot plants.

95. Ti-plasmid from T-DNA of *Agrobacterium* has been modified to be used as vector for plants.

96. (d) Disarming the plasmid DNA

97. Retrovirus

98. (ii) DNA is a hydrophilic molecule that is why, it cannot cross cell membranes.

99. Competent cell

100. (c) Treatment with divalent cation followed by heat shock.

101. Pore

102. (b) Reaction mixture was heated to 60°C for few seconds.

103. Gene gun is the odd one out as it is a direct method of gene transfer while others are indirect method of gene transfer.

104. Microinjection

105. Gold or tungsten

106. Virulence

107. True

108. (c) III and IV are incorrect.

109. The correct sequence is I, III, VI, II, IV, VII and V.

110. Nucleic acid

111. A-2, B-1, C-3

112. 4 (RNA, lipids, proteins and polysaccharides)

113. Ribonuclease

114. Chilled ethanol

115. Spooling

116. False. Fragmentation of DNA is facilitated by incubation with restriction enzymes.

117. Agarose gel electrophoresis

118. PCR

119. *A*–Denaturation, *B*–Annealing of primers, *C*–Extension of primers.

120. 4 (DNA template, primer, *Taq* polymerase and *d*NTPs).

121. (c) Both statements I and II are true.

122. Denaturation

123. *Thermus aquaticus*

124. False. In PCR the *Taq* polymerase extends the primers by adding dNTPs.

125. 1 billion

126. True
127. PCR
128. (a) II → I → IV → V → III
129. True
130. Recombinant protein
131. Bioreactors
132. Continuous
133. False. In continuous culturing technique, a larger biomass lead to higher yield of recombinant proteins.
134. Exponential
135. Sparged stirred-tank bioreactor
136. (d) Fresh media is constantly poured into bioreactor to replace used media which is discarded. The stirrer in a stirred tank reactor functions by facilitating even mixing and O_2 availability throughout the bioreactor.
137. Bubbles increase the oxygen transfer area and facilitate the mixing of culture media.
138. (i) *A*-Acid / Base inlet for pH control, *B*-Steam inlet for sterilisation, *C*-Foam braker, *D*-Flat bladed impeller, *E*-Culture broth.
(ii) Simple stirred tank bioreactor
(iii) Impeller
139. (c) Aeration and homogenisation.
140. *A*- Agitator, *B* - Uninterrupted O_2 supply, *C*- Foam breaker, *D* - To withdrawl of small samples, *E* - Sparger, *F* - Prevents a whirlpool effect that could impede proper mixing.
141. Downstream processing
142. Safety and functionality of drugs
143. (c) Both statements I and II are true.

Assertion-Reason Questions

1. (b) Both A and R are true, but R is not the correct explanation of A.
For creating recombinant plasmid it is necessary to cut the plasmid and foreign DNA with the same restriction enzyme so that the same sticky ends can make the ligation process easier.
2. (d) A is false, but R is true. A can be corrected as
Agarose gel electrophoresis allows separating DNA fragments based on their molecular size.
3. (a) Both A and R are true and R is the correct explanation of A.
4. (d) A is false, but R is true. A can be corrected as
Non-recombinants produce blue colonies, while the recombinants produce white colonies.
5. (b) Both A and R are true, but R is not the correct explanation of A.
To allow the host cells take up the recombinant plasmid, the cells are treated with a divalent cations because the cations neutralise the negative charge on DNA and allow it to be taken up by the cell.
6. (c) A is true, but R is false. R can be corrected as
Plant cells can be degraded by cellulase enzymes which makes the isolation easier.
7. (a) Both A and R are true and R is correct explanation of A.
8. (a) Both A and R are true and R is the correct explanation of A.
9. (b) Both A and R are true, but R is not the correct explanation of A.
In a sparged stirred type bioreactor sterile air bubbles are sparged, to supply oxygen to the cells growing in the media.
10. (c) A is true, but R is false. R can be corrected as
Downstream processing and quality control testing vary from one product to another.

Case Based Questions

1. (i) (b) (ii) (c) (iii) (c)
2. (i) (d) (ii) (c) (iii) (a)

Competition Edge Up

1. (b)	**2.** (b)	**3.** (a)	**4.** (a)
5. (a)	**6.** (b)	**7.** (c)	**8.** (a)
9. (a)	**10.** (c)	**11.** (a)	**12.** (d)
13. (b)	**14.** (d)	**15.** (a)	

Chapter-10

Biotechnology and Its Applications

1. 4 (Waste treatment, bioremedation, genetically modified crops and energy generation).
2. False. Downstream processing aims to purify the organic compound or recombinant proteins obtained by biotechnological processes.
3. Green revolution
4. Use of agrochemicals like fertilisers, pesticides, etc.
5. Organic farming
6. False. Using conventional breeding methods, we cannot increase the yield of crops with the existing varieties.
7. (c) Both statements I and II are true.
8. (b) Meristerm
9. (a) Somatic hybrids
10. (d) Somatic hybrids are genetically dissimilar to the parent plants.
The naked protoplast of plant cells retain the cell membrane.
11. Genetically Modified Organisms (GMOs).
12. False. As a result of genetically modified crops, chemical use on an agricultural lands have gone down significantly in some crops (with little or no change on others).
13. True
14. Golden rice
15. Production of insect resistance.
16. They have *Bt* toxin produced by *cry* gene.
17. *Bacillus thuringiensis*
18. Lepidoptera
19. Bacteria
20. A-2, B-3, C-1
21. (i) Introduce natural insect resistance in plants.
22. (i) Toxic insecticidal
(ii) Protoxin
23. The alkaline pH of the insect's gut is responsible for activation of the inactive protoxin as it reaches the target insect's body.
24. Creating pores in mid gut epithelial cells that cause swelling and lysis of cell.
25. False. *Bt* toxins are insect group specific.
26. *cry*
27. 5 (Cotton, corn, rice, potato and soyabean).
28. *cry* IAb

29. (d) Both b and c
30. *Meloidogyne incognitia*
31. RNA interference
32. False. RNAi is a method of cellular defence in all eukaryotic organisms.
33. (a) The *ds*RNA in RNAi is complementary to the the pathogen *m*RNA and thus silences them.
34. Gene silencing
35. RNA virus.
36. Translation of *m*RNA.
37. *Agrobacterium tumefaciens.*
38. False. *Agrobacterium* vectors are used to introduce nematode specific genes in host plants.
39. False. RNAi is a strategy to produce plants with pest resistance.
40. Tobacco
41. Silencing of specific *m*RNA
42. 30, genetic engineering
43. 3 (Insulin, growth hormone and α-1-anti-tyrpsin).
44. Diabetes mellitus
45. False. Insulin extracted from animal source is not as effective as that secreted in human body.
46. Allergic reactions
47. *Escherichia coli*
48. C-peptide
49. Eli Lilly
50. (a) A and B chains
51. False. Mature insulin consists of two polypeptide chains.
52. (c) Both statements I and II are true
53. Disulphide bridges
54. (d) Combining of chains A and B by hydrogen bonding between them.
55. The correct sequence is I → III → IV→ V → II → VI.
56. *A*-Proinsulin, *B*-A-peptide, *C*-B-peptide, *D*-Free, C-peptide
57. Chains-A and B are essential for the formation of mature insulin.
58. Assembly of both newly synthesised polypeptide chains.
59. Gene therapy
60. False. Correction of genetic disorders involves the replacement of non-functional genes.
61. Adenosine Deaminase (ADA) deficiency
62. The diseases are all caused due to genetic disorders.
63. Immune system
64. (a) I and III
65. Lymphocytes
66. Bone marrow
67. True
68. 2 (Retroviruses and cosmids
69. (c) Retrovirus
70. Because genetically modified lymphocytes have limited lifespan.
71. (i) Gene therapy can be a permanent cure for ADA deficiency disorder if gene producing ADA is introduced at early embryonic stages.
72. Conventional
73. ECG is odd one out. Rest all are molecular diagnostic techniques.
74. Polymerase Chain Reaction
75. Enzyme Linked Immuno-sorbent Assay.
76. PCR test
77. I, II and III
78. Probe
79. Autoradiography
80. (c) Cloned cells had muted version of the gene.
81. Antigen-antibody interaction
82. Transgenic animals
83. 4 (Rabbits, pigs, sheep, fish).
84. Mice
85. True
86. *Bt* tobacco is odd one out as it is a transgenic plant. Others are transgenic animals.
87. 4 (Cancer, cystic fibrosis, rheumatoid arthritis and Alzheimer's disease).
88. Emphysema
89. False. The first transgenic cow is Rosie.
90. Human α-lactalbumin
91. Transgenic mice and monkeys both are used to check vaccine safety.
92. (a) A-3, B-2, C-4, D-1
93. True
94. Genetic Engineering Approval Committee
95. GEAC
96. (i) This is because there is danger of entry of virus or toxins with new transgenic crops.
97. True
98. Biopatent
99. False. Patents are granted only for novel inventions.
100. 3(Turmeric, rice and neem).
101. (b) Tulsi
102. Indian Basmati with semi-dwarf variety.
103. 200,000
104. Biopiracy
105. Indian patents bill

Assertion-Reason Questions

1. (d) A is false, but R is true. A can be corrected as
Micropropagation techniques can be used to develop genetically similar plants.
2. (a) Both A and R are true, and R is the correct explanation of A.
3. (c) A is true, but R is false. R can be corrected as
The *Bt* toxins are produced as inactive protoxins and become activated by the alkaline pH of the insect gut.
4. (b) Both A and R are true, but R is not the correct explanation of A.
Plants can be protected from nematode pathogen by using RNA interference and *Agrobacterium* vectors by creating *ds* RNA that binds and silences target *m*RNA of the nematode.
5. (d) A is false, but R is true. A can be corrected as

Insulin as a pro-hormone contains an additional stretch of C-peptide which is absent in the mature form.

6. (a) Both A and R are true and R is the correct explanation of A.
7. (c) A is true, but R is false. R can be corrected as
Transgenic animals are developed by introducing DNA that codes for α-1 antitrypsin to treat emphysema.
8. (a) Both A and R are true and R is the correct explanation of A.

Case Based Questions

1. (i) (b) (ii) (a) (iii) (b)
2. (i) (b) (ii) (b) (iii) (a)

Competition Edge UP

1. (c) **2.** (c) **3.** (a) **4.** (b)
5. (a) **6.** (d) **7.** (d) **8.** (b)
9. (c) **10.** (b)

Chapter-11

Organisms and Populations

1. Population ecology
2. 8/20 = 0.4 offspring per lotus per year.
3. Sex ratio
4. Age pyramid
5. *A*-Stable, *B*-Declining
6. *A* - Post-reproductive
B - Reproductive
C - Pre-reproductive
7. (c) Pyramid A has equal number of young or pre-reproductiove and reproductive individuals
8. Pug marks and fecal pellets
9. Population density
10. Population density
11. False. The size of a population for any species is not a static parameter.
12. (c) Both statements I and II are true
13. Mortality
14. A-Immigration, B-Natality, C-Mortality
15. (a) 1040
16. A-2, B-1, C-3
17. $N_{t+1} = N_t \ [(B+I)-(D+E)]$
18. Increase
19. Immigration, birth rate
20. A-2, B-4, C-1, D-3
21. Exponential model and logistic model
22. Unimpeded
23. $\frac{dN}{dt} = (b-d) \times N$
24. 'r' or intrinsic rate of natural increase.
25. True
26. J-shaped curve
27. $N_t = N_0 \ e^{rt}$
28. Exponentially
29. Competition
30. Carrying capacity
31. Lag, deceleration, carrying capacity.
32. False 'K' stands for carrying capacity in the Verhulst-Pearl logistic growth equation.
33. True
34. Sigmoid
35. $\frac{dN}{dt} = rN\left(\frac{K-N}{K}\right)$
36. *A*-Exponential growth
B-Logistic growth
37. Logistic growth
38. (b) C
39. (a) I, II and IV
40. High
41. Pacific salmon fish, bamboo
42. Option (iii) is incorrect. It can be corrected as
Small-sized but many offspring oysters and pelagic fishes, etc., produce large number of small-sized offspring.
43. Constraints, biotic, abiotic
44. Organic, inorganic
45. False. Organisms cannot live in isolation in nature.
46. Interaction of populations of two different species.
47. (i) Beneficial interaction
(ii) Neutral interaction
48. Competition
49. True
50. Commensalism
51. *A*–Mutualism, *B*–0
C – +, *D*–Parasitism/Predation
52. Competition is odd one out. Rest of options share a common character that the interacting species live closely together.
53. True
54. Energy
55. True
56. Prickly pear cactus
57. Biological
58. Predators
59. (c) Hinders the energy transfer process
60. Monarch butterfly
61. The butterfly acquires the chemical during its caterpillar stage by feeding on a poisonous weed.
62. (b) The loss of invertebrates in the absence of starfish in the Pacific coast was due to loss of predation which leads to competition between the two prey species.
63. Phytophagous
64. *Acacia* and *Cactus*
65. *Calotropis*
66. (b) *Calotropis* produces highly poisonous cardiace glycocides
67. Chloroquine is odd one out. Rest of the options are chemical substances produced by plant as defence against grazers.
68. True
69. True
70. False. Abingdon tortoise in Galapagos island became extinct due to competition with goats.
71. A-2, B-1, C-3, D-4
72. True
73. (i) *Balanus*, (ii) *Chathamalus*
74. False. Herbivores are more affected than carnivores by competition.
75. Competitive exclusion principle
76. (c) Both statements I and II are true.
77. Resource partitioning
78. (a) Competitive release
79. A-2, B-3, C-1
80. True
81. Digestive system, adhesive organs and suckers.
82. Two
83. Ectoparasites.
84. Fluke. All others are ectoparasite.
85. *Cuscuta*
86. (d) *Plasmodium*

87. The female mosquito needs blood for reproduction and not for nutrition. It does not bite human for its meal.

88. True

89. Lice, copepods, ticks, *Cuscuta*

90. Brood parasitism

91. (b) Commensalism

92. A-3, B-4, C-1, D-2

93. Lichens

94. Mycorrhizae

95. Pollen and nectar

96. True

97. Oviposition

98. *Ophrys*

99. True

100. (b) The female wap uses the fig plants for ovipositon and in turn pollinates the flowers.

101. (a) A-2, B-1, C-4, D-3

Competition Connect

1. Ecology

2. Organisms → Populations → Communities → Biomes.

3. True

4. A-2, B-1, C-4, D-3

5. Tropical rain forest, Deciduous forest, Desert, Sea coast.

6. Plant is odd one out. Rest of the options are major abiotic factors.

7. Light is odd one out. Rest of the options are biotic components of a habitat.

8. Natural selection

9. Decreases

10. False. Average temperature exceeds 100°C in deep sea thermal vents.

11. Canada and Germany

12. Moisture

13. Temperature

14. True

15. Water

16. Inland water < Sea water < Hypersaline lagoons.

17. (i) Sea water, (ii) Inland water

18. (b) A few organisms can tolerate and thrive in a wide range of temperature and are eurythermal.

19. (a) Stenothermal and euryhaline respectively

20. A-2, B-3, C-1, D-4

21. Low light

22. (a) Trees, shrubs, herbs

23. Photoperiod, foraging, migratory.

24. UV is harmful

25. Climate, weathering.

26. Percolation, water holding capacity

27. Types of animal is odd one out. Rest of the options are the factors that determine the vegetation in that area.

28. Aquatic

29. Homeostasis

30. Regulators

31. Osmoregulation

32. Partial regulators

33. (c) Both statements I and II are true.

34. True

35. Winter

36. False. Plants do not have a mechanism to maintain internal temperature.

37. All birds and mammals

38. False. 99% of animals are conformers which are also referred as ectotherms.

39. Conformers

40. (c) Snake, crocodile fish, frog

41. Energetically

42. Shrews and humming bird.

43. Surface area

44. Larger

45. More

46. The small animals have a larger surface area relative to their volume. They lose body heat very fast when it is cold outside, then they have to expend much energy to generate body heat through metabolism.

47. Migration and suspension

48. *A* - Internal level
B - External level
C - Conformers
D - Partial regulators

49. (c) Both statements I and II are true

50. Keoladeo National Park (Rajasthan)

51. True

52. Dormancy

53. Hibernation

54. Aestivation

55. A-2, B-3, C-1

56. Diapause

57. Adaptation

58. Morphological, physiological and behavioural

59. (i) Behavioural
(ii) Physiological
(iii) Physiological
(iv) Morphological

60. Physiological adaptation

61. To meet its water requirement.

62. (c) Long and muscular legs

63. (i) Water is obtained as a byproduct.
(ii) Concentrating urine to reduce amount of water in excretion.

64. Minimise, transpiration

65. Desert plants, e.g. cactus

66. Phylloclade, spines.

67. (a) In *Opuntia* photosynthesis is performed by flattened stems during daytime and the leaves are reduced to spine.

68. True

69. Allen's rule

70. Blubber, insulator

71. Altitude sickness

72. (i) Increasing RBCs production
(ii) Increasing breathing rate.

73. Higher RBCs

74. Crushing pressure

75. False. Desert lizard lacks the physiological condition to deal with high temperature of their habitat, but manage to keep their body temperature fairly constant by behavioural means.

76. (c) Both statements I and II are true

Assertion-Reason Questions

1. (a) Both A and R are true and R is the lorrect explanation of A.

2. (a) Both A and R are true and R is the correct explanation of A

3. (a) Both A and R are true and R is the correct explanation of A.

4. (d) A is false, but R is true. A can be corrected as
Natality rate and immigration are the positive attributes that causes an increase in population density.

5. (b) Both A and R are true, but R is not the correct explanation of A. If food and resources become unlimited, a population shows geometric growth or exponential growth as these factors check or control the population of a place.

6. (a) Both A and R are true and R is the correct explanation of A.
7. (b) Both A and R are true, but R is not the correct explanation of A.
   Exotic species when introduced in an area can become invasive and spread faster due to absence of any predators that feed on them.
8. (c) A is true, but R is false. R can be corrected as
   Quinines are produced by plants as a defence strategy against grazing animals.
9. (d) A is false, but R is true. A can be corrected as
   In the association between sea anemone and clown fish, only the clown fish is benefitted while the sea anemone remains unaffected.
10. (a) Both A and R are true and R is the correct explanation of A.

Case Based Questions

1. (i) (c) (ii) (c) (iii) (a)
2. (i) (b) (ii) (a) (iii) (c)

Competition Edge Up

1. (c) 2. (d) 3. (d) 4. (b)
5. (a) 6. (d) 7. (d) 8. (d)
9. (d) 10. (b) 11. (b) 12. (a)

Chapter-12

Ecosystem

1. Functional, physical environment
2. Terrestrial and aquatic ecosystems.
3. Estuary is odd one out as it is an aquatic ecosystem whereas the rest three are terrestrial ecosystems.
4. Crop fields and aquarium.
5. Biotic and abiotic components.
6. Identification, enumeration
7. (b) Stratification
8. Top, grasses.
9. 4 (Productivity, decomposition, energy flow, nutrient cycling).
10. True
11. *A*- Abiotic components
    B- Autotrophic components
    C- Zooplanktons
    D- Fungi, bacteria and flagellates
12. (i) Water
    (ii) Autotrophs
    (iii) Decomposers
13. Decomposition and mineralisation
14. Unidirectional, higher, heat.
15. $gm^{-2}\ yr^{-1}$
16. Net Primary Productivity (NPP).
17. (c) 400 (kcal m^{-2}) yr^{-1}
18. (c) Both statements I and II are true
19. A-3, B-1, C-4, D-2
20. 4 (Plant species habitat, environmental factors, nutrient availability, photosynthetic capacity of plants).
21. False. Primary productivity of different ecosystem varies and oceans havs low productivity despite occupying 70% of the surface.
22. 55 billion tons
23. Decomposition
24. Earthworm
25. Inorganic substances is odd one out as it is the end product of decomposition.
26. Detritus
27. Detritivores
28. (b) Inorganic materials by the process of leaching precipitates into unavailable salts.
29. False. Humus is highly resistant to microbial action and undergoes decomposition at slower rate.
30. Humus
31. (b) High rate of decomposition
32. (i) V → I → II → III → IV
    (ii) 3 (I, II, V)
    (iii) 2 (III, IV)
33. A-3, B-4, C-1, D-2, E-5
34. Decomposition cycle in terrestrial ecosystem.
35. Oxygen, chemical composition, climatic
36. (a) High chitin composition
37. Nitrogen and sugars in detritus
38. Temperature and soil moisture
39. Anaerobiosis is the odd one out as it inhibits decomposition whereas the other two factors favour decomposition.
40. (d) Decomposition of the detritus is reduced under anaerobic conditions.
    Presence of lignin and chitin in the detritus lowers decomposition rate.
41. True
42. Inhibits
43. Deep sea hydrothermal ecosystem
44. Photosynthetically Active Radiation
45. 2-10%
46. Unidirectional
47. False. Ecosystems are not exempted from the second law of thermodynamics as they need a constant supply of energy to synthesise the molecules.
48. Producers
49. Food chain
50. Producers
51. (a) Energy cannot be trapped in a consumer forever as it is passed on to the next trophic levels or released when an organism dies.
52. True
53. A-3, B-2, C-1
54. 3 (Insects, birds, mammals).
    Molluscs are the herbivores in aquatic ecosystem.
55. Tertiary consumers
56. (d) III and IV
57. Grazing Food Chain
58. (i), i.e. Grass → Goat → Man
59. Producers
60. Detritus Food Chain
61. Organic matter
62. Fungi and bacteria
63. Saprotrophs
64. Grazing, detritus
65. (d) The major flow of energy takes place through DFC and not by GFC
66. (a) Trophic level III, Secondary consumer, primary carnivore.
67. Food webs
68. True
69. 4 (i) Plants → Cow → Lion
    (ii) Plants → Goat → Lion
    (iii) Plants → Grasshopper → Frog
    (iv) Plants → Goat → Man

70. Trophic level

71. (i) *A*–First trophic level, *D*–Fourth trophic level
(ii) Phytoplanktons, grass, trees
(iii) Herbivores
(iv) *C*, i.e. secondary consumers
(v) Second

72. False. The amount of energy decreases at successive trophic levels.

73. Standing crop

74. Biomass

75. (c) I, III and IV

76. (i) Grazing food chain
(ii) 10%. According to Lindemann, only 10% of available energy at a trophic level passes to the next level. The rest of energy is either consumed or dissipated.
(iii) 5 kJ. In the given diagram, top carnivora is present at fourth trophic level and each level receives only 10% energy from the lower trophic level.

Plants 5000 kJ → Herbivores 500 kJ → Carnivores 50 kJ → Top carnivores 5 kJ

(iv) True

77. (a) 1000 J

78. Ecological pyramids

79. Standing crop is odd one out as it is not studied through ecological pyramids.

80. Producers

81. (d) At the base

82. True

83. Functional level

84. Upright

85. Pyramid of numbers in grassland ecosystem.

86. Inverted pyramid of numbers.

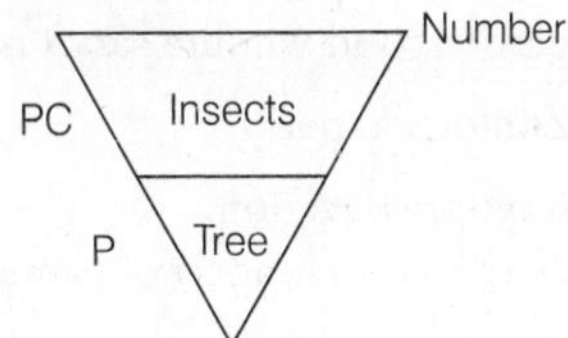

87. *B*. Spindle-shape, because number of the smaller birds will be more than the tree and the population of large birds would be lesser than that of smaller birds.

88. (d) Snakes feeding on rats in a grassland.

89. Decrease

90. *A*, i.e. inverted pyramid because standing crop of phytoplanktons is lesser than that of zooplanktons.

91. Inverted

92. *A*-Pyramid of energy is always upright.

93. 4 (Inverted pyramid of number, upright pyramid of biomass, inverted pyramid of biomass, spindle-shaped pyramid of number). Inverted pyramid of energy is never found because some energy is always lost as heat at each trophic level.

94. Chain, web

95. Saprophytes

Assertion-Reason Questions

1. (d) A is false, but R is true. A can be corrected as
The consumers are represented by the zooplanktons that dwell at the bottom of a pond ecosystem.

2. (a) Both A and R are true and R is the correct explanation of A.

3. (d) A is false, but R is true. A can be corrected as
Detritivores are involved in the fragmentation step of decomposition process.

4. (b) Both A and R are true, but R is not the correct explanation of A.
Only a small fraction of the solar energy is passed to trophic levels two and three as plants can capture only 2-10% of the Photosynthetically Active Radiation (PAR).

5. (c) A is true, but R is false. R can be corrected as
Only 10 % of the energy can be transferred from one trophic level to the other.

6. (d) A is false, but R is true. A can be corrected
All ecological pyramids are not upright like the pyramid of biomass in a sea is inverted.

7. (a) Both A and R are true and R is the correct explanation of A.

Case Based Questions

1. (i) (c) (ii) (c) (iii) (c)
2. (i) (c) (ii) (a) (iii) (d)

Competition Edge Up

1.	(c)	**2.**	(d)	**3.**	(a)
4.	(b)	**5.**	(b)	**6.**	(b)
7.	(a)	**8.**	(d)	**9.**	(a)
10.	(b)	**11.**	(c)	**12.**	(c)

Chapter-13

Biodiversity and Conservation

1. Ants, orchids

2. Ecologist, evolutionary

3. Diversity

4. Edward Wilson

5. Genetic, species, ecological

6. False. A single species can show high diversity at the genetic level over its distributional range.

7. *Rauwolfia vomitoria*, concentration, reserpine

8. 50,000

9. False. More than 1000 genetically different varieties of mango are found in India.

10. Species diversity

11. (b) There are more than 28,000 species of fishes.

12. Ecosystem

13. True

14. (d) *Rauwolfia vomitoria*–Genetic diversity

15. International Union for Conservation of Nature and Natural Resources.

16. 1.5 million

17. Temperate

18. 7 million

19. False. Based on current species inventories, about 70% of total recorded species are animals while 22% are of plants.

20. (i) A-2, B-1, C-3
(ii) 70

21. (c) C – Reptile, D – Amphibian

22. False. The number of species of fishes is equal to the combined total of species of birds amphibians, reptiles and mammals.

23. (c) Both statements I and II are true.
24. (i) A-2, B-4, C-1, D-3
(ii) Prokaryotes
25. Microbial
26. 8.1%
27. 12
28. 22%
29. Latitudinal gradient
30. 23.5° N to 23.5°S
31. A-3, B-1, C-4, D-2
32. IV → III → I → II
[56] [105] [1200] [1400]
33. False. Equador forest has up to 10 times more species of vascular plants as compared to midwest forest of the USA.
34. Equador
35. Amazonian rainforest
36. A-3, B-1, C-4, D-5, E-2
37. True
38. (c) Frequent glaciation in tropical latitudes
39. 4 (Less seasonal and more constant, environment more solar energy, niche specialisation, higher productivity).
40. (c) III and IV are incorrect
41. Alexander von Humboldt, South America
42. (i) I - Species richness
II - CA^Z
III - $Z \log A$
(ii) False. Species richness increases with increasing explored area within a region, but up to a limit.
(iii) 4 (Angiosperm plants, birds, bats, freshwater fishes).
43. (a) 0.6 to 1.2
44. *S*–Species richness
C–Y-intercept
Z–Regression coefficient
45. Frugivorous birds in tropical forest is odd one out because its *Z*-value range is 0.6-1.2.
For other listed taxa, *Z*-value ranges from 0.1 to 0.2.
46. 1.15
47. $\log S = 0.8 + 0.3 \times 4$
$= 0.8 + 1.2 = 2.0$
48. True
49. Stable
50. Variable productivity is odd one out, because a stable community does not show too much variations in productivity from year to year.
51. False. David Tilman proposed that higher number of species show less year to year variation in total biomass.
52. (a) Biomass
53. David Tilman
54. Paul Ehrlich
55. Species
56. (a) In the famous analogy by Paul Ehrlich, the rivets of the plane represented species in an ecosystem.
57. Key species
58. Yes
59. II, As loss of rivets of wings-I (key species) is of major concern because they drive aeroplane signifying (here) major ecosystem functions.
60. 2000, birds
61. Red list
62. Vertebrates-338, Invertebrates-359, Plants-87
63. A-2, B-4, C-1, D-3
64. Tiger
65. Amphibians
66. Endangered
67. IV → II → I → III
(12%) (23%) (31%) (32%)
68. Five
69. Sixth, faster, human
70. Decline, lowered, increased.
71. The Evil Quartet
72. Habitat loss and fragmentation
73. Soyabeans, grasslands, beef cattle, small fragments
74. 2 (Stellar's sea cow and passenger pigeon). Rest two are invasive species.
75. Invasive weed species
76. African catfish or *Clarias gariepinus.*
77. (d) Reduced reproductive ability of the native species.
78. False. Co-extinction results due to the obligatory relationship between species.
79. A-3, B-1, C-2, D-4
80. Conservation
81. Pollination is odd one out as it is an example of broadly utilitarian, while other three are the examples of narrowly utilitarian.
82. Bioprospecting
83. (d) Both (a) and (c)
84. Broadly utilitarian.
85. A-3, B-1, C-2
86. True
87. *In situ*
88. Endemic species
89. Low species richness is an odd one out because hotspots are characterised by high species richness.
90. 34
91. Three
92. Madagascar is a hotspot, but not in India.
93. Two, high, mass extinction
94. (c) Only selected species in the entire area of the national park are conserved.
95. *In situ* conservation
96. III → I → II
[14 (now 18)] [90] [448]
97. Sacred groves
98. Last refuges
99. False. Sacred groves help in *in situ* conservation of wildlife and threatened plants.
100. A-4, B-1, C-2, D-3
101. *Ex situ* conservation
102. False. In *ex situ* conservation, threatened species are protected outside their natural habitat in special setting.
103. Zoological parks, botanical gardens and wildlife safari parks.
104. Zoological parks
105. Cryopreservation
106. *In vivo* conservation of gametes
107. *In vitro*, tissue culture, seed banks.

108. 1992

109. Rio de Janeiro

110. (i) Conservation of biodiversity.
(ii) Sustainable utilisation of benefits of biodiversity.

111. 2002, global, regional, local.

Assertion-Reason Questions

1. (d) A is false, but R is true. A can be corrected as
A high degree of genetic diversity is observed in *Rauwolfia vomitoria* in the Himalaya regions.
2. (a) Both A and R are true and R is the correct explanation of A.
3. (b) Both A and R are true, but R is not the correct explanation of the A.
Tropics have a greater species diversity of the world than the temperate regions because there is greater availability of solar energy in the tropics which increases productivity.
4. (c) A is true, but R is false. R can be corrected as
A plot between species richness of a place and area is a rectangular hyperbola.
5. (d) A is false, but R is true. A can be corrected as
The rivet popper hypothesis explains why species extinction can cause the ecosystem to collapse.
6. (c) A is true, but R is false. R can be corrected as
Breaking of habitats into fragments can be caused by various human activities like pollution, clearing land for cultivation and rearing livestock.
7. (b) Both A and R are true, but R is not the correct explanation of assertion. Extinction of one species can drive the extinction of another in a process called co-extinction if the two species are associated with one another in an obligatory way.
8. (a) Both A and R are true and R is the correct explanation of A.
9. (a) Both A and R are true and R is the correct explanation of A.
10. (d) A is false, but R is true. A can be corrected as
Ex situ conservation is offered to a species that needs urgent measures for protection.

Case Based Questions

1. (i) (b) (ii) (c) (iii) (c)
2. (i) (c) (ii) (d) (iii) (a)

Competition Edge Up

1. (d)	**2.** (a)	**3.** (b)	**4.** (d)
5. (b)	**6.** (d)	**7.** (b)	**8.** (a)
9. (d)	**10.** (a)	**11.** (c)	**12.** (c)
13. (c)	**14.** (b)	**15.** (d)	**16.** (b)